RxPrep®

Y0-BZY-403

THE REVIEW PROGRAM TRUSTED BY TOP EMPLOYERS

Thank you for purchasing the 2012 Edition of the Rx-Prep Course Book. We are confident it will help you ace your licensure exams.

RxPrep study materials are the only source used by the top 4 chains – and many colleges and professional organizations.

Our materials focus on must-know drug information. They were developed by board-certified, clinical pharmacists with years of experience.

We know what's important. Some students prepare for their exams using only our course book and do well. Others find the full program essential.

and the quiz bank (see special pricing for those who purchased the course book in the box).

We are here to help you. Our on-line students get unlimited clinical support – if you don't understand something, email us and you will get a call or email response within 24 hours. In addition, our online students can enjoy playing our Face-book drug trivia game and earn gift cards – it's a way to relieve a little of the pressure.

The Proven Way to Do Well

WATCH the complete online video lectures, which correlate with the chapters in your text.

STUDY by highlighting or taking notes on the points we emphasize that you need to review. It's all there.

TEST yourself with the 2,200 question online quiz. You should score 100% on each quiz section – the quiz questions are basic, fundamental knowledge.

$118 off the online course and quiz bank for students purchasing the 2012 Edition of the RxPrep Course Book

Use the promotional code GAX7

RxPrep has created a **complete program that is all you need** to prepare for your exams. Thousands of students pass each year using this program, which consists of the course book, the online lectures

RXPREP TEXT + ONLINE COURSE + QUIZ BANK:

The proven method to MASTER the material before you test!

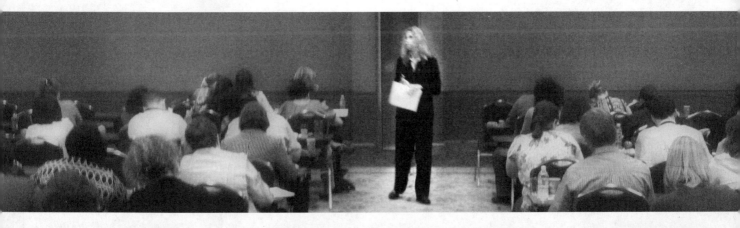

RXPREP COURSE BOOK
2012 EDITION

K. Shapiro, PharmD, BCPS

S. Brown, PharmD, MBA, BCPS

Cover design by Creativeshoebox.com

Book design by Media Arts International

TABLE OF CONTENTS

1. Exam Overview 1
   NAPLEX® Overview 1
   Test Taking Tips 3
   How to Use this Book 5
   CPJE Pointers – for CA exam takers 6
2. Calculations 8
3. Compounding Requirements & Terminology 61
4. Pharmacokinetics & Drug Formulations 68
5. Biostatistics & Pharmacoeconomics 74
6. Pharmacogenomics 90
7. Drug Allergies, ADRs & ADR Reporting 96
8. Medication Errors, Patient Safety, and the Joint Commission 105
9. FDA (U.S.) Drug Development Process 130
10. Natural Products & Vitamins 133
11. Drug Interactions 140
12. Renal Disease and Dosing Considerations 153
13. Drug Use in Pregnancy 164
14. Drug References 170
15. Disposal of Prescription Drugs 175
16. Infectious Diseases 181
17. Immunization 236
18. Human Immunodeficiency Virus (HIV) 253
19. Hepatitis and Liver Disease 273
20. Diabetes 286
21. Thyroid Disorders 310
22. Osteoporosis & Hormone Therapy 319
23. Contraception 334
24. Pain 346
25. Migraine 368
26. Rheumatoid Arthritis (RA) & Systemic Lupus Erythematosus (SLE) 375
27. Gout 389
28. Hypertension 395
29. Dyslipidemia 415

30. Heart Failure 430
31. Anticoagulation 447
32. Chronic Angina 463
33. Acute Coronary Syndromes 472
34. Antiarrhythmics 481
35. Pulmonary Arterial Hypertension (PAH) 496
36. Asthma 502
37. COPD 523
38. Smoking Cessation 530
39. Allergic Rhinitis, Cough & Cold 538
40. Cystic Fibrosis 548
41. Oncology 552
42. Anemia 579
43. Transplant/Immunosuppression 588
44. Intravenous Drugs, Fluids & Antidotes 597
45. Depression 609
46. Schizophrenia/Psychosis 624
47. Bipolar Disorder 635
48. Parkinson Disease 645
49. Alzheimer's Disease 653
50. Attention Deficit Hyperactivity Disorder (ADHD) & Stimulant Agents 658
51. Anxiety 666
52. Insomnia 671
53. Epilepsy/Seizures 677
54. Multiple Sclerosis 692
55. Stroke 698
56. Gastroesophageal Reflux Disease (GERD) 704
57. Peptic Ulcer Disease (PUD) 715
58. Constipation & Diarrhea 723
59. Inflammatory Bowel Disease (IBD) 729
60. Erectile Dysfunction 738
61. Benign Prostatic Hyperplasia (BPH) 744
62. Overactive Bladder 750
63. Glaucoma, Allergic Conjunctivitis, Other Opthalmics & Otics 755
64. Motion Sickness 763
65. Common Skin Conditions 766
66. Weight Loss 777
67. Appendix 780
    Top Selling Drugs 780
    Common Laboratory Values 784
    Common Medical Abbreviations 786

EXAM OVERVIEW

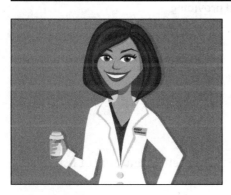

Introduction

This section includes four topics:

- NAPLEX® Overview

- Test Taking Tips

- How to Use this Book

- CPJE Pointers – for CA exam takers

NAPLEX® Overview

The NAPLEX® exam blueprint (outline) is effective for anyone taking the exam after March, 2010. This is available on the board's website at www.nabp.net. Please review the complete blueprint on the website. Below is a summary of the blueprint:

The first section is "Safe and Effective" use and is the majority of the exam (56%).

- These are largely asked in a patient-case format. You will need to identify aberrant labs, medical histories, medication use history – and recognize appropriate or inappropriate therapy options.

- This section includes expected dosing options, regimens, and formulations. Pharmaco-economic factors may be important: if a patient cannot afford a drug and a less-expensive, but valid option is available, you'll need to recognize it. Is the physician choosing a drug based on poor study data? This is an important area for pharmacists; manufacturers can entice clinicians to use their new, expensive drugs – but our job is to review study data and <u>protect</u> the <u>patient</u>. Occasionally, new drugs are lifesavers, but many times new agents are copy-cat drugs (similar to older agents) or are not superior to less-expensive, existing options. Review our pharmacoeconomics section for more information.

- Also included is the ability to monitor patient outcomes (is the dose level correct, is the patient responding well?). Be able to choose correct monitoring tests. Improving medication adherence and recommending better treatment options are tested on as well.

The second section is safe and accurate preparation and dispensing of medications (33%).

- This includes calculations, including nutritional requirements and basic TPN calculations. Flow rates for drugs administered by IV infusion should be reviewed, along with drug concentrations, and the other general calculations in the section. <u>If you do not know the calculations well in this text</u> (which are standard pharmacy calculations) <u>you are not likely to do well.</u>

- Trade/generics are tested, along with common dosage forms. See our tips on which drugs to review below. Be able to use PK parameters and quality assurance information to identify appropriate interchange, identify information regarding storage, packaging, handling, administration, and medication disposal. Some equipment questions may be asked (pumps, etc.)

The third section requires assessment, recommendations, and providing health care information to promote public health (11%).

- Know your drug reference sources.

- Be able to read simple study summaries and interpret the data.

- Review emergency care and vaccinations.

- Review basic information regarding dietary supplements.

- Review self-care products and durable medical equipment, and self-monitoring of health status by the patient.

NAPLEX® is a computer-adaptive exam that consists of 185 multiple-choice questions. Of these, 150 questions are used to calculate your test score.

- The majority of the questions are asked in a scenario-based format (such as patient profiles with accompanying questions). There are also stand alone questions. The exam is moving towards more stand-alone questions.

- The exam time is 4 hours and 15 minutes with an optional 10-minute break after approximately 2 hours. Any other breaks that are needed will be subtracted from the total testing time.

- On the day of the exam, arrive 30 minutes prior to your appointment to get signed in (fingerprints will be taken, you will need 2 forms of ID, etc.)

- If you arrive 30 minutes or later than your scheduled appointment, and are refused admission to sit for the exam, you will be required to forfeit your appointment.

- A computer-adaptive exam assesses the answer to a given question in order to determine the level of difficulty to be selected for the following question. If you answer a question correctly, the computer will select a more difficult question from the test pool in an appropriate content area. If you answer a question incorrectly, an easier question will be selected by the computer. <u>If you miss a simple calculation you will get a relatively simple problem next and you may not accumulate enough points to pass.</u>

- The computer-adaptive format requires that ALL test questions be answered in the order in which they are presented. Therefore, you can NOT skip questions or go back to questions.

- Be sure to look at the website: www.nabp.net and take the pre-test prior to sitting for the exam. It is $50 and you can take it up to two times. Many students score poorly on the pre-test, and better on the actual exam. However, it gives a feel for how the cases look and for this reason is useful. The cases in our book (at the end of most of the therapeutics chapters) are also designed to be similar to exam-style cases.

Test Taking Tips

Study the top selling drugs (group them together; you'll see all the statins are there, many ACE Is, etc) – and focus on the doses for the common agents. We have bolded most of them in this text.

- For example, with beta blockers, focus on the dosing for atenolol, metoprolol, carvedilol (IR and CR) and propranolol (special uses). For loops, furosemide (1st); for thiazides, HCTZ, chlorthalidone. For NSAIDs, know dosing for ibuprofen, naproxen, and celecoxib.

Many times, the counseling and safety considerations will be similar for all agents in a particular class; therefore, if you know trade/generics, you can identify the SEs, ADRs, etc. for the group.

There are exceptions where individual agents have differences.

For example, propranolol (lipophilic, non-selective), carvedilol (not beta-1 selective), SSRI's (fluoxetine is most activating and is taken in the AM), some have more DI's (fluvoxamine, then fluoxetine, then paroxetine) otherwise SEs are similar. Study for the group, along with the individual exceptions.

When reading the case, write down the allergies, abnormal labs and major enzyme inducers/inhibitors. They are there for a reason.

- You will have a dry erase board – take time to write these things down – so they are in your mind when looking at the questions.

Know the major drug interactions – use our drug interactions section.

Focus on the common, chronic conditions first (diabetes, hypertension, lipids, pain, geriatric conditions, asthma/COPD, psych, common ID, common OTC), basic calculations and contraception.

- These usually make up a good bulk of the questions.

Study the drugs that pharmacists manage such as anticoagulation (warfarin, heparin, enoxaparin), infectious disease, coronary conditions, seizures, etc.

- Pharmacists write the questions for the exam. You should be studying material developed by practicing pharmacists – they'll know what is important.

When studying specialty topics (HIV, oncology, others), focus on the areas that each pharmacist should know (not what the specialists know).

- Know trade/generics of common oncology agents that are dispensed in the community setting.

- Know major toxicities of chemo drugs and how to prevent or mitigate them.

- Know how to manage the side effects of chemo agents (N/V, ESA use).

- For HIV, know commonly used agents, major toxicities and SEs, current guidelines, prophylaxis of OI's.

Make educated choices and have confidence

If you don't know the answer, narrow it down to 2 options, and then choose what seems most likely, focusing on <u>safety</u> issues first.

Example:

1. Ibuprofen can cause
   - *a.* Headache
   - *b.* GI irritation
   - *c.* Gastrectasis
   - *d.* Peripheral neuropathy
   - *e.* Phlebitis

- Almost all analgesics (not DHE) can cause rebound headaches – technically, this answer is correct. But don't choose it – choose the more obvious choice of GI irritation. Some people will choose gastrectasis – because it sounds scary and they may not be sure what it is!

If the answer seems too simple or obvious – that's likely because you know it.

Review the foundation topics at the beginning of this book, and study them first before the therapeutics, which begin with ID. These include:

- Key Drug References

- Immunizations

- Biostatistics and Pharmacoeconomics

- Medication Safety

<u>Review the Drug Interaction pages in this book</u>. You will see there are several key drugs that have significant interactions. Several key inducers and inhibitors. If you see a problem "substrate" drug or inducer or inhibitor, look for an interaction. Review carefully the additive drug interactions, including additive CNS effects, bleeding risk, QT prolongation, and the others – often, one drug alone may not be a problem, but when others with similar toxicities are taken together, and/or the doses are high, the pharmacist should notice the risk.

You don't need to answer every question correctly. You will realize that you answered a question wrong – after you have passed it. Some will freeze.

- Don't –forget about it and move on.

When you are studying, use time efficiently. Do not study for more than 45-50 minutes. Do some type of physical activity in short breaks. Do not study passively – use colleagues, write, talk.

Be sure you know how to provide patient counseling

- Talk to patients about how to monitor for S/Sx of side effects/ADR's at home (e.g., liver impairment, hyperkalemia, etc.). Counseling in this text appears after the drug tables.

- Be sure to know device techniques and administration techniques (MDI's, eye drops, insulin pen, etanercept injection (SC), Epi pen, nasal inhalers, etc.). We demonstrate most of these in the online video lectures.

Safety is key. Of all things, pharmacy licensure exams want to make sure we "do no harm."

Do not panic or worry excessively. This will not benefit you in your studies nor in the exam. Be confident. Stay positive. This is not a rocket science exam. But, there is a lot to know. Take time to learn well. If you get to feeling low think of some kooky person you know who has passed and realize you can do it too! If you are not sure if you have mastered key material, check your retention of key points with the matching quiz bank section at www.rxprep.com. If you are missing these questions (which are basic, must-know knowledge) you may wish to consider using the online video course which will help your understanding and, consequently, your retention.

How to Use this Book

This book is designed as a companion to our live or online courses. You can register for a review program at www.rxprep.com.

If you are using the book as a stand-alone, here are some pointers:

- If an item is bolded it is a key drug and if it is underlined it is essential information.

- Not all essential information is designated. Use the top seller list in the appendix as a guide to must-know drugs. You will also be tested on drugs that are not top sellers, but have safety considerations. Hospital drugs that are essential are not on the top seller list.

- This book is complete; you do not need to have a myriad of additional resources. In this version (2012) we have expanded the calculations by 50% to help students master the math – make sure you can do these well. The calculations in this text represent must-know math for pharmacists. Read our pointers on how to answer math questions.

- This text has "foundation" type material in the beginning of the text that is increasingly important in pharmacy, such as pharmacoeconomics and medication errors. Do not skip these chapters. It is best to review everything up to ID first.

- Many key drugs have counseling points after the "box" that outlines the drug. Review the counseling points; for example, if a drug causes "hepatotoxicity" the counseling points will include symptoms that the patient should notice if the liver is failing. The counseling, therefore, provides a review of key adverse effects, and may be representative of questions. Counseling is included for essential drugs – that is, none of the counseling information is superfluous.

- At the end of many of the core chapters are patient cases with practice questions. These are designed to be somewhat similar to NAPLEX® style cases – either in a written format, or the profile you might see on a pharmacy computer. The cases are designed to review key drugs points and should not be missed.

- You may wish to take the self-assessment quiz bank that is available on our website at www.rxprep.com. If you get 80%, it is not enough, as these questions are designed to test the most basic drug competency knowledge. Again, the knowledge in these questions, including calculations, should be at 100%. If you get something wrong right it down and learn it. If you are not scoring well on a section it means that you need to go back and review that material. The quiz bank for 2012 will have over 2,200 basic knowledge questions. The exam has more – which means, do not miss this information.

- If you notice anything that seems unusual or have a question please feel free to email us off the website and we will respond promptly. Our goal is to provide the best review source and to help in your journey towards becoming a safe, knowledgeable pharmacist.

- A special note to parents: if there are children in the house, any loving parent will be listening for them. This is good – but makes it difficult to focus on studying! Studying for a board exam requires a dedicated mind. You may need to make arrangements with your family to get out of the house and prepare with study partners, or go to an environment with fewer distractions than will be present in the home. Studying in a coffee shop or a library can be helpful. During the spring exam season students can "connect" with study partners using the RxPrep Facebook page.

CPJE Pointers – for CA exam takers

CPJE is about 80% clinical and about 20% law. Do not ignore the law; these are the straight forward questions and if you miss them you may not accrue enough points. You need a source to study the CA-specific law that is "readable" (much law material is not) and current.

- For law study we recommend these sources:

  - A Guide to California Community Pharmacy Law 7th Edition (2009-2011), by Dr. Fred G. Weissman, PharmD, J.D, *PLUS the* Supplement to the 7th Edition. The book and supplement can be purchased on our website at www.rxprep.com or from the USC Bookstore (same price). Dr. Weissman is planning to issue the 8th Edition sometime mid-year in 2012.

❑ Review the Community and Hospital Self Assessment Form prior to taking the exam – the points on this form should be clear before you sit for licensure. This is a check-off list that the Pharmacist-in-Charge completes every other (odd) year to ensure that the pharmacy is board-compliant. It is a nice way to check that you know these basic law requirements (such as how to store controlled drugs, legal requirements to store off-site, etc.). The form is available on the board website; click on the tabs in this order: Licensees/Pharmacists/Forms.

■ There are practice questions in the exam handbook that are available on the website. The handbook is also sent out once you have registered for the exam.

■ <u>Make sure you have reviewed the topics on the exam blueprint</u>. Note that there are important medication safety topics included, such as ADCs and NPSGs. Partly because of this, we put quite a bit of emphasis into the medication safety chapter in this text book. These topics are covered in our online course, and in our live programs in California.

■ You may wish to take (and get 100% – these are all basic information) the self-assessment quiz bank that is available on our website. We have included the material in the practice questions in the exam handbook in the quiz questions, but you should also do the practice quiz in the exam handbook because the questions are worded differently.

Best wishes for your CPJE preparation.

CALCULATIONS

Abbreviations Used in Prescriptions

ABBREVIATION	MEANING		ABBREVIATION	MEANING
ss	one-half		mL	milliliter
ac	before meals		NTE	not to exceed
pc	after meals		MDI	metered-dose inhaler
gtt, gtts	drop, drops		q	every
au	each ear		qd	every day
as	left ear		qod	every other day
ad	right ear		PO	by mouth or orally
ATC	around the clock		NPO	nothing by mouth
hs	at bedtime		IV	intravenous
bid	twice a day		IVP	intravenous push
tid	three times a day		IVPB	intravenous piggy back
qid	four times a day		ID	intradermal
biw	two times a week		IM	intramuscular
tiw	three times a week		subc, subq, SC, SQ	subcutaneous
os	left eye		ung	ointment
od	right eye		top	topically
ou	each eye		WA	while awake
qs	sufficient quantity		prn	as needed
qs ad	a sufficient quantity to make		stat	immediately
NR	no refills		SL	sublingual
c or w/	with		sup or supp	suppository
s or w/o	without		PR	per rectum
inj	injection		BM	bowel movement
X	times		N/V or N & V	nausea and vomiting

Equivalent Measurements

MEASUREMENT	EQUIVALENT
tsp (t)	5 mL
tbsp (T)	15 mL
1 fl oz	30 mL (approx.); 29.6 mL (actual)
1 cup	8 oz
1 pint (16 oz)	473 mL
1 quart	2 pints; 946 mL
1 gallon	4 quarts; 3,785 mL
1 kg	2.2 pounds
1 oz	28.4 g
1 pound	454 g
1 in	2.54 cm
1 grain (gr)	65 mg (approx); 64.8 mg (actual)
% (w/v)	g/100 mL
% (v/v)	mL/100 mL
% (w/w)	g/100 g

Metric Conversions

PREFIX	DEFINITION
kilo	1,000 (one thousand), as in kg
deci	1/10 (one-tenth), as in dL
milli	1/1,000 (one-thousandth), as in mL
micro	1/1,000,000 (one-millionth), as in mcg
nano	1/1,000,000,000 (one-billionth), as in ng

Labeling Instructions

- Begin with an instructive word (such as: Take, Place, Unwrap, Insert, Inhale).

- Follow with the quantity and dosage form (such as: 1 capsule).

- Follow by the location (such as: by mouth, rectally, vaginally, under tongue).

- Follow with the frequency (such as: daily, twice daily, at meals and bedtime).

- Finish with any noted instructions (such as: for pain, for cholesterol, on an empty stomach).

CPJE Students Only

Note in California the 2011 new prescription label requirements include changes to the label layout such as 16 phrases of directions for use. When applicable and consistent of that of the prescriber, these phrases should be used on the prescription label. Please refer to pages 20-23 of *A Guide To California Community Pharmacy Law*, Supplement to the 7th edition 2009-2011, by Fred G. Weissman, Pharm.D., J.D. or, the law statement on the board website.

Practice Problems

1. Choose the correct wording for the prescription label:

Joe Brown, MD
927 Deep Valley Drive
Ontario, California
Phone 333-5555

Name _Patty Johnson_____   Date _March 8, 2008_____

Address _58 Pine Oak Avenue_____

Vicodin 5/500 mg #12

Sig: i-ii tabs PO q 4-6 hrs prn pain X 2 days. NTE 6/d.

REFILL O 1 2 3 4 5 6	DEA NO.
Physician Signature	DATE

---

    a. Take 1-2 tablets by mouth every 4-6 hours as-needed for pain for 2 days. Do not exceed 6 tablets per day.

    b. Take up to 2 tablets by mouth every 4-6 hours as-needed for pain. Do not exceed 6 tablets per day.

    c. Take 1-2 tablets by mouth every 4-6 hours as-needed for pain. NTE 6 tablets per day.

    d. Take 1-2 tablets by mouth every 4-6 hours for pain. Do not exceed 6 tablets per day.

    e. Take 1-2 tablets by mouth up to 6 times daily as-needed for pain for 2 days. Do not exceed 6 tablets per day.

The correct answer is (A). Note that this prescription is using a daily maximum APAP dose of 3,000 mg/day (with the 500 mg dose). This is the component with the higher risk of toxicity (liver toxicity).

2. Choose the correct wording for the prescription label:

Joe Brown, MD
927 Deep Valley Drive
Ontario, California
Phone 333-5555

Name ___Patty Johnson_____ Date ___March 8, 2008_____

Address ___58 Pine Oak Avenue_____

Keflex 500 mg PO 1 po ac and hs.

REFILL O 1 2 3 4 5 6	DEA NO.
Physician Signature	DATE

[handwritten margin notes: ac = before meals; 3 meals + 1 @bedtime]

   a. Take one capsule four times daily: with meals and at bedtime.
   b. Take one capsule by mouth four times daily: with meals and at dinnertime.
   c. Take one capsule by mouth four times daily: with meals and at snack time.
   d. Take one capsule by mouth four times daily: with meals and at bedtime.
   e. Take one capsule by mouth four times daily: before meals and at bedtime.

The correct answer is (E). The patient should be counseled to finish all of the medication even if they start feeling better.

---

3. A pharmacist receives a prescription for "APAP 5 gr supp #6 1 PR prn temperature > 102 degrees". Choose the correct wording for the prescription label:

[handwritten margin note: 1gr = 65mg]

   a. Insert 1 suppository as needed when temperature is greater than 102 degrees.
   b. Unwrap and insert 1 suppository rectally as needed for a temperature greater than 102°.
   c. Take 500 mg of APAP suspension as needed 6 times per day for a temperature greater than 102°.
   d. Take 6 suppositories vaginally as needed for a temperature greater than 102°.
   e. Insert 500 mg of APAP into the rectum as needed for a fever greater than 102°.

The correct answer is (B). It is important to tell patients exactly how to take a medication. Five grains is 325 milligrams (65 mg x 5 mg/grain).

CALCULATING THE CORRECT DOSE FOR A PRESCRIPTION

Instructions to perform with each calculations problem in order to increase accuracy:

■ Check your math. Time permitting, double-check the calculations. It is very easy to make mistakes that you will catch when repeating the calculations.

- Place your answer directly into the equation used to solve the problem as another accuracy check. An example with a ratio conversion practice problem:

$$\frac{5\,g}{100\,g} = \frac{X\,g}{1{,}000\,g} \quad X = 50\,g$$

Check: 5/100 = 0.05; 50/1,000 = 0.05

If setting up a ratio, make sure the units, (and route and drug if applicable) in the numerators match, and then check that everything matches in the denominators as well.

- Read the question again after solving the problem to be certain you have answered with correct units (g or mg, mEq, mL or L, etc.).

- Make sure you are answering the question. The next problem illustrates that the problem may have more than one step, and you want to be careful to get to the right step to get to the requested response.

4. In the following prescription, the pharmacist dispensed 3 oz to Mrs. Chernoff. How many days of therapy will the patient be short?

Joe Brown, MD
927 Deep Valley Drive
Ontario, California
Phone 333-5555

Name _Jane E. Chernoff_____ Date _June 28, 2009_____

Address __33 Walden Rd. N Falls_____

TMP/SMX 40-200 mg/5 mL
Sig: 1 tsp PO BID x 10 days, until all taken.

REFILL O 1 2 3 4 5 6	DEA NO.
Physician Signature	DATE

---

    a. 10 mL
    b. 90 mL
    c. 1 day
    d. 9 days
    e. None of the above

The correct answer is (C). Use caution with calculations where a step of the answer (but not the final step) will be a selection. Always go back and read the question prior to selecting your response.

- 5 mL (per dose) x 2 times/day x 10 days = 100 mL needed

- Quantity dispensed: 3 oz x 30 mL/oz = 90 mL dispensed

- Difference: Quantity needed – Quantity dispensed = 100 mL – 90 mL = 10 mL

- Each tsp (t) is 5 mL. She needs 2 tsp (t) daily, which is 10 mL. She is 1 day short for her course of therapy.

---

5. How many milliliters (mL) of Mylanta suspension are contained in each dose of the prescription below?

PRESCRIPTION	QUANTITY
Belladonna Tincture	10 mL
Phenobarbital	60 mL
Mylanta susp. qs. ad	120 mL
Sig. 5 mL BID	

The total prescription is 120 mL; 10 mL belladonna, 60 mL of phenobarbital, and 50 mL of Mylanta.

120 – 60 – 10 = 50mL

$$\frac{50 \text{ mL Mylanta}}{120 \text{ mL total}} = \frac{X \text{ mL}}{5 \text{ mL dose}} \quad X = 2.08 \text{ mL/dose}$$

After solving the problem, read the question again to be certain you have answered the question with the correct units (mL per dose).

---

6. You have tablets that contain 0.25 mg of levothyroxine per tablet. You are crushing the tablets and mixing with glycerol and water for a 36 pound child. How many levothyroxine tablets will be needed to compound the following prescription?

PRESCRIPTION	QUANTITY
Levothyroxine Liq.	0.1 mg/mL
Disp.	60 mL
Sig. 0.01 mg per kg PO BID	

$$60 \text{ mL total} \times \frac{0.1 \text{ mg}}{\text{mL}} = 6 \text{ mg of levothyroxine needed}$$

$\frac{0.1 mg}{mL} \times 60 = 6 mg \times \frac{1 \ tab}{0.25 mg}$

$$6 \text{ mg levo} \times \frac{1 \text{ tab}}{0.25 \text{ mg}} = 24 \text{ tabs of levothyroxine needed}$$

24 Labs

Note: You can also solve many problems by <u>dimensional analysis</u>, a process of placing all of the arithmetical terms into one equation where all the units cancel out except the units of the desired answer. The use of dimensional analysis consolidates the multiple arithmetical steps into a single step. For the problem above, solving by dimensional analysis:

$$\frac{1 \text{ tab}}{0.25 \text{ mg}} \quad X \quad \frac{0.1 \text{ mg}}{\text{mL}} \quad X \quad \frac{60 \text{ mL}}{} \quad = 24 \text{ tabs of levothyroxine needed}$$

After solving the problem, read the question again to be certain you have answered the question with the correct units (tablets).

---

7. How many milligrams of codeine will be contained in each capsule?

PRESCRIPTION	QUANTITY
Codeine Sulfate	0.6 g
Guaifenesin	1.2 g
Caffeine	0.15 g
M. ft. caps. no. 24	
Sig. One capsule TID prn cough	

Begin by converting to the unit requested in the answer (mg).

$$0.6 \text{ g Codeine} \quad X \quad \frac{1,000 \text{ mg}}{1 \text{ g}} \quad = 600 \text{ mg of codeine for the total prescription}$$

The prescription order is for 24 capsules: 600 mg total /24 caps = 25 mg/capsule

After solving the problem, read the question again to be certain you have answered the question with the correct units (mg per capsule).

---

8. A physician writes an order for aminophylline 500 mg IV , dosed at 0.5 mg per kg per hour for a patient weighing 165 pounds. There is only theophylline in stock. How many milligrams (mg) of theophylline will the patient receive per hour?

$$\frac{0.5 \text{ mg Amino}}{\text{kg/hr}} \quad X \quad \frac{1 \text{ kg}}{2.2 \text{ pounds}} \quad X \quad 165 \text{ pounds} \quad = 37.5 \text{ mg/hr Aminophylline}$$

To get the theophylline dose, multiply by 0.8. Therefore, 37.5 mg/hr x 0.8 = 30 mg/hr of theophylline. You must know how to convert between aminophylline and theophylline.

After solving the problem, read the question again to be certain you have answered the question with the correct units (mg per hour).

---

9. How many milliliters of hydrocortisone liquid 40 mg/mL will be needed to prepare 30 grams of a 0.25% cream?

■ 0.25% cream = 0.25 g/100 g = 250 mg/100 g = 2.5 mg/1 gram.

$$\frac{2.5 \text{ mg}}{1 \text{ gram}} \quad X \quad 30 \text{ grams for Rx} \quad = \quad 75 \text{ mg needed}$$

$$75 \text{ mg } \quad X \quad \frac{1 \text{ mL}}{40 \text{ mg}} \quad = \quad \underline{1.875 \text{ mL needed}}$$

After solving the problem, read the question again to be certain you have answered the question with the correct units (mL).

---

10. How many grains of aspirin will be contained in each capsule? Round to the nearest tenth.

PRESCRIPTION	QUANTITY
Aspirin	6 g
Phenacetin	3.2 g
Caffeine	0.48 g
No. 20 caps	
Sig. One capsule Q6H prn pain	

$$6 \text{ g ASA } \quad X \quad \frac{1,000 \text{ mg}}{1 \text{ g}} \quad X \quad \frac{1 \text{ gr}}{65 \text{ mg}} \quad = 92.3 \text{ grains}$$

We have 92.3 grains per 20 capsules. 92.3 gr/20 capsules = 4.6 grains/capsule

After solving the problem, read the question again to be certain you have answered the question with the correct units (grains per capsule).

PROPORTIONS

A proportion is the expression of the equality of two ratios. Given any three values of a proportion, it is easy to calculate the fourth. You must keep the same units in the numerator as well as in the denominator (and keep the route, and drug, the same in each as well if they are in the problem).

$$\frac{a}{b} = \frac{c}{d}$$

---

11. If one 10 mL vial contains 0.05 g of diltiazem, how many milliliters should be administered to provide a 25 mg dose of diltiazem?

First, convert grams to milligrams: 0.05 gram of diltiazem x 1,000 mg/1 gram = 50 mg

Use proportions to calculate the number of mL for a 25 mg dose:

$$\frac{50 \text{ mg}}{10 \text{ mL}} = \frac{25 \text{ mg}}{X \text{ mL}} \quad X = 5 \text{ mL dose}$$

12. If phenobarbital elixir contains 18.2 mg of phenobarbital per 5 mL, how many grams of phenobarbital would be used in preparing a pint of the elixir?

First, convert milligrams to grams. Usually, it is best practice to convert to the units required in the answer when you begin the problem.

- 18.2 mg x 1 gram/1,000 mg = 0.0182 g

$$\frac{0.0182 \text{ g}}{5 \text{ mL}} = \frac{X \text{ g}}{473 \text{ mL}} \quad X = \underline{1.72 \text{ g}}$$

---

13. A cough syrup contains 4 g of brompheniramine maleate per liter. How many milligrams are contained in a teaspoonful (t) dose of the elixir?

- 4 g x 1,000 mg/1 gram = 4,000 mg per 1 liter

- 1 L = 1,000 mL, therefore 4,000 mg per 1,000 mL

- 1 teaspoonful (t) = 5 mL

Solve using proportions.

$$\frac{4,000 \text{ mg}}{1,000 \text{ mL}} = \frac{X \text{ mg}}{5 \text{ mL}} \quad X = \underline{20 \text{ mg}}$$

---

14. A patient is to receive acyclovir 5 mg/kg every 8 hours. What daily dose should a 110 pound female receive?

Begin by converting the patients weight in pounds (lbs) to kilograms (kg)

- 2.2 pounds = 1 kg

- 110 pounds x 1 kg/2.2 pounds = 50 kg

$$\frac{5 \text{ mg}}{1 \text{ kg}} = \frac{X \text{ mg}}{50 \text{ kg}} \quad X = 250 \text{ mg} \times 3 \text{ doses} = \underline{750 \text{ mg/d}}$$

---

15. A patient weighing 110 kg is to receive 0.25 mg/kg per day amphotericin B (reconstituted and diluted to 0.1 mg/mL) by IV infusion. What volume of solution is required to deliver the daily dose?

Begin by calculating the total daily dose (mg) for this patient.

$$\frac{0.25 \text{ mg}}{1 \text{ kg}} = \frac{X \text{ mg}}{110 \text{ kg}} \quad X = 27.5 \text{ mg daily}$$

Solve the problem by calculating the total daily volume (mL) of reconstituted amphotericin B solution (0.1 mg per mL) needed per day.

$$\frac{27.5 \text{ mg}}{X \text{ mL}} = \frac{0.1 \text{ mg}}{1 \text{ mL}} \quad X = \underline{275 \text{ mL daily dose}}$$

PERCENTAGE PREPARATIONS

Percent weight-in-volume (% w/v) is expressed as g/100 mL. Percent volume-in-volume (% v/v) is expressed as mL/100 mL. Percent weight-in-weight (% w/w) is expressed as g/100 g.

---

16. How many grams of NaCl are in 1 liter of normal saline (NS)?

Normal saline (NS) = 0.9% (w/v) NaCl solution

Remember (w/v) is always expressed as grams per 100 mL, therefore NS contains 0.9 g NaCl per 100 mL of solution.

$$\frac{0.9 \text{ g}}{100 \text{ mL}} = \frac{X \text{ g}}{1,000 \text{ mL}} \qquad X = 9 \text{ g} \checkmark$$

---

17. Digoxin injection is supplied in ampules of 500 mcg per 2 mL. How many milliliters must a nurse administer to provide a dose of 0.2 mg?

First, convert 500 mcg to mg: 500 mcg x 1 mg/1,000 mcg = 0.5 mg.

$$\frac{0.5 \text{ mg}}{2 \text{ mL}} = \frac{0.2 \text{ mg}}{X \text{ mL}} \qquad X = 0.8 \text{ mL}$$

---

18. If 200 capsules contain 500 mg of an active ingredient, how many milligrams of the active ingredient will 76 capsules contain?

$$\frac{200 \text{ caps}}{500 \text{ mg}} = \frac{76 \text{ caps}}{X \text{ mg}} \qquad X = 190 \text{ mg}$$

---

19. A metered dose inhaler provides 90 micrograms of albuterol sulfate with each inhalation. The canister provides 200 inhalations. If the patient uses the entire canister, how many total milligrams will the patient have received?

200 inhalations x 90 mcg/inhalation = 18,000 micrograms

$$\frac{18,000 \text{ mcg}}{1,000} = 18 \text{ milligrams}$$

---

20. An elixir of ferrous sulfate contains 220 milligrams of ferrous sulfate in each 5 milliliters. If each milligram of ferrous sulfate contains the equivalent of 0.2 milligrams of elemental iron, how many milligrams of elemental iron would be in each 5 milliliters of elixir?

Ferrous sulfate ($FeSO_4$) contains 20% elemental iron (Fe); this is given in the problem which states that 1 milligram has 0.2 milligrams of elemental iron, which is 20%.

$$\frac{0.2 \text{ mg Fe}}{1 \text{ mg FeSO}_4} = \frac{X \text{ mg Fe}}{220 \text{ mg FeSO}_4} \qquad X = 44 \text{ mg Fe}$$

21. How many grams of NaCl are in 1 Liter of ½ NS?

$$\frac{0.45\ g}{100\ mL} = \frac{X\ g}{1{,}000\ mL} \qquad X = 4.5\ g$$

If NS is 0.9 grams/100 mL, then ½ NS will be 0.45 grams/100 mL.

---

22. A penicillin V 250 mg tablet equals 400,000 units of penicillin activity. A patient is taking penicillin V 500 mg tablets QID for 7 days. How much penicillin activity (units) will this patient receive?

If 250 mg contains 400,000 units, then 500 mg contains 800,000 units. The patient is taking 4 tablets daily, for 7 days (or 28 total tablets), at 800,000 units each.

$$\frac{800{,}000\ units}{1\ tab} = \frac{X\ units}{28\ tabs} \qquad X = 22{,}400{,}000\ units$$

---

23. A 45 milliliter nasal spray delivers 20 sprays per milliliter of solution. Each spray contains 1.5 mg of active drug. How many milligrams of drug are contained in the 45 mL package?

First, add up the amount of drug per mL: 1.5 mg drug/spray x 20 sprays/mL = 30 mg/mL.

$$\frac{30\ mg}{mL} = \frac{X\ mg}{45\ mL} \qquad X = 1{,}350\ mg$$

---

24. Oral potassium chloride 20% solution contains 40 mEq of potassium per 15 milliliters of solution. A patient needs 25 mEq of potassium daily. What is the amount, in milliliters, of 20% potassium chloride that the patient should take?

$$\frac{40\ mEq}{15\ mL} = \frac{25\ mEq}{X\ mL} \qquad X = 9.375\ mL$$

---

25. How many grams of dextrose are in 500 mL of D5W?

$$\frac{5\ g}{100\ mL} = \frac{X\ g}{500\ mL} \qquad X = 25\ g$$

---

26. A 10 gram packet of potassium chloride provides 20 mEq of potassium and 4 mEq of chloride. How many grams of powder would provide 8 mEq of potassium?

$$\frac{10\ g}{20\ mEq} = \frac{X\ g}{8\ mEq} \qquad X = 4\ g$$

27. How many grams of triamcinolone should be used in preparing the following prescription?

PRESCRIPTION	QUANTITY
Triamcinolone (w/v)	5%
Glycerin qs	60 mL
Sig. Two drops in right ear	

$$\frac{5\ g}{100\ mL} = \frac{X\ g}{60\ mL} \quad X = 3\ g$$

28. If 1,250 g of a solution contains 80 g of drug, what is the percentage strength (w/w) of the solution?

$$\frac{80\ g}{1,250\ g} = \frac{X\ g}{100\ g} \quad X = 6.4\ g,\ which\ is\ 6.4\%$$

29. A mouth rinse contains 1/12% (w/v) of chlorhexidine gluconate. How many grams of chlorhexidine gluconate should be used to prepare 18 liters of mouth rinse?

- 1/12 % = 0.083 grams per 100 mL (w/v).

- 18 L x 1,000 mL/L = 18,000 mL

$$\frac{0.083\ g}{100\ mL} = \frac{X\ g}{18,000\ mL} \quad X = 14.9\ g$$

30. A pharmacist dissolves 6 metronidazole tablets, each containing 250 mg, into an ointment liquid base to prepare 60 mL of a topical solution. What is the percentage strength (w/v) of metronidazole in the prescription?

- 6 tablets x 250 mg/tab = 1,500 mg, or 1.5 grams

$$\frac{1.5\ g}{60\ mL} = \frac{X\ g}{100\ mL} \quad X = 2.5\ g,\ which\ is\ 2.5\% \ ✓$$

RATIO STRENGTH

Ratio strength is a way to express concentrations of weak solutions or liquid preparations (as in 1:5,000).

31. Express 0.04% as a ratio strength.

$$\frac{0.04}{100} = \frac{1\ part}{X\ parts} \quad X = 2,500.\ Ratio\ strength\ is\ 1:2,500$$

You can go back to 0.04% by taking 1/2500 x 100; try it. Or, this can be solved as a ratio, as seen in problem 33.

32. What is the percentage strength of imiquimod in the prescription?

PRESCRIPTION	QUANTITY
Imiquimod 5% cream	15 g
Xylocaine	20 g
Hydrophilic ointment	25 g

First, calculate the amount of imiquimod in the prescription. 5% is 5 g/100 g X 15 g = 0.75 grams of imiquimod.

The total weight of the prescription is 60 g (15 g + 20 g + 25 g).

$$\frac{0.75 \text{ g}}{60 \text{ g}} = \frac{X \text{ g}}{100 \text{ g}} \quad X = 1.25 \text{ g/100 g, which is } \underline{1.25\%}$$

33. Express 1:4,000 as a percentage strength.

$$\frac{1 \text{ part}}{4,000 \text{ part}} = \frac{X}{100} \quad X = 0.025, \text{ which is } \underline{0.025\%}$$

PARTS PER MILLION (PPM)

Parts indicate amount proportions. Parts per million (ppm) and parts per billion (ppb) are commonly used to quantify strengths of very dilute solutions. It is defined as the number of parts of the drug per 1 million (or 1 billion) parts of the whole. 1 PPM is equivalent to 1 mg/L of water. If you are given a bottle labeled 30 PPM, this is the same as 30 mg/L or 0.03 g/L or 0.003 g/100 mL or 0.003%.

34. Express 0.00022% w/v as PPM.

$$\frac{0.00022 \text{ g}}{100 \text{ mL}} = \frac{X \text{ g}}{1,000,000} \quad X = 2.2 \text{ PPM}$$

35. Express 30 ppm of copper in solution as a percentage.

$$\frac{30}{1,000,000} = \frac{X \text{ g}}{100 \text{ mL}} \quad X = 0.003\%$$

36. Express 5 ppm of iron in water as a percentage.

$$\frac{5}{1,000,000} = \frac{X \text{ g}}{100 \text{ mL}} \quad X = 0.0005\%$$

If asked to express something in PPB (parts per billion), you divide by 1,000,000,000 (9 zeros).

BODY MASS INDEX (BMI)

BMI is a measure of body fat based on height and weight that applies to adult men and women. A primary health problem is overweight and obesity which substantially increases the risk of morbidity from hypertension, dyslipidemia, diabetes, coronary heart disease, stroke, gallbladder disease, osteoarthritis and others. Higher body weights are also associated with increases in all-cause mortality. BMI is a useful measure of body fat, but the BMI can over-estimate body fat in persons who are muscular, and can under-estimate body fat in frail elderly and others who have lost muscle mass. Waist circumference is used concurrently. If most of the fat is around the waist, there is a higher disease risk. High risk is a waist size > 35 inches for women or > 40 inches for men..

Underweight can be a problem if a person is fighting a disease such as a frail, hospitalized patient with an infection. BMI is calculated as follows:

$$BMI = \frac{weight\ (kg)}{height\ (m^2)}$$

Alternatively, BMI can be calculated using the following formula:

$$BMI = \frac{weight\ (pounds)}{height\ (in)^2} \times 704.5$$

BMI Classifications

SCORE	CLASSIFICATION
< 18.5	Underweight
18.5-24.9	Normal weight
25-29.9	Overweight
> 30	Obese

37. **A male comes to the pharmacy and tells you he is 6'7" tall and 250 pounds. His waist circumference is 43 inches. Calculate his BMI. Is the patient underweight, normal weight, overweight, or obese?**

- Convert weight: 250 pounds/2.2 = 113.6 kg

- Convert height: 6'7" = 79" x 2.54 cm/inch = 200.66 cm.

- 200.66 cm = 2 m (divide cm by 100 to get the height in meters)

$$BMI\ (kg/m^2) = \frac{113.6}{2^2} = 28.4,\ \text{which is overweight.}$$

38. Calculate the BMI for a male who is 6′ tall and weighs 198 lbs. Is the patient underweight, normal weight, overweight, or obese?

$$\text{BMI (pounds/in}^2) \ = \ \frac{198 \text{ pounds}}{(72 \text{ in})^2} \ \times \ 704.5 \ = \ 26.9, \text{ which is overweight.}$$

IDEAL BODY WEIGHT (IBW)

IBW is the healthy (ideal) weight for a person (neither too thin nor too heavy). Some medications which are hydrophilic do not distribute much into fat and should be dosed on IBW to prevent giving the patient too much drug. <u>Although this is not one of the simpler formulas, it is generally known by pharmacists, as is the creatinine clearance formula below, and may not be provided.</u>

- IBW (males) = 50 kg + (2.3 kg)(each inch > 5 feet)

- IBW (females) = 45.5 kg + (2.3 kg)(each inch > 5 feet)

Renal Function and Creatinine Clearance (CrCl) Estimation

A normal range of serum creatinine is approximately 0.6 to 1.2 mg/dL. A creatinine above this range indicates that the kidneys are not functioning properly. However, the values can appear normal when renal function is compromised. The dosing example using the Cockcroft-Gault equation below will show a normal creatinine level in a patient with reduced renal function.

Creatinine is a break-down product produced when muscle tissue makes energy. If the kidneys are declining and cannot clear (excrete) the creatinine, the creatinine level will increase in the blood and the creatinine clearance (CrCl) will decrease. This tells us that the concentration of drugs that are renally cleared will also increase and a dose reduction may be required.

The patient should be assessed for <u>dehydration</u> if the creatinine value is elevated. Dehydration can cause both the serum creatinine (SCr) and the blood, urea, nitrogen (BUN) values to increase. Generally, a BUN:SCr ratio > 20 indicates dehydration. Correcting the dehydration will reduce both BUN and SCr, and can prevent or treat acute renal failure. In actual practice signs of dehydration will be assessed, including decreased urine output, tachycardia, tachypnea, dry skin/mouth/mucous membranes, lack of skin tenting (skin does not bounce back when pinched into a fold) and possibly fever. Dehydration is usually caused by diarrhea, vomiting, and lack of adequate fluid/electrolyte intake. High fever and lack of sweating capacity can be contributory.

39. Looking at the laboratory values below, is this patient experiencing dehydration?

	NORMAL RANGE	PATIENT'S RANGE
BUN	7-25 mg/dL	54
Creatinine	0.6-1.2 mg/dL	1.8

Yes, the BUN:SCr ratio is 54/1.8 = 30. Since 30 > 20, the BUN is disproportionately elevated relative to the creatinine, meaning the patient is dehydrated and should receive fluids.

---

40. Nancy is receiving a furosemide infusion at 5 mg/hr. The nurse notices her urine output has decreased in the last hour. Laboratory values are drawn and the patient has a SCr 1.5 mg/dL and a BUN 26 mg/dL. The nurse wants to know if she should stop the furosemide infusion due to the patient becoming dehydrated. Is this patient dehyrated?

No, the BUN:SCr ratio is 26/1.5 = 17.3, which is < 20. Continue to monitor the patient. This question, by itself, has little meaning since the patient's previous BUN and SCr values are not given as reference points, but the question about dehydration can still be answered.

THE COCKCROFT-GAULT EQUATION

This formula is used commonly by pharmacists to estimate renal function. It is not commonly used, however, in very young children, ESRD or when renal function is fluctuating rapidly. There are different methods used to estimate renal function in these circumstances. This formula should be known, as it is commonly used in practice.

$$\text{CrCl} = \frac{140 - (\text{age of patient})}{72 \times \text{SCr}} \times \text{wt in kg} \ (\times 0.85 \text{ if female})$$

For obese patients, the adjusted body weight (AdjBW) may be preferable. As mentioned above, the IBW is commonly used for drugs that are hydrophilic, such as aminoglycosides, theophylline and others. If the actual weight is used, a drug that primarily stays in the blood compartment and does not distribute into fat may be overdosed.

CRCL (ML/MIN)	INTERPRETATION
60-90	mild renal insufficiency
30-59	moderate renal insufficiency
15-29	severe renal insufficiency
< 15	kidney failure (or dialysis)

41. An 87 year-old female patient (height 5'4", weight 103 pounds) is placed on levofloxacin, dosing per pharmacy. Her labs include BUN 22 mg/dL and SCr 1 mg/dL. Choose the correct dosing regimen using the following chart.

CRCL	≥ 50 ML/MIN	20-49 ML/MIN	< 20ML/MIN
Levofloxacin Dose	500 mg Q 24 hours	250 mg Q 24 hours	250 mg Q 48 hours

First, convert weight to kg: 103 pounds x 1 kg/2.2 pounds = 46.8 kg

$$\text{CrCL} = \frac{140 - 87}{72 \times 1} \times 46.8 \ (\times 0.85) = 29 \text{ mL/min. The correct dose is 250 mg Q 24H.}$$

42. A 34 year-old male (height 6'7", weight 227 pounds) is hospitalized after a motor vehicle accident. He develops a *P. aeruginosa* infection. The physician orders tobramycin 2 mg/kg IV Q8H. Calculate the tobramycin dose using the patient's IBW. Round to the nearest 10 milligrams.

- IBW (males) = 50 kg + (2.3 kg x height in inches over 5 feet)

- IBW = 50 kg + (2.3 x 19 in) = 93.7 kg

- Tobramycin 2 mg/kg x 93.7 kg = <u>187 mg</u>, round to 190 mg IV Q8H.

---

43. A 45 year-old male (height 6'1", weight 177 pounds) has HIV and is being started on tenofovir, emtricitabine and efavirenz therapy. His laboratory values include K⁺ 4.4 mEq/L, BUN 40 mg/dL, SCr 1.8 mg/dL, and CD4 count of 455 cells/mm³. Based on the chart information below, what is the correct dose of tenofovir for this patient?

CRCL	≥ 50 ML/MIN	30-49 ML/MIN	10-29 ML/MIN	< 10 ML/MIN
Tenofovir Dose	300 mg daily	300 mg Q 48 hours	300 mg Q 72-96 hours	300 mg weekly

- First, convert weight to kg: 177 pounds x 1 kg/2.2 pounds = 80.5 kg

$$\text{CrCL} = \frac{140 - 45}{72 \times 1.8} \times 80.5 = \underline{59 \text{ mL/min}}. \text{ The correct dose is 300 mg daily.}$$

---

44. An 82 year-old female patient weighing 155 pounds is hospitalized with a nosocomial pneumonia which is responding to treatment. Her current antibiotic medications include ceftazidime, imipenem and vancomycin. Her morning laboratory values include K⁺ 4.0 mEq/L, BUN 60 mg/dL, SCr 2.7 mg/dL, and glucose 222 mg/dL. Based on the chart information below, what is the correct dose of imipenem for this patient?

CRCL	≥ 71 ML/MIN	41-70 ML/MIN	21-40 ML/MIN	≤ 20 ML/MIN
Imipenem Dose	500 mg IV Q6H	500 mg IV Q8H	250 mg IV Q6H	250 mg IV Q12H

- First, convert weight to kg: 155 pounds/2.2 = 70.5 kg

$$\text{CrCL} = \frac{140 - 82}{72 \times 2.7} \times 70.5 \, (0.85) = \underline{17.9 \text{ mL/min}}. \text{ The correct dose is } \underline{250 \text{ mg IV Q12H}}.$$

---

45. A female patient is to receive 5 mg/kg/d of theophylline, dosed on IBW. The patient is 5'7" and weighs 243 pounds. Calculate the theophylline dose the patient should receive.

- IBW (females) = 45.5 kg + 2.3 (every inch over 5 feet)

- IBW (females) = 45.5 kg + 2.3 (7) = 61.6 kg

- Theophylline 5 mg/kg x 61.6 kg = <u>308 mg</u>

- Check if there were any instructions in the problem regarding rounding.

SPECIFIC GRAVITY (SG)

Specific gravity is the ratio of the density of a substance to the density of water. SG can be important for calculating IV medications, in compounding, and in urinalysis for use in diagnosis. Water has a specific gravity of 1. 1 gram water = 1 mL water. Substances that have a SG < 1 are lighter than water. Substances that have a SG > 1 are heavier than water. SG does not have units.

$$SG = \frac{weight\ (g)}{volume\ (mL)}$$

---

46. What is the weight of 750 mL of concentrated acetic acid (SG=1.2)?

$$1.2 = \frac{X\ g}{750\ mL} \qquad X = 900\ g$$

Check the answer: 900 g/750 mL = 1.2

---

47. How many mL of polysorbate 80 (SG = 1.08) are needed to prepare a prescription that includes 48 g of the surfactant/emulsifier (polysorbate)?

$$1.08 = \frac{48\ g}{X\ mL} \qquad X = 44.44\ mL$$

Check the answer: 48 g/44.44 mL = 1.08

---

48. What is the specific gravity of 150 mL of glycerin weighing 165 grams?

$$SG = \frac{165\ g}{150\ mL} \qquad SG = 1.1$$

Check the answer: 150 mL x 1.1 = 165 g

---

49. Nitroglycerin has a specific gravity of 1.59. How much would 1 quart weigh?

- 1 pint = 473 mL. One quart = 2 pints, or 946 mL.

$$1.59 = \frac{X\ g}{946\ mL} \qquad X = 1,504\ g$$

Check the answer: 1,504 g/946 mL = 1.59

Note that the SG is equivalent to the density in g/mL. If asked for the density (for example in the above problem), it would be 1.59 g/mL.

BODY SURFACE AREA (BSA)

BSA is the measured surface of the body. BSA is sometimes used to dose chemotherapy and in pediatrics. Currently, BSA is used less frequently than previously (dosing by weight is used more commonly), but it may still be used with certain medications. Note that the units are in m². There are a few variations in the way BSA is calculated. If you calculate BSA using this formula, you might need to choose an answer that is close (a few digits away) from your answer. If given a certain formula, use it.

$$BSA\ (m^2) = \sqrt{\frac{Ht\ (cm) \times Wt\ (kg)}{3{,}600}}$$

---

50. A patient has a weight of 58 kg and height of 152.4 cm. What is the patient's BSA?

$$BSA\ (m^2) = \sqrt{\frac{152.4 \times 58}{3{,}600}} = \underline{1.57\ m^2}$$

FLOW RATES

Intravenous infusions are commonly used to deliver medications in many settings including hospitals. Flow rates are used to calculate the volume or amount of drug a patient will receive over a given period of time. An order can specify the rate of flow of intravenous fluids in milliliters per minute, drops per minute, amount of drug (e.g. mcg/hour), or as the total time to administer the entire volume of the infusion (e.g., give over 8 hours).

---

51. The pharmacist has an order for heparin 25,000 units in 250 mL D5W to infuse at 1,000 units/hour. What is the infusion rate in mL/hour?

First, calculate units per mL: 25,000 units/250 mL = 100 units/mL

Second, since there are 100 units in each mL and 1,000 units/hour are delivered to the patient, the pump should be programmed for an infusion rate of 10 mL/hr.

$$\frac{1\ mL}{100\ units} \times \frac{1{,}000\ units}{hour} = 10\ mL/hour$$

---

52. The pharmacist has an order for heparin 25,000 units in 250 mL D5W to infuse at 1,000 units/hour. How much time will be needed to infuse the entire bag?

$$25{,}000\ units \times \frac{1\ hr}{1{,}000\ units} = 25\ hours$$

You may need to calculate how many drops will be administered per minute (or per hour). The problem would state the number of drops/mL, which depends on the infusion set.

---

53. An infusion set delivers 15 drops/mL. The heparin infusion is running at 10 mL/hr. How many drops/hr will the patient receive?

$$\frac{15\ drops}{1\ mL} \times \frac{10\ mL}{hr} = 150\ drops/hr$$

54. A nurse is hanging a 4% lidocaine solution for a patient. If the dose is 6 mg/min, how many hours will a 250 mL bag last?

$$\frac{1 \text{ hr}}{60 \text{ min}} \times \frac{1 \text{ min}}{6 \text{ mg}} \times \frac{1{,}000 \text{ mg}}{1 \text{ g}} \times \frac{4 \text{ g}}{100 \text{ mL}} \times 250 \text{ mL} = \underline{27.8 \text{ hours}}$$

55. An order is written for 10 mL of a 10% calcium chloride injection and 10 mL of multivitamin injection (MVI) to be mixed with 500 mL of D5W. The infusion is to be administered over 6 hours. The IV set delivers 15 drops/mL. What should be the rate of flow in drops/minute to deliver this infusion?

Total volume of the infusion = 500 mL (D5W) + 10 mL (CaCl$_2$) + 10 mL (MVI) = 520 mL

$$\frac{15 \text{ gtts}}{\text{mL}} \times \frac{520 \text{ mL}}{6 \text{ hr}} \times \frac{1 \text{ hr}}{60 \text{ min}} = \underline{21.67 \text{ gtts/min}}$$

56. An intravenous infusion contains 2 mL of a 1:1,000 solution of epinephrine and 250 mL of D5W. At what flow rate, in mL/min, should the infusion be administered to provide 0.3 mcg/kg/min of epinephrine to an 80 kg patient?

- 1:1,000 = 0.1% (w/v) = 0.1 g/100 mL or 100 mg/100 mL. 1 mg/1 mL x 2 mL = 2 mg Epi in the 2 mL

The patient is 80 kg x 0.3 mcg/kg/min = 24 mcg/min

$$\frac{252 \text{ mL}}{2 \text{ mg}} \times \frac{1 \text{ mg}}{1{,}000 \text{ mcg}} \times \frac{24 \text{ mcg}}{\text{min}} = \underline{3 \text{ mL/min}}$$

57. A patient is to receive argatroban at a dose of 2 mcg/kg/min. The pharmacy mixes a concentration of 100 mg argatroban in 250 mL of D5W. The patient weighs 85 kg. How many mL/hour should the nurse infuse to provide the desired dose? Round to the nearest whole number.

First, determine the amount of drug needed based on body weight:

- 2 mcg/kg/min x 85 kg = 170 mcg/min

Then, calculate mL/hr:

$$\frac{250 \text{ mL}}{100 \text{ mg}} \times \frac{1 \text{ mg}}{1{,}000 \text{ mcg}} \times \frac{170 \text{ mcg}}{\text{min}} \times \frac{60 \text{ min}}{\text{hr}} = \underline{25.5 \text{ mL/hr, rounded up to 26 mL/hr}}$$

STRENGTH ADJUSTMENTS

Often, the strength of a concentration must be increased or decreased. Or, a new quantity (volume) is required. This formula can be used to change the strength or volume. Be careful: the units on each side must match and one or more may need to be changed, such as mg to gram, or vice-versa.

- $Q_1 \times C_1 = Q_2 \times C_2$

- Q_1 = old quantity

- C_1 = old concentration

- Q_2 = new quantity

- C_2 = new concentration

---

58. How many mL of a 1:2,500 (w/v) solution of aluminum acetate can be made from 100 mL of a 0.2% solution?

- 1:2,500 is converted to a percentage by making it into a fraction and multiplying by 100:

- 1:2,500 = 1/2,500 x 100 = 0.04%

- $Q_1 \times C_1 = Q_2 \times C_2$

- 100 mL x 0.2% = Q_2 x 0.04%

- Q_2 = 500 mL

---

59. Using 20 g of a 9% Boric Acid ointment base, the pharmacist will manufacture a 5% ointment. How much diluent is required?

Note the difference from the previous problem where the calculation provided the total volume. Here, you will get the final quantity (weight) but are asked how much diluent should be added to make the final weight.

- 20 g x 9% = Q_2 x 5%; Q_2 = 36 g total.

- Then take 36 g – 20 g (already present) = 16 g diluent required

---

60. How many grams of petrolatum (diluent) should be added to 250 g of a 20% ichthammol ointment to make a 7% ointment?

- 250 g x 20% = Q_2 x 7%; Q_2 = 714.3 g total

- 714.3 g – 250 g present = 464.3 g petrolatum required

---

61. What is the ratio strength (w/v) of 50 mL containing a 1:20 (w/v) ammonia solution diluted to 1,000 mL?

- 1:20 is converted to a percentage by making it into a fraction and multiplying by 100:

- 1:20 = 1/20 x 100 = 5%

- 50 mL x 5% = 1,000 mL x C_2

- C_2 = 0.25% = 1:400

62. If 1 gallon of a 20% (w/v) solution is evaporated to a solution with a 50% (w/v) strength, what will be the new volume (in mL)?

- 3,785 mL x 20% = Q_2 x 50%

- Q_2 = 1,514 mL ⟍

ALLIGATION

Alligation is used to obtain a new strength (percentage) that is between two strengths that the pharmacist has in stock. Occasionally, no math is required to solve this type of problem if the strength needed is exactly in the middle of the 2 strengths that are given.

63. Measure out 100 g of a 50% hydrocortisone powder using the 25% and 75% in stock.

- Use 50g of the 75%, and 50g of the 25% (total is 100 grams).

If the prescription calls for an ingredient that is pure, the concentration (higher) is 100%. If you are given a diluent, such as petrolatum, lanolin, alcohol, "ointment base", etc., the concentration of the diluent (lower) is 0%.

---

64. You are asked to prepare 80 g of a 12.5% ichthammol ointment. You have 16% and 12% ichthammol ointments in stock.

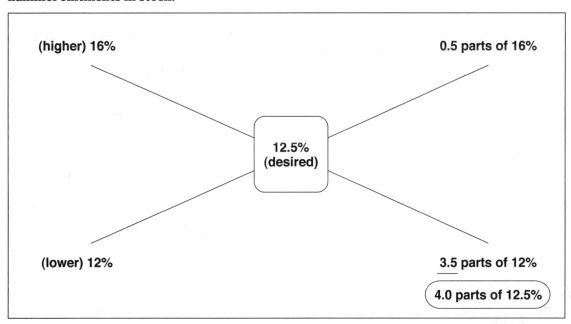

- Add the parts to find the total # of parts (4 parts in this problem).

- Divide by the total weight (80 g) by the number of parts to get the weight per part: 80 g/4 parts = 20 g per part.

  - ⟍ ❑ 0.5 parts x 20 g = 10 g of the 16% ichthammol ointment

  - ⟍ ❑ 3.5 parts x 20 g = 70 g of the 12% ichthammol ointment

- ⟍ The end product provides 80 g of a 12.5% ichthammol ointment.

65. You are asked to prepare 1 gallon of tincture containing 5.5% iodine. The pharmacy has 3% iodine tincture and 8.5% iodine tincture in stock. How many mL of each 3% and 8.5% iodine tincture should be used? (Use 1 gallon = 3,785 mL)

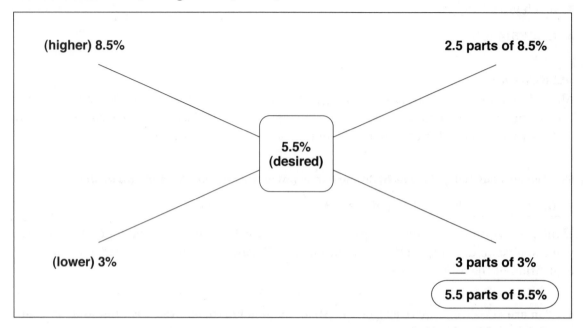

- Add the parts to find the total # of parts (5.5 parts in this problem).

- Divide by the total volume (3,785 mL) by the number of parts to get the volume per part: 3,785 mL/5.5 parts = 688.2 mL per part.

- 2.5 parts x 688.2 mL = 1,720 mL of the 8.5% iodine tincture

- 3 parts x 688.2 mL = 2,065 mL of the 3% iodine tincture

The end product provides 3,785 mL of a 5.5% iodine tincture.

HALF-LIFE (T$_{1/2}$)

The half-life is the amount of time required for the drug concentration to decrease by 50%. In nuclear pharmacy, the half-life refers to the time required for half the drug to decay. Usually, we refer to the concentration remaining in the body, which may have been reduced by hepatic metabolism or renal excretion. The formula is provided here, but we provide an example without exponents.

$t_{1/2} = 0.693/k_e,$ where k_e = elimination rate constant

---

66. A patient receives 200 mg of a drug with a half-life of 5 hrs. How much of the drug still remains in the patient after 10 hours?

- 10 hrs = 2 half-lives:

- 200 mg /2 = 100 mg (amount of drug left after one half-life)

- 100 mg /2 = 50 mg is left after 10 hours (2 half-lives)

67. A patient with renal failure received 1 gram of vancomycin on 3/21 at 1300. The peak was taken 1 hour later and was 26.8 mg/L. On 3/24 at 1400, the concentration was taken and was 13.4 mg/L and a 1 g dose was given at the same time. The desired trough is 10-15 mg/L. When should the patient receive the next 1 gram dose? Assume the renal clearance stays constant.

    a. 1 day

    b. 3 days

    c. 4 days

    d. 6 days

    e. Not enough information is provided

The correct answer is (D), 6 days.

The half-life is ~3 days. (The concentration decreased from 26.8 to 13.4 in 3 days).

When the 2nd dose was given, the concentration was 13.4 mg/L. Add the 26.8 mg/L you expect from the new dose: 13.4 + 26.8 = new concentration of 40.2 mg/L.

- 40.2 mg/L divided by 2 = 20.1 mg/L in 3 days

- 20.1 mg/L divided by 2 = 10.1 mg/L is left after 6 days. Since the trough should be 10-15 mg/L, a 1 g dose should be given about every 6 days. In practice the level would likely be checked earlier (such as on day 5) to avoid a subtherapeutic level. The renal function is an estimate, and may fluctuate.

---

68. From the graph below, what is the half-life of Drug A?

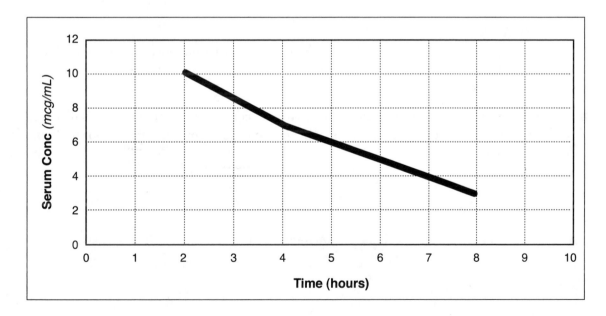

Answer: 4 hours

TOTAL PARENTERAL NUTRITION (TPN)

Total parenteral nutrition provides all of the patient's daily nutritional requirements. Components of a TPN include fluids, dextrose, amino acids, vitamins, minerals, trace elements, electrolytes, lipids and sometimes medications (e.g. insulin). TPN is given parenterally, usually through a catheter into a central vein (↓ risk phlebitis). Examples of central catheters are Hickman and Groshong lines, or a PICC ("pick") line, which is inserted peripherally (through a vein, and then threaded to the vena cava). PICC lines are commonly used for TPN, long-term antibiotic therapy and for chemotherapy drugs which would cause phlebitis or other damage if administered directly into a vein.

NORMAL DIET COMPONENT	TPN COMPONENT
Protein (fish, meat, soy)	Amino acids
Carbohydrates (bread, rice)	Dextrose (glucose)
Fat	Lipids
Vitamins	Multivitamin infusion (MVI)
Minerals	Electrolytes and trace elements

General Rule: "If the gut works, use it."

TPN INDICATIONS

- Patients requiring long-term (> 7 days) supplemental nutrition because they are unable to receive daily requirements through oral or enteral feedings. There is no justification for TPN < 4 days.

- Patients with severe gut dysfunction due to various conditions, such as Crohn's disease, ulcerative colitis, bowel obstruction, short bowel syndrome from surgery, etc. (or patients who are NPO).

This chart provides the calories/gram for the major TPN components a <u>pharmacist is required to know</u>:

COMPONENT	UNITS
Dextrose*	3.4 kcal/g
Amino Acids	4 kcal/g
Lipids**	9 kcal/g
10% lipid emulsion	1.1 kcal/mL
20% lipid emulsion	2 kcal/mL

*Carbohydrates in TPN are given as dextrose monohydrate, which has 3.4 kcal/gram (glucose has 4.0 kcal/gram).

**Lipid emulsions contain glycerol, so they are not straight 9 kcal/g as if they were pure fat and the calories are calculated per mL of the formulation used.

DETERMINING FLUID NEEDS

Fluid requirements are often calculated 1st in the TPN. Enough (but not too much) fluid needs to be given to maintain adequate hydration. Daily fluid needs can be calculated using this formula:

When weight > 20 kg: 1,500 mL + (20 mL)(Wt in kg - 20 kg)

Alternatively, some institutions estimate adult fluid need using a general guideline of 30-40 mL/kg/day. The TPN should be tailored to the patient. If the patient has problems with fluid accumulation (such as heart failure, renal dysfunction, etc.) the amount of fluid they can handle will be reduced. Fluid volume from medications (including IVPBs) should be included.

---

69. GG is a 57 year old female admitted to the hospital with bowel obstruction. She is made NPO and will be at least several days. The decision was made to start TPN. She weighs 65 kg and is 5'6". Calculate her daily fluid needs.

- 1,500 mL + (20 mL)(65 kg - 20 kg) = 2,400 mL/day

CALCULATING PROTEIN CALORIES

Typical protein requirements for a non-stressed, ambulatory patient are 0.8-1 g/kg/day. Protein requirements increase as the patient is placed under stress, which is defined as the illness severity. The more severely ill, the greater the protein requirements will be per day. In very sick, hospitalized patients, protein requirements can be as high as 2 g/kg/day.

CONDITION	PROTEIN REQUIREMENTS
Ambulatory, non-hospitalized (non-stressed)	0.8-1 g/kg/day
Hospitalized, or malnourished	1.2-2 g/kg/day

70. MK is a 62 year old female who has been admitted with enteritis and pneumonia. She has a history of ulcerative Crohn's and COPD. The staff gastroenterologist has ordered TPN therapy, to be prepared by pharmacy. She is 158 pounds, 5'4". Calculate her protein requirements using her actual weight. She is hospitalized and should receive 1.5 g/kg/day of protein.

First, convert pounds to kg. 158 pounds x 1 kg/2.2 lbs = 71.8 kg

Then, calculate the protein requirements. 71.8 kg x 1.5 g/kg/day = 108 g protein/day.

---

71. PP is a 46 year old male (207 pounds, 5'11") who has been admitted for bowel resection surgery. Post surgery, he is to be started on TPN therapy. The physician wants the patient to receive 1.3 g/kg/day of protein. Calculate his protein requirements using his actual weight.

First, convert lbs to kg. 207 lbs x 1 kg/2.2 pounds = 94.1 kg

Then, calculate protein requirements. 94.1 kg x 1.3 g/kg/day = 122 g protein/day.

CALCULATING NON-PROTEIN CALORIES - TOTAL ENERGY EXPENDITURE (TEE) AND BASAL ENERGY EXPENDITURE (BEE)

The basal energy expenditure (BEE) is the total energy expenditure in the resting state exclusive of eating and activity. It is estimated separately in male and female subjects using the Harris-Benedict equations (it can also be estimated in adults at 15-25 kcal/kg/day).Harris-Benedict equations:

- BEE (males): 66.47 + 13.75(weight in kg) + 5.0(height in cm) - 6.76(age in years)

- BEE (females): 655.1 + 9.6(weight in kg) + 1.85(height in cm) - 4.68(age in years)

Total energy expenditure (AKA total daily expenditure or TDE) is a measure of basal energy expenditure plus excess metabolic demands as a result of stress, the thermal effects of feeding, and energy expenditure for activity. TEE = BEE x activity factor x stress factor. Once the BEE is calculated, calculate the TEE by taking the BEE calories and multiplying by the appropriate activity factor and stress factor. This will INCREASE the calories required. Energy requirements are extra non-protein calorie sources needed only in severely ill patients (including this hospitalized, elderly patient). Protein calories are reserved for muscle building, rather than for energy requirements.

The activity factor is either 1.2 if confined to bed (non-ambulatory), or 1.3 if out of bed (ambulatory). Commonly used stress factors are listed in the table:

STATE OF STRESS	STRESS FACTOR
Minor surgery	1.2
Infection	1.4
Major trauma, sepsis, burns up to 30% BSA	1.5
Burns over 30% BSA	1.5-2

72. Using the Harris-Benedict equation, calculate the resting non-protein caloric requirement for a major trauma patient (stress factor 1.5) who is a 66 year old male, weighing 175 pounds and measures 5′10″ in height. Activity factor is 1.2

- Height = 70″ x 2.54 cm/inch = 177.8 cm. Weight 175 pounds x 1 kg/2.2 pounds = 79.5 kg.

- BEE (males): 66.47 + 13.75(weight in kg) + 5.0(height in cm) - 6.76(age in years)

- BEE = 66.47 + 13.75(79.5) + 5(177.8) - 6.76(66)

- BEE = 66.47 + 1,093.13 + 889 - 446.16 = 1,602.44 kcal/day

The BEE can be estimated using 15-25 kcal/kg (adults). You may want to check your calculations by using the estimates and seeing if the numbers are close. In this case, an estimation using 20 kcal/kg/day would provide 1,590 kcal/day (close to 1,602.44 kcal/day as above).

---

73. Using the total energy expenditure equation, calculate the total non-protein caloric requirement for the patient above (stress factor is 1.5, activity factor is 1.2). Round to the nearest whole number.

- TEE = BEE x activity factor x stress factor

- TEE = 1,602.44 x 1.2 x 1.5 = 2,884 kcal/day

---

74. A 25 year old female major trauma patient survives surgery and is recovering in the surgical intensive care unit. The medical team wants to start TPN. She is 122 pounds, 5′ 7″ with some mild renal impairment. Calculate her BEE using the Harris Benedict equation and her TEE non-protein caloric requirements (stress factor = 1.7 and activity factor =1.2)

- Height = 67″ x 2.54 cm/inch = 170 cm. Weight 122 lbs x 1 kg/2.2 pounds = 55.5 kg.

- BEE (females): 655.1 + 9.6(weight in kg) + 1.85(height in cm) - 4.68(age in years)

- BEE = 655.1 + 9.6(55.5) + 1.85(170) - 4.68(25)

- BEE = 655.1 + 532.8 + 314.5 - 117 = 1,385 kcal/day

- TEE = BEE x activity factor x stress factor

- TEE = 1,385 x 1.2 x 1.7 = 2,825 kcal/day

CALCULATING AMINO ACIDS

Amino acids are the source of proteins in a TPN. Amino acids are used to build muscle mass and are not usually counted as an energy source in critically ill patients because they are catabolic. Amino acids come in stock preparations of 5%, 8.5%, 10% and 15%. The daily protein requirements calculated will need to be multiplied by the concentration of amino acids. It may be useful to calculate what percentage of the total TPN calories come from the protein.

---

75. If the pharmacy stocks *Aminosyn* 8.5%, how many mL will be needed to provide 108 g of protein?

$$\frac{8.5\ g}{100\ mL} = \frac{108\ g}{X\ mL} \qquad X = 1,271\ mL$$

76. How many calories are provided by 108 grams of protein?

$$\frac{4 \text{ kcal}}{g} \quad x \quad 108 \text{ g} \quad = \quad 432 \text{ kcal of protein}$$

77. The pharmacy stocks *Aminosyn* 10%. A patient requires 122 grams of protein per day. How many mL of *Aminosyn* will the patient need?

$$\frac{10 \text{ g}}{100 \text{ mL}} = \frac{122 \text{ g}}{X \text{ mL}} \quad X = 1,220 \text{ mL}$$

78. JR is requiring 1.4 g/kg/day of protein and the pharmacy stocks *Aminosyn* 8.5%. JR is a 55 year old male (wt. 189 pounds, ht. 6'0") who is confined to bed (activity factor 1.2) due to his current infection (stress factor 1.5) Calculate the amount of *Aminosyn*, in milliliters, JR should receive.

First, convert weight to kg. 189 pounds x 1 kg/2.2 pounds = 86 kg

Next, calculate protein requirements. 1.4 g/kg/day x 86 kg = 120 g/day

Then, calculate the amount of *Aminosyn* (mL) needed. Note the activity factor and stress factor are not required to calculate the protein requirements.

$$\frac{8.5 \text{ g}}{100 \text{ mL}} = \frac{120 \text{ g}}{X \text{ mL}} \quad X = 1,411 \text{ mL}$$

79. JR is receiving 97 grams of protein in an *Aminosyn* 8.5% solution on day 8 of his hospitalization. How many calories are provided by this amount of protein?

$$\frac{4 \text{ kcal}}{g} \quad x \quad 97 \text{ g} \quad = \quad 388 \text{ kcal of protein}$$

80. TE is a 35 year old female who is receiving 325 grams of dextrose, 85 grams of amino acids, and 300 mL of 10% lipids via her TPN therapy. What percentage of calories is provided by the protein content?

First, calculate the calories from all sources; dextrose, amino acids, and lipids.

Dextrose

$$\frac{3.4 \text{ kcal}}{g} \quad x \quad 325 \text{ g} \quad = \quad 1,105 \text{ kcal of dextrose}$$

Protein

$$\frac{4 \text{ kcal}}{g} \quad x \quad 85 \text{ g} \quad = \quad 340 \text{ kcal of protein}$$

Lipids

$$\frac{1.1 \text{ kcal}}{mL} \quad x \quad 300 \text{ mL} \quad = \quad 330 \text{ kcal of fat}$$

Then, add up the total calories from all the sources. 1,105 + 340 + 330 = 1,775 kcal

Finally, calculate the percent of protein.

$$\frac{340 \text{ kcal}}{1,775 \text{ kcal}} \times 100 = \underline{19\%}$$

CALCULATING DEXTROSE

Dextrose is the source of carbohydrates in a TPN. The standard distribution of non-protein calories is 70-85% as carbohydrate (dextrose) and 15-30% as fat (lipids). Dextrose comes in concentrations of 5%, 10%, 20%, 30%, 50% and 70%. The higher concentrations are used for TPN. When calculating the dextrose, do not exceed 4 mg/kg/min (some use 7 g/kg/day). This is a conservative estimate of the maximum amount the liver can handle.

---

81. Using 50% dextrose in water, how many mL are required to fulfill a TPN order for 405 g of dextrose?

$$\frac{50 \text{ g}}{100 \text{ mL}} = \frac{405 \text{ g}}{X \text{ mL}} = \underline{810 \text{ mL}}$$

---

82. DF, a 44 year old male, is receiving 1,235 mL of D30W, 1,010 mL of *Aminosyn* 8.5%, 200 mL of *Intralipid* 20% and 50 mL of electrolytes/minerals in his TPN. How many calories from dextrose is DF receiving from the TPN? (Round to the nearest whole number)

$$\frac{30 \text{ gram}}{100 \text{ mL}} \times \frac{1,235 \text{ mL}}{\text{day}} \times \frac{3.4 \text{ kcal}}{\text{gram}} = \underline{1,260 \text{ kcal/day}}$$

$$\frac{30}{100} = \frac{x}{1235} \qquad x \times \frac{3.4 \text{ kcal}}{g} = \boxed{}$$

---

83. A pharmacy is preparing a TPN order for 280 g of dextrose. How many mL of dextrose are required if the concentration of dextrose is 20%?

$$\frac{20 \text{ g}}{100 \text{ mL}} = \frac{280 \text{ g}}{X \text{ mL}} \qquad X = \underline{1,400 \text{ mL}}$$

---

84. WC, a 57 year old male, is receiving 1,145 mL of D30W, 850 mL of *Aminosyn* 8.5%, and 350 mL of *Intralipid* 10% in his TPN therapy. What percentage of the non-protein calories are represented by dextrose?

First, calculate the non-protein calories (dextrose and lipids).

Dextrose

$$\frac{3.4 \text{ kcal}}{g} \times \frac{30 \text{ g}}{100 \text{ mL}} \times 1,145 \text{ mL} = \underline{1,168 \text{ kcal}}$$

Lipids

$$\frac{1.1 \text{ kcal}}{\text{mL}} \times 350 \text{ mL} = \underline{385 \text{ kcal}}$$

Then, add up the calories from these non-protein sources. 1,168 + 385 = \underline{1,553 kcal}

Finally, calculate the percent from dextrose.

$$\frac{1{,}168 \text{ kcal}}{1{,}553 \text{ kcal}} \quad x \quad 100 \;=\; 75\%$$

---

85. AH is receiving 640 mL of D50W in her TPN. How many calories does this provide?

$$\frac{50 \text{ gram}}{100 \text{ mL}} \quad x \quad \frac{640 \text{ mL}}{\text{day}} \quad x \quad \frac{3.4 \text{ kcal}}{\text{gram}} \;=\; 1{,}088 \text{ kcal}$$

CALCULATING LIPIDS

Lipids are the source of fat in a TPN. The standard distribution of non-protein calories is 70-85% as carbohydrate (dextrose) and 15-30% as fat (lipids). Lipids are available as 10% or 20% emulsions. 10% lipid emulsions provide 1.1 kcal/mL and 20% lipid emulsions provide 2 kcal/mL. Do not exceed 2.5 g/kg/day. Lipids do not need to be given daily, especially if the triglycerides are high. Patients receiving lipids should have their triglycerides monitored. If lipids are given once weekly, then divide the total calories by 7 to determine the daily amount of fat the patient receives. Lipid emulsion cannot be filtered through 0.22 micron filters; filters are not used.

---

86. A patient is receiving 500 mL of 10% lipids. How many calories is the patient receiving from the lipids?

$$\frac{1.1 \text{ kcal}}{\text{mL}} \;=\; \frac{X \text{ kcal}}{500 \text{ mL}} \qquad X = 550 \text{ kcal}$$

---

87. The total energy expenditure (TEE) for a patient is 2,435 kcal/day. The patient is receiving 1,446 kcal from dextrose and 810 kcal from protein. How many kcal should be provided by the lipids?

TEE refers to the non-protein calories. Therefore, 2,435 kcal (total) - 1,446 kcal (dextrose) = 989 kcal remaining. 989 kcal should be provided by the lipids.

---

88. Using a 20% lipid emulsion, how many mL are required to meet 989 calories?

$$\frac{2 \text{ kcal}}{\text{mL}} \;=\; \frac{989 \text{ kcal}}{X \text{ mL}} \qquad X = 494.5 \text{ mL}$$

---

89. A patient is receiving 660 mL of 10% *Intralipid* on Saturdays along with his normal daily TPN therapy of 1,420 mL of D20W, 450 mL *Aminosyn* 15%, and 30 mL of electrolytes. What is the daily amount of calories provided by the lipids?

$$\frac{1.1 \text{ kcal}}{\text{mL}} \;=\; \frac{X \text{ kcal}}{660 \text{ mL}} \qquad X = 726 \text{ kcal. Need to divide by 7days} = 103.7 \text{ kcal/day}$$

If asked to round to the nearest whole number, the answer would be 104 kcal/day.

90. A patient is receiving 360 mL of 20% lipids. How many calories is the patient receiving from the lipids?

$$\frac{2 \text{ kcal}}{\text{mL}} = \frac{X \text{ kcal}}{360 \text{ mL}} \quad X = 720 \text{ kcal}$$

91. A TPN order calls for 475 calories to be provided by lipids. The pharmacy has 10% lipid emulsion in stock. How many mL should be administered to the patient?

$$\frac{1.1 \text{ kcal}}{\text{mL}} = \frac{475 \text{ kcal}}{X \text{ mL}} \quad X = 431.8 \text{ mL}$$

DETERMINING THE AMOUNT OF ELECTROLYTES

Sodium Considerations

Sodium is the principal <u>extra</u>cellular cation. Sodium may need to be reduced in renal dysfunction or cardiovascular disease, including hypertension. Sodium chloride comes in many concentrations, such as 0.9% NS, 0.45%, and others. Sodium chloride 23.4% is used for TPN preparation and contains 4 mEq/mL.

Sodium can be added to the TPN as either sodium chloride or sodium acetate. If a patient is acidotic, sodium acetate should be added. Sodium acetate is converted to sodium bicarbonate and may help correct the acidosis. A patient may require a certain quantity of mEq from the acetate and also may need an additional amount from the sodium chloride formulation. Or, they may get sodium chloride alone.

92. The pharmacist is going to add 80 mEq of sodium to the TPN; half will be given as sodium acetate (2 mEq/mL) and half as <u>sodium chloride</u> (4 mEq/mL). How many mL of sodium chloride will be needed?

40 mEq will be provided by the NaCl.

$$\frac{4 \text{ mEq}}{\text{mL}} = \frac{40 \text{ mEq}}{X \text{ mL}} \quad X = 10 \text{ mL}$$

POTASSIUM, CALCIUM AND PHOSPHATE CONSIDERATIONS

Potassium is the principal <u>intra</u>cellular cation. Potassium may need to be reduced in renal or cardiovascular disease. Potassium can be provided by potassium chloride (KCl) or potassium phosphate (K Phos). <u>The normal range for serum potassium is 3.5-5.0 mEq/L (pharmacists know this value).</u>

Calcium is important for many functions including cardiac conduction, muscle contraction, and bone homeostasis. The normal serum calcium level is 8.5-10.5 mg/dL. Almost half of serum calcium is bound to albumin. Low albumin will lead to an incorrect calcium concentration. If albumin is low (< 3.5 g/dL), calcium levels will need to be corrected with this equation prior to the addition of calcium into the TPN:

$$Ca_{corrected} = (calcium_{reported(serum)}) + [(4.0 - albumin) \times (0.8)]$$

93. Calculate the corrected calcium for a patient with the following lab values:

LAB	VALUE
Calcium	7.6 mEq/L (normal range 8.5 – 10.5 mEq/L)
Albumin	1.5 g/dL (normal range 3.5 – 5 g/dL)

- $Ca_{corrected} = (calcium_{reported(serum)}) + [(4.0 - albumin) \times (0.8)]$

- $Ca_{corrected} = (7.6) + [(4.0 - 1.5) \times (0.8)] = \underline{9.6\ mEq/L}$

Phosphorus (or phosphate, PO_4) is present in DNA, cell membranes, ATP, acts as an acid-base buffer, and is vital in bone metabolism. Phosphate and calcium need to be added carefully, or they can bind together and precipitate, which can cause which can cause a pulmonary emboli. This can be fatal. The following considerations can help reduce the risk of a calcium-phosphate precipitate:

- Choose <u>calcium gluconate</u> over calcium chloride ($CaCl_2$) due to being less reactive and lower risk (Calcium chloride has 3X more elemental calcium than calcium gluconate).

- Add phosphate first, and calcium should be added near the end to take advantage of the maximum volume of the TPN formulation.

- The calcium and phosphate added together should not exceed 45 mEq/L. You will need this conversion to calculate: 1 mmol = 2 mEq.

- Maintain a proper pH to eliminate binding and refrigerate the bag once prepared (TPNs are kept in the unit refrigerator until they are hung).

An additional safety consideration involves ordering the correct dose of phosphate. Phosphate can be ordered as potassium or sodium salts. The two forms do not provide equivalent amounts of phosphate. The order should be written in mmol (of phosphate), followed by the type of salt form (potassium or sodium).

94. The pharmacist has calculated that a patient requires 30 mmol of phosphate and 80 mEq of potassium. The pharmacist has potassium phosphate 3 mmol of phosphate with 4.4 mEq of potassium/mL vials and potassium chloride 2 mEq/mL vials in stock. How much potassium phosphate and how much potassium chloride will be required to meet the patient's needs?

First, calculate the phosphate required (since potassium comes along with the phosphate in the potassium-phosphate solution):

$$\frac{3\ mmol\ Phosphate}{mL} = \frac{30\ mmol\ Phosphate}{X\ mL} \qquad X = 10\ mL\ K\text{-}Phos$$

Each mL of the potassium phosphate (K-Phos) supplies 4.4 mEq of potassium. Calculate the amount of potassium the patient received from the 10 mL of K-Phos:

- 10 mL x 4.4 mEq/mL = 44 mEq potassium

The remaining potassium will be provided by KCl:

- 80 mEq K required – 44 mEq potassium (from K-Phos) = 36 mEq to be obtained from the KCl.

$$\frac{2 \text{ mEq K}^+}{\text{mL}} = \frac{36 \text{ mEq K}^+}{\text{X mL}} \qquad X = \underline{18} \text{ mL KCl}$$

---

95. A patient is to receive 8 mEq of calcium. The pharmacy has calcium gluconate 10% in stock which provides 0.465 mEq/mL. How many mL of calcium gluconate should be added to the TPN?

$$\frac{1 \text{ mL}}{0.465 \text{ mEq Ca}^{2+}} \times 8 \text{ mEq Ca}^{2+} = 17.2 \text{ mL calcium gluconate}$$

---

96. In the above problem, the patient is receiving 30 mmol of phosphate and 8 mEq of calcium in a total volume of 2,400 mL. There are 2 mEq PO_4/mmol. Confirm that the calcium and phosphorus added together do not exceed 45 mEq/L.

First, calculate mEq from the phosphate.

$$\frac{2 \text{ mEq PO}_4}{\text{mmol}} \times 30 \text{ mmol PO}_4 = 60 \text{ mEq phosphate}$$

Then, add the phosphate to the calcium. 60 mEq phosphate + 8 mEq calcium = 68 mEq.

The final volume of the TPN is 2,400 mL, or 2.4 L. 68 mEq/2.4 L = 28.33 mEq/L, which is less than 45 mEq/L.

Questions 97 - 106 relate to TPN order below.

97. A pharmacy receives the following TPN order. Calculate the amount, in mL, of dextrose 70% that should be added to the TPN. Round to the nearest mL.

ITEM	QUANTITY
Dextrose 70%	250 g
Amino acids	50 g
Sodium chloride	44 mEq
Sodium acetate	20 mEq
Potassium	40 mEq
Magnesium sulfate	12 mEq
Phosphate	18 mmol

TPN order Continued

ITEM	QUANTITY
Calcium	4.65 mEq
MVI-12	5 mL
Trace elements-5	1 mL
Vitamin K-1	0.5 mg
Famotidine	10 mg
Regular insulin	20 units
Sterile water qs ad	960 mL

$$\frac{70 \text{ g}}{100 \text{ mL}} = \frac{250 \text{ g}}{X \text{ mL}} \qquad X = 357 \text{ mL of dextrose}$$

---

98. Using amino acids 10%, calculate the amount of amino acids that should be added to the TPN.

$$\frac{10 \text{ g}}{100 \text{ mL}} = \frac{50 \text{ g}}{X \text{ mL}} \qquad X = 500 \text{ mL}$$

---

99. Calculate the amount of sodium chloride 23.4% (4 mEq/mL) that should be added to the TPN.

$$\frac{4 \text{ mEq}}{\text{mL}} = \frac{44 \text{ mEq}}{X \text{ mL}} \qquad X = 11 \text{ mL}$$

**This concentration of NaCl is hypertonic (> 9%) and is a high-alert drug due to heightened risk of patient harm when dosed incorrectly.

---

100. Calculate the amount of sodium acetate 16.4% (2 mEq/mL) that should be added to the TPN.

$$\frac{2 \text{ mEq}}{\text{mL}} = \frac{20 \text{ mEq}}{X \text{ mL}} \qquad X = 10 \text{ mL}$$

---

101. Using the potassium phosphate (each mL contains 3 mmol of phosphate AND 4.4 mEq of potassium) vials in stock, calculate the amount of potassium phosphate that should be added to the TPN.

$$\frac{3 \text{ mmol Phosphate}}{\text{mL}} = \frac{18 \text{ mmol Phosphate}}{X \text{ mL}} \qquad X = 6 \text{ mL K-Phos}$$

102. The TPN contains 6 mL of potassium phosphate (3 mmol of phosphate/mL with 4.4 mEq of potassium/mL). The daily potassium requirement is 40 mEq. How much potassium chloride (2 mEq/mL) should be added to the TPN?

First, calculate the amount of K$^+$ already in the TPN.

$$\frac{4.4 \text{ mEq K}^+}{\text{mL}} \times 6 \text{ mL} = 26.4 \text{ mEq K}^+$$

Total K$^+$ needed is 40 mEq. 40 mEq - 26.4 mEq = 13.6 mEq still needed.

$$\frac{2 \text{ mEq K}^+}{\text{mL}} = \frac{13.6 \text{ mEq K}^+}{X \text{ mL}} \qquad X = 6.8 \text{ mL KCL}$$

103. The TPN order calls for 4.65 mEq of calcium. The pharmacy has calcium gluconate 10% (0.465 mEq/mL) in stock. How many mL of calcium gluconate 10% should be added to the TPN?

$$\frac{0.465 \text{ mEq Ca}^{2+}}{\text{mL}} \times \frac{4.65 \text{ mEq Ca}^{2+}}{X \text{ mL}} \qquad X = 10 \text{ mL calcium gluconate 10\%}$$

104. The TPN calls for 18 mmol of phosphate and 4.65 mEq of calcium (provided by 10 mL of calcium gluconate 10%, as calculated in the previous problem) in a total volume of 960 mL. There are 2 mEq PO$_4$/mmol. Confirm that the calcium and phosphorus added together do not exceed 45 mEq/L.

First, calculate mEq from the phosphate.

$$\frac{2 \text{ mEq PO}_4}{\text{mmol}} \times 18 \text{ mmol PO}_4 = 36 \text{ mEq phosphate}$$

Then, add the phosphate to the calcium. 36 mEq phosphate + 4.65 mEq calcium = 40.65 mEq. The final volume of the TPN is 960 mL, or 0.96 L. 40.65 mEq/0.96 L = 42.3 mEq/L, which is less than 45 mEq/L.

105. Calculate the amount of magnesium sulfate (4 mEq/mL) that should be added to the TPN.

$$\frac{4 \text{ mEq}}{\text{mL}} = \frac{12 \text{ mEq}}{X \text{ mL}} \qquad X = 3 \text{ mL magnesium sulfate}$$

106. What percentage of the total calories from the above TPN are represented by the protein component?

First, calculate the total calories.

Dextrose

$$\frac{3.4 \text{ kcal dextrose}}{g} \times 250 \text{ g dextrose} = 850 \text{ kcal of dextrose} \checkmark$$

Protein

$$\frac{4 \text{ kcal protein}}{g} \quad x \quad 50 \text{ g protein} = 200 \text{ kcal of protein} \quad \checkmark$$

Total calories = 850 + 200 = 1,050 kcal. Now, calculate the amount of calories from protein.

$$\frac{200 \text{ kcal}}{1,050 \text{ kcal}} \quad x \quad 100 = 19\%$$

Determine The Grams Of Nitrogen Contained In The Protein

- There is 1 g of nitrogen (N) for each 6.25 g of protein. Or, to calculate the grams of nitrogen in a certain weight of protein, divide the protein grams by 6.25.

- In the above problem there are 50 grams of protein, which is divided by 6.25:

- 50 g/6.25 = 8 grams of nitrogen

Calculate The Non-Protein Calories To Nitrogen (NPC:N) Ratio

- This is determined by dividing the non-protein calories (dextrose plus lipids) by the nitrogen.

- In the above example, the non-protein calories are only the glucose, since there were no lipids in the formula. The glucose calories are 850 kcal. Divide the 850 by 8 (the grams of nitrogen) to get a non-protein to nitrogen ratio of 106.

- A normal ratio is 150-250, but the ratio is much lower in a patient with severe stress it is much lower (90-125:1).

ADD-IN MULTIVITAMINS, TRACE ELEMENTS, AND INSULIN

Multivitamins: There are 4 fat-soluble vitamins (A, D, E and K) and 9 water-soluble vitamins (thiamine, riboflavin, niacin, pantothenic acid, pyridoxine, C, folic acid, B12, biotin) in the standard MVI-13 mixture. The MVI-12 mixture does not contain vitamin K since certain patients may need less or more of this vitamin. If patients are using warfarin the INR will need to be monitored.

Trace Elements

The standard mix includes zinc, copper, chromium and manganese (and may include selenium). Manganese and copper should be withheld in severe liver disease. Chromium, molybdenum and selenium should be withheld in severe renal disease. Iron is not routinely given in a TPN.

Insulin

Many TPNs contain insulin, usually half what the person is expected to require per day, supplemented by a sliding scale. A minimum dose to add is 10 units, and is increased by 10 unit increments. It is important to avoid adding too much insulin. Half the previous day's sliding scale can be used as a safe amount.

ENTERAL NUTRITION

Enteral nutrition (EN) provides food into the enteric system (GI tract) through a tube placed in the nose, stomach, or small intestine. Several advantages of EN over TPN include less cost associated with EN, using the gut which prevents atrophy and other problems, and a lower risk of complications. The most common risk associated with enteral feeding is aspiration which can lead to pneumonia. Enteral feedings can cause drug interactions. The general rule for preventing drug/enteral feeding interactions is to hold the feedings one hour before or two hours after the drugs listed below, and any others thought to pose a problem. Some drugs may require further separation.

Tube feeds do not, by themselves, provide enough water. Water is given in addition to the tube feeds. If fluid intake is inadequate, it will be uncomfortable for the patient and put them at risk for complications such as hypernatremia.

Drug-Nutrient interactions with enteral feedings (most common problems):

- Warfarin: many enteral products bind warfarin, resulting in low INRs and the need for dose adjustments.

- Fluoroquinolone and tetracycline antibiotics: these drugs chelate with metals, including calcium, magnesium, and iron, which reduces drug availability.

- Phenytoin *(Dilantin suspension)*: is often reduced when the drug binds to the protein component, leading to less free drug availability and sub-therapeutic levels. Separate tube feeds by 2 hours.

Tube names

- A tube in the nose to the stomach is called a nasogastric (NG) or nasoenteral, tube.

- A tube that goes through the skin into the stomach is called a gastrostomy, or percutaneous endoscopic gastrostomy (PEG, or G) tube.

- A tube into the small intestine is called a jejunostomy, or percutaneous endoscopic jejunostomy (PEJ, or J) tube.

OSMOLARITY

Osmolarity is the measure of total number of particles (or solutes) per liter (L) of solution, or milliosmoles/Liter (mOsmol/L). Solutes can be either ionic (such as NaCl, which dissociates into 2 solutes in solution, Na^+ and Cl^-) or non-ionic, which do not dissociate (such as glucose and urea). The term for osmolarity when used to refer to the solute concentration in body fluids is tonicity, and solutions are thus isotonic (osmolarity the same as blood which is ~ 300 mOsmol/L), hypotonic or hypertonic.

If the osmolarity is higher in one cellular component, it will cause water to move from the lower to higher concentration of solutes. If a TPN solution is injected with a higher osmolarity than blood, fluid will flow into the vein, resulting in edema, inflammation, phlebitis and possible thrombosis. Another common area of concern, besides IV infusions, are eye drops, since the drop will cause discomfort (puckering, from too few solutes), or be washed out by tears (from too many solutes).

Some compounds for which it may be useful to know dissociations include:

■ Sodium acetate ($NaC_2H_3O_2$) dissociates into 2 particles

■ Calcium chloride ($CaCl_2$) dissociates into 3 particles

■ Sodium citrate ($Na_3C_6H_5O_7$) dissociates into 4 particles

Osmolarity Calculations

Use this formula to find the mOsmol/L.

$$\text{mOsmol/L} = \frac{\text{Wt of substance (g/L)}}{\text{MW (g)}} \times (\text{\# of species}) \times 1{,}000$$

■ Add up the number of particles into which the compound dissociates.

■ Calculate the number of grams of the compound present in 1 L.

■ Find the Molecular Weight (M.W.).

---

107. What is the osmolarity of normal saline (0.9% NaCl)? M.W. = 58.5 g

NaCl dissociates into 2 particles; Na^+ and Cl^-.

Convert compound (NaCl) into the proper units.

$$\frac{0.9\text{ g}}{100\text{ mL}} = \frac{X\text{ g}}{1{,}000\text{ mL}} \qquad X = 9\text{ g}$$

$$\text{mOsmol/L} = \frac{9\text{ g/L}}{58.5\text{ g}} \times 2 \times 1{,}000 = 308\text{ mOsmol/L}$$

---

108. What is the osmolarity of D5W? M.W. = 180 g

Dextrose does not dissociate and is counted as 1 particle.

$$\frac{5\text{ g}}{100\text{ mL}} = \frac{X\text{ g}}{1{,}000\text{ mL}} \qquad X = 50\text{ g}$$

$$\text{mOsmol/L} = \frac{50\text{ g/L}}{180\text{ g}} \times 1 \times 1{,}000 = 278\text{ mOsmol/L}$$

---

109. A solution contains 373 mg Na^+ ions per liter. How many milliosmoles are represented in the solution? M.W. = 23 g

First, convert the units to match the formula.

$$\frac{373\text{ mg}}{L} \times \frac{1\text{ g}}{1{,}000\text{ mg}} = 0.373\text{ g/L}$$

$$\text{mOsmol/L} = \frac{0.373\text{ g/L}}{23\text{ g}} \times 1 \times 1{,}000 = 16.2\text{ mOsmol/L}$$

110. Calculate the osmolar concentration, in milliosmoles, represented by 1 liter of a 10% (w/v) solution of anhydrous dextrose (M.W. = 180) in water. Round to the nearest tenth.

$$\frac{10\ g}{100\ mL} = \frac{X\ g}{1,000\ mL} \qquad X = 100\ g$$

$$mOsmol/L = \frac{100\ g/L}{180\ g} \times 1 \times 1,000 = 555.6\ mOsmol/L$$

---

111. How many milliosmoles of CaCl$_2$ (M.W.= 147) are represented in 150 mL of a 10% (w/v) calcium chloride solution? Round to the nearest whole number.

$$\frac{10\ g}{100\ mL} = \frac{X\ g}{150\ mL} \qquad X = 15\ g$$

$$mOsmol/L = \frac{15\ g}{147\ g} \times 3 \times 1,000 = 306\ mOsmol$$

---

112. A solution contains 200 mg Ca$^+$ ions per liter. How many milliosmoles are represented in the solution? M.W = 40 g

$$mOsmol/L = \frac{0.2\ g/L}{40\ g} \times 1 \times 1,000 = 5\ mOsmol/L$$

ISOTONICITY

Osmolarity is the measure of total number of particles (or solutes) per liter (L) of solution. Tonicity is a term used for the osmolarity of body fluids. When solutions are prepared they need to be as close to isotonic as possible. In pharmacy, the term hypotonic is used, rather than hypo-osmotic, and hypertonic, rather than hyperosmotic. Isotonicity is most commonly used when preparing eye drops.

Since isotonicity is related to the number of particles in solution, we have to determine the dissociation factor, symbolized by the letter i, for the compound (drug). Non-ionic compounds do not dissociate and will have a dissociation factor, i, of 1. The graph below shows the dissociation factors (i) based on number of ions.

NUMBER OF DISSOCIATED IONS	DISSOCIATION FACTOR, i
2	1.8
3	2.6
4	3.4
5	4.2

Body fluids are often described as having an osmotic pressure equivalent to 0.9% sodium chloride. Compounds (drugs) have "sodium chloride equivalents", or "E values". The amount of the sodium chloride equivalent from a given compound must be measured to know how much additional sodium chloride is required to make the final product isotonic. Here is the formula for calculating the E value of a compound:

$$E = \frac{(58.5)(i)}{(MW\ of\ drug)(1.8)}$$

Isotonicity calculations require the pharmacist to know that NaCl has a molecular weight (MW) of 58.5 and a dissociation factor of 1.8 – we need these figures since we are going to compare the contribution of our compound to NaCl – and then add enough NaCl to make the solution equivalent to the body fluid. The reason we compare the compound to NaCl is because NaCl is the major determinate of the isotonicity of our body fluid. We will put in our compound (drug) and end up with a tonicity lower than normal saline. The next step after adding the compound is to add enough NaCl to make the solution isotonic. Here are a few steps to follow when calculating isotonic solutions:

1. Calculate the amount of sodium chloride equivalents represented by the compound(s) in the prescription (multiply the E value by the weight).

2. Calculate the amount of NaCl alone that would make the final product isotonic.

3. Subtract step 1 from step 2 to determine the additional amount of NaCl needed.

Isotonicity Calculations

113. **Calculate the E value for mannitol (M.W. = 182). Round to the nearest hundredth.**

$$\frac{(58.5)(i)}{(MW\ of\ drug)(1.8)} = \frac{58.5\ (1)}{182\ (1.8)} = 0.18$$

---

114. **Calculate the E value for potassium iodide, which dissociates into 2 particles (M.W. = 166). Round to two decimal places.**

$$\frac{(58.5)(i)}{(MW\ of\ drug)(1.8)} = \frac{58.5\ (1.8)}{166\ (1.8)} = 0.35$$

---

115. **Physostigmine salicylate (M.W. = 413) is a 2- ion electrolyte, dissociating 80% in a given concentration. Calculate its sodium chloride equivalent. Round to two decimal places.**

$$\frac{(58.5)(i)}{(MW\ of\ drug)(1.8)} = \frac{58.5\ (1.8)}{413\ (1.8)} = 0.14$$

116. The E-value for ephedrine sulfate is 0.23. How many grams of sodium chloride are needed to make the following prescription?

PRESCRIPTION	QUANTITY
Ephedrine sulfate	0.4 g
Sodium chloride	q.s.
Purified water qs	30 mL
Make isotonic soln.	
Sig. For the nose.	

Step 1. Determine amount of sodium chloride represented from ephedrine sulfate.

- 0.4 g x 0.23 (E value) = 0.092 g of sodium chloride

Step 2. Determine how much NaCl would make the product isotonic.

$$\frac{0.9 \text{ g}}{100 \text{ mL}} = \frac{X}{30 \text{ mL}} \quad X = 0.27 \text{ g}$$

Step 3. Subtract step 1 from step 2.

0.27 g - 0.092 g = 0.178 g of NaCl are needed to make an isotonic solution

---

117. You receive an order for 10 mL of tobramycin 1% ophthalmic solution. You have tobramycin 40 mg/mL solution. Tobramycin does not dissociate and has a M.W. of 468. Find the E value for tobramycin and determine the amount of NaCl needed to make the solution isotonic. Round to two decimal places.

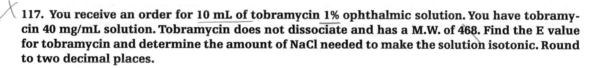

$$E = \frac{(58.5)(i)}{(MW \text{ of drug})(1.8)} = \frac{58.5 (1)}{468 (1.8)} = 0.07, \text{ which is the "E value" for tobramycin.}$$

The "E value" for tobramycin is 0.07. The recipe asks for 10 mL of 1% solution.

Step 1. Determine amount of sodium chloride represented from tobramycin.

$$\frac{1 \text{ gram}}{100 \text{ mL}} = \frac{X}{10 \text{ mL}} \quad X = 0.1 \text{ gram, or } 100 \text{ mg} \qquad 0.01 \times 10 = 0.1$$

100 mg x 0.07(E value) = 7 mg

Step 2. Determine how much NaCl would make the product isotonic (if that is all you were using).

$$\frac{0.9 \text{ gram}}{100 \text{ mL}} = \frac{X}{10 \text{ mL}} \quad X = 0.09 \text{ grams, or } 90 \text{ mg}$$

Step 3. Subtract step 1 from step 2. You are using tobramycin, so you do not need all the NaCl – subtract out the equivalent amount of tonicity provided by the tobramycin, which is 7 mg.

90 mg - 7 mg = 83 mg (83 mg additional sodium chloride are needed to make an isotonic solution)

We can also calculate how much of the original stock solution is required. We have a solution that is 40 mg/mL. We need 10 mL of a 1% solution. We calculated above that we need 100 mg to provide 10 mL of a 1% solution.

$$\frac{40 \text{ mg}}{1 \text{ mL}} = \frac{100 \text{ mg}}{X \text{ mL}} \qquad X = 2.5 \text{ mL of the original stock solution.}$$

MILLIMOLES (MMOL)

A mole is the molecular weight of a substance in grams, or g/mole. A millimole is 1/1,000 of the molecular weight in grams, or 1/1,000 of a mole. For monovalent species, the numeric value of the milliequivalent and millimole are identical.

Helpful equation

$$\frac{g}{\text{mole}} = \frac{X \text{ g}}{1 \text{ mole}}$$

---

118. How many millimoles of sodium phosphate (M.W. = 138) are present in 90 g of the substance?

$$\frac{138 \text{ g}}{\text{mole}} = \frac{90 \text{ g}}{X \text{ mole}} \qquad X = 0.652 \text{ moles, which is 652 mmol}$$

---

119. How many millimoles of calcium chloride (M.W. = 147) are represented in 147 mL of a 10% (w/v) calcium chloride solution?

Step 1: Calculate the amount (g) of $CaCl_2$ in 147 mL of 10% $CaCl_2$ solution.

$$\frac{10 \text{ g}}{100 \text{ mL}} = \frac{X \text{ g}}{147 \text{ mL}} \qquad X = 14.7 \text{ g}$$

Step 2: Calculate the moles of $CaCl_2$ in 147 mL of 10% $CaCl_2$ solution.

$$\frac{147 \text{ g}}{\text{mole}} = \frac{14.7 \text{ g}}{X \text{ mole}} \qquad X = 0.1 \text{ mole}$$

Step 3: Solve the problem by converting moles to millimoles; 0.1 mole x 1,000 = 100 mmol

MILLIEQUIVALENTS (MEQ)

Drugs can be expressed in solution in different ways;

- Milliosmoles refers to the number of particles in solution.

- Millimoles refers to the molecular weight (MW).

- Milliequivalents represent the amount in milligrams (mg) of a solute equal to 1/1,000 of its gram equivalent weight, taking into account the valence of the ions. Like osmolarity, the quantity of particles is important – but so is the electrical charge. Based on atomic weight and valence of the species, 1 mEq is represented by 1 mg of hydrogen.

To count the valence, divide the compound into its positive and negative components, and then count the number of either the positive or the negative charges. Some common compounds and their valence include:

- calcium chloride $(CaCl_2)$ = 2

- magnesium sulfate $(MgSO_4^{2-})$ = 2

- ferrous sulfate $(FeSO_4^{2-})$ = 2

- potassium chloride (KCl^-) = 1

- ammonium chloride (NH_4Cl) = 1 (the valence is counted as the bond between the ammonia NH4 and the chlorine atom)

- sodium acetate $(NaC_2H_3O_2)$ = 1 (the valence is counted as the bond between the acetate and the sodium atom)

mEq formula

$$mEq = \frac{mg \times valence}{MW}$$

---

120. A 20 mL vial is labeled potassium chloride (2 mEq/mL). How many grams of potassium chloride are present? (M.W. of KCl = 74.5 g)

20 mL x 2 mEq/mL = 40 mEq KCl total

$$mEq = \frac{mg \times valence}{MW}$$

$$40\ mEq = \frac{mg \times 1}{74.5} = 2,980\ mg,\ which\ is\ 2.98\ g$$

Note if you are asked to convert KCl liquid to tablets, you can use simple proportion since KCl 10% = 20 mEq/15 mL. For example, if someone is using Klor-Con 20 mEq BID, the total daily dose is 40 mEq, and if you convert to KCl 10%, you would solve this equation to get 30 mL required dose:

$$\frac{40\ mEq}{X\ mL} = \frac{20\ mEq}{15\ mL}$$

---

121. How many milliequivalents of potassium chloride are present in a 12 mL dose of a 10% (w/v) potassium chloride elixir? (M.W. = 74.5 g) Round the answer to 1 decimal place.

$$\frac{10\ g}{100\ mL} = \frac{X\ g}{12\ mL} \quad X = 1.2\ g,\ or\ 1,200\ mg$$

$$mEq = \frac{1,200\ mg \times 1}{74.5} = 16.1\ mEq$$

122. Calculate the milliequivalents of a standard ammonium chloride 21.4 mg/mL sterile solution in a 500 mL container (M.W. = 53.5 g)

- 21.4 mg/mL x 500 mL = 10,700 mg

$$mEq = \frac{10,700 \text{ mg} \times 1}{53.5} = 200 \text{ mEq}$$

---

123. A solution contains 0.04% w/v of Ca²⁺ ions. Express this concentration in milliequivalents per liter. (M.W. of Ca²⁺ = 40 g)

$$\frac{0.04 \text{ g}}{100 \text{ mL}} = \frac{X \text{ g}}{1,000 \text{ mL}} \qquad X = 0.4 \text{ g} \times 1,000 = 400 \text{ mg}$$

$$mEq/L = \frac{400 \text{ mg} \times 2}{40} = 20 \text{ mEq/L}$$

---

124. How may milliequivalents of sodium are in a 50 mL vial of sodium bicarbonate 8.4%? (M.W. = 84 g).

$$\frac{8.4 \text{ g}}{100 \text{ mL}} = \frac{X \text{ g}}{50 \text{ mL}} \qquad X = 4.2 \text{ g} \times 1,000 = 4,200 \text{ mg}$$

$$mEq = \frac{4,200 \text{ mg} \times 1}{84} = 50 \text{ mEq}$$

TEMPERATURE CONVERSIONS

Fahrenheit to Celsius

Minus 32 from the temperature, then divide by 1.8

Example: 88°F = (88-32)/1.8 = 31.1°C

Celsius to Fahrenheit

Multiply the temperature by 1.8, then add 32.

Example 26°C = (26 x 1.8) +32 = 78.8°F

CALCIUM CARBONATE TO CALCIUM CITRATE TABLET CONVERSION

Calcium carbonate (*Oscal, Tums*, etc) has acid-dependent absorption and should be taken with meals. Calcium carbonate is a dense form of calcium and contains 40% elemental calcium. A tablet that advertises 500 mg of elemental calcium weighs 1,250 mg. If 1,250 mg is multiplied by 0.40 (which is 40%) it will yield 500 mg elemental calcium.

Calcium citrate (*Citracal*, etc) has acid-independent absorption and can be taken with or without food. Calcium citrate is less dense and contains 21% elemental calcium. A tablet that advertises 315 mg calcium weighs 1,500 mg. If 1,500 mg is multiplied by 0.21 (or 21%), it will yield 315 mg elemental calcium. This is why the larger calcium citrate tablets provide less elemental calcium per tablet.

---

 125. A patient is taking 3 calcium citrate tablets daily (one tablet, TID). Each weighs 1,500 mg total (non-elemental) weight. She wishes to trade her calcium tablets for the carbonate form. If she is going to use 1,250 mg carbonate tablets (by weight), how many tablets will she need to take to provide the same total daily dose?

- 1,500 x 0.21 x 3 = 945 mg elemental calcium, daily.

Each of the carbonate tablets (1,250 mg x 0.4) = 500 mg per tablet. She would need 2 tablets to provide the same dose. Calcium absorption increases with lower doses. The tablets should be taken with two different meals.

CBC AND CBC WITH DIFFERENTIAL

When a CBC is ordered it usually contains these components (for ranges refer to the Appendix).

- RBCs (red blood cells or erythrocytes) have an average life span of 120 days.

- WBCs (white blood cells or leukocytes) are important for fighting infections. When WBC count is low, it is called leukopenia. When the WBC count is high, it is called a leukocytosis (and generally indicates an infection).

- Hgb, hemoglobin

- Hct, hematocrit

- Platelets (Plt) have an average life span of 7-10 days. A low platelet count is called thrombocytopenia.

- MCV, mean corpuscular volume

- MCH, mean corpuscular hemoglobin

- MCHC, mean corpuscular hemoglobin concentration

- RDW, red cell distribution width

When a CBC with differential is ordered, the types of WBCs are analyzed, and would include the percentage of polymorphonuclear neutrophils ("segs" or "polys"), band neutrophils ("bands"), lymphocytes, monocytes, eosinophils (an increase may indicate inflammation or a parasite infection), and basophils.

ABSOLUTE NEUTROPHIL COUNT (ANC)

Neutrophils make up most of the WBCs and represent the primary cells that fight infection. A low absolute neutrophil count (ANC) indicates higher infection risk. This can be caused by drugs (most commonly chemotherapy agents), clozapine, carbamazepine and others.

The normal range for the ANC is 2,200-8,000/microliter. The microliter may be written as mm³, or µL, but we are attempting to avoid this designation for safety reasons. A level < 2,000 is high-risk; for example, clozapine cannot be refilled if the ANC is < 2,000. A level < 1,000 is very high-risk for developing an infection.

A neutropenic patient should be watched for signs of infection, including fever, shaking, general weakness or flu-like symptoms. Precautions to reduce infection risk, such as proper hand-washing and avoiding others with infection, should be followed.

Calculating the ANC
Multiply the WBC by the percentage of neutrophils (the segs plus the bands).

Example Problems

126. A patient is being followed up at the oncology clinic today after her first round of chemotherapy 1 week ago. A CBC with differential is ordered and reported back as WBC = 14.8 x 10^3 cells/mm^3, segs are 10%, bands are 11%. Calculate this patient's ANC.

- Segs = 10% Bands = 11%

- 14,800 x (0.1 + 0.11) = 14,800 x 0.21 = ANC of <u>3,108</u>

127. A patient is taking clozapine and is at the clinic for a routine visit. Today's labs include WBC = 4,300 with 48% segs and 2% bands. Calculate this patient's ANC.

- Segs = 48% Bands = 2%

- 4,300 x (0.48 + 0.02) = 4,300 x 0.5 = ANC of <u>2,150</u>

BASIC METABOLIC PANEL (BMP)/COMPREHENSIVE METABOLIC PANEL (CMP)

The BMP is 8 tests (see Appendix for values) and includes sodium, potassium, CO_2 (bicarbonate), chloride, calcium, BUN, creatinine and glucose.

A CMP is 14 tests. All the tests in the BMP are included, plus the proteins Tbili and albumin and the liver tests ALT, AST, Alk Phos (alkaline phosphatase) and bilirubin. The CMP used to be called the Chem 12.

ACIDS, BASES, PH, IONIZATION AND BUFFERS

An <u>acid</u> is a compound that dissociates, releasing protons into solution. Once the proton is released, the compound is now a conjugate base. For example, HCl in solution is an acid and dissociates (giving up the proton) into H^+ and Cl^-. A <u>base</u> picks up, or binds, the proton. For example, NH_3^- is a base that can pick up a proton and become NH_4^+.

<u>The pH refers to the acidity or basicity of the solution.</u> As a solution becomes <u>more acidic (the concentration of protons increases), the pH decreases.</u> Conversely, when the <u>pH increases, protons decrease, and the solution is more basic, or alkaline.</u> Pure water is neutral at a pH of 7, and blood, with a pH of 7.4, is slightly alkaline. Stomach acid has a pH of ~2, is therefore acidic, with many protons in solution.

The pKa is the pH at which half the compound is protonated, and half is not protonated.

Acid-Base reactions are equilibrium reactions; there is always some drug moving back and forth between the acid and base state. You can use the pKa and the pH to determine if the compound is acting as an acid or a base.

A 'strong' acid means that you get 100% dissociation and a 'weak' acid means you get very limited dissociation. Any time you are given a pKa, it always refers to the acid form losing a proton to give the base form, thus, it is a 'weak acid'.

If you were given the 'pKb' then you would say, 'weak base' simply because of the definitions of the two terms.

If the pH is greater than the pKa, more of the acid is ionized, and more of the conjugate base is un-ionized.

If the pH is the same as the pKa, the ionized and un-ionized forms are equal.

If the pH is less than the pKa, more of the acid is un-ionized, and more of the conjugate base is ionized.

The percentage of drug in the ionized versus un-ionized state is important because an ionized drug is soluble but cannot cross lipid membranes. An un-ionized drug is not soluble but can cross the membranes and reach the proper receptor site. Most drugs are weak acids. They are soluble, and then can pick up a proton to cross the lipid layer.

A buffer is used to minimize fluctuations in pH so if a strong acid or a strong base enters the solution it is absorbed by the buffer – rather than interacting with a drug or protein and causing it to be destroyed. Buffers consist of a weak acid and its salt and a weak base and its salt. Water is a buffer and acts as a weak acid or base and looks like this:

$A\text{-}H$		H_2O		H_3O^+		A^-
Acid	+	Base	⇔	Conjugate Acid	+	Conjugate Base

It may be necessary to calculate the pH of a solution. This will require using the Henderson-Hasselbalch equation for either a weak acid or weak base.

Weak acid

$$pH = pK_a + \log (salt/acid)$$

Weak base

$$pH = pK_w - pK_b + \log(base/salt)$$

where pKw = 14

pH NOTES

A lower pH means more hydronium ions ($H3O+$, or $H+$) in solution and is therefore more acidic. A higher pH is more basic and has less hydronium ions and more hydroxide ($OH-$) ions in solution. The pH of 7 is said to be neutral. Blood is just slightly alkaline with a pH that should stay between 7.35-7.45.

128. What is the pH of a solution prepared to be 0.5 M sodium citrate and 0.05 M citric acid (pKa for citric acid = 3.13)?

pH = pKa + log (salt/acid)

pH = 3.13 + log (0.5M/0.05M)

pH = 3.13 + log(10)

pH = 3.13 + 1

pH = 4.13

---

129. What is the pH of a solution prepared to be 0.4 M ammonia and 0.04 M ammonium chloride (pKb for ammonia = 4.76)?

pH = pKw – pKb + log (base/salt)

pH = (14) - 4.76) + log (0.4/0.04)

pH = 9.24 + log (10)

pH = 9.24 + 1

pH = 10.24

Some Compounding Examples

---

130. A prescription reads as follows: Prepare lidocaine HCl 2% w/v; qs with pure water to 120 mL. How much lidocaine is required to make the prescription?

$$\frac{2\ g}{100\ mL} = \frac{X\ g}{120\ mL} = X = 2.4\ g$$

The weight of drug required is 2.4 g. Weigh the drug, place in a beaker, add water to the 120 mL line, stir, and place into a container labeled: Lidocaine 2% solution, 120 mL.

Common steps for compounding an ointment or cream:

- Weigh or measure the active ingredient/s

- If you are using a dry powder or granules, you will need to triturate with the pestle to reduce particle size

- Levigate on an ointment slab with a metal spatula (unless you are mixing metal ions, then use a plastic spatula)

- Package into a tube or jar

---

131. A prescription reads as follows: Prepare 150 g of a 3% coal tar preparation. How much petrolatum will be needed to make the prescription?

$$\frac{3\ g}{100\ g} = \frac{X\ g}{150\ g} \quad X = 4.5\ g$$

150 g (total weight) – 4.5 g (active ingredient) = 145.5 g petrolatum

ALIQUOT MEASUREMENT

Aliquots are used when you need to make a preparation but cannot weigh out the small amount needed directly since the scale is not accurate to such a small degree. This problem is solved with aliquots.

<u>Note on balances:</u> The sensitivity requirement (SR) of a balance determines the minimum amount of drug that can be weighed accurately. In school calculation courses, a torsion scale is often used that has an SR of 6. We will use this type of common scale in our examples. To calculate the minimum weighable quantity (MWQ) that can be weighed accurately, take the SR of the scale, which is 6, and divide by the percentage of error (0.05). The percentage of error is generally 5% (0.05), but some problems may suggest to use other percentages of error.

$$MWQ = \frac{SR — Sensitivity\ req.}{0.05}$$

If the balance has an SR of 6 mg, the MWQ = 6 mg/0.05 = 120 mg, which is the least weighable amount (you can weigh at or above the MWQ).

Aliquot Steps

1. Calculate the MWQ (as mentioned above).

2. Select a multiple of the desired quantity that can be weighed with the required precision.

3. Dilute the multiple quantity with an inert substance (lactose is commonly used; check patient is not lactose intolerant).

4. Weigh the aliquot portion of the dilution that contains the desired quantity.

Aliquot Capsule Example

132. A prescription calls for 10 capsules, each containing 0.5 mg lorazepam. A torsion balance has a SR of 6 mg. Explain how you would weigh 5 mg of lorazepam with an accuracy of ± 5%, using lactose as the diluent.

1. Calculate the MWQ.

$$mwQ = \frac{6}{0.05}$$

■ SR/0.05 = 6 mg/0.05 = 120 mg

2. Select a multiple of the desired quantity that can be weighed with the required precision.

Select a multiple of 5 that can be weighed with the desired accuracy. For this scale, we cannot weigh less than 120 mg. We need to find a multiple of 5 that will give us 120 mg (or preferably a little over 120 mg). In this case, 5 x 25 = 125 mg of lorazepam.

3. Dilute the multiple quantity with an inert substance. This will give us the quantity of the total dilution.

■ 120 mg (the aliquot) x 25 = 3,000 mg (drug + lactose = dilution).

4. Weigh the aliquot portion of the dilution that contains the desired quantity.

Weigh 1/25 of dilution (3,000 mg), or 120 mg of dilution (the aliquot), which will contain 5 mg of drug (answer).

You have calculated the total amount of the dilution. We don't need this much, but the purpose of doing this was to get the exact amount of drug (5 mg) in each 120 mg aliquot portion. Now, calculate the actual amount required in the prescription, and use 1 aliquot portion (120 mg of the trituration) to get the 5 mg of lorazepam.

---

133. What is the total amount of lactose needed for the aliquot in the above prescription?

- 3,000 mg dilution - 125 mg lorazepam = 2,875 mg lactose

---

134. A prescription calls for 10 capsules, each containing 0.5 mg lorazepam and each weighing a total of 200 mg. A torsion balance has a SR of 6 mg. Explain how would you prepare this prescription.

Calculate the total weight of the capsules = 200 mg x 10 capsules = 2,000 mg

Calculate the weight of lactose (diluent) required.

- 2,000 mg (total weight) – 120 mg (aliquot that contains 5 mg of the active drug) = 1,880 mg lactose

Here is how the prescription can now be completed:

Prepare the Aliquot
Weigh 125 mg of lorazepam.

Weigh 2,875 mg lactose (from the example problem above).

Mix (triturate) the lorazepam and lactose together.

Remove 120 mg of the dilution. This aliquot contains the 5 mg of lorazepam needed.

Prepare the Capsules
Weigh 1,880 mg lactose and mix with the 120 mg aliquot.

This results in a 2,000 mg total mixture, of which 5 mg is the lorazepam, and 1,995 mg is lactose.

Divide this into 10 capsules containing 200 mg; each capsule will contain 0.5 mg of lorazepam.

Aliquot Liquid Example

135. Prepare 100 mL of a solution containing 0.2 mg/mL of clonidine.

Calculate the total weight of active drug required.

0.2 mg/mL x 100 mL = 20 mg clonidine

Choose your solvent. In this case we will use water. Water is the usual solvent, but there are others, including ethanol and glycerol.

Choose a volume for the aliquot. The volume must include enough solution so that the drug will dissolve. A compound's solubility can be found in the Merck Index or Remington's. Choose a small amount that will dissolve the drug. Do not exceed the total volume in the prescription.

For this example, we will choose 5 mL which will dissolve 20 mg of clonidine. The concentration is calculated as follows:

We are using the same scale, which has a MWQ of 120 mg. We cannot weigh out 20 mg of clonidine with this scale, but need a multiple of 20 that is close to 120 mg. Since 20 x 6 = 120 exactly, we can weight out 120 mg of clonidine.

Using ratio proportion, calculate the total volume of solution to be prepared.

$$\frac{120 \text{ mg clonidine}}{X \text{ mL solution}} = \frac{20 \text{ mg clonidine}}{5 \text{ mL}} \qquad X = 30 \text{ mL solution}$$

This means that you have 120 mg of clonidine in the 30 mL solution. Each 5 mL aliquot contains 20 mg clonidine. This is exactly the amount of clonidine you need for the entire prescription. You will prepare this 30 mL of solution. Then, draw up 5 mL of this solution to provide your total amount of active drug and qs to 100 mL to complete the prescription. Here are the remaining steps itemized:

Prepare the Aliquot

- Weigh 120 mg clonidine.

- Dissolve the clonidine in water and qs to 30 mL. You cannot add 30 mL of water, since the clonidine will contribute to the 30 mL. Rather, add water to the 30 mL line.

- Remove 5 mL of the solution. This aliquot contains the 20 mg of clonidine needed.

Prepare the Prescription

- Place the 5 mL aliquot into a beaker.

- Add water (qs) to 100 mL to complete the prescription. You have 20 mg in 100 mL, or 0.2 mg/mL. This is the concentration stated on the prescription, which should be recorded on the dispensed product.

Aliquot Problems

136. A prescription calls for 15 capsules, each containing 1 mg doxazosin. A torsion balance has an SR of 6.5 mg. Explain how you would weigh 15 mg of doxazosin with an accuracy of ± 5%, using lactose as the diluent.

1. Calculate the MWQ.

- SR/0.05 = 6.5 mg/0.05 = 130 mg   130 x 10 = 1300

2. Select a multiple of the desired quantity that can be weighed with the required precision.

Select a multiple of 15 that can be weighed with the desired accuracy. For this scale, we cannot weigh less than 130 mg. We need to find a multiple of 15 that will give us 130 mg (or preferably a little over 130 mg). In this case, we are going to use 10. 15 mg x 10 = 150 mg of doxazosin.

3. Dilute the multiple quantity with an inert substance.

- 130 mg (the aliquot) x 10 = 1,300 mg (dilution).

4. Weigh the aliquot portion of the dilution that contains the desired quantity.

Weigh 1/10 of dilution (1,300 mg), or 130 mg of dilution (the aliquot), which will contain 15 mg of doxazosin (answer).

---

137. A prescription calls for 5 mg bromocriptine mesylate. A torsion balance has a SR of 4 mg. Explain how you would weigh 5 mg of bromocriptine mesylate with an accuracy of ± 5%, using lactose as the diluent.

1. Calculate the MWQ.

- SR/0.05 = 4 mg/0.05 = 80 mg

2. Select a multiple of the desired quantity that can be weighed with the required precision.

Select a multiple of 5 that can be weighed with the desired accuracy. For this scale, we cannot weigh less than 80 mg. We need to find the minimum multiple of 5 that will give us 80 mg (or preferably more than 80 mg). In this case, we are going to use 20. 5 x 20 = 100 mg of bromocriptine mesylate.

3. Dilute the multiple quantity with an inert substance.

- 80 mg (the aliquot) x 20 = 1,600 mg (dilution).

4. Weigh the aliquot portion of the dilution that contains the desired quantity.

Weigh 1/20 of dilution (1,600 mg), or 80 mg of dilution, which will contain 5 mg of bromocriptine mesylate (answer).

COMPOUNDING REQUIREMENTS & TERMINOLOGY

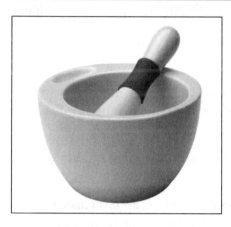

Compounding calculations are in the calculations chapter.

Compounding versus FDA-approved drugs

Compounding is different from manufacturing since it is patient-specific (ordered by a prescriber for the patient) and regulated by the state boards of pharmacy. For example, a prescriber designates specific percentages of hormone cream for an individual female patient. Or, a hospitalized patient is getting powders prepared since she cannot swallow pills.

- <u>Beyond use dates</u> must be applied to each product, using either the USP guidelines, or a reasonable date that allows time for the patient to use the drug but will not cause any of the individual ingredients to lose potency.

- The recipe must be kept in a log book (see next section).

- Advertisement of compounded products is not permitted.

- Compounded products do not have NDC numbers.

- In contrast, <u>FDA-approved and regulated drugs must have an approved NDA, must be produced under Good Manufacturing Practices (GMP), have NDC numbers, and carry a set expiration date</u> (provided to the pharmacy).

General compounding rules

- Compounding space should be separate and away from dispensing section.

- Ideally, use only USP or NF chemicals from FDA-inspected manufacturers.

- 4 logs must be in pharmacy: compounding formulas and procedures, compounded item log, equipment maintenance records (includes refrigerator and freezer temp logs), record of ingredients purchased.

- Procedure detail must be enough so the procedure can be duplicated, and must include all names, lot #'s, quantities, order of mixing, expiration or "beyond use" date (never more than 6 months), and any special storage instructions.

- Product label must include generic or chemical name of active ingredients, strength or quantity, pharmacy lot number, beyond-use date, and any special storage requirements.

- Capsule label must include mcg or mg/capsule.

- Liquid strength should be in concentration (e.g. 125 mg/5 mL), or percentage.

- The coining of short names for marketing or convenience (e.g., *Johnson's Solution*) is strongly discouraged.

- Purified water (not tap water) is used. Purified water is also used for rinsing equipment.

- If you are compounding a prescription that calls for alcohol and the type is not specified, use USP 95% ethyl alcohol.

SELECTED NOTES ON STERILE COMPOUNDING

- The following products must be sterile: injections, inhalations, wound and cavity irrigation baths, eye drops and eye ointments. Water used in preparation must be sterile water for injection, or bacteriostatic water for injection.

- Sterile compounding requires personnel trained in aseptic techniques, air quality testing and product sterility testing.

- If the product is an injectable, the preparation hood must be either an ISO class 5 (class 100) laminar air flow hood within a ISO class 7 (class 10,000) clean room (with positive air pressure differential relative to adjacent areas) or an ISO class 5 (class 100) clean room with positive air pressure differential relative to adjacent areas or a barrier isolator that provides a ISO class 5 (class 100) environment for compounding.

- Clean room garb (low-shedding coverall, head cover, face mask and shoe covers) is required and should be put on and taken off outside the designated area. Hand, finger and wrist jewelry is not allowed. Head and facial hair have to out of the way (tied up) and covered.

- When preparing cytotoxic agents, gowns and gloves are worn. All cytotoxic agents must be labeled "cytotoxic agents – dispose of properly" and disposal and spill policies kept in the pharmacy.

- Sterile and non-sterile areas must be separate.

Compounding Equipment Used in a Community Pharmacy

BALANCE

2 types required: torsion balance, and if compounding routinely, a top-loading electronic balance

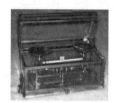

Torsion balance

Electronic balance

MEASURING DEVICES

When measuring, select a device equal to or slightly larger than the amount to be measured.

- If the volume to be measured is viscous use a syringe, rather than a cylinder. If the volume is less than 1 ml, use a micropipette.

- Liquids in a container curve up, therefore measure at the bottom of the meniscus.

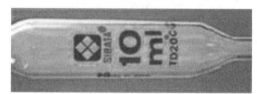

Pipette

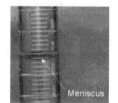

Measure from bottom of meniscus

MORTAR & PESTLE

Minimum of 2 types: 1 glass and 1 Wedgewood or porcelain (ceramic). Wedgewood or porcelain is used most commonly and is best for reducing particle size of dry powders and crystals. Porcelain has a smoother surface than Wedgewood and is preferred for blending powders or pulverizing soft materials. If Wedgewood is used for powders or crystals, first coat the inside with lactose to fill in the crevices.

Glass is used for liquids and chemicals that are oily or will stain the porcelain, including many chemotherapeutics.

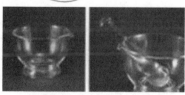

Glass mortar & pestle

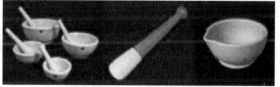

Ceramic mortar and pestle

SURFACES & SPATULAS

Glassine weighing paper (as opposed to bond paper) should be used for weighing ointments, creams and some dry chemicals.

Parchment ointment paper is convenient and easy to clean, but cannot be used for creams or other aqueous mixtures because the paper will absorb water – use a slab instead.

Generally, large metal (stainless steel) spatula blades are used, but small spatula blades (< 6 inches) can be used for removing product from the large spatula and putting it into the jar.

Plastic spatulas should be used for chemicals (e.g., potassium, iodine) that can react with stainless steel blades.

Compounding Terminology and Ingredients

LEVIGATION

The process of reducing the size of a particle of a solid by triturating it in a mortar or spatulating it on an ointment slab with a small amount of liquid in which the solid is not soluble. The goal is to transfer it from a solid to a paste-like substance utilizing a levigating agent. This incorporates the solid into a cream or ointment base. It also makes the solid more uniform throughout the base and gets rid of the gritty feeling.

- The levigation agent must be miscible with the ointment base.

- Mineral oil is good to use for levigating a hydrophobic ointment such as white petrolatum.

- If heat is used (to mix things easier) the use should be limited and the ingredient with the higher melting point should be heated. Otherwise, undesired chemical reactions could occur.

- A water bath will help prevent over-heating.

TRITURATION

Reducing substances to fine particles by rubbing them with a mortar and pestle, or on an ointment slab.

EXTEMPORANEOUS

A compound prepared without a specific formula from an official compendium and made especially to fill the needs of a specific patient.

EMOLLIENTS

An emollient is a single agent that is used to soften and smooth the skin. A moisturizer is sometimes referred to as an emollient, but the term emollient is used for single agents, and moisturizers often have coloring, scents, and other ingredients added. (Astringents tighten the skin.)

EMULSIONS AND EMULSIFIERS

Emulsions are a two-phase system of two immiscible liquids, one of which is dispersed through the other as small droplets. They can be oil in water, or water in oil. Emulsifiers (or emulgent) is used to stabilize the emulsion. Emulsifiers are usually surfactants (or wetting agents) that reduce surface tension so that the 2 substances can move closer to each other. Emulsions are immiscible (they do not form a suspension – which means the two liquids stay separate when you combine them).

- Emulsifiers include acacia, agar, pectin, lipophilic esters of sorbitan (*Arlacel* and *Span*) and the hydrophilic esters (*Myrj* and *Tween*).

- The Continental or dry gum method of preparing an emulsion uses oil, purified water and gum (such as acacia) in the ratio of 4:2:1.

- The hydrophilic-lipophilic balance (HLB) number determines how much surfactant will be required to form the mixture together.

OINTMENTS AND CREAMS

 LCO

Lotions, creams and ointments are all oil in water preparations. Lotions have the most water, followed by creams (which are therefore thicker), followed by ointments (the most oil of the three). Consequently, ointments provide the best skin barrier but are thick to apply and can be difficult to wash off. These are semisolid dosage forms used externally on the skin or mucous membranes. They have good skin penetration and adhere well. They are packaged in jars or in tubes. Many ointments are medicated (e.g., coal tar ointment for psoriasis, diaper rash ointment).

- Ointment bases which are oleaginous and hydrocarbon-based do not absorb water, are occlusive and do not wash off with water. An example is white petrolatum.

- An absorption ointment base is similar in that they are occlusive and do not wash off with water, but do absorb water. Examples are lanolin, *Aquaphor* and *Aquabase*.

- Water-in-oil emulsions include *Eucerin, Nivea* and rose water ointment.

- Oil-in-water emulsions. *Cetaphil, Dermabase, Keri lotion, Lubriderm* and hydrophilic ointment.

GELS

Gels are used as thickeners. They have a solid and a liquid that are dispersed evenly throughout a material (the suspension is inter-penetrated by the liquid). Example – *BenzaClin* acne gel.

- Common gels used as thickeners are the alginates (including Na^+, K^+, Ca^{2+} alginate), agar, carrageenan and gelatin.

SOLUTIONS

Solutions are liquid preparations of soluble chemicals dissolved in solvents such as water, alcohol, or propylene glycol. When alcohol is used as a solvent, the pharmacist should consider effects on the patient, and if the alcohol may interact with medications.

SUSPENSIONS

A two phased-system of a finely divided solid in a liquid medium. The drug must be uniformly dispersed in the medium. Suspending agents:

- Natural hydrocolloids, including acacia, alginic acid, gelatin, guar gum, alginate, xanthan gum

- Semi-synthetic hydrocolloids, including methylcellulose

- Synthetic hydrocolloids, including carbomers and polyvinyl alcohol

- Clays, including bentonite and veegum

SUPPOSITORIES

Suppositories are solid dosage forms used to deliver medicine into the rectum, vagina or urethra.

- The base must be compatible with the medication, it must not melt too quickly (in your hands while inserting), must be stable and must not have a disagreeable look or scent.

- Examples are acetaminophen suppository (good for feverish infant who is not eating or is vomiting), hemorrhoid suppository (rectum), mesalamine rectal suppository (used to treat distal disease – the suppository provides medication where the disease is located, and avoids systemic toxicity – mesalamine also comes as an enema), and vaginal suppositories of antifungal medication for vaginal candida infections.

- Suppositories bypass the oral route and avoid first-pass metabolism. Commonly used bases are cocoa butter, glycerin, hydrogenated vegetable oils, and polyethylene glycol.

SYRUPS

Syrups are concentrated, aqueous preparations of sugar or sugar-substitute, medicinal agents, or flavoring in water, such as cough syrups.

ELIXIRS

Elixirs are clear, sweetened, hydroalcoholic solutions suitable for water insoluble drugs, such as mouthwashes.

LOZENGES/TROCHES

Lozenges are called troches and deliver drug to the oral mucosa. They can also be used for patients who have trouble swallowing, as the material dissolves in the mouth. Clotrimazole troches *(Mycelex)* is an antifungal troche that dissolves in the mouth and is used to treat oral thrush. Troches are made in molds, with any flavorings or coloring added right before the mold is filled.

CAPSULES

Capsules are unit doses made in soluble shells of gelatin. Unpleasant drug tastes and odors can be masked by the gelatin shell. They are made by triturating the powders to a small particle size, mixing by geometric dilution, and calculating the weight needed to fill a capsule.

Hard gelatin capsules: largest is 000, the smaller the size the higher the number.

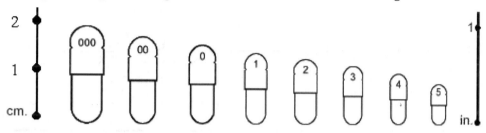

TABLETS

In large-scale manufacturing, the formulation that is often the least expensive to make (and the most common dispensed in everyday practice) are compressed tablets. Tablets may contain excipients (also called binders) that hold the tablet together. Capsules may also use similar ingredients as fillers. Sorbitol is used (particularly in chewables as it is sweet). Sorbitol can cause considerable GI distress in some patients with IBS; it has laxative properties. If lactose is used, this will present a problem for patients with lactose-intolerance.

4

PHARMACOKINETICS & DRUG FORMULATIONS

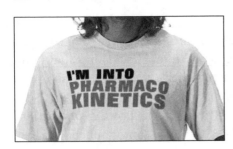

Pharmacokinetics

Pharmacokinetics (PK) determines what happens to the drug in the body. (Pharmacodynamics is the study of what the drug does to the body.)

PK involves these elements: dissolution, absorption, distribution, metabolism, and excretion.

DISSOLUTION

This applies to oral formulations; if the drug does not break up (dissolve) in the gut, it cannot be absorbed. All, or part, will be excreted in the feces. Drugs can bind with other compounds, which will prevent complete dissolution and may reduce the amount absorbed. Drugs can be destroyed in the gut. The primary pathway of drug degradation in the gut is hydrolysis (lysis with water). One part of the compound takes the proton (H+) and the other takes the hydroxyl group (OH-). Most drugs dissolve in an acidic medium (in the gut) and are absorbed (mostly) in the small intestine. In order to increase tablet dissolution the chemist could increase the tablet's surface area. The rate of dissolution is described by the Noyes–Whitney equation.

① hydrolysis

ABSORPTION

The amount absorbed is the fraction, or percentage of the drug that enters the body. This is determined by the drug's bioavailability, which is called F. The bioavailability of an oral formulation is compared to the amount available if the drug were given by intravenously. When a drug is given IV, the full dose is received (F = 100%). In oral intake, some of the drug can stay in the gut and be excreted in the feces. For example, bisphosphonates stick to other compounds easily and have very poor oral absorption (< 10%). An IV bisphosphonate requires a much lower dose, since oral absorption is bypassed.

If active transport is involved, the drug requires energy to move the drug across the membrane, and may move against the concentration gradient. Since there is more drug in the gut initially (after the medicine is swallowed) than is present in the serum, most drugs are absorbed into the body passively by moving down the concentration gradient. Most drug absorption occurs in the small intestine, since the surface is covered by villi and microvilli and provides a large surface area for absorption. Enteric coated formulations dissolve in the more basic environment of the small intestine.

Distribution

Distribution is the dispersion, or passage of the drug throughout the body. Lipophilic compounds are uncharged, and can pass more easily through lipid membranes. Most drugs are weak acids and can pick up a proton to become uncharged. Polar, charged compounds (such as aminoglycosides) cannot pass easily through cell walls. More of the drug will stay in the blood compartment, which is one reason why aminoglycosides are nephrotoxic.

Small changes in protein binding can cause large changes in drug distribution. The most significant protein involved in drug binding is albumin. Changes in albumin (normal range 3.5-5 g/dL) will cause changes in the amount of bound drug. For example, the reported level of phenytoin will need to be adjusted if the albumin is low, or below < 3.5. Phenytoin is highly-protein bound, and if the albumin is low, the phenytoin concentration will be higher than shown by the total serum level. Or, one highly protein-bound drug may displace another, resulting in elevated concentration of the other drug. Phenytoin, if displaced, can result in toxicity (nystagmus, diplopia, ataxia, confusion). Warfarin is also highly protein-bound.

Metabolism

See the Drug Interactions chapter for further discussion on hepatic metabolism. If a drug is subject to first-pass metabolism, it goes through the liver prior to reaching the systemic circulation. The liver (along with drug-metabolizing enzymes in the gut wall) can extract, or pull out, a portion of the drug by changing the drug's structure. This results in less drug being available for therapeutic benefit (or more drug if a pro-drug is hepatically metabolized to the active form.)

Drugs can also be affected by enzyme inducers (which decrease drug concentration) or enzyme inhibitors (which increase drug concentration). Since about three-quarters of all drugs undergo hepatic metabolism, it is important to recognize when the liver is not functioning well, and which drugs are likely to be affected.

Excretion

Excretion involves the elimination of the drug (out of the body, which can be renally, or back into the gut and through the feces, etc.) The elimination half life (t½) is the time it takes for the plasma concentration to ↓ 50%. After 4-5 half-lives, the elimination is considered complete. See the t½ examples in the calculations chapter. More on renal excretion is provided in the renal dosing chapter.

Drug Formulation Considerations

It may be necessary to choose whether or not a drug comes in a specific formulation. It is difficult to memorize all the various formulations, but consider that it takes money to develop unique dosing forms. If a drug is available in something unusual – there has to be a market for the formulation or the manufacturer would not have spent money to develop a novel method of delivery. <u>Think about who would need the drug in that form to help remember the various formulations.</u>

Dysphagia, trouble swallowing large capsules or tablets (small children)

Patients with swallowing difficulty (elderly, frail, dementia, stroke, young children, etc.) may need a formulation other than a traditional tablet or capsule. Tablets that <u>dissolve in the mouth</u> (orally disintegrating (or dissolving, or dispersable) tablets, or ODT) are available for many drugs that are used in elderly patients: dementia drugs such as donepezil *(Aricept ODT)*, memantine comes as solution *(Namenda* solution), the Parkinson drug ODT form of carbidopa-levodopa *(Parcopa)*, the antidepressant mirtazapine *(Remeron SolTab* – an ODT) – this medication is often given to frail elderly due to the side effect profile (sedation and increased appetite), among others.

Rivastigmine, a dementia drug, comes in a patch formulation that makes it easy to give to a person with dementia – it is applied once daily. Some patients with dysphagia need to grind up tablets – be careful patients do <u>not grind up long-acting</u> formulations. Medications that come as beads in capsules can sometimes be sprinkled on a small amount of soft food or mixed with beverages. Typically these are long-acting beads – if they sit in applesauce or pudding the liquid will ruin the slow release. Instruct patients to consume right after they sprinkle. Children can have trouble swallowing some tablets or capsules and montelukast *(Singulair* – used for asthma or allergies) comes in packets that can be sprinkled on food. Valproate, used for seizures in children, also comes as a sprinkle-filled capsule. Many of the ADHD medications can be sprinkled on applesauce or pudding – since young children may have difficulty swallowing tablets or capsules. Lisdexamfetamine *(Vyvanse)*, a popular ADHD drug, comes in a small capsule that can be opened so the parent can mix the contents in a small amount of water. Like *Concerta*, it is designed to be small to make it easier for younger people to swallow. Both are designed to be hard to abuse; see the ADHD chapter for more details on the design.

Nausea

If a medication <u>causes nausea it is easier to tolerate if it comes as a dissolving form</u>. The medical condition itself may be causing nausea – and it would be worsened by administering medications that cause additional nausea.

Migraine medications come in various formulations because nausea is common with these types of headaches. Rizatriptan *(Maxalt MLT)* and Zolmitriptan *(Zomig ZMT)* are both ODTs. The primary side effect of the acetylcholinesterase inhibitors used for dementia is nausea – and the *Aricept ODT* or the *Exelon* patch could be helpful. Patches for any formulation bypass the oral route. [As an interesting aside, most medications that are dosed at night are dosed QHS due to sedation – but donepezil is dosed at night so the nausea is lessened during the day.] Suppositories may be useful to avoid the GI route and reduce any GI complaint. IV is another option. If a hospitalized patient is vomiting, they will primarily receive the IV route.

Many drugs that cause stomach upset come in long-acting formulations – if less of the drug is released initially (versus disintegrating in the stomach all at once), stomach upset (nausea, abdominal pain, sometimes diarrhea) can be lessened. Metformin XR is a key example – this can be dosed with dinner and once daily – both are helpful to reduce daytime stomach upset.

STAT onset needed!

If the condition causes pain onset FAST then it may be required to bypass the oral route – oral absorption requires at least ½ an hour, and usually an hour, for onset. Sumatriptan (*Imitrex STAT dose*, *Sumavel DosePro)* is used by many patients who require fast onset for acute migraine pain. Fentanyl sublingual forms are used for acute breakthrough pain in patients being treated for cancer. Injections provide fast relief and are frequently used in acute care settings for treating severe pain, such as with the use of patient controlled analgesia (PCA) devices. Sublingual (SL) formulations work faster than oral absorption and drugs that are designed to work faster by SL absorption include fentanyl (for breakthrough cancer pain), buprenorphine, some of the hypnotics, and others.

Nonadherence

If a patient is likely to forget their medicine, or refuses to take it, it is useful to choose a formulation that can be dosed less frequently. Not all long-acting tablets are once daily, however – some are BID. Some of the psychosis medications have been formulated in long-acting formulations to enable caregivers to administer the drug less frequently. Haloperidol comes as the *Haldol decanoate*, which is given every 4 weeks. Paliperidone comes in a monthly injection. Risperidone in the *Risperdal Consta* injection is a 2-week formulation. Another 2-week formulation is the older antipsychotic fluphenazine (*Prolixin decanoate*). Divalproex comes in a sprinkle formulation that can be used on food for patients with bipolar who require a mood stabilizer – this way, they may not be aware they have received the drug. This formulation is also used for seizure control in children who cannot swallow capsules or tablets.

School-time dosing

Many of the stimulant medications that are used for ADHD are designed to avoid noon-time dosing (and to provide a more steady drug response). If a child has to go to the nurse's office to get the dose, they are stigmatized, and may have to wait in line (with the children getting inhalers, or insulin) and miss playtime. In addition they may need a little bit of medication to get them going in the morning (IR) so they are alert in homeroom, and more later (via a long-acting formulation) to carry them throughout the day. *Concerta* comes in the *OROS* deliver system that provides both IR/ER release – and there are others that provide a similar delivery. Methylphenidate comes in a patch (*Daytrana*) that is applied each morning (to the hip) to provide a steady release of medication throughout the day.

Long-acting formulations

These are useful to primarily permit once-daily dosing but are not always once-daily, and may help with side effects such as reduced GI upset or reduced dry mouth (for example, from long-acting anticholinergics used for OAB). When a drug delivery is spread-out (in a more even, smooth delivery), side effects are generally lessened since the "peak" is lower. Side effects occur more readily when more of the drug is available to interact with the wrong receptors. Patches generally cause decreased side effects due to slow delivery.

Certain drugs are designed as slow release to avoid irritation to the GI lining. Or, they may be enteric-coated. Do not crush or chew any drug that has the following suffix that indicates it is a long-acting formulation: XR, ER, LA, SR, CR, CRT, SA, TR, TD, or have 24 in the name, or the ending –cont (for controlled release, such as *MS Contin* or *Oxycontin*), or timecaps or sprinkles.

Note the danger: There are certain drugs that, if crushed, could KILL the patient! These include opioids – where a 24H dose could be released in less than an hour. Be sure to look for the suffix and counsel. There are a few long-acting formulations that can be cut at the score line – but still NOT crushed, such as *Toprol XL*.

Suppositories

Mesalamine comes in a suppository because the disease is often present in the distal portion of the intestine. There is no reason to expose the patient to the drug systemically if the disease is local. With a mesalamine suppository (or enema) the diseased area is treated and the patient suffers less side effects. Suppositories are useful if nausea is present. They can also provide stat relief – including for constipation. Glycerin suppositories are useful to treat (not prevent) constipation in small children and elderly. Bisacodyl suppository is another fast-relief option for constipation. The bisacodyl suppository is to treat constipation (when a bowel movement is needed now) versus the tablet, which is generally dosed QHS in order for the patient to have a bowel movement the following morning. Suppositories are used for either local or systemic drug delivery.

Marketing formulations that may not provide benefit

Sometimes long-acting formulations, or other formulations, are released only because the drug went generic and the manufacturer is looking to retain market share. *Paxil CR* was promoted to help with GI side effects when paroxetine generic became available – but the IR formulation does not usually cause much stomach problems. Most patients using *Ambien CR* would find the same benefit with zolpidem generic. The new higher dose *Aricept* was promoted when donepezil went generic, but the higher dose does not provide noticeable benefit for the majority of patients.

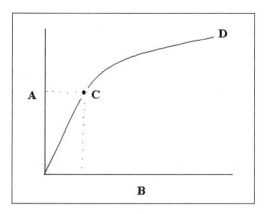

First-Order Kinetics

The lower left corner of the chart (up to point C) indicates first-order kinetics. The absorption of <u>most drugs follows first-order kinetics</u>. The amount of drug given is proportional to the increase seen in plasma concentration.

In first-order kinetics, <u>the more drug given, the higher the drug concentration</u>.

MICHAELIS-MENTEN KINETICS

Michaelis-Menten, or saturable kinetics, begins as first-order, but when the metabolism becomes saturated, the concentration increases rapidly. Drugs with this type of kinetics begin as first-order kinetics, but can change to zero order once a certain dose is reached and metabolizing enzymes are saturated. In zero order elimination, <u>the elimination rate is independent of the drug's concentration</u>. At this point, toxicity can result. <u>Phenytoin, theophylline and voriconazole</u> have this type of saturable kinetics (see figure).   P v T

<u>With saturable kinetics, a small increase in dose may result in a large increase in drug concentration</u>.

Michaelis-Menten kinetics – example

A patient has been using phenytoin 100 mg three times daily. The phenytoin level was taken and found to be 9.8 mcg/mL. The physician increased the dose to 100 mg with breakfast and lunch, and 200 mg with dinner. The patient started to slur her words, felt fatigued and returned to the physician's office. The level was retaken and found to be 18.7 mcg/mL.

The most likely explanation for the increase in phenytoin level is that although first-order kinetics took place initially, when the dose was increased, the metabolism became saturated, and the level increased dramatically, as shown above in the Michaelis-Menten diagram.

5

BIOSTATISTICS & PHARMACOECONOMICS

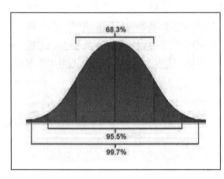

Biostatistics

BACKGROUND

Health care is changing rapidly. As pharmacists, the "drug experts," it is our responsibility to review and evaluate literature assessing safety, effectiveness and economic issues concerning new drugs and innovative uses of current medications. Journal articles and other publications present clinical data, using statistical methods and tools to answer research questions and aid in clinical guideline development and consensus statements on how best to treat conditions. While there are a few types of studies that do not require statistical analysis (e.g. case studies, case series), most robust studies are based on statistical analysis.

DESCRIPTIVE STATISTICS

Descriptive statistics are designed to give us a general view of the data and provide simple summaries. One of the most common ways to evaluate data is to analyze its distribution. Measures of central tendency estimate the "center" of a distribution of values, or the point around which the numbers cluster. There are three main ways of estimating central tendency; the mean, the median and the mode. Although they all estimate the "center," the answers obtained can be quite different.

Mean

The mean is the average value of a sample distribution. It is found by adding up the values in a list, and dividing by the number of items. The mean will reflect (or be sensitive to) the outlying values – which may not be representative of the norm. For example, in the list 2-3-4-3-4-2-9, the outlier is 9, and the mean would capture an effect from this value. The mean is used for continuous data.

Median

The median is the value in the middle of the list – to find it, arrange all the observations in numerical order (lowest to highest) and pick the middle value. Half of the values will be above the median, and half will be below. If the list contains an even number of values, then select the 2 values in the middle and add them together and divide by 2 to get the median. The outliers are not reflected in the median value – which can be far away from the central value. Another term for the median is the 50th percentile, which means that 50% of the values are smaller and the other 50% are larger. If a student is ranking a professor, and the class is small, the median would be more appropriate to choose than the mean. If 1 or 2 students just don't like the topic, they will rank the professor low. By choosing the value in the middle, you would avoid the angry outlier's effect on the data. Median values better represent data that is skewed. When the mean and the median values are very different, the data is skewed. Median values can be used with both continuous and ordinal, or ranked, data.

Mode

The mode is the value that occurs most frequently.

Range

The range is the difference between the highest and the lowest values.

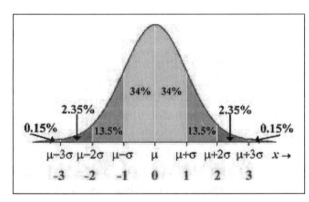

Normal Distribution

A "normal" distribution is also known as a bell shaped, or Gaussian, curve. Generally, clinical studies rely on "sample" populations that appear to be representative of the population of interest. When we look at a sample, we do not have the entire population, and are forced to estimate. When the population group is large, the distribution approximates a normal curve (see picture) where μ is the mean, and σ is the standard deviation (SD). In a Gaussian or normal distribution, the mean, mode and median would all be the same value and would look like the figure above. Notice the curve is symmetric around the mean and the skew is zero.

Standard Deviation (SD)

The standard deviation shows how much variation, or dispersion, there is from the mean. The closer the numbers cluster around the mean, the smaller the standard deviation. If the SD is small (low), this would lead one to infer that the drug being studied had a similar effect on most subjects. SD is expressed in the same units as the data, is used for data that is normally distributed, is always a positive number, and can be used for continuous data only. In a normal distribution, roughly 68% of the values are within 1 SD from the mean and 95% are within 2 standard deviations.

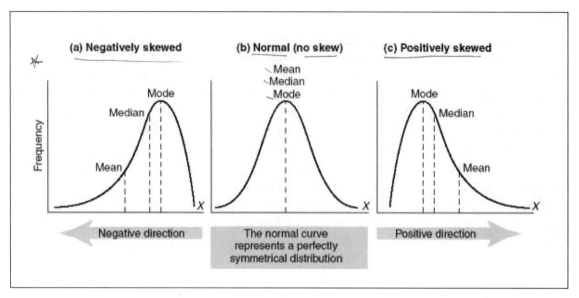

Skewness

Data that does not have a normal distribution is said to be skewed data. The asymmetric data can be skewed to the right or skewed to the left. Data that is skewed to the right has a positive skew (curve C in figure above) and data that is skewed to the left has a negative skew (curve A in figure above). The direction of the skew refers to the direction of the longer tail, not to the bulk of the data or curve hump.

Confidence Interval

In studies we come up with estimates for different variables. How valid is the estimate? This can be determined by looking at the confidence interval (CI). In biostatistics, we use CIs commonly to help determine the validity of the mean (or average) of the data. The confidence interval tells us that there is a given probability that the population's mean value is contained within the interval. For example, if a study reports that the mean weight of newborns is 3.18 kg, with a 95% confidence interval 2.93-3.43 kg, there is a 95% chance that the true population mean (if you had various data sets) would fall within the range, and there is a 5% chance that the true population mean would fall outside this range. In this example the CI is reported at 95%, which can also be written as having a probability of 0.95.

Null Hypothesis, H_o

The null hypothesis states that there is no difference between the two groups (Drug A = Drug B). A study would try to disprove this assertion by testing for a statistically significant difference between Drug A and Drug B (this is called the alternate hypothesis or H_A). If the study data indicated Drug A ≠ Drug B, the null hypothesis would be rejected.

Alternative Hypothesis, H_A

The alternative hypothesis states that there IS a difference between the two arms of the trial (Drug A ≠ Drug B). If you reject the null hypothesis (H_o), you are accepting the alternative hypothesis.

p-value

The p-value measures the likelihood of the null hypothesis being true. In simple terms, it is the probability that the result was obtained by chance. Generally, a p-value of < 0.05 (and sometimes < 0.01, depending on the trial design) indicates statistical significance. If the p-value is less than 0.05 then there is less than a 5% probability that the result was obtained by chance.

Conversely, there is a high probability the result was not obtained by chance and we can state that the conclusion is "statistically significant." When statistical significance is obtained with a proper p-value, it enables us to reject the null hypothesis.

Note that a measure of statistical significance is not the same as "clinical significance". For example, if a blood pressure drug lowers SBP by 3 mmHg, it may be statistically significant (with a p-value < 0.05) versus the placebo, but clinically it will not be used since other drugs lower BP to a greater degree. It would not be "clinically significant" because it doesn't measure up to other drugs and would not have a useful clinical benefit.

Type I error

A type I error occurs when the null hypothesis is true, yet it is rejected in error. Said another way, it was concluded that there was a difference between two groups when, in fact, there was none. The probability of a type I error is represented by the Greek letter, alpha (α). Commonly, α is set to 0.05, which means that 5% of the time the null hypothesis will be rejected in error. When we choose the p-value of < 0.05, for statistical significance, we accept the fact that this error will occur < 5% of the time. It is also known as a false positive (e.g. a court finds an innocent person guilty and sends them to jail). Type 1: null (+) → when is −

Type II error

A type II error occurs when the null hypothesis is false, yet it is accepted in error. Said another way, it was concluded that there was no difference when, in fact, there was one. It may also be known as a false negative (e.g. a court finds a criminal not guilty and sets them free). The probability of making a type II error is represented by the Greek letter, beta (β). Beta is a measure of sensitivity. Sensitivity relates to the test's ability to identify positive results.

Statistical Power

Power of a statistical test is the probability that the test will reject the null hypothesis when the null hypothesis is false (that it will not make a type II error). As the power increases, the chance of a type II error occurring decreases. Therefore, power is equal to $1-\beta$. A higher statistical power means that we can be more certain that the null hypothesis was not rejected incorrectly. The power of a study is determined by several factors, including the sample size, the number of events (MIs, strokes, deaths, etc.), and the statistical significance criterion used.

Relative Risk (RR)

The relative risk is the probability of an event occurring in the exposed group versus a non-exposed (or control) group. It is expressed as a fraction or percentage of the risk to the control group. A relative risk of 1 indicates no difference between comparison groups. A RR < 1 means that the intervention reduced the risk of the outcome. RR is simply a ratio of risks in the 2 groups. For example, if disease progression occurred in 28% of placebo-treated patients and in 16% of metoprolol-treated patients, then the ratio is 16/28, or 0.57. In other words, subjects treated with metoprolol were only 57% as likely as placebo-treated patients to have disease progression. This term can be important when we are looking at results from drug trials. For example, the conclusion of a clinical trial reports that Drug A had a relative risk reduction of MIs of 50%, versus placebo. If the study had 10,000 subjects, and there were 4 MIs in the placebo group and 2 MIs in the drug group, it is accurate that the relative risk was reduced 50%. However, the absolute risk (see below) of MI was small. By reporting only the relative risk, the value of the drug may be over-rated.

Relative Risk Reduction (RRR)

The relative risk reduction (RRR) is 1-RR. Using the example above, 1- 0.57 = 0.43; meaning there is a 43% risk reduction in disease progression in patients being treated with metoprolol. Expressing the result as a relative risk reduction may be more intuitively understandable. RR and RRR are limited in that these data do not reflect how important, or large, the treatment effect really is in the population at-large. They only provide a measure of what the risk of an event is in one group compared to the risk of that event in a comparison group.

Absolute Risk Reduction (ARR)

Absolute risk reduction is the absolute difference in outcome rates between the treatment and control groups. Using the example with metoprolol, 28% - 16% = 12%. The ARR is 12%. Therefore, for every 100 patients enrolled, metoprolol reduced disease progression by 12%. When considering the example above with 4 MIs in the placebo group versus 2 MIs in the drug group, the absolute risk reduction would be 0.04%, assuming each group contained 5,000 subjects.

Number Needed to Treat (NNT)

This is 1/ARR. The number needed to treat represents the number of people who would need to be treated with the intervention in order to prevent 1 adverse event. Using the example above, 1/0.12 = 8.3 (round up to 9 since you cannot divide a person into fractions). Therefore, for every 9 patients who received metoprolol, you would expect disease progression to be prevented in one patient. The NNT puts the results of a trial in a clinically relevant context. When the treatment or exposure causes harm (e.g. cigarette smoking, *Vioxx*, etc), the term NNT does not work and it is more accurate to report as "the number needed to harm."

Odds Ratio (OR)

The odds ratio is the ratio of the odds of an event occurring in the treatment group to the odds of an event occurring in the control group. In a group of 100 smokers, 40 people developed lung CA while 60 people do not. In a similar group of 100 non-smokers, lung CA developed in 10 people. The odds of a smoker developing lung CA would be 40/60 = 0.66, whereas the odds of a non-smoker developing lung CA would be 10/90 = 0.11. The odds ratio is then 0.66/0.11, or 6. An odds ratio of 1 indicates no difference between groups. When the event rate is small, odds ratios are very similar to the relative risk.

Correlation

Correlation is a measure of the relation between two variables. The direction and magnitude of the linear correlation can be quantified with a correlation coefficient. The most widely-used type of correlation coefficient is the Pearson Correlation Coefficient, abbreviated r. Its value ranges from -1 to 1. If the coefficient is 0, then the two variables do not vary together at all (no correlation). If the coefficient is positive, the 2 variables tend to increase or decrease together. If the coefficient is negative, the 2 variables are inversely related, that is, as one variable decreases, the other variable increases. If the coefficient is 1 or -1, the two variables vary together completely, that is, a graph of the data points forms a straight line.

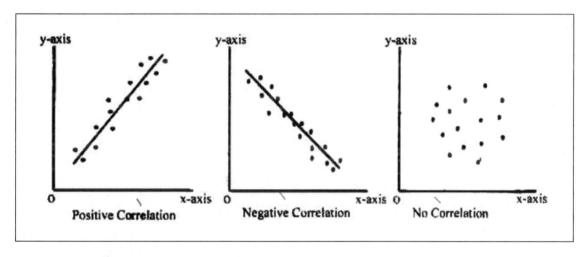

VARIABLES

A dependent variable is the outcome of interest, which should change in response to some intervention. An independent variable is the intervention, or what is being manipulated. For example, aspirin is compared against placebo to see if it leads to a reduction in coronary events. The dependent variable (or outcome of interest) is the number of coronary events while the independent variable (the intervention) is aspirin.

TYPES OF DATA

Discrete Data

Discrete data can have only a limited, or finite, set of values (i.e., not continuous) and can assume only whole numbers. There are 2 types of discrete data:

Nominal Data

Consists of categories, where the order of the categories is arbitrary (e.g., marital status, gender, ethnicity).

Ordinal Data

Consists of ranked categories, where the order of the ranking is important. However, the difference between categories cannot be considered to be equal. These are usually scoring systems that are ranked by severity (e.g., Apgar score, Likert scales, NYHA functional class) but cannot be measured/quantified. There is no consistent correlation between the rank and the degree of severity. For example, a trauma score of 4 does not necessarily mean you are twice as ill as a trauma score of 2.

Continuous Data

Can take an infinite number of possible values (such as height, weight, A1C, blood pressure) within a defined range. Continuous data can include fractional data (e.g. A1C of 7.3%).

Interval data

Has equal distances between the values, but the zero point is arbitrary (e.g. Celsius temperature scale).

Ratio Data

Has equal intervals between values and a meaningful zero point (e.g., height, weight).

Parametric vs. Non-parametric

Parametric statistics make the assumption that the data being evaluated are distributed in a normal, or Gaussian, distribution. Interval and ratio data are parametric, and are used with parametric tools in which distributions are predictable and often normally distributed. Nominal and ordinal data are non-parametric, and do not assume any particular distribution. Examples of non-parametric tests include the chi-squared test and Spearman's rank correlation coefficient. Whether the data is discrete or continuous is important because the type of data will determine the type of test used to analyze the data.

Additional Descriptive Terminology with Clinical Trials

PLACEBO

A placebo is made to look exactly like a real drug but is made of an inactive substance, such as a starch or sugar. Placebos are now used only in research. A placebo administered to study participants serves as a reference to distinguish the true effects of an active drug from anticipatory or coincidental effects. Placebos are used in clinical trials to "blind" people to their treatment allocation and to minimize bias. Placebos should be indistinguishable from the active intervention (the actual drug) to ensure adequate blinding.

STUDY DESIGN TYPES

Observational Study

An observational study is a study in which scientific observation is made under precisely defined conditions in a systematic and objective manner. Often the event to be observed cannot be controlled by the experimenter. It is called observational because the tactic is to observe the effect in the general population, in a non-controlled environment. In epidemiological research, where the researcher applies statistical methods to analyze patterns of occurrence of disease and its association with other events within a population, observational studies are done to better understand the origins or mode of transmission of the disease.

Case-Control Study

Case control studies compare groups retrospectively. They seek to identify possible predictors of outcome and are useful for studying rare diseases or outcomes. They are often used to generate hypotheses that can then be studied via a prospective cohort or other studies. The case-control studies are used to identify factors that may contribute to a medical condition by comparing subjects who have that condition (the cases) with patients who do not have the condition (the controls) but are otherwise similar. For example, did subjects exposed to statins have a higher incidence of liver damage? One advantage to this type of study is ease of data collection, which may be obtained by reviewing individual patient cases or clinic databases already in existence. There is a risk of selection bias in this type of review since clinics may accept only older or more seriously ill patients.

Cohort Study

Cohort studies are used to study incidence, causes, and prognosis. Because they measure events in chronological order, they can be used to distinguish between cause and effect. A cohort is a group of people who share a common characteristic or experience within a defined period (e.g. year born, exposure to pollutant/drug/vaccine, having undergone a certain procedure, etc.). A cohort study follows the cohort over time (longitudinal) and the outcomes are compared to a subset of the group who were not exposed to the intervention, such as a drug (e.g., the Framingham studies). One advantage to a large cohort study is the ability to observe occurrences of rare conditions. Cohort studies may be prospective in design (they are carried out into the future) but can be done retrospectively as well.

Cross-Sectional Study

Cross sectional studies are used to determine prevalence. They are relatively quick and easy but do not permit distinction between cause and effect. Cross sectional studies examine the relationship between diseases (or other health related outcomes) and other variables of interest at a single point in time. Sometimes these studies are the only practicable method of studying instances where a randomized controlled trial might be unethical, e.g. incidence of heart disease in people who have smoked for a given period of time vs. nonsmokers after the same period.

Controlled Clinical Trial

A study group is compared to one or more control (comparison) groups in a controlled setting. The setting can be controlled in many ways. "Blinding" on the part of the subjects and researchers reduces bias, as does randomization, or random allocation to a treatment arm. Single blinding means that the subjects do not know if they received the active drug or placebo. Double-blinding means that neither the subjects nor the researchers know which subjects received the active drug and which received the placebo. The gold standard for clinical drug trials is a randomized, placebo-controlled, double-blinded, multicenter trial with adequate statistical power.

Cross-Over Trial

In cross over trials the subjects, upon completion of a course of treatment, are switched to another course of treatment. For example, for a comparison of drugs A and B, half the participants are randomly allocated to receive them in the order A, B and half to receive them in the order B, A. The stage in a crossover trial when the first treatment is withdrawn and before the second treatment is given is called a washout period, and is designed to attempt to reduce any effect from the 1st stage of the trial on the 2nd stage of the trial. In this type of study, the patient serves as their own control.

Clinical trials may not provide "real life" comparisons

Patients in clinical trials, regardless of the type of trial, are not reflective of those treated in everyday clinical practice. Patients in clinical trials tend to be younger, more compliant with therapy, more likely to reach target doses of the drug and do so more quickly than in everyday practice. They are not as likely to have as complex a presentation as real-life patients. For example, practitioners may be using a drug that is cleared renally and, in clinical trials, patients with significant renal dysfunction may have been excluded. Therefore, we do not know how to use the drug safely in this patient population.

Meta-Analysis

The statistical analysis of primary research combining the results of different, but related studies, and using statistical methodology to integrate the results. This type of study can be useful to pool smaller trials into a larger group for analysis (e.g. Cochrane reviews). However, there are many potential flaws in this type of pooled data. For example, the populations studied can differ, there can be different lengths of treatment and the inclusion and exclusion criteria may differ. The differences in the trials will confound the results of the meta-analysis. For example, a meta-analysis that looked at the effects of different studies of *Echinacea* for cold prevention compared studies that used different parts of the *Echinacea* plant, which was harvested at different seasons, and used in patients with different definitions of cold symptoms. Therefore, it was difficult to conclude if the result of the meta-analysis was valid.

Pharmacoeconomics

BACKGROUND

Health care costs in the United States rank among the highest of all industrialized countries. In 2009 (the most recent data available), total health care expenditures reached 2.5 trillion dollars, which translates to an average of $8,086 per person, or about 17.6% of the nation's gross domestic product (up from 16.6% in 2008). This increase continues to outpace inflation and the growth in national income and is not sustainable. The increasing costs have resulted in a need to understand how our limited resources can be used most effectively and efficiently in the care of our patients and society as a whole. Therefore, it is necessary to scientifically evaluate the costs and outcomes of interventions such as drug therapy.

PHARMACOECONOMICS

Pharmacoeconomics, or Pharmaceutical Economics, is a collection of descriptive and analytic techniques for evaluating pharmaceutical interventions (drugs, devices, procedures, etc.) in the health care system. Pharmacoeconomic research identifies, measures, and compares the costs (direct, indirect and intangible) and consequences (clinical, economic and humanistic) of pharmaceutical products and services. Various research methods can be used to determine the impact of the pharmaceutical product or service. These methods include cost-effectiveness analysis, cost-minimization analysis, cost-utility analysis, and cost-benefit analysis, among others. Pharmacoeconomics is often termed health outcomes research particularly when a process or clinical/care pathway is evaluated (not a medication).

Clinicians and other decision makers can use these methods to evaluate and compare the total costs and consequences of pharmaceutical products and services. When looking at certain analyses, it is important to consider whose interests are being taken into account. What may be viewed as cost-beneficial for society or for the patient may not be cost-beneficial for hospital administrators and/or hospital employees (e.g. a shorter length of stay when a longer length of stay is fully reimbursed).

Drug costs and benefits can be rationally analyzed via the use of pharmacoeconomic analysis and the development of "decision trees" that can guide prescribing in a fiscally responsible manner. Decision pathways should not bypass the guidelines, if available, that provide the evidence-based treatment approach to managing the condition. They should support the evidence, but in a fiscally responsible manner.

Pharmacists are on the front-line for considering whether drugs are worth the cost by using various pharmacoeconomic analyses. The ECHO model (Economic, Clinical and Humanistic Outcomes) is used to determine pharmacoeconomic benefit and is used to incorporate these elements:

- Economic outcomes are the direct, indirect and intangible costs of the drug compared to a medical intervention.

- <u>C</u>linical outcomes are the medical events that occur as a result of the treatment or intervention.

- <u>H</u>umanistic <u>O</u>utcomes, or patient-reported outcomes, are the consequences of the disease or treatment as reported by the patient or caregiver (patient satisfaction, quality of life).

PHARMACOECONOMIC METHODOLOGIES AND COSTS

Costs

The majority of pharmacoeconomic methods require proper identification of the costs involved with an intervention. Costs can be categorized into 4 types:

<u>Direct medical costs</u>: medications, medication administration, hospitalizations, clinic visits, emergency room visits, nursing services

<u>Direct non-medical costs</u>: travel costs (gas, bus, hotel stays for family), child care services (for children of patients)

<u>Indirect costs</u>: loss of productivity for patient (and possibly of caregiver)

<u>Intangible costs</u>: pain and suffering, anxiety, weakness

Cost-Effectiveness Analysis

Cost-effectiveness analysis (CEA) is defined as a series of analytical and mathematical procedures that aid in the selection of a course of action from various alternative approaches. Inputs are usually measured in dollars and outputs are used measured in natural units (e.g. LDL values in mg/dL, clinical cures, length of stay). <u>The main advantage of this method is that the outcomes are easier to quantify when compared to other analyses, and clinicians and decision makers are familiar with these types of outcomes since they are similar to outcomes seen in clinical trials. Therefore, CEA is the most common methodology seen in the literature today. A disadvantage of CEA is the inability to directly compare different types of outcomes</u>. For example, one cannot compare the cost effectiveness of implementing a diabetes program with implementing an asthma program where the outcome units are different (e.g. blood glucose values versus asthma exacerbations). It is also difficult to combine two or more outcomes into one value of measurement (e.g. comparing one chemotherapeutic agent that prolongs survival but has significant side effects to another chemotherapeutic agent that has less effect on prolonging survival and has fewer side effects).

The idea behind the use of a cost-effectiveness analysis is to supplement the randomized clinical trials. From the clinical trials, the drug has demonstrated safety and efficacy. With a cost-effectiveness analysis, health care providers can decide where, if at all, the drug fits into the decision tree for a specific condition. They may decide, in some cases, not to use the drug at all (even if a mortality benefit is present) due to high cost and a limited budget. These types of decisions have political ramifications but still need to happen in order to use the limited healthcare dollar rationally.

Cost-Minimization Analysis

Cost-minimization analysis (CMA) is used when two or more interventions have already demonstrated equivalency in outcomes and the costs of each intervention are being compared. CMA measures and compares the input costs and assumes outcomes are equivalent. For example, two ACE-inhibitors, captopril and lisinopril, are considered therapeutically equivalent in the literature but the acquisition cost (the price paid for the drug) and administrative costs may be different (captopril is administered TID and lisinopril is administered once daily). A CMA would look at "minimizing costs" when multiple drugs have equal efficacy and tolerability. Another example of CMA is looking at the same drug regimen given in two different settings (e.g. hospital versus home health care). CMA is considered the easiest analysis to perform. However, the use of this method is limited given it can only compare alternatives with the same outcome.

Cost-Benefit Analysis

Cost-benefit analysis (CBA) is a systematic process for calculating and comparing benefits and costs of an intervention in terms of monetary units. CBA consists of identifying all the benefits from an intervention and converting them into dollars in the year that they will occur. Also, the costs associated with the intervention are identified and are allocated to the year when they occur. Then, all costs are discounted back to their present day value. Given that all other factors remain constant, the program with the largest present day value of benefits minus costs is the best economic value. In CBA, both benefits and costs are expressed in terms of dollars and are adjusted to their present value. This can be difficult when having to measure the benefits and then assigning a dollar amount to that benefit. For example, when measuring the benefit of patient quality of life, not only is it difficult to measure, but is also very difficult to assign a dollar value to this outcome. One advantage to using CBA is the ability to determine if the benefits of the intervention exceed the costs of implementation. CBA can also be used to compare multiple programs whether the outcomes are similar or unrelated, as long as the outcome measures can be converted to dollars.

Cost-Utility Analysis

Cost-utility analysis (CUA) is a specialized form of CEA that includes a quality-of-life component associated with morbidity using common health indices such as quality-adjusted life years (QALYs) and disability-adjusted life years (DALYs). With CEA, you can measure the quantity of life (years gained) but not the "quality" or "utility" of those years. In a CUA, the intervention outcome is measured in terms of quality-adjusted life-year (QALY) gained. QALY takes into account both the quality (morbidity) and the quantity (mortality) of life gained. CUA measures outcomes based on years of life that are adjusted by utility weights, which range from 1 for "perfect health" to 0 for "dead". These weights take into account patient and society preferences for specific health states; however, there is no consensus on the measurement, since both patient and society preferences may vary based on culture. An advantage of CUA is that different types of outcomes and diseases with multiple outcomes of interest can be compared (unlike CEA) using one common unit, like QALY. Also, CUA combines morbidity and mortality into one unit without having to place a dollar value on it (unlike CBA). Outcome units may also be expressed as quality-adjusted life months (QALMs) and healthy-year equivalents (HYEs).

FOUR BASIC PHARMACOECONOMIC METHODOLOGIES

METHODOLOGY	COST MEASUREMENT UNIT	OUTCOME UNIT
Cost-effectiveness analysis	Dollars	Natural units (life-years gained, mmHg blood pressure, mg/dL LDL, etc.)
Cost-minimization analysis	Dollars	Assumed to be equivalent in comparative groups
Cost-benefit analysis	Dollars	Dollars
Cost-utility analysis	Dollars	Quality-adjusted-life-year (QALY) or other utilities

Practice Case

A major clinical trial has just been published in *NEJM* evaluating a new drug (Drug X) to the current standard of care drug (Drug Y) in patients presenting with MIs to the emergency department. The study was a prospective, open-label, randomized, multicenter trial in 3,600 patients (1,800 patients in each arm). Partial results of the trial are found below.

OUTCOMES AT 30 DAYS

ENDPOINTS	DRUG X	DRUG Y	P-VALUE
Primary Endpoints			
Death, MI, and urgent revascularization	166 (9.2%)	218 (12.1%)	0.045
Major Bleeding	89 (4.9%)	99 (5.5%)	0.1
Secondary endpoints			
Strokes	13 (0.7%)	11 (0.6%)	0.48
Blood Transfusions	49 (2.7%)	72 (4.0%)	0.02
Revascularization	47 (2.6%)	35 (1.9%)	0.18

QUESTIONS

1. Looking at the results of the trial above, which of the following statements is correct?

   a. Drug Y has demonstrated a statistically significant benefit over Drug X in reducing death, MI, urgent revascularization and major bleeding.

   b. Drug X has demonstrated a statistically significant benefit over Drug Y in reducing death, MI, urgent revascularization and major bleeding.

   c. Drug Y has demonstrated a statistically significant benefit over Drug X in reducing death, MI, and urgent revascularization but not in reducing major bleeds.

   d. Drug X has demonstrated a statistically significant benefit over Drug Y in reducing death, MI, and urgent revascularization but not in reducing major bleeds.

   e. There is no statistical difference between Drug X and Drug Y in the primary endpoints.

2. Which of the following statements below are true regarding the clinical trial results above?

   a. Strokes, transfusions and revascularization all met statistical significance.

   b. Drug X resulted in statistically significantly fewer strokes than Drug Y.

   c. Drug X resulted in more clinically significant major bleeding than Drug Y.

   d. Drug X resulted in statistically significantly fewer revascularizations than Drug Y.

   e. None of the above statements are true.

3. In the trial above, which of the following parameter changes would make this data subject to less bias?

    a. Single center
    b. Allowing only one gender type
    c. Cohort study
    d. Non-randomized
    e. Double blind

4. In the trial above, what is the absolute risk reduction in death, MI, and urgent revascularization?

    a. 0.4%
    b. 1.5%
    c. 2.9%
    d. 9.2%
    e. 12.1%

5. In the trial above, what is the relative risk of major bleeding requiring blood transfusions?

    a. 0.24
    b. 0.52
    c. 0.67
    d. 0.89
    e. 0.94

Questions 6-15 do not relate to the case.

6. Students took a statistics course in pharmacy school. When the class was completed, the students ranked the course on a scale of 1 to 5, with 1 corresponding to the worst topic possible, and 5 to the most desirable. What type of variable is described above?

    a. Normal distribution
    b. Ordinal
    c. Nominal
    d. Ratio
    e. Correlation

7. A trial is conducted between 2 different beta blockers, referred to as Drug A and Drug B. The null hypothesis is that both drugs will be equal in their effects on lowering BP. The study concluded that the effects of Drug A were better than Drug B in lowering BP (p-value < 0.01). Which of the following statements is correct?

    a. We can accept the null hypothesis.
    b. We can reject the null hypothesis.
    c. There is a 10% chance that Drug A is superior.
    d. There is a 0.1% chance that Drug B is superior.
    e. This trial did not reach statistical significance.

8. Correlation in a clinical trial describes:

    a. The ability of 1 or more variables to predict another
    b. The relationship between 2 variables
    c. Nominal data
    d. Confounding variables
    e. A cause and effect relationship

9. Which of the following statements concerning a Type I error is correct?

    a. A type I error means that the null hypothesis is accepted in error.
    b. A type I error means that the null hypothesis is rejected in error.
    c. A type I error means failing to reject the null hypothesis in error.
    d. A type I error means that the null hypothesis is accepted.
    e. A type I error is a beta error.

10. Which of the following statements concerning case-control studies are correct?

    a. They are usually retrospective.

    b. They include cases without the intervention.

    c. The researcher analyzes individual patient cases.

    d. A and B are correct.

    e. All of the above are correct.

11. Which of the following statements regarding the median is correct?

    a. It the value in the middle of an ordered list.

    b. In a Gaussian distribution, it is the same as the mean.

    c. It is not sensitive to outliers.

    d. A and B are correct.

    e. All of the above.

12. Choose the best description of the purpose of a pharmacoeconomic analysis:

    a. To measure and compare the costs and outcomes of drug therapy and other medical interventions.

    b. To reduce health care expenditures by limiting medication use to only those who need it most.

    c. To get the best treatments available to as many people as possible.

    d. To examine the indirect costs of medical care in each medical specialty within hospitals, clinics, and outpatient surgery centers.

    e. To reduce the pharmacy drug budget within a hospital setting as a way to control health care costs.

13. Choose the example that represents direct medical costs:

    a. Lost productivity

    b. Quality of life

    c. Cost of taking the bus to the hospital

    d. Nursing services

    e. Pain and suffering

14. A pharmacist is conducting an analysis to determine the best way to manage patients with diabetes based on A1C values. Three treatment regimens will be evaluated based on costs and effects on A1C reduction. Choose the type of analysis the pharmacist should perform:

    a. A cost-utility analysis

    b. A cost-minimization analysis

    c. A cost-effectiveness analysis

    d. A cost-benefit analysis

    e. Any of the above

15. A pharmacist is considering which intravenous vasodilator should be preferred at his institution. He has narrowed his search down to two agents. Each drug provides similar health benefits and similar tolerability. The pharmacist will base his decision on drug acquisition, administration, and monitoring costs. The pharmacist should use the following analysis to decide which intravenous vasodilator should be added to his institution's formulary:

    a. A cost-utility analysis

    b. A cost-minimization analysis

    c. A cost-effectiveness analysis

    d. A cost-benefit analysis

    e. Any of the above

ANSWERS

1-d, 2-e, 3-e, 4-c, 5-d, 6-b, 7-b, 8-b, 9-b, 10-e, 11-e, 12-a, 13-d, 14-c, 15-b

6

PHARMACOGENOMICS

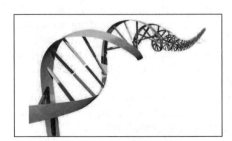

Background

Pharmacogenomics is the science which examines in-herited variations in genes that dictate drug response, and explores ways that the variations can be used to predict whether a patient will have a good response to a drug, a bad response, or no response at all. It deals with the influence of genetic variations on drug response by correlating gene expression or single-nucleotide polymorphisms (SNPs) with the drug's efficacy or toxicity. In this manner, drug therapy can be optimized with respect to the patients' genotype. Pharmacogenomics can be used to determine who is more likely to develop a serious adverse event (e.g., abacavir) or who will derive benefit from a medicine [e.g., trastuzumab *(Herceptin)]*. At the present time, few drugs require pharmacogenomic testing, but the field is growing. The goal is to provide "personalized medicine" in which drugs and drug combinations are optimized for each individual's unique genetic makeup.

SINGLE NUCLEOTIDE POLYMORPHISMS (SNPS)

SNPs are the most common genetic variations in DNA. SNPs are single-base differences that exist between 2 individuals. Nucleotide substitution results in two possible alleles. An allele is one of the different forms of a specific sequence in DNA. Two identical alleles make up a homozygous genotype. Two different alleles make up a heterozygous genotype. The phenotype is the observable trait that results from the gene expression. Right now, there is a race to catalog as many of the genetic variations (the SNPs) found within the human genome as possible.

Polymorphisms in Genes for Drug-Metabolizing Enzymes

A polymorphism is a variation in the DNA that is too common to be due merely to a new mutation, and is present in at least 1% of the population. An example is the CYP 2D6 extensive-metabolizer (EM) and poor-metabolizer (PM) phenotypes. Another example is the expression of the HLA-B*1502 allele, which, if present, gives the recipient a 10% chance of having a severe skin reaction if they use carbamazepine, including toxic epidermal necrolysis (TEN) or Stevens Johnson syndrome (SJS) – these can both be fatal. Although anyone can get a severe skin reaction from carbamazepine, there is a much higher risk if the HLA-B*1502 allele is present. Among patients from Asian descent, there is a 10-15% risk of carrying this gene. All patients of Asian descent must be tested for this variation prior to the start of carbamazepine therapy.

Another important example in pharmacy is the link between abacavir and the HLA-B*5701 allele, which if present, puts the patient at higher risk for a severe, multi-organ hypersensitivity reaction.

A beneficial effect of a specific genotype is found with trastuzumab *(Herceptin)*. In breast cancer cases, amplification of the HER2/neu oncogene is linked with disease recurrence and a worse prognosis. Trastuzumab is a monoclonal antibody that interferes with the HER2/neu receptor. If a patient is positive for the HER2/neu oncogene, they are potential candidates for trastuzumab therapy.

The intended application of pharmacogenomics research include identifying responders and nonresponders to medications, avoiding adverse events, optimizing drug doses, and avoiding unnecessary healthcare costs. In the future, it is hoped that a rapid test of a patient's DNA will provide a genetic profile and enable the prescriber to avoid drugs with risk or choose drugs that would provide the most benefit.

The table below begins with drugs where genetic testing is routinely done and/or required according to the labeling of these drugs. Following this list are the drugs known to have genetic risk, but where standardized testing is not yet routine. This list continues to grow as the science evolves in this area.

DRUGS WITH REQUIRED GENETIC TESTING & DRUGS WITH KNOWN OR POSSIBLE GENETIC RISK FACTORS

DRUG	USED TO TREAT	TESTING	REACTION/PACKAGE WARNINGS
Drugs with Required Genetic Testing			
Abacavir *(Ziagen)* abacavir+lamivudine *(Epzicom)* abacavir +zidovudine+ lamivudine *(Trizivir)*	HIV	Test for HLA-B*5701 If positive, drug cannot be used.	Hypersensitivity to abacavir is a multi-organ clinical syndrome usually characterized by 2 or more of these signs and symptoms: ■ Fever ■ Rash ■ Gastrointestinal (nausea, vomiting, diarrhea, or abdominal pain) ■ Constitutional (generalized malaise, fatigue, or achiness) ■ Respiratory (dyspnea, cough, or pharyngitis) Discontinue as soon as a hypersensitivity reaction is suspected.

Drugs with Required Genetic Testing & Drugs with Known or Possible Genetic Risk Factors Continued

DRUG	USED TO TREAT	TESTING	REACTION/PACKAGE WARNINGS
Carbamazepine *(Tegretol, Tegretol XR)*	Seizures, other occasional uses	Test for HLA-B*1502 if of Asian ancestry. If positive, do not use unless benefit clearly outweighs risk.	Serious dermatologic reactions with positive HLA-B*1502 alelle, including Toxic Epidermal Necrolysis (TEN) and Stevens-Johnson Syndrome (SJS), have occurred.
Trastuzumab *(Herceptin)*	Breast and gastric cancer	HER2/neu oncogene	HER2/neu over-expression required for use
Crizotinib *(Xalkori)*	Metastatic non-small cell lung cancer (NSCLC)	Anaplastic lymphoma kinase (ALK) - positive	Crizotinib is a kinase inhibitor indicated for the treatment of patients with locally advanced or metastatic non-small cell lung cancer (NSCLC) that is anaplastic lymphoma kinas (ALK)-positive as detected by an FDA-approved test
Vemurafenib *(Zelboraf)*	Metastatic melanoma	BRAFV600E mutation	Vemurafenib is a kinase inhibitor for patients with unresectable or metastatic melanoma with BRAF-V600E mutation as detected by an-FDA approved test. This agent is not recommended in patients with wild-type BRAF melanoma.
Cetuximab *(Erbitux)*/ panitumumab *(Vectibix)*	Colorectal cancer	K-ras mutations	K-ras mutations indicate a poor response to therapy. These agents will not work in patients with colorectal cancer who have a K-ras mutation (~40% of patients). Package inserts state that there is no benefit in patients with K-ras mutations in codon 12 or 13.
Maraviroc *(Selzentry)*	HIV	Tropism testing, using the Trofile test, must be conducted to identify patients appropriate for the use of maraviroc.	Adult patients infected with only CCR5-tropic HIV-1 should use maraviroc. Do not use in patients with dual/mixed or CXCR-4-tropic HIV-1 disease as efficacy was not demonstrated in a Phase 2 trial of this patient population.

Drugs with Required Genetic Testing & Drugs with Known or Possible Genetic Risk Factors Continued

DRUG	USED TO TREAT	TESTING	REACTION/PACKAGE WARNINGS

Drugs with Known or Possible Genetic Risk Factors

DRUG	USED TO TREAT	TESTING	REACTION/PACKAGE WARNINGS
Phenytoin (*Dilantin*)	Seizures	Test for HLA-B*1502 if of Asian ancestry. If positive, do not use unless benefit clearly outweighs risk.	Strong association between the risk of developing Stevens-Johnson Syndrome (SJS) and Toxic Epidermal Necrolysis (TEN) and the presence of the HLA-B*1502 allele.
Atomoxetine (*Strattera*)	ADHD	Poor metabolizers of 2D6 may have exaggerated response (5 fold increase) to drug due to reduced rate of metabolism. No recommendation, but use caution.	Atomoxetine concentrations have been measured at 5-fold higher concentrations in poor metabolizers versus extensive metabolizers. This can lead to an increase in adverse effects like decreased appetite, insomnia, sedation, depression, tremor, early morning awakening, pruritus, and mydriasis.
Allopurinol (*Zyloprim*)	Gout	Increased risk of severe cutaneous reactions with HLA-B*5801 No recommendations for testing.	Discontinue at 1st appearance of skin rash or other signs which may indicate an allergic reaction. In some instances, a skin rash may be followed by more severe hypersensitivity reactions such as exfoliative, urticarial, and purpuric lesions, as well as SJS, (and/or generalized vasculitis, irreversible hepatotoxicity, and, on rare occasions, death).
Codeine	Pain, cough	Extensive metabolizers of 2D6 may have exaggerated response to drug due to extensive conversion to morphine metabolite. No recommendation, but use caution – 2D6 extensive metabolizers are common.	Over-production of morphine can result in CNS effects, including an ↑ risk of respiratory depression. Use extreme caution in lactating women as most opioids are excreted in breast milk. While use may be acceptable in small amounts, the risk to the infant must be considered. Do not use codeine (in *Tylenol #3*, others), since rapid metabolizers of the CYP 450 2D6 enzyme will produce excessive amounts of morphine, which could be fatal to the infant.

Drugs with Required Genetic Testing & Drugs with Known or Possible Genetic Risk Factors Continued

DRUG	USED TO TREAT	TESTING	REACTION/PACKAGE WARNINGS
Warfarin (Coumadin, Jantoven) See Warfarin Pointers Below	Clot Prevention	From package insert: Identification of risk factors for bleeding and certain genetic variations in CYP2C9 and VKORC1 in a patient may increase the need for more frequent INR monitoring and the use of lower warfarin doses.	Increased bleeding risk. Loss-of-function alleles, CYP2C9*2 and CYP2C9*3, can lead to an increased risk of bleeding. If not testing, use caution by selecting a low starting dose, increasing slowly, and frequent INR monitoring – especially at initiation. If the test indicates variations, a safer starting dose can be calculated.
Azathioprine and Mercaptopurine	Solid organ cancers and leukemia	Monitor for TPMT (thiopurine methyltransferase)	Patients with a genetic deficiency of TPMT may have ↑ risk of myelosuppressive effects; those patients with low or absent TPMT activity are at risk for severe myelotoxicity
Irinotecan (Camptosar)	Colon cancer and other cancers	May test for the UGT1A1*28 allele (homozygous vs. heterozygous carriers)	Patients homozygous for the UGT1A1*28 allele are at risk of neutropenia; initial one-level dose reduction should be considered. Heterozygous carriers of the UGT1A1*28 allele may also be at risk, however, most patients tolerate normal starting doses

WARFARIN POINTERS

Warfarin consists of two racemic isomers – an S-isomer and an R-isomer. The S-isomer is 3-5 times more potent than the R-isomer. The S-isomer is metabolized by CYP 2C9, and a reduction in the ability of this enzyme to metabolize warfarin will result in slow metabolism. If lower doses are not used, bleeding risk is increased. The CYP 2C9*2 and the CYP 2C9*3 alleles are loss-of function alleles, therefore, associated with more bleeding. CYP 2C9*2 allele may lead to a 30% reduction in metabolism of warfarin whereas the CYP 2C9*3 allele may lead to a 90% reduction in metabolism. Patients who are homozygous are the *3 allele have the greatest risk of bleeding.

The 2nd variation resulting in an increased bleeding risk is a variation in the VKORC1 gene. In the VKORC1 SNP, the common G allele is replaced with the A allele. Patients with the 'A haplotype' produce less VKORC1 and will require a lower dose of warfarin.

With the patient's genetic information, the warfarin starting dose can be more accurately determined. Genetic testing has been simplified by the availability of the several outside companies that test for these variations; however, testing is not yet routinely performed nor has testing been adequately validated. In warfarin initiation, proceed cautiously and monitor the INR frequently.

Practice Questions

1. A 15 year-old girl of Asian ancestry presents with a seizure disorder. The physician plans to initiate carbamazepine therapy, but first orders genetic testing in order to determine if she is at an increased risk for the following adverse drug reaction:

   a. Gastrointestinal bleeding
   b. Hemorrhage
   c. Serious skin reactions
   d. Neuropathy
   e. Tendon rupture

2. Which of the following alleles is the one tested for before initiating carbamazepine therapy?

   a. HLA-B *5701
   b. HLA-B *1502
   c. HLA-B *5801
   d. HLA-B *1501
   e. TPMT activity

3. Trastuzumab is indicated in cancers with an overexpression of this gene:

   a. AKT
   b. C-erb/B-2
   c. N-Myc
   d. HER2+
   e. BRCA2

4. A patient was started on warfarin 5 mg once daily. She presents to the clinic 2 weeks later and is found to have an INR of 4.7 with excessive oral bleeding when she brushes her teeth. Which of the following most likely describes the patient's genotype?

   a. Slow metabolizer of CYP 2C9
   b. Rapid metabolizer of CYP 2C9
   c. Slow metabolizer of CYP 3A4
   d. Rapid metabolizer of CYP 3A4
   e. Rapid metabolizer of CYP 2D6

5. Which of the following statements regarding abacavir is correct?

   a. Testing for HLA-B*5701 is recommended on initiation or re-initiation of therapy
   b. If the testing is positive for HLA-B*5701, abacavir cannot be used
   c. Do not let your abacavir run out
   d. This drug can be taken with or without food
   e. All of the above

ANSWERS

1-c, 2-b, 3-d, 4-a, 5-e

7

DRUG ALLERGIES, ADRs & ADR REPORTING

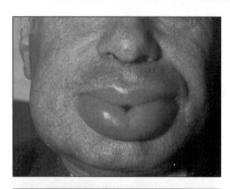

Reference

FDA MedWatch program, available at: http://www.fda.gov/Safety/MedWatch/default.htm

WHAT IS IT? A SIDE EFFECT? AN ADVERSE EFFECT? AN ALLERGY? ANAPHYLAXIS?

ADVERSE DRUG REACTIONS: SIDE EFFECTS, ADVERSE EVENTS AND MEDWATCH REPORTING

Side effects or adverse events are <u>not generally avoidable</u> and can <u>occur in anyone with normal doses</u> (although higher doses can increase the side effect severity). <u>Side effects are more common and generally less severe</u> (such as orthostatic hypotension from doxazosin) while <u>adverse events are known complications of a drug but are generally rarer and more severe</u> (such as rash from lamotrigine).

[Note: do not mix these up with medication errors, which are due to someone doing something incorrectly, such as giving the wrong drug to a patient. Medication errors are an important area and are discussed in the Medication Safety chapter.]

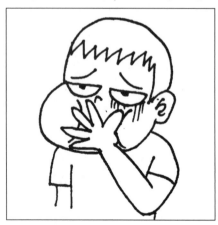

Most adverse drug reactions are characterized as "type A" which means that they are dose-dependent and predictable from the drug's pharmacology. For example, if a patient starts doxazosin at 1 mg QHS they will have much less orthostatic hypotension and dizziness than if they began the medication at a 4 mg dose; thus, this drug is slowly titrated upward to reduce the severity of the side effects. Type B reactions [which are idiosyncratic – this means a particular patient has an independent peculiar reaction (or hypersensitivity) to the drug] are not predictable from the known pharmacology of the drug and the reaction is determined by patient-specific susceptibility factors.

Although side effects or adverse effects can occur in anyone, we need to consider that they may be more likely if a drug is given to a patient at high risk for a certain condition. For example, anyone taking an aminoglycoside for longer than a few days would expect to suffer some degree of renal damage. However, if a patient with impaired renal function receives an aminoglycoside they would be more susceptible to further damage sooner.

- Side effects, adverse events (and allergies, which are discussed below) should be reported to the FDA's MedWatch program. This is called an adverse event reporting system (AERS) that provides a central collection for problem caused by drugs. [Note that vaccines are an exception that are not reported under AERS; vaccine adverse drug reactions are reported under a different program called VAERS; this is described in the immunization section.]

- The FDA conducts Phase IV (post-marketing safety surveillance programs) for approved drug and therapeutic biologic products and collates the reports to better understand the drug safety profile in a real world setting. When drugs are tested in trials, high-risk patients are typically excluded. Yet, in real life settings high risk patients are often included. If a drug causes a reaction in 1 out of every 3,000 people you might not even see the reaction appear in a smaller clinical trial. This is why community-based adverse event reporting is critical.

Example of "real life" adverse event incidence versus that in a clinical trial setting

When spironolactone was studied in heart failure patients during the RALES trial, patients with renal insufficiency or elevated potassium levels were excluded due to the known risk of additional hyperkalemia from the use of spironolactone. The drug was found to have benefit in advanced heart failure patients and doctors in the community began to use it in their heart failure patients. In this real life setting, patients with renal insufficiency or elevated potassium were occasionally prescribed spironolactone, and arrhythmias and sudden death due to hyperkalemia were reported.

- Reporting is voluntary. Healthcare professionals and patients may also report adverse events to the drug manufacturer, who is required by law to send the report to the FDA's MedWatch program. The MedWatch form that is used for reporting is included at the end of this section. We can also call in or report online via the link provided at the top of this section. MedWatch is not only used to report problems with drugs; it is also used for reporting problems with biologics, medical devices and some nutritional products and cosmetics.

- If the FDA receives enough reports that a drug caused a particular problem they may require that the product's drug information, such as the package insert or labeling, be changed. In especially risky cases they will issue safety alerts to prescribers, usually before the labeling is changed.

Example of a side effect that was added to the package insert many years after the drug had been released due to the ADR reports received by the FDA

Oseltamivir *(Tamiflu)* was initially released without any warning of unusual behavior in children. The FDA received enough reports that they issued a warning to prescribers in 2006. After many more reports, in 2008, the FDA required the drug company to update the prescribing information to include a precaution about hallucinations, confusion and other strange behavior in children.

Example of a posting on the FDA website of a drug that is being monitored under Phase IV

DRUG	USAGE	ADVERSE EVENTS	NOTES
Savella (Milnacipran) NDA 022256	For management of fibromyalgia.	Adverse event reports of elevated blood pressure and heart rate, possibly more severe than reflected in the labeling were identified.	FDA is continuing to evaluate these issues to determine if the current labeling, which includes these events in the Warnings and Precautions section, is adequate.

- Vaccine adverse drug reactions are reported to the Vaccine Adverse Event Reporting System (VAERS). This is described further in the Immunization chapter.

CHARACTERIZING AN ADVERSE DRUG REACTION

In order to properly characterize an adverse reaction, sensitivity to a drug or a true drug allergy, pharmacists need to ask the right questions. When patients report an "allergy" to a drug these questions can help place the reaction into the proper context:

- What reaction occurred (was it a mild rash, a severe rash with blisters, trouble breathing?)

- When did it occur? (about how old were you?)

- Can you use similar drugs in the same class (for example, if they report an allergy to penicillin, have they ever used *Keflex*?)

- Ask and include any food allergies and latex allergies in the patient record. Latex allergies should be recorded since some drugs require tubing, have latex vial stoppers, or require gloves for administration.

Drug Side Effects (or Sensitivities) that are NOT Allergies: Stomach Upset/ Nausea, MILD Rash, Photosensitivity

STOMACH UPSET/NAUSEA

Stomach upset or nausea is often incorrectly reported as an allergy. The reaction should be listed on the patient profile because the drug bothered the patient and, if possible, the drug should be avoided in the future, but this is not an allergy and should not prevent drugs in the same class from being used. For example, many patients get stomach upset from codeine (but not hydrocodone or other drugs in the morphine class) or from erythromycin (but not azithromycin or other macrolides).

Example of stomach upset due to codeine being reported incorrectly as a drug allergy:

Carmen received acetaminophen 300 mg-codeine 30 mg *(Tylenol #3)* for pain relief after a dental extraction several years ago. Carmen got very nauseated from the medicine. When Carmen was admitted to the hospital for a left hip replacement, she reported to the intake coordinator that she was "allergic" to codeine. The intake coordinator did not attempt to clarify the reaction. The hospital's pain management protocol calls for hydromorphone in a patient-controlled analgesic device for post-op pain control. The physician used a less desirable option for pain control due to the reported allergy.

MILD RASH

Opioids can commonly cause histamine-induced skin rash or itching, particularly in the in-patient setting post-op when opioid-naïve patients are receiving the medication or non-naïve patients are receiving higher-than-normal dosing. This reaction can be reduced or avoided if the patient is pre-medicated with an antihistamine before use, such as diphenhydramine.

PHOTOSENSITIVITY

Many drugs can cause photosensitivity, which requires limiting sun exposure and using sunscreens that block both UVA (causes aging, skin cancer) and UVB (causes sunburn). Sunscreens that cover both UVA and UVB are labeled broad-spectrum. The drugs that most commonly cause sun sensitivity are sulfa antibiotics and tetracyclines. Some other drugs that can cause this problem are NSAIDs, metronidazole, isoniazid, quinolones, azole antifungals, some of the HIV medications (including ritonavir), diuretics, isotretinoin (oral) and almost all of the topical acne drugs (most notably the retinoids).

[Note that there is a different type of skin reaction that occurs when sunlight causes the drug to become toxic; this is an allergic reaction and is rare. The reaction looks like a bad sunburn on only sun-exposed skin.]

Another sensitivity that some people have is to the iodine in contrast dyes. This reaction can cause itching, flushing and a drop in blood pressure, but is not technically a true allergy.

NSAIDs can cause issues with either sensitivity or true allergy; these are discussed in the next section.

TRUE DRUG ALLERGIES

Penicillins and sulfonamides cause the most drug allergies. For a true drug allergy to occur the person must have taken the drug previously. Initial exposure will cause IgE production, which primes the body to release excessive histamine at the next drug exposure.

SYMPTOMS OF AN ALLERGIC REACTION

- Skin rash or urticaria (hives – which is a rash with itchy, raised bumps)

- Wheezing or other breathing problems

- Swelling

- Drop in blood pressure, dizziness

If the reaction is mild the only action that may be required is to stop the drug. In more severe cases antihistamines are used to counteract the histamine-release that causes swelling and rash. Steroids, and occasional NSAIDs, can be used to decrease swelling. Severe swelling may necessitate a steroid injection. Epinephrine may be needed to keep the airways open. In cases with severe constriction of the airways ventilator support may be required.

Often the drug that caused the reaction can be replaced with another drug. Rarely this is not possible and desensitization may be recommended. This requires administering the drug in a medical setting with increasing amounts until the patient can tolerate the needed dose. "Patch testing" is occasionally used to try and determine possible rash reactions, including severe skin reactions such as toxic epidermal necrolysis (TENS), but the tests do not always work and the research on patch testing is inconsistent.

Anaphylaxis

Anaphylaxis is a severe, life-threatening allergic reaction that occurs seconds to minutes after taking the drug. Anaphylaxis can occur after an initial exposure and subsequent immune response, but some drugs can cause anaphylaxis with the first exposure.

SIGNS/SYMPTOMS OF ANAPHYLAXIS

- Swelling, with or without urticaria

- Bronchoconstriction, difficulty breathing, pulmonary edema

- Light headedness or dizziness, confusion

- Nausea, vomiting

- Sudden drop in blood pressure, with or without loss of consciousness

- Shock, with possible organ damage

HOW TO TREAT ANAPHYLAXIS

If a patient has an anaphylactic reaction, they will need to go to the ER right away (or call 911) and receive an epinephrine injection +/- diphenhydramine and IV fluids. Milder reactions (primarily itching/rash/swelling) can be treated with oral or injectable diphenhydramine. Do not put a pillow under a patient's head because this makes it more difficult to get air into the lungs. Do not attempt to put anything into their mouth.

Swollen airways can be quickly fatal and patients who have had such a reaction should carry injectable epinephrine (EpiPen, Twinject), if they may be at future risk. Their emergency kit should include diphenhydramine tablets (25 mg) and emergency contact information.

EpiPen Injection Instructions

- Grasp the epinephrine shot injector in one fist with the black tip pointing down. Do not touch the black tip. (Color may be different.)

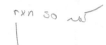

- With the other hand, pull off the cap.

- Hold the tip close to your outer thigh. Swing and jab the tip into your outer thigh (through clothing if necessary). The injector should be at a 90-degree angle to your thigh.

- Keep the injector in your outer thigh while you slowly count to 5.

- Remove the injector and rub the area where the medicine entered your skin.

- Look at the black tip: If the needle is showing, you received the dose. If not, you need to repeat steps 3 through 5. It is normal for most of the liquid to be left in the injector. Do not try to inject the remaining liquid.

- After the shot, press the needle against a hard surface to bend the needle back. Put the injector back in its case, needle first. Do not put the gray activation cap back on the injector.

- Take the antihistamine tablet in your allergy kit.

- Anyone with serious allergies to food or drugs should wear a *Medic Alert* bracelet. These are available in the pharmacy, and link the patient and reactions to a 24-hour information line. Patients with serious allergies and medical conditions (including hypoglycemia that may require glucagon) should wear this type of identification.

Drug Classes that Can Cause Allergic Reactions

BETA LACTAM ALLERGY

Penicillin is a beta lactam antibiotic and there are many related compounds in this family, including nafcillin, oxacillin, ampicillin, amoxicillin, ticarcillin, piperacillin and others. Anyone who is allergic to one of the penicillins should be presumed to be allergic to all penicillins and should avoid the entire group, unless they have been specifically evaluated for this problem.

Cephalosporins are closely related to penicillin. People with a history of penicillin allergy have a small risk of having an allergic reaction to a cephalosporin. It is prudent on the exam to avoid any beta lactam with a stated allergy to another, unless there is no alternative agent.

SULFA ALLERGIES

These are most commonly reported with sulfamethoxazole (SMX, in *Bactrim, Septra),* and the patient should avoid using sulfapyridine, sulfadiazine and sulfisoxazole. "Non-arylamine" sulfonamides (thiazide diuretics, loop diuretics, sulfonylureas, acetazolamide, zonisamide and celecoxib) usually do not cross react with a SMX allergy, but on the exam you will likely have to recognize the reaction. Since the cross-reactivity between SMX and thiazides and loops is very small, the reaction is usually not considered when the need for these drugs is present – but the patient should be aware to watch for a possible reaction. There are other sulfa-type groups that also have low cross-reactivity. Sulfites or sulfate allergies do not cross react with a sulfonamide allergy.

OPIOID ALLERGY

Opioid allergies and cross-reactivity is described in detail in the pain section. Fentanyl (*Duragesic*), meperidine (*Demerol*) and methadone (*Dolophine*) do not cross-react with opioids of the morphine-type. However, they each have safety considerations and can <u>only</u> be used in select groups of patients (see pain chapter). Meperidine is in the same chemical class as fentanyl (and alfentanyl) and could cross-react.

BREATHING DIFFICULTIES AND NSAIDS

Reactions to NSAIDs, including aspirin, can be either a drug sensitivity (which can cause rhinitis, mild asthmatic type reactions or skin reactions) or a true allergic reaction. If a true allergy is present the patient will experience urticaria and angioedema, and occasionally anaphylaxis. COX-2 selective NSAIDs are used clinically, but on licensing exams it may be prudent to avoid all NSAIDs.

PEANUT/SOY ALLERGY

A food allergy that is important for pharmacists to know is a peanut allergy, since soy is used in some medications. Peanuts and soy are in the same family and can have cross-reactivity. Parents of children with peanut allergies should be trained in CPR. An *EpiPen* may need to be kept within close reach. Most likely, a reaction will be due to consuming peanuts or soy unknowingly in food products. Drugs to avoid with peanut allergy:

- Ipratropium/albuterol (*Combivent*) – new formulation *Combivent Respimat* does not contain soy or CFCs.

- Clevidipine *(Cleviprex)*

- Propofol (*Diprivan*)

- Progesterone in *Prometrium*

EGG ALLERGY

If a patient has a true allergy to eggs (which means they cannot enjoy birthday cake), they cannot use:

- Seasonal and H1N1 influenza shots or nasal mists, and a few other vaccines (described in the immunizations chapter, which includes a few other possible allergans in vaccines.) In some cases the flu vaccines may be given in a medical setting because the amount of egg protein in the vaccine is very small and reactions are rare, but as of December 2011 the contraindication is still present.

- Clevidipine *(Cleviprex)*

- Propofol (*Diprivan*)

U.S. Department of Health and Human Services

MEDWATCH

The FDA Safety Information and
Adverse Event Reporting Program

For VOLUNTARY reporting of
adverse events, product problems and
product use errors

Page ____ of ____

Form Approved: OMB No. 0910-0291, Expires: 10/31/08
See OMB statement on reverse.

FDA USE ONLY

Triage unit
sequence #

A. PATIENT INFORMATION

1. Patient Identifier	2. Age at Time of Event, or Date of Birth:	3. Sex	4. Weight
In confidence		☐ Female ☐ Male	_____ lb or _____ kg

B. ADVERSE EVENT, PRODUCT PROBLEM OR ERROR

Check all that apply:

1. ☐ Adverse Event ☐ Product Problem (e.g., defects/malfunctions)
   ☐ Product Use Error ☐ Problem with Different Manufacturer of Same Medicine

2. Outcomes Attributed to Adverse Event
   (Check all that apply)

☐ Death: _____ (mm/dd/yyyy)   ☐ Disability or Permanent Damage

☐ Life-threatening   ☐ Congenital Anomaly/Birth Defect

☐ Hospitalization - initial or prolonged   ☐ Other Serious (Important Medical Events)

☐ Required Intervention to Prevent Permanent Impairment/Damage (Devices)

3. Date of Event (mm/dd/yyyy)   4. Date of this Report (mm/dd/yyyy)

5. Describe Event, Problem or Product Use Error

6. Relevant Tests/Laboratory Data, Including Dates

7. Other Relevant History, Including Preexisting Medical Conditions (e.g., allergies, race, pregnancy, smoking and alcohol use, liver/kidney problems, etc.)

C. PRODUCT AVAILABILITY

Product Available for Evaluation? (Do not send product to FDA)

☐ Yes ☐ No ☐ Returned to Manufacturer on: _____ (mm/dd/yyyy)

D. SUSPECT PRODUCT(S)

1. Name, Strength, Manufacturer (from product label)

#1 _____

#2 _____

2.	Dose or Amount	Frequency	Route
#1			
#2			

3. Dates of Use (If unknown, give duration) from/to (or best estimate)

#1 _____

#2 _____

4. Diagnosis or Reason for Use (Indication)

#1 _____

#2 _____

5. Event Abated After Use Stopped or Dose Reduced?

#1 ☐ Yes ☐ No ☐ Doesn't Apply

#2 ☐ Yes ☐ No ☐ Doesn't Apply

8. Event Reappeared After Reintroduction?

#1 ☐ Yes ☐ No ☐ Doesn't Apply

#2 ☐ Yes ☐ No ☐ Doesn't Apply

6. Lot #	7. Expiration Date
#1	#1
#2	#2

9. NDC # or Unique ID

E. SUSPECT MEDICAL DEVICE

1. Brand Name

2. Common Device Name

3. Manufacturer Name, City and State

4. Model #	Lot #	5. Operator of Device
Catalog #	Expiration Date (mm/dd/yyyy)	☐ Health Professional ☐ Lay User/Patient
Serial #	Other #	☐ Other: _____

6. If Implanted, Give Date (mm/dd/yyyy)   7. If Explanted, Give Date (mm/dd/yyyy)

8. Is this a Single-use Device that was Reprocessed and Reused on a Patient?
   ☐ Yes ☐ No

9. If Yes to Item No. 8, Enter Name and Address of Reprocessor

F. OTHER (CONCOMITANT) MEDICAL PRODUCTS

Product names and therapy dates (exclude treatment of event)

G. REPORTER (See confidentiality section on back)

1. Name and Address

Phone #   E-mail

2. Health Professional?	3. Occupation	4. Also Reported to:
☐ Yes ☐ No		☐ Manufacturer ☐ User Facility ☐ Distributor/Importer

5. If you do NOT want your identity disclosed to the manufacturer, place an "X" in this box: ☐

FORM FDA 3500 (10/05)   Submission of a report does not constitute an admission that medical personnel or the product caused or contributed to the event.

ADVICE ABOUT VOLUNTARY REPORTING

Detailed instructions available at: http://www.fda.gov/medwatch/report/consumer/instruct.htm

Report adverse events, product problems or product use errors with:

- Medications *(drugs or biologics)*
- Medical devices *(including in-vitro diagnostics)*
- Combination products *(medication & medical devices)*
- Human cells, tissues, and cellular and tissue-based products
- Special nutritional products *(dietary supplements, medical foods, infant formulas)*
- Cosmetics

Report product problems - quality, performance or safety concerns such as:

- Suspected counterfeit product
- Suspected contamination
- Questionable stability
- Defective components
- Poor packaging or labeling
- Therapeutic failures (product didn't work)

Report SERIOUS adverse events. An event is serious when the patient outcome is:

- Death
- Life-threatening
- Hospitalization - initial or prolonged
- Disability or permanent damage
- Congenital anomaly/birth defect
- Required intervention to prevent permanent impairment or damage
- Other serious (important medical events)

Report even if:

- You're not certain the product caused the event
- You don't have all the details

How to report:

- Just fill in the sections that apply to your report
- Use section D for all products except medical devices
- Attach additional pages if needed
- Use a separate form for each patient
- Report either to FDA or the manufacturer *(or both)*

Other methods of reporting:

- 1-800-FDA-0178 -- To FAX report
- 1-800-FDA-1088 -- To report by phone
- www.fda.gov/medwatch/report.htm -- To report online

If your report involves a serious adverse event with a device and it occurred in a facility outside a doctor's office, that facility may be legally required to report to FDA and/or the manufacturer. Please notify the person in that facility who would handle such reporting.

If your report involves a serious adverse event with a vaccine call 1-800-822-7967 to report.

Confidentiality: The patient's identity is held in strict confidence by FDA and protected to the fullest extent of the law. FDA will not disclose the reporter's identity in response to a request from the public, pursuant to the Freedom of Information Act. The reporter's identity, including the identity of a self-reporter, may be shared with the manufacturer unless requested otherwise.

The public reporting burden for this collection of information has been estimated to average 36 minutes per response, including the time for reviewing instructions, searching existing data sources, gathering and maintaining the data needed, and completing and reviewing the collection of information. Send comments regarding this burden estimate or any other aspect of this collection of information, including suggestions for reducing this burden to:

Department of Health and Human Services	*Please DO NOT*	*OMB statement:*
Food and Drug Administration - MedWatch	*RETURN this form*	*"An agency may not conduct or sponsor, and a*
10903 New Hampshire Avenue	*to this address.*	*person is not required to respond to, a collection of*
Building 22, Mail Stop 4447		*information unless it displays a currently valid*
Silver Spring, MD 20993-0002		*OMB control number."*

U.S. DEPARTMENT OF HEALTH AND HUMAN SERVICES
Food and Drug Administration

FORM FDA 3500 (10/05) (Back)   Please Use Address Provided Below -- Fold in Thirds, Tape and Mail

---

DEPARTMENT OF HEALTH & HUMAN SERVICES

Public Health Service
Food and Drug Administration
Rockville, MD 20857

Official Business
Penalty for Private Use $300

BUSINESS REPLY MAIL

FIRST CLASS MAIL   PERMIT NO. 946   ROCKVILLE MD

MEDWATCH
The FDA Safety Information and Adverse Event Reporting Program
Food and Drug Administration
5600 Fishers Lane
Rockville, MD 20852-9787

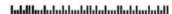

MEDICATION ERRORS, PATIENT SAFETY, AND THE JOINT COMMISSION

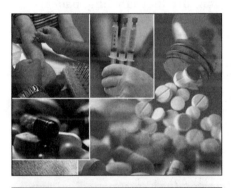

GUIDELINES/REFERENCES

Institute for Safe Medication Practices, www.ismp.org

Cohen, Michael R (2007). *Medication Errors*. Washington DC: American Pharmacists Association.

Joint Commission, www.jointcommission.org

MMWR Guideline for Hand Hygiene in Health-Care Settings October 25, 2002, 51(RR16);1-44.

CDC Guideline for Isolation Precautions: Preventing Transmission of Infectious Agents in Healthcare Settings, 2007.

We gratefully acknowledge the help of Melissa A. McAuley, PharmD, mmcauley@ismp.org, Institute for Safe Medication Practices (ISMP), Horsham, PA in preparing this section.

Background

Awareness of the prevalence of medical errors increased after the release of a study from the Institute of Medicine (IOM), *To Err is Human* (2000), which found that up to 98,000 Americans die each year in U.S. hospitals due to preventable medical errors. These numbers understated the problem because they did not include preventable deaths due to medical treatments outside of hospitals. Since the release of the IOM study, there has been a greater focus on the quality of healthcare provided in the U.S. and the need to reduce medical errors, which are preventable. As pharmacists we are most concerned with errors involving medications.

This chapter begins with an overview of medication errors, followed by specific measures to limit medication errors in the community and institution settings. Included is a discussion of two types of medication devices that have important benefits but known safety risks – patient controlled analgesic devices (PCAs) and automated dispensing cabinets (ADCs).

Patient safety includes reducing infection risk. Essential methods to reduce infections, such as proper hand-washing technique, enforcing universal precautions and using safe injection technique are included. The chapter concludes with a discussion of the Joint Commission, which provides accreditation for healthcare facilities. A primary focus of the Joint Commission is patient safety.

DEFINITION OF A MEDICATION ERROR

A medication error means that someone (the prescriber, pharmacist, nurse, or even the patient) did something that was not correct, such as administering the wrong drug, strength, route, or dose of the medication, confusing look-alike/sound-alike drugs, incorrectly calculating a dose; or making an error when prescribing, transcribing, dispensing, administering or monitoring a medication. The most common medication errors are giving the wrong medication or the wrong dose to a patient.

> The formal definition of a medication error developed by the National Coordinating Council on Medication Error Reporting and Prevention (NCCMERP) is "any preventable event that may cause or lead to inappropriate medication use or patient harm while the medication is in the control of the health care professional, patient, or consumer. Such events may be related to professional practice, health care products, procedures, and systems, including prescribing; order communication; product labeling, packaging, and nomenclature; compounding; dispensing; distribution; administration; education; monitoring; and use."

Do not confuse medication errors with adverse drug reactions – these are generally not avoidable although they may be more likely if the drug is given to a patient at high risk for certain complications.

Example of an adverse drug reaction (not a medication error)

A 55-year old female had a history of herpes zoster. She has no other known medical conditions. The patient reported considerable "shingles pain" that "run from my back through my left breast." The physician prescribed pregabalin. The patient returned to the physician with complaints of ankle swelling, which required drug discontinuation.

This problem would <u>not</u> be attributable to a medication error made by the physician who prescribed pregabalin or by the pharmacist who dispensed it. Although this drug can cause fluid retention, it does not occur with everyone and there is no way to know in advance if the patient would suffer this problem.

WHO IS MOST RESPONSIBLE FOR ERRORS: THE INDIVIDUAL OR THE "SYSTEM?"

Experts in medication safety concur that the most common cause of medication errors is not individual error but <u>problems with the design of the medical system itself</u>. Currently, instead of blaming the "lousy pharmacist" or the "lousy technician" (or the prescriber), health care professionals should find ways to improve the system in order to reduce the chance that the error will occur again. The idea is to design systems so that mistakes are not as likely or can be captured before reaching the patient.

Example of how medication errors should NOT be handled

A young man graduated from pharmacy school shortly after the release of the IOM report. He was a top student, a class leader and was well-liked by co-workers. During his first year of practice as a licensed pharmacist he dispensed the wrong strength of phenobarbital tablets for a 10 year-old child. The child was overdosed and hospitalized for several days. Fortunately, the child recovered. The pharmacist was fired by his employer and subsequently suffered from a lack of self-confidence and depression. Eventually, he returned to pharmacy in a different practice setting.

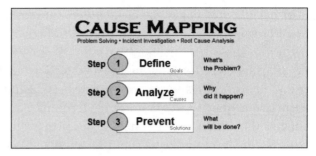

Root cause and FMEA analyses are used by many industries, including pharmacy.

ROOT CAUSE ANALYSIS TO PREVENT FUTURE ERRORS

One reason the error described above occurred is because the pharmacy stored two strengths of phenobarbital tablets next to each other on the shelf. The technician who pulled the medication grabbed the wrong bottle and the pharmacist missed the error during the check. Errors like this can be prevented from occurring again when the contributing factors are made known and appropriate prevention strategies are employed. <u>A root cause analysis (RCA) investigates an event that has already occurred (it is retrospective)</u>. It looks back at the sequence of events that led to the error. <u>The information obtained in the analysis is used to design changes that will hopefully prevent future errors</u>.

Findings from the RCA (the identification of the factors that contributed to the event and led to a "<u>sentinel event</u>" – the unexpected occurrence involving death or serious physical or psychological injury, or risk thereof) can be applied proactively to analyze and improve processes and systems before they breakdown again.

The RCA can be of enormous value in capturing both the big-picture perspective and the details of the error. They facilitate system evaluation, analysis of need for corrective action, and tracking and trending. <u>Targeting corrective measures at the identified root causes is the best way to prevent similar problems from occurring in the future</u>. However, it is recognized that complete prevention of recurrence by a single intervention is not always possible. Thus, <u>RCA is often considered to be a repetitive process, and is frequently viewed as a continuous quality improvement (CQI) tool.</u>

After an analysis of the various factors contributing to the error described above, changes were implemented to make it much more difficult for anyone to make the same mistake. These included the following:

- Alerts regarding safety concerns with this medication (and others labeled as "high alert") were built into the computer system. Pharmacists are now required to acknowledge and accept or reject high doses in the system.

- The pharmacy now requires that the bottles of phenobarbital tablets and the suspension be placed in separate <u>high-alert medication bins</u> that are labeled with a warning to double check the dosage.

Pharmacists now flag these medications for mandatory patient education/counseling at the point of sale.

An analysis can also be done <u>prospectively</u> to identify pathways that could lead to errors and to identify ways to reduce the error risk. <u>Failure Mode and Effects Analysis (FMEA) is a proactive method</u> used to reduce the frequency and consequences of errors. FMEA is used to analyze the design of the system in order to evaluate the potential for failures, and to determine what potential effects could occur when the medication delivery system changes in any substantial way or if a potentially dangerous new drug will be added to the formulary.

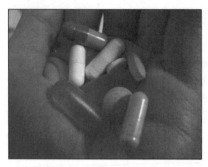

Medical Error Classification: Errors of Omission and Errors of Commission

ERRORS OF OMISSION

An error of omission means leaving something out that is needed for safety, such as missed instructions, or failure to provide a dose at the required time. For example, consider the drug chloral hydrate, which is occasionally used in children as a pre-operative sedative. There have been instances of overdose (some with fatalities) due to incorrect dosing and incorrect administration. It is critical that the pharmacist check that the mg/kg dose is reasonable and help to ensure that the correct dose is given by providing an oral dosing syringe or measuring cup, with instructions, to the parent. If the pharmacist does not provide the measuring device with clear instructions (an error of omission) the parent may be receiving doses for several procedures in one bottle and could mistakenly provide the entire bottle of syrup prior to one procedure. Another example of omission: if hydrochlorothiazide is dispensed when the combination of hydrochlorothiazide/lisinopril was prescribed, the omission of lisinopril is an error of omission even though hydrochlorothiazide was dispensed correctly.

Example of an error of omission

A physician prescribed warfarin 5 mg to a 70 year-old frail female with atrial fibrillation, heart failure and renal insufficiency. The bottle label was incorrectly prepared as warfarin 5 mg Q daily. Neither the technician who typed the label nor the pharmacist who checked the label noticed that the dosing schedule had not been provided on the prescription. The physician had intended to instruct the patient to begin the medication at 1/2 tablet daily, but had left this off the instructions and did not inform the patient or her caregiver. The patient took one tablet daily for ten days and reported to the medical office. The INR was measured at 4.8. Fortunately, the patient did not have any noticeable bleeding and the dosage was decreased.

ERRORS OF COMMISSION

An error of commission means that something was done incorrectly, such as prescribing bupropion to a patient with a history of epilepsy or dispensing sulfamethoxazole to a patient with a sulfa allergy.

Example of an error of commission

Manuel is a 38 year-old male patient with a creatinine clearance of 24 mL/min. He is an inpatient in the amputation unit. Manuel's tissue sample is positive for gram positive cocci. The physician ordered vancomycin 1 gram IV Q 8 hours. The pharmacist approved the order and the patient received the medication, at this dose, for the next two days. He suffered further renal damage. This is considered an error of commission because the vancomycin was dosed too high for a patient with reduced clearance.

REPORTING MEDICATION ERRORS

Medication errors, preventable adverse drug reactions, close calls, or hazardous conditions should be reported. We report medication errors so that changes can be made to the system to prevent

> **Those who cannot remember the past are condemned to repeat it.**
> *Poet and Philosopher George Santayana 1863-1952*

similar errors in the future. Without reporting, such events may go unrecognized and thus important epidemiological and preventive information would be unavailable.

In a community pharmacy, the staff member who discovers the error should immediately report it to the corporate office or in the case of an independently owned pharmacy, the owner, who is involved with the quality assurance program (also called quality improvement). These are mandated by many state boards of pharmacy and have the purpose (in the words of the California state board) "to develop pharmacy systems and workflow processes designed to prevent medication errors." Error investigations need to take place quickly – often as soon as within 48 hours of the incident so that the sequence of events remains clear to those involved. Many states mandate the ethical requirement that errors be reported to the patient and their prescriber as soon as possible.

In a hospital setting, the staff member should report a medication error through the hospital's specific medication event reporting system. Many medication error reporting systems within hospitals are electronic, however some hospitals may still maintain a paper reporting system. The hospital's pharmacy and therapeutics (P&T) committee should be informed of the error as well as the Medication Safety Committee. The P&T committee is required to record errors and responses to The Joint Commission (TJC). The Joint Commission is primarily involved with promoting safety and is described later in this chapter.

REPORTING TO ORGANIZATIONS THAT SPECIALIZE IN ERROR PREVENTION

The Patient Safety and Quality Improvement Act of 2005 (Patient Safety Act) authorized the creation of Patient Safety Organizations (PSOs) to improve the quality and safety of health care delivery in the U.S. The Patient Safety Act encourages clinicians and health care organizations to voluntarily report and share quality and patient safety information without fear of this information being used in legal proceedings.

The Agency for Healthcare Research and Quality (AHRQ) administers the provisions of the Patient Safety Act and the Patient Safety Rule dealing with PSO operations. More information regarding PSOs can be found at the Agency for Healthcare Research and Quality website (http://www.pso.ahrq.gov/).

Organizations that specialize in error prevention can analyze the system-based causes of the errors and make recommendations to others who can learn from the mistakes. Every pharmacist should make it a practice to read medication error reports in order to use this history to improve their own practice settings. Information sources include the Institute for Safe Medication Practices (ISMP) newsletters which have information about medication-related errors, adverse drug reactions, as well as recommendations that will help reduce the risk of medication errors and other adverse drug events at the practice site. ISMP's medication error report analysis and adverse drug reaction monthly articles in the journal *Hospital Pharmacy* is available free of charge for hospital pharmacists.

The ISMP National Medication Error Reporting Program (MERP) is a confidential national voluntary reporting program that provides expert analysis of the system causes of medication errors and disseminates recommendations for prevention.

On the ISMP website (www.ismp.org) medication errors <u>and</u> close calls can be reported. Click on "Report Errors." Professionals and consumers should be encouraged to report medication errors using this site even if the error was reported internally.

Example of a close call that should be reported

A pain specialist pharmacist worked at a large county hospital. She was asked to provide a pain consult for a patient hospitalized due to pneumonia. The patient had been taking oxycodone immediate release 20 mg on an as-needed basis for chronic pain. She used 6-7 tablets daily and remained in significant pain. At 10:00 the pharmacist went to the bedside, conducted a pain assessment and wrote an order to discontinue the current pain medication. She replaced the oxycodone with morphine controlled-release 60 mg Q 12 hours, with a lower dose of morphine immediate-release as-needed. At 16:00 the pharmacist went to check on the patient and saw that a feeding tube had been inserted. She panicked and ran to find the nurse and the patient's medication administration record. Fortunately, the nurse was an experienced practitioner who knew not to crush a long-acting opioid. The nurse had contacted the physician for a replacement order.

If this close call was reported, the hospital would have the opportunity to implement procedures to avoid this situation in the future. At this hospital nursing students often administer medications with little supervision. By reporting this "close call" the hospital was provided an opportunity to intervene and avoid a potentially fatal mistake in the future.

Other organizations involved in helping to reduce medication errors and promote patient safety are The American Society of Health-System Pharmacists (ASHP), The National Coordinating Council for Medication Error Reporting and Prevention (NCC MERP) and the Agency for Healthcare Research and Quality (AHRQ).

Common Methods Used to Reduce Medication Errors

PATIENT PROFILES

Pharmacies should maintain current patient profiles that include all prescription drugs, over the counter (OTC) medications, and anything else the patient is taking such as natural products and other supplements. Allergies and the type of allergic reaction (i.e., rash, lip swelling) should be recorded. See the drug allergy chapter for pointers on proper documentation. The most common use of the profile is to check for allergies and drug interactions, but it can also be used for monitoring appropriateness of therapy, checking for polypharmacy (polypharmacy means "many drugs" and refers to problems that can occur when a patient is taking more medications than are necessary) and assessing patient compliance with their medication regimen. Patient disease-state information and diagnosis is also important information in order to check the appropriateness of medication selection and dosage.

Example of polypharmacy discovered by a review of a patient's profile

Jessica is a 52 year-old female with a history of bipolar II disorder, anxiety, insomnia and restless leg syndrome. She is using olanzapine 10 mg Q AM, fluoxetine 20 mg QHS, zolpidem 10 mg QHS and ropinirole 1 mg QHS. The pharmacist recording the patient's profile asked about the patient's general health and was told that since the initiation of olanzapine therapy eighteen months ago the patient's weight has increased by 8 pounds and she was told recently that her blood glucose and LDL cholesterol are high. The pharmacist considers the possibility that the olanzapine is typically sedating (and might be moved to QHS dosing) and the fluoxetine is typically activating (and might be moved to QAM dosing). Perhaps if this was done the patient might not require a hypnotic. The pharmacist also asked about the patient's sleep schedule and whether the restless leg began after the initiation of fluoxetine therapy. The physician is considering the addition of diabetes and hypertension medications. The pharmacist informs the physician that the metabolic changes may be due to the olanzapine therapy and has suggested an alternative. (Hopefully, these suggestions are not all implemented concurrently.)

MEDICATION THERAPY MANAGEMENT

The example above may have been discovered during a more comprehensive review through the process of medication therapy management (MTM). This is a program mandated under the Medicare drug benefit (Medicare Part D) to promote safe and effective medication use. Medicare's drug benefit (Part D) provides outpatient prescription drug coverage for anyone with Medicare. It is available only through private companies. At a minimum, beneficiaries targeted for MTM include members with multiple chronic conditions who are taking multiple Part D drugs and are likely to incur annual costs for covered Part D drugs that exceed a predetermined level. Computer databases are used to identify patients with certain high-risk conditions (such as heart failure or uncontrolled diabetes) who are generally using many medications (some systems tag patients taking 9 or more chronic medications daily) and assign a pharmacist (preferably) to review profiles for proper use. This program is a Medicare requirement and therefore the majority of MTM programs exist within Medicare-funded health care plans. MTM may also apply to populations outside of Medicare, including patients less than 65 years of age.

The pharmacist can form a partnership with the patient and prescriber to remedy any issues or lapses. Often, these reviews identify missed therapy such as lack of an ACE I or ARB in patients with diabetes, missing beta blocker therapy post-MI, missing bisphosphonate therapy with high-dose chronic steroids, among others, since these are easily searchable in databases. A popular MTM initiative is to improve non-adherence in heart failure patients due to the high-rate of ED visits due to decompensated heart failure. MTM is also used to identify cost-savings, by promoting switches to generics or more affordable brands, or by suggesting patient assistance programs or low income subsidies for eligible members.

DRUG UTILIZATION REVIEWS (DURs)

The Medicaid Drug Utilization Review (DUR) Program was created by the Omnibus Budget Reconciliation Act (OBRA) of 1990. The main emphasis of the program is to promote patient safety by an increased review and awareness of outpatient prescribed drugs.

It accomplishes these tasks through the following means:

- Retrospective analysis of patient drug usage, physician prescribing, and pharmacy dispensing activities.

- Identification and review of critical patient profiles.

- Regular reporting of activities and important findings to Medicaid providers and pharmacies.

- Awareness campaigns for new pharmaceutical products and techniques.

- Research studies into drug-related trends and the application of those studies into cost-savings plans.

States were encouraged by enhanced federal funding to design and install point-of-sale electronic claims management systems that interface with their Medicaid Management Information Systems (MMIS) operations. The annual report requirement provides an excellent measurement tool to assess how well patient safety, provider prescribing habits and dollars saved (by avoidance of problems such as drug-drug interactions, drug-disease interactions, therapeutic duplication, and over-prescribing by providers.)

RETROSPECTIVE ANALYSIS

Retrospective DURs can be done individually (such as with an MTM review) or, more commonly, with a system-wide review using aggregate data. The retrospective DUR program involves reviews of patient drug history profiles generated from medical assistance paid claims data by a panel of active practicing physicians and pharmacists. DURs used to be performed more commonly but they are still done and can serve a useful purpose, such as a DUR conducted in a healthcare group to determine which physician's handwriting contributes to the most prescribing errors, or which prescribers use the highest percentage of branded drugs, when less-expensive alternatives are available.

Example of a drug utilization review by the state of Wyoming

In 2010 many regions in the U.S. experienced fiscal restraints, including the state of Wyoming, which has high costs due to ED visits. The state wished to reduce the prevalence of ED admits due to asthma exacerbations. The state conducted a DUR of asthma medication adherence and found that adherence rates of asthma medications declined during pregnancy, although the medication was covered under the state's low income medication plan. Through further follow-up the researchers discovered that the primary reason many women decreased asthma medication adherence during pregnancy was due to safety concerns. Based on the data provided by the DUE the state initiated a campaign to increase awareness of the health risks associated with discontinuation of asthma medications during pregnancy.

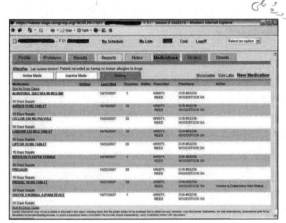

MEDICATION RECONCILIATION

Medication reconciliation refers to the process of avoiding inadvertent inconsistencies and or medication errors such as omissions, duplications, dosing errors or drug interactions <u>across transitions in care</u>.

<u>This is accomplished by reviewing the patient's complete medication regimen at the time of admission, transfer, and discharge and comparing it with the regimen being considered for the new setting of care</u>. Though most often discussed in the hospital context, medication reconciliation can be equally important in ambulatory care, as many patients receive prescriptions from more than one outpatient provider.

In 2005, medication reconciliation was named as National Patient Safety Goal number 8 by the Joint Commission.

Example of the benefit of medication reconciliation

Ann is an 82 year-old female. Her only medication for the previous ten years has been amlodipine 10 mg Q daily. Ann recently developed influenza. She began to have trouble breathing and was taken to the hospital. It was discovered that Ann had pneumonia and new-onset atrial fibrillation. She was prescribed diltiazem, dabigatran and digoxin. Ann was discharged to transitional care and received the new medications plus the previous medication amlodipine. The consultant pharmacist conducted a medication review to reconcile the medications and, after discussion with the physician on the patient's rate control, the pharmacist wrote an order to discontinue the diltiazem.

MEDICATION GUIDES

Medication Guides (or MedGuides) present <u>important adverse events</u> that can occur with over 300 medications. MedGuides are <u>FDA-approved patient handouts</u> and are considered part of the drug's labeling. If a medication has a MedGuide, it should be dispensed with the original prescription and with each refill. Some medications dispensed while inpatient require MedGuides and these should be available to the patient or family upon request. It is not necessary to dispense them to inpatients routinely as the patient is being monitored. MedGuides are required for many individual agents and some entire classes of medications (including anticonvulsants, antidepressants, NSAIDs and the ADHD stimulants and atomoxetine.)

CONSUMER MEDICATION INFORMATION (CMI) LEAFLETS

Consumer medication information (CMI) leaflets for all prescription medicines are voluntarily provided with new prescriptions by retail pharmacies. The leaflets explain how the medicine works, as well as providing practical advice on how and when to take it, common side effects and potential interactions.

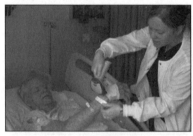

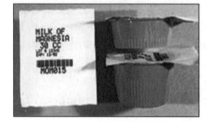

BAR CODING

Bar coding may be the <u>most important medication error reduction tool</u> in the arsenal right now. The bar code <u>follows the drug through the medication use process</u> to make sure it is being properly stocked (such as in the right space in the pharmacy or in the right pocket in the dispensing cabinet), through compounding (if required), and to the patient. The bar code is used at the bedside to identify that the correct drug (by scanning the code on the drug's packaging) is going to the right patient (via scanning the patient's wristband) and confirms that the dose is being given at the right time. The nurse may have a badge bar code that can track who administered the dose. Bar codes are now on many pumps and can prevent the errors involving medications being given IV that are not meant to be administered in this manner. The FDA requires bar coding on medications with (minimally) the drug's national drug code (NDC) number. It may also include other items, such as the lot number and expiration date.

LOOK-ALIKE, SOUND-ALIKE MEDICATIONS

Confusing drug names is a common cause of medication errors. Poor handwriting and similar product labeling aggravate the problem of pulling a look-alike or sound-alike agent instead of the intended medication. Computer systems are being built with alerts to attempt to double-check that the correct medication is being ordered or withdrawn, such as the warning on some of the automated dispensing cabinets: This is DILAUDID. Did you want hydroMORPHONE? (to avoid confusions with morphine).

Drugs that are easily mixed up should be labeled with tall man letters (e.g., CeleXA, CeleBREX). Several studies have shown that highlighting sections of drug names using tall man letters can help distinguish similar drug names, making them less prone to mix-ups. ISMP, FDA, The Joint Commission, and other safety-conscious organizations have promoted the use of tall man letters as one means of reducing confusion between similar drug names. If receiving an oral order for a drug that is easily confused with another be sure to repeat the drug name back, with spelling if useful, to the prescriber. It may be possible to remove a drug that is easily confused with another from the institution's formulary.

The FDA's and ISMP's approved Tallman lettering information is available at: http://www.ismp.org/tools/tallmanletters.pdf

DO NOT USE ERROR-PRONE ABBREVIATIONS, SYMBOLS, AND DOSAGE DESIGNATIONS

Abbreviations are unsafe and contribute to many medical errors. The Joint Commission standards include recommendations against the use of unsafe abbreviations. The ISMP's list of error-prone abbreviations, symbols, and dosage designations (attached at the end of this chapter) includes those on the Joint Commission's do-not-use list (designated by **). Try writing the number 5.0 on a lined paper and you can see how easily the number could be mistaken for 50; this is why trailing zeros (after a whole number) are not permitted. Leading zeros are required because it would be easy to miss a decimal point placed before a number (such as .5) if the leading zero was not present (the correct way to write this is 0.5). The other items on the list are important enough that it is almost misleading to give one example – such as the long history of mix-ups between morphine and magnesium and resultant fatalities. Review this list carefully. If abbreviations are used within an institution (such as a hospital) they must not be on that institution's unapproved abbreviation list (and not include any on the Joint Commission's do-not use list). The unapproved abbreviations list is supposed to be kept readily accessible in the unit and may be placed at the back of the patient chart. It is best to attempt to avoid abbreviations entirely.

The ISMP's list of error-prone abbreviations that is provided at the end of this chapter is available at: http://www.ismp.org/tools/errorproneabbreviations.pdf

INDICATIONS FOR USE ON PRESCRIPTIONS

An indication for use that is written on the prescription (such as lisinopril 10 mg once daily for hypertension) helps us assure appropriate prescribing and drug selection. If the pharmacist does not know what the medication is being used for they should ask the patient or contact the prescriber. Indications provide information in order to appropriately provide counseling to a patient. In this example, the pharmacist can inform the patient this medication is to help keep their blood pressure at the right level and they can make sure the patient is aware of the blood pressure goal. The retail pharmacist should open the bag, open the vial and show the patient the medication (this can be tricky; lisinopril comes in various tablet sizes and colors – hopefully the same generic manufacturer can be chosen). Also, many pharmacies now provide the tablet description on the patient label. The patient should be instructed always to read this description so they are sure that what is in the vial looks like the description provided on the label. The patient is now equipped to monitor their condition and to help catch a dispensing error if one occurs. The pharmacist who has educated the patient on their blood pressure goal (or any other therapeutic goal) has helped improve the patient's health.

MEASUREMENTS SHOULD BE IN THE METRIC SYSTEM

<u>Measurements should be kept in the metric system only</u>. Prescribers should use the metric system to express all weights, volumes and units.

PROVIDE INSTRUCTIONS ON PRESCRIPTIONS; AVOID USING "AS DIRECTED"

Using <u>the term "as directed" is not acceptable</u> on prescriptions because the patient often has no idea what this means and the pharmacist cannot verify a proper dosing regimen. Occasionally, this term is used on the bottle along with a separate dosing calendar, such as with warfarin. It would be preferable to write "use per instructions on the dosing calendar" since the patient may not understand how to take the medication and may not be aware that a separate dosing calendar exists.

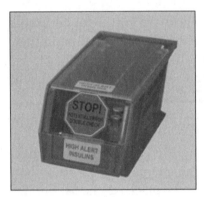

SPECIAL BINS AND LABELING FOR HIGH ALERT DRUGS

<u>Drugs that bear a heightened risk of causing significant patient harm when used in error should be designated as "High Alert"</u>. Any drug that is high risk for significant harm if dispensed incorrectly can be placed in a medication bin that provides a visual alert to the person pulling the medication. The bin can be labeled with warnings and include materials (placed inside the bin) that should be dispensed with the drug (such as oral syringes or MedGuides). In the hospital setting certain drugs are classified as "high alert" and these can be placed in bins labeled with dispensing requirements.

There are many drugs considered high-alert, including insulin and oral hypoglycemics, opioids, anticoagulants, antiarrhythmics, anesthetics, chemotherapeutics, injectable KCl, phosphate, magnesium and saline at concentrations greater than 0.9%.

Use the ISMP "high alert" list to determine which medications require special safeguards to reduce the risk of errors. It is available at: http://www.ismp.org/tools/highalertmedications.

DO NOT RELY ON MEDICATION PACKAGING FOR IDENTIFICATION PURPOSES

Look-alike packaging can contribute to errors. If unavoidable, separate look-alike drugs in the pharmacy and units, or repackage.

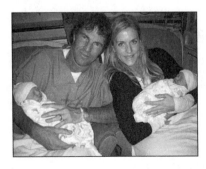

Example of an error due to misidentification of a dose based on the packaging

The intravenous catheters of three neonates in a NICU unit in Los Angeles were flushed with the adult therapeutic dose of heparin (10,000 units/mL) rather than the heparin flush dose of 10 units/mL. This accident did not result in fatalities although two of the babies required protamine. Three babies died from a similar incident the previous year at a different hospital. The overdose was administered because the nurse thought she had used the lower dose of heparin due to multiple system failures.

Due to the high risk associated with heparin overdose, high concentration heparin vials should not be present in patient care areas. Instead, therapeutic doses should be sent by the pharmacy department.

CODE BLUE

Code Blue refers to a patient requiring emergency medical care, typically for cardiac or respiratory arrest. The overhead announcement will provide the patient's location. The code team will rush to the room and begin immediate resuscitative efforts.

USE SAFE PRACTICES FOR EMERGENCY MEDICATIONS/CRASH CARTS

Staff must be properly trained to handle emergencies and use crash cart medications. The medications should be unit dose and age-specific, including pediatric-specific doses. A weight-based dosing chart can be placed in the trays used in the pediatric units. If a unit dose medication is not available it is best to have prefilled syringes and drips in the cart as much as possible because it is easy to make a mistake under the stress of a code. The emergency medications should be stored in sealed or locked containers in a locked room and replaced as soon as possible after use (through a cart exchange so that the area is not left without required medications). Monitor the drug expiration dates. Trained pharmacists should be present at codes when possible.

DEDICATE PHARMACISTS TO THE ICU, PEDIATRIC UNITS AND EMERGENCY DEPARTMENTS

These are units with a high incidence of avoidable errors and pharmacists in the units reduce errors. Dosing for very young children is challenging. Medications are usually packaged for adults and need to be prepared in different volumes or concentrations when used in the very young. The calculations are pediatric-specific and errors can multiply. Children are usually less able to physiologically tolerate a medication error due to developing renal, immune and hepatic functions.

ORGANIZE EDUCATIONAL PROGRAMS

Staff education programs such as "in-services" should be provided whenever new (dangerous) drugs are being used in the facility, if there are procedure changes, to discuss medical errors and prevention and if there are new therapeutic guidelines. Hopefully the information is unbiased and is not being provided in a skewed manner by drug company representatives. Many hospitals now limit the use of pharmaceutical companies to provide drug education (with meals to entice participation) due to the inherent bias.

DEVELOP AND USE STANDARD PROTOCOLS

Standard protocols for high-risk drugs increase the rate of appropriate prescribing based on published recommended guidelines and reduce the chance of errors due to inappropriate prescribing. The Joint Commission requires that standard order flow sheets should exist for all antithrombotics. The standard order sheet should include instructions for initial doses of warfarin and other high-risk antithrombotics, monitoring for bleeding, using appropriate antidotes, monitoring for HIT with heparin and discontinuing heparin if HIT is suspected. The prescriber should be required to justify any order outside the protocol and a pharmacist should approve the request.

IMPLEMENT COMPUTERIZED PRESCRIBER ORDER ENTRY (CPOE)

Computerized physician/provider order entry is a computer system that allows direct entry of medical orders by prescribers. Directly entering orders into a computer has the benefit of reducing errors by minimizing the ambiguity of hand-written orders. A much greater benefit is seen with the combination of CPOE and clinical decision support tools. Clinical guidelines and patient labs can be built-into the CPOE system and alerts can notify a prescriber if the drug is inappropriate, or if labs indicate the drug could be unsafe (such as a high potassium level and a new order for a potassium-sparing agent). CPOE can include standard order flow sheets. In addition to medication orders, CPOE is used for laboratory orders and procedures.

EDUCATE PATIENTS AND THEIR FAMILIES

Patients can play a vital role in preventing medication errors when they have been encouraged to ask questions and seek satisfactory answers about their medications before drugs are dispensed at a pharmacy. If a patient questions any part of the medication dispensing process, whether it is about the drug's appearance, or dose, or something else, the pharmacist must be receptive and responsive (not defensive). All patient inquiries should be thoroughly investigated before the medication is dispensed. The written information about the medications should be at a reading level that is comprehensible.

It may be necessary to provide pictograms or other means of instruction to patients who do not speak English or are unable to read English. In certain communities there is a high percentage of patients who are functionally illiterate, which may include many native English speakers. An inability to understand written English has no correlation with intelligence and does not imply an inability to understand simple instructions; it is still necessary for pharmacists to ensure that these patients understand how to use their medications safely.

MONITOR FOR DRUG-FOOD INTERACTIONS

Check for drug-food interactions routinely and have nutrition involved with this effort when drugs with a high rate of food interactions (such as warfarin) are ordered.

FOLLOW REQUIREMENTS FOR RISK EVALUATION AND MITIGATION STRATEGIES (REMS) DRUGS

REMS is an FDA program that requires specified training and various restrictions (patient requirements, user registries, etc.) on certain drugs. Examples include the clozapine patient registry, the APPRISE program for erythropoietin use in oncology, the iPLEDGE program for isotretinoin, and others. In 2011 the FDA began new REMS to reduce the misuse of long-acting opioids, which covers a lot of drugs (morphine extended-release, fentanyl patches, hydromorphone, oxycodone and oxymorphone, methadone and buprenorphine.) The list of REMS drugs keeps growing. When working your way through this book note the many drugs that have prescribing qualifications.

Patient Controlled Analgesic (PCA) Device Overview and Safety Concerns

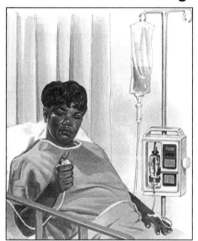

Opioids are effective agents used for moderate to severe post-surgical pain and are the mainstay of treatment. These may be administered through PCA devices. PCAs allow the patient to treat pain quickly (there is no need to call the nurse and wait for the dose to arrive.) They allow the administration of small doses, which helps reduce side effects (particularly over-sedation). However, as some patients will be opioid-naïve or receiving higher-than-normal doses post-surgically, anti-emetics or anti-histamines may be required. PCA drug delivery can mimic the pain pattern more closely and provide good pain control. Increasingly, the PCA is administered with anesthetics for a synergistic benefit in pain relief.

PCAs HAVE IMPORTANT SAFETY CONSIDERATIONS

- The devices can be complex and require set-up and programming. This is a significant cause of preventable medication errors. PCAs should be used only with well-coordinated health care teams.

- Patients may not be appropriate candidates for PCA treatment. They should be cooperative and should have a cognitive assessment prior to using the PCA to ensure they can follow instructions.

- Friends and family members should not administer PCA doses. This is a Joint Commission requirement.

- PCAs do not frequently cause respiratory depression, but the risk is still present. Advanced age, obesity and concurrent use of CNS depressants (in addition to higher opioid doses) increases risk.

WITH PCAs IT IS IMPORTANT TO FOLLOW THESE SAFETY STEPS

- Limit the opioids available in floor stock. Use standard orders (set drug dosages, especially for opioid-naïve patients) so that drugs are not over-dosed.

- Educate staff about HYDROmorphone and morphine mix-ups.

- Implement PCA protocols that include double-checking of the drug, pump setting, and dosage.

- The concentration on the <u>Medication Administration Record (MAR)</u> should match the PCA label.

- Use <u>bar-coding</u> technology. Some infusion pumps incorporate bar-coding technology. Scanning the barcode on the PCA bag would help ensure the correct concentration is entered during PCA programming. It will also ensure that the right patient is getting the medication.

- Assess the patient's <u>pain, sedation and respiratory rate</u> on a scheduled basis.

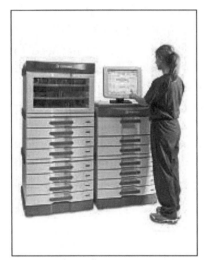

Automated Dispensing Cabinet Overview and Safety Concerns

Most pharmacy interns will have seen automated dispensing cabinets (ADCs) while on clinical rotations. Common names are *Pyxis, Omnicell* and *AccuDose.* Over half of the hospitals in the U.S. now use ADCs. In about half of these, the ADCs have replaced patient cassettes that had to be filled at least once daily and exchanged.

ADCs PROVIDE PRACTICAL BENEFITS

The drug inventory and medication can be automated when drugs are placed into the cabinet and removed. Controlled drug security can be improved (versus the previous method of keeping the controlled drugs locked in a metal cabinet or in a drawer in the nurses' station.) The drugs are easily available at the unit and do not require individual delivery from the pharmacy. ADCs provide alerts, usage reports and work well with bar-coding.

The Institute for Safe Medication Practices published *Guidance on the Interdisciplinary Safe Use of Automated Dispensing Cabinets* that discusses ways to avoid errors. The ISMP also has a "checklist" that institutions can use to make sure that they meet safe use recommendations.

ADCs HAVE IMPORTANT SAFETY CONSIDERATIONS

- Stocking errors, such as a drug being placed in an incorrect drawer or bin, can lead to the wrong drug being dispensed. (Bar code scanning can be used to make sure that the correct drug is being placed into the ADC or dispensed.)

- The wrong drug can be selected from the screen or ADC.

- The wrong dose can be selected from the screen.

- Errors can occur due to overrides that are not subject to a pharmacist's prospective order review.

METHODS TO IMPROVE ADC SAFETY

- <u>The Joint Commission requires that the pharmacist review the order before the medication can be removed from the ADC for a patient, except in special circumstances.</u> The override function should be limited to true emergencies and all overrides should be investigated.

- The most common error associated with ADC use is giving the wrong drug or dose to a patient. The patient medication administration records (MARs) should be accessible to practitioners while they are removing medications from the ADC. <u>Bar code scanning improves ADC safety.</u> The drug can be scanned to make sure it is going into the right place into the cabinet and can ensure that the right drug is being pulled. Prior to administration the patient's wrist band can be scanned to make sure the drug is going to the right patient.

- <u>Look-alike and sound-alike medications should be stored in different locations within the ADC.</u> Using computerized alerts, ideally pop-ups that require a confirmation, when medications with high potential for mix-up in a given setting are selected, can help reduce error risk. For example, to minimize morphine and hydromorphone confusion risk, the ADC screen may prompt, "This is DILAUDID. Is that correct?" whenever hydromorphone is selected.

- Certain medications should not be put into the ADCs, including warfarin and high-dose narcotics (such as hydromorphone 10 mg/mL and morphine 20 mg/mL.)

- Do not let nurses put medications back into the medication compartment because it might be placed in the wrong area; it is best to have a separate draw for all "returned" medications.

- If the machine is in a busy, noisy environment, or in one with poor lighting, errors increase. The ISMP recommendations for ADC safety suggest a careful evaluation of the unit prior to planning for installation or upgrades. Distractions undermine safety, in any setting. Distractions should be reduced when stocking or removing medications from ADCs. For example, answering cell phones while performing high-stakes activities impairs accuracy. Social exchanges with colleagues, patients, and family members should not occur at the ADC.

The California board specifically states that all drugs that are stocked in the ADC are restocked by a pharmacist or by an intern or technician working under the supervision of a pharmacist. Removable pockets or drawers transported between the pharmacy and a stocking facility must be transported in a secure tamper-evident container.

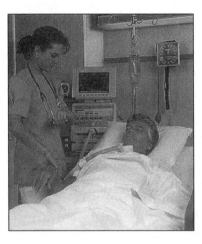

Infection Control in Hospitals

Nearly two million infections occur in hospitals annually – about one infection for every twenty patients. It is somewhat incredulous that so many patients enter hospitals for treatment of a condition and contract a different condition at the same facility.

The organisms in healthcare settings are highly pathogenic – this means that resistant bacteria are in the hospitals because that is where the sickest patients are and certain organisms grow in hospital settings, such as pseudomonas in the moist environment of the ventilator.

Hospital infections cause avoidable illness and death and add enormous financial costs. The worst part of this sad state of affairs is that many of these infections are preventable if proper techniques (which are often simple measures) are followed. Many states now require hospitals to report infection rates and Medicare has begun to refuse reimbursement for hospital-acquired infections that are largely avoidable.

COMMON TYPES OF HOSPITAL (NOSOCOMIAL) ACQUIRED INFECTIONS

- Urinary tract infections, from indwelling catheters (very common), remove the catheter as soon as possible) – preventing catheter associated infections is a new Joint Commission National Patient Safety Goal (NPSG) in 2012.

- Blood stream infections from IV lines (central lines have the highest risk) & catheters

- Surgical site infections (see the section on antibiotic prophylaxis in the ID chapter)

- Decubitis ulcers

- Hepatitis

- *Clostridium difficile*, other GI infections

- Pneumonia (mostly due to ventilator use), bronchitis

HAND HYGIENE

Many hospital infections are spread by hospital worker's hands and numerous studies show that proper hand hygiene reduces the spread of nosocomial infection. Patients are often carriers of resistant bacteria, including MRSA and VRE. Alcohol-based hand rubs (gel, rinse or foam) are considered more effective in the healthcare setting than plain soap or antimicrobial soap and water. Review the conditions below in which soap and water are preferable. Do not wear jewelry under gloves – these harbor bacteria and can tear the gloves. Keep fingernails clipped short and clean.

Antimicrobial hand soaps that contain chlorhexidine (*Hibiclens,* others) may be preferable to soap and water to reduce infections in healthcare facilities. Triclosan may also be better but this compound gets into the water supply and has environmental concerns.

When to Wash Hands

- Before entering and after leaving patient rooms.

- Between patient contacts if there is more than one patient per room.

- Before and after removing gloves (new gloves with each patient).

- Before handling invasive devices, including injections.

- After coughing or sneezing.

- Before handling food and oral medications.

Use Soap and Water (not alcohol-based rubs) in these situations

- Before eating.

- After using the restroom.

- Anytime there is visible soil (anything noticeable on the hands).

- After caring for a patient with diarrhea or known *C. difficile* or spore forming organisms – alcohol-based hand rubs have poor activity against spores.

- Before caring for patients with food allergies.

Soap and Water Technique

- Wet both sides of hands, apply soap, rub together for at least 15 (slow) seconds.

- Rinse thoroughly.

- Dry with paper towel and use the towel to turn off the water.

Alcohol-Based Hand Rubs Technique

- Use enough gel (2-5 mL or about the size of a quarter).

- Rub hands together until the rub dries (15-25 seconds).

- Hands should be completely dry before putting on gloves.

It is important to properly clean surfaces, including bed rails, eating trays, and other room surfaces. Health care professionals should be careful not to be sources of infection from contaminated clothing (including white coats and ties). Organisms that spread via surface contact include VRE, *C. difficile*, noroviruses and other intestinal tract pathogens.

UNIVERSAL PRECAUTIONS

In 1985, largely because of the HIV epidemic, isolation practices in the United States were altered dramatically by the introduction of a new strategy for isolation precautions, which became known as universal precautions (UP). (See recommendations for post-exposure prophylaxis in the HIV chapter.)

Blood is the single most important source of HIV, hepatitis, and other bloodborne pathogens in the occupational setting. Infection control efforts for bloodborne pathogens must focus on preventing exposures to blood as well as on delivery of hepatitis B (HBV) immunization. Although lower risk, there is still a chance of infection from other bodily fluids and universal precautions also apply to semen and vaginal secretions, tissues and to the following fluids: cerebrospinal fluid (CSF), synovial fluid, pleural fluid, peritoneal fluid, pericardial fluid and amniotic fluid.

A mask that covers both the nose and the mouth, and goggles or a face shield are worn by hospital personnel during procedures and patient care activities that are likely to generate splashes or sprays of blood, body fluids, secretions, or excretions in order to provide protection of the mucous membranes of the eyes, nose, and mouth from contact transmission of pathogens. Contaminated gloves, clothing or other equipment should be placed in appropriately labeled bags or containers.

As much as possible we should try to protect ourselves, colleagues and patients with vaccination. There are vaccinations for Hepatitis B and influenza, but none at present for Hepatitis C and HIV.

VACCINES FOR HEALTH CARE WORKERS

Hepatitis B

OSHA mandates that health care workers be vaccinated for Hepatitis B. Refer to the hepatitis and immunizations chapters for more information.

Influenza

Health care workers, including community and hospital pharmacists, should receive an annual (fall) influenza vaccine. This is especially important to reduce infection risk to others. Refer to the immunization chapter for more information.

PATIENT ISOLATION

Patients can be placed in isolation if they are high risk for getting an infection (such as bone marrow transplant patients) or if they have a highly contagious infection (such as VRE or tuberculosis).

Patients in isolation have clear signs outside their rooms. There should be a specific isolation cart outside the room with the required gown, gloves, or mask to be put on before entering the room. Regulated waste should be placed in closeable, leak proof containers and be appropriately labeled or color-coded. Even contaminated laundry has rules regulating management. It should be handled as little as possible and only when using personal protective equipment. It should be bagged at the location where it was used without any sorting or rinsing, and bagged in labeled or color-coded bags.

SAFE INJECTION PRACTICES

Outbreaks involving the transmission of blood borne pathogens or other microbial pathogens to patients (and occasionally to healthcare workers) continue to occur due to unsafe injection technique. The majority of safety breaches involve the reuse of syringes in multiple patients, contamination of IV bags with used syringes, failure to follow basic injection safety when administering IV medications and inappropriate care or maintenance of glucometer equipment that is used on multiple patients.

The following practices ensure safe injection practice:

- <u>Never reinsert used needles into a multiple-dose vial or solution container</u> (whenever possible, <u>use of single-dose vials is preferred over multiple-dose vials</u>, especially when medications will be administered to multiple patients.)

- Needles used for withdrawing blood or any other body fluid, or used for administering medications or other fluids should preferably have "engineered sharps protection" which reduces the risk of an exposure incident by a mechanism such as drawing the needle into the syringe barrel after use.

- To avoid contamination to the patient, <u>never touch the tip or plunger of a syringe.</u>

- Disposable needles contaminated with drugs, chemicals or blood products should never be removed from their original syringes unless no other option is available. <u>Throw the entire needle/syringe assembly (needle attached to the syringe) into the red plastic sharps container.</u>

- Never remove a needle by unscrewing it.

- Used disposable needles/sharps should be discarded immediately after use <u>without recapping</u> into a sharps container (a <u>non</u>-reusable <u>plastic</u> container that is puncture resistant, leak proof on the sides and bottom, properly labeled and closable).

- Sharps containers should be easily accessible, replaced routinely, and not allowed to overfill. <u>Never compress or "push down" on the contents of any sharps container.</u>

- If someone is stuck with a needle the proper department at the facility should be contacted immediately.

IV MEDICATION PREPARATION AND LAMINAR FLOW HOODS

Medications given intravenously bypass the protective mechanisms of the skin barrier and gastrointestinal tract. About half of medications given in the hospital setting are given IV. If the medication is contaminated the patient will suffer severe adverse effects and possible death.

Hoods are ventilation devices used to keep sterile compounded or parenteral drugs free of contaminants, and are used to keep the pharmacy area free of noxious fumes. Laminar flow means that the air is moving in an uninterrupted, constant stream. The air is drawn through a High Efficiency Particulate Air (HEPA) filter that catches particulates. The air is may be directed horizontally toward the user, as shown in the picture. Some laminar flow hoods move the air vertically. HEPA filters remove 99.97% of all air particles 0.3 mm or larger. This keeps the workspace area free of contaminants. The cabinet is stainless steel with a smooth design to keep out contaminants and is designed to reduce the risk of joints and other spaces where spores might accumulate.

Laminar Flow Hood Technique and Safety

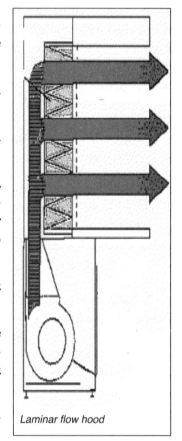

- Do not place objects lined up in front of each other in a laminar flow hood or the flow of air is interrupted. Items are placed side by side.

- Use a mask that covers the nose and mouth when working in the hood.

- Miscellaneous items (calculators, pens) should not be put in the hood.

- Any sterile component or supply (syringes, needles, ampules, etc.) should only be opened and/or removed from their packaging within the laminar-flow workspace. Do not tear paper open, it should be peeled open. Do not touch the syringe tip and plunger, even with gloved fingers.

- Preparation has to be at least six inches back from the front of the hood.

- The hood is kept operating continuously and all surfaces are cleaned prior to use from the back to the front. If for any reason the hood is turned off it should be turned on for at least 30 minutes prior to use and thoroughly cleaned.

- Since contamination can cause death, any product whose purity is in doubt should be discarded.

Laminar flow hood

Vertical flow hoods (also called biological safety cabinets or chemotherapy hoods) blow air from the top down to maintain sterility and to protect the pharmacist or technician preparing the medication from breathing in dangerous fumes. They are used for chemotherapy.

THE JOINT COMMISSION ON ACCREDITATION OF HEALTHCARE ORGANIZATIONS (JOINT COMMISSION, OR TJC)

The Joint Commission is an independent, not-for-profit organization that accredits and certifies more than 17,000 health care organizations and programs in the U.S. including hospitals, health care networks, long term care facilities, home care organizations, office-based surgery centers and independent laboratories. The Joint Commission focuses on the highest quality and safety of care and sets standards that institutions must meet to be accredited. An accredited organization must undergo an on-site survey at least every three years and surveys can be unannounced.

National patient safety goals (NPSGs) are set annually by the Joint Commission for different types of health care settings in order to improve patient safety. Hospital NPSGs include the following:

Reduce the likelihood of harm associated with anticoagulant therapy.

There are many elements to this goal, including the requirement to use standardized dosing protocols, monitoring INRs, using programmable pumps for heparin, and providing education to patients and families.

Maintain and communicate accurate patient medication information.

This includes medication reconciliation, providing written information to the patient and conducting discharge counseling.

Comply with the Centers for Disease Control (CDC) hand hygiene guidelines.

Proper hand hygiene technique as described previously.

Implement evidence-based practices to reduce health-care associated infections.

These include recommendations to reduce the likely sources of infection, such as from urinary catheters and ventilators.

Use at least two patient identifiers when providing care, treatment and services.

There have been countless medication errors (and surgical misadventures) due to patient misidentification. Two identifiers (such as name and medical record number) must be verified prior to administering medications, blood or blood components, taking lab samples or providing any treatment or procedure.

Conclusion

We are in an age where medication delivery is becoming more accountable and poor safety routines are no longer acceptable. Proactive assessment of safe medication use involves pharmacists at every step. Fortunately, we are over twenty years into the process and there is now a wide range of resources and information available to help us provide improved medication safety.

ISMP's List of *Error-Prone Abbreviations, Symbols,* and *Dose Designations*

The abbreviations, symbols, and dose designations found in this table have been reported to ISMP through the ISMP National Medication Errors Reporting Program (ISMP MERP) as being frequently misinterpreted and involved in harmful medication errors. They should **NEVER** be used when communicating medical information. This includes internal communications, telephone/verbal prescriptions, computer-generated labels, labels for drug storage bins, medication administration records, as well as pharmacy and prescriber computer order entry screens.

Abbreviations	Intended Meaning	Misinterpretation	Correction
μg	Microgram	Mistaken as "mg"	Use "mcg"
AD, AS, AU	Right ear, left ear, each ear	Mistaken as OD, OS, OU (right eye, left eye, each eye)	Use "right ear," "left ear," or "each ear"
OD, OS, OU	Right eye, left eye, each eye	Mistaken as AD, AS, AU (right ear, left ear, each ear)	Use "right eye," "left eye," or "each eye"
BT	Bedtime	Mistaken as "BID" (twice daily)	Use "bedtime"
cc	Cubic centimeters	Mistaken as "u" (units)	Use "mL"
D/C	Discharge or discontinue	Premature discontinuation of medications if D/C (intended to mean "discharge") has been misinterpreted as "discontinued" when followed by a list of discharge medications	Use "discharge" and "discontinue"
IJ	Injection	Mistaken as "IV" or "intrajugular"	Use "injection"
IN	Intranasal	Mistaken as "IM" or "IV"	Use "intranasal" or "NAS"
HS	Half-strength	Mistaken as bedtime	Use "half-strength" or "bedtime"
hs	At bedtime, hours of sleep	Mistaken as half-strength	
IU**	International unit	Mistaken as IV (intravenous) or 10 (ten)	Use "units"
o.d. or OD	Once daily	Mistaken as "right eye" (OD-oculus dexter), leading to oral liquid medications administered in the eye	Use "daily"
OJ	Orange juice	Mistaken as OD or OS (right or left eye); drugs meant to be diluted in orange juice may be given in the eye	Use "orange juice"
Per os	By mouth, orally	The "os" can be mistaken as "left eye" (OS-oculus sinister)	Use "PO," "by mouth," or "orally"
q.d. or QD**	Every day	Mistaken as q.i.d., especially if the period after the "q" or the tail of the "q" is misunderstood as an "i"	Use "daily"
qhs	Nightly at bedtime	Mistaken as "qhr" or every hour	Use "nightly"
qn	Nightly or at bedtime	Mistaken as "qh" (every hour)	Use "nightly" or "at bedtime"
q.o.d. or QOD**	Every other day	Mistaken as "q.d." (daily) or "q.i.d. (four times daily) if the "o" is poorly written	Use "every other day"
q1d	Daily	Mistaken as q.i.d. (four times daily)	Use "daily"
q6PM, etc.	Every evening at 6 PM	Mistaken as every 6 hours	Use "daily at 6 PM" or "6 PM daily"
SC, SQ, sub q	Subcutaneous	SC mistaken as SL (sublingual); SQ mistaken as "5 every;" the "q" in "sub q" has been mistaken as "every" (e.g., a heparin dose ordered "sub q 2 hours before surgery" misunderstood as every 2 hours before surgery)	Use "subcut" or "subcutaneously"
ss	Sliding scale (insulin) or ½ (apothecary)	Mistaken as "55"	Spell out "sliding scale;" use "one-half" or "½"
SSRI	Sliding scale regular insulin	Mistaken as selective-serotonin reuptake inhibitor	Spell out "sliding scale (insulin)"
SSI	Sliding scale insulin	Mistaken as Strong Solution of Iodine (Lugol's)	
i/d	One daily	Mistaken as "tid"	Use "1 daily"
TIW or tiw	3 times a week	Mistaken as "3 times a day" or "twice in a week"	Use "3 times weekly"
U or u**	Unit	Mistaken as the number 0 or 4, causing a 10-fold overdose or greater (e.g., 4U seen as "40" or 4u seen as "44"); mistaken as "cc" so dose given in volume instead of units (e.g., 4u seen as 4cc)	Use "unit"
UD	As directed ("ut dictum")	Mistaken as unit dose (e.g., diltiazem 125 mg IV infusion "UD" misinterpreted as meaning to give the entire infusion as a unit [bolus] dose)	Use "as directed"

Dose Designations and Other Information	Intended Meaning	Misinterpretation	Correction
Trailing zero after decimal point (e.g., 1.0 mg)**	1 mg	Mistaken as 10 mg if the decimal point is not seen	Do not use trailing zeros for doses expressed in whole numbers
"Naked" decimal point (e.g., .5 mg)**	0.5 mg	Mistaken as 5 mg if the decimal point is not seen	Use zero before a decimal point when the dose is less than a whole unit
Abbreviations such as mg. or mL. with a period following the abbreviation	mg mL	The period is unnecessary and could be mistaken as the number 1 if written poorly	Use mg, mL, etc. without a terminal period

ISMP's List of *Error-Prone Abbreviations, Symbols,* and *Dose Designations* (continued)

Dose Designations and Other Information	Intended Meaning	Misinterpretation	Correction
Drug name and dose run together (especially problematic for drug names that end in "l" such as Inderal40 mg; Tegretol300 mg)	Inderal 40 mg Tegretol 300 mg	Mistaken as Inderal 140 mg Mistaken as Tegretol 1300 mg	Place adequate space between the drug name, dose, and unit of measure
Numerical dose and unit of measure run together (e.g., 10mg, 100mL)	10 mg 100 mL	The "m" is sometimes mistaken as a zero or two zeros, risking a 10- to 100-fold overdose	Place adequate space between the dose and unit of measure
Large doses without properly placed commas (e.g., 100000 units; 1000000 units)	100,000 units 1,000,000 units	100000 has been mistaken as 10,000 or 1,000,000; 1000000 has been mistaken as 100,000	Use commas for dosing units at or above 1,000, or use words such as 100 "thousand" or 1 "million" to improve readability

Drug Name Abbreviations	Intended Meaning	Misinterpretation	Correction
To avoid confusion, do not abbreviate drug names when communicating medical information. Examples of drug name abbreviations involved in medication errors include:			
ARA A	vidarabine	Mistaken as cytarabine (ARA C)	Use complete drug name
AZT	zidovudine (Retrovir)	Mistaken as azathioprine or aztreonam	Use complete drug name
CPZ	Compazine (prochlorperazine)	Mistaken as chlorpromazine	Use complete drug name
DPT	Demerol-Phenergan-Thorazine	Mistaken as diphtheria-pertussis-tetanus (vaccine)	Use complete drug name
DTO	Diluted tincture of opium, or deodorized tincture of opium (Paregoric)	Mistaken as tincture of opium	Use complete drug name
HCl	hydrochloric acid or hydrochloride	Mistaken as potassium chloride (The "H" is misinterpreted as "K")	Use complete drug name unless expressed as a salt of a drug
HCT	hydrocortisone	Mistaken as hydrochlorothiazide	Use complete drug name
HCTZ	hydrochlorothiazide	Mistaken as hydrocortisone (seen as HCT250 mg)	Use complete drug name
MgSO4**	magnesium sulfate	Mistaken as morphine sulfate	Use complete drug name
MS, MSO4**	morphine sulfate	Mistaken as magnesium sulfate	Use complete drug name
MTX	methotrexate	Mistaken as mitoxantrone	Use complete drug name
PCA	procainamide	Mistaken as patient controlled analgesia	Use complete drug name
PTU	propylthiouracil	Mistaken as mercaptopurine	Use complete drug name
T3	Tylenol with codeine No. 3	Mistaken as liothyronine	Use complete drug name
TAC	triamcinolone	Mistaken as tetracaine, Adrenalin, cocaine	Use complete drug name
TNK	TNKase	Mistaken as "TPA"	Use complete drug name
ZnSO4	zinc sulfate	Mistaken as morphine sulfate	Use complete drug name

Stemmed Drug Names	Intended Meaning	Misinterpretation	Correction
"Nitro" drip	nitroglycerin infusion	Mistaken as sodium nitroprusside infusion	Use complete drug name
"Norflox"	norfloxacin	Mistaken as Norflex	Use complete drug name
"IV Vanc"	intravenous vancomycin	Mistaken as Invanz	Use complete drug name

Symbols	Intended Meaning	Misinterpretation	Correction
ʒ	Dram	Symbol for dram mistaken as "3"	Use the metric system
♏	Minim	Symbol for minim mistaken as "mL"	
x3d	For three days	Mistaken as "3 doses"	Use "for three days"
> and <	Greater than and less than	Mistaken as opposite of intended; mistakenly use incorrect symbol; "< 10" mistaken as "40"	Use "greater than" or "less than"
/ (slash mark)	Separates two doses or indicates "per"	Mistaken as the number 1 (e.g., "25 units/10 units" misread as "25 units and 110" units)	Use "per" rather than a slash mark to separate doses
@	At	Mistaken as "2"	Use "at"
&	And	Mistaken as "2"	Use "and"
+	Plus or and	Mistaken as "4"	Use "and"
°	Hour	Mistaken as a zero (e.g., q2° seen as q 20)	Use "hr," "h," or "hour"

**These abbreviations are included on The Joint Commission's "minimum list" of dangerous abbreviations, acronyms, and symbols that must be included on an organization's "Do Not Use" list, effective January 1, 2004. Visit www.jointcommission.org for more information about this Joint Commission requirement.

www.ismp.org

FDA (U.S.) DRUG DEVELOPMENT PROCESS

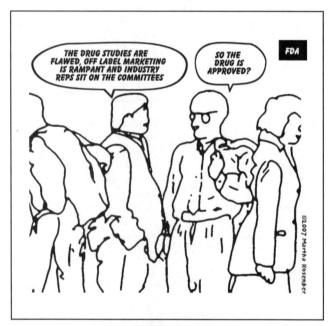

REFERENCE

http://www.fda.gov/drugs/developmen-
tapprovalprocess/default.htm

Overview

The U.S. drug approval process is overseen by the Food and Drug Administration's (FDA) Center for Drug Evaluation and Research (CDER). The FDA is an important organization in safeguarding public health. A notable example that emphasizes this point was the refusal of Dr. Frances Oldham Kelsey to approve thalidomide as an antiemetic for use in pregnancy. In the 1950's and 60's thalidomide was given to pregnant women in other countries, and caused thousands of cases of severe birth defects including missing long bones. This case is considered one of the worst examples of medication-induced tragedy. Fortunately, the American consumer was largely protected by the heroic action of one FDA administrator.

The information below is for prescription drugs. For OTC products, a manufacturer either begins with the NDA process described below or submits an OTC monograph. Each OTC drug monograph is a "recipe book" covering acceptable ingredients, doses, formulations, labeling, and, in some cases, testing parameters.

For prescription drugs, the drug approval process begins with pre-clinical (animal) research, which is followed by an Investigational New Drug (IND) application. [Or, if the company is requesting approval of a generic drug they file an Abbreviated New Drug Application (ANDA)].

Federal law requires an IND in place before a drug is transported or distributed across state lines. Because a manufacturer will want to ship the investigational drug to clinical investigators in many states, it must seek an exemption from that legal requirement. The IND is the means through which the sponsor technically obtains this exemption from the FDA. The clinical trial process follows and is outlined in a chart. Note that each phase includes safety analysis.

Phase I studies focus on the safety and pharmacology of a compound. Low doses of the compound are given to a small group of healthy volunteers who are closely supervised. In cases of severe or life-threatening illnesses, volunteers with the disease may be used.

Phase II studies examine the effectiveness of a compound. Patients without complications and co-morbidities are often selected for a trial to reduce the number of confounding variables that may influence the trial results. Enrolling healthier individuals allows the potential benefit of the drug to be more clearly demonstrated. It is common in phase 2 trials to have 3 or 4 arms of the study; each investigating different doses for the best therapeutic benefit and minimal side effect profile.

After phase II, the manufacturer meets with the FDA to pave way for the "pivotal trials." Phase III trial designs must obtain FDA approval before enrollment can begin. During phase III, researchers try to confirm previous findings in a larger population. These studies usually last from 2 to 10 years and typically involve thousands of patients across multiple sites.

After Phase III, the manufacturer files a New Drug Application (NDA). Once the NDA is filed, the FDA has one year to review all the data and provide its decision to the manufacturer/researcher. The NDA can either be approved or rejected, or the FDA may request further study before making a decision. Following acceptance, the FDA can also request that the manufacturer conduct additional post-marketing studies (AKA phase IV). Fast-track approval (decision from the FDA is expected within 6 months) may be given to agents that show promise in treating serious, life-threatening medical conditions for which no other drug either exists or works well.

Importance of Phase IV

For some drugs the total drug approval process is limited to a few hundred patients – while in others, such as cardiovascular drugs, tens of thousands of subjects can be included. If a drug is tested in a relatively small number of patients, the complete safety profile may be missed. Even in larger trials, safety issues may be missed due to the exclusion of certain patient types. The FDA may request a post-marketing, or phase IV, study to examine the risks and benefits of the new drug in a different population or to conduct special monitoring in a high-risk population. The phase IV study can also be used to assess such issues as the longer term effects of drug exposure, to optimize the dose for marketing, to evaluate the effects in pediatric patients, or to examine the effectiveness of the drug for additional indications.

PHASE	PURPOSE	SUBJECTS	SCOPE	LENGTH OF TIME
I	Safety profile and dosing range, PK/PD, open label, often 1 center, may not be done in the US	Can be healthy volunteers or patients with illness	20-80 subjects	6-12 months
II	Safety and efficacy (dose response) IIa – proof of concept; pilot study, etc. IIb- well-controlled target population	Used in intended population	100-300 patients	1-2 years
III	Safety and efficacy at the dose and schedule you are seeking approval (package labeling) IIIb – post NDA –submission trial looking at additional indications	Subjects with indications the drug is seeking	Hundreds to thousands of patients	2-3 years
IV	New indications, QOL, surveillance studies	Subjects with indications the drug is seeking	Hundreds to thousands	1-5 years

For changes to an existing drug, the Supplemental New Drug Application (SNDA) is used. These changes include:

- Labeling changes

- New dose

- New strength

- New manufacturing process

NATURAL PRODUCTS & VITAMINS

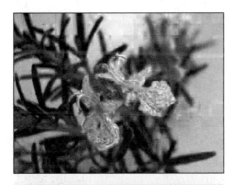

REFERENCE

Natural Medicines Database, available at www.naturaldatabase.com

Shapiro, K. Natural Products: A Case-Based Approach for Health Care Professionals, APhA, Washington, D.C. 2007.

Background

Natural product use has a long history of traditional use among native cultures and has become popular today. Many patients supplement their diet or prescription medicines with vitamins or natural products. Natural product is an umbrella term that includes herbals (plant products), vitamins and many substances that are not plant-derived but exist in nature, such as glucosamine from shellfish.

Most natural products act as either mild drugs or are harmless. Pharmacists have accessible sources to check for drug interactions, safety concerns, dosage by indication, and quality. Some natural products pose health risks. A few top safety concerns include manufacturing quality, safety and effectiveness, and the use of a few select agents that can pose specific problems in certain patients:

- <u>Manufacturing may not follow good manufacturing practices (GMP);</u> pharmacists need to help consumers choose a reputable product. In recent years quality companies have put in place programs that will put a seal of approval on products made by a company following good manufacturing practices. The website consumerlab.com is useful to help choose a reputable product – this is an independent testing service that analyzes the content of many popular supplements.

- <u>A dietary supplement manufacturer does not have to prove a product's safety and effectiveness before it is marketed.</u> For example: late-night TV ads are promoting a thyroid product to help with low energy and fatigue. Perhaps some patients need a thyroid supplement, but this requires lab testing. If people who do not need thyroid hormone take it, they can become hyperthyroid and be subject to cardiovascular and other health risks. The product quality may be poor – this can be a particular issue with thyroid hormone which may contain prions that can carry mad cow disease. Last but not least, the product used in this example is expensive. Generic levothyroxine, a safer alternative, is pennies per tablet.

- Three areas of particular safety concern are natural products that increase bleeding risk, interactions between prescription drugs and St. John's wort and natural products that may be hepatotoxic.

  ❑ <u>Ginkgo biloba and other agents that can ↑ bleeding risk</u>

  ❑ Ginkgo biloba <u>increases bleeding risk</u> with <u>no effect on the INR</u>. Other natural products that can also pose a risk include bromelains, danshen, dong quai (this product may ↑ INR), vitamin E, evening primrose oil, high doses of fish oils, garlic, ginseng, glucosamine, grapefruit, policosanol, and willow bark.

  ❑ <u>Enzyme induction by St. John's wort</u>: this herbal is a "broad-spectrum" inducer and cannot be used with oral contraceptives, transplant drugs, warfarin, among others. St. John's wort induces 3A4 >> 2C9 > 1A2. See the Drug Interactions chapter for more information.

  ❑ <u>Natural products may be hepatotoxic</u> (chaparral, comfrey, kava). If liver enzymes are elevated, check with the patient – sometimes the use of "tea blends" or mixtures can be contributory.

SAFETY/FINANCIAL COMMENTS ON HOMEOPATHIC PRODUCTS AND MEDICAL FOODS

<u>Homeopathic Products: Homeopathy is based on "the law of similars" or the concept that "like is cured by like."</u> This is the belief that giving very small amounts of the illness (so dilute that the original substance cannot be measured) will protect the patient or cure them of an illness. Most evidence does not support validity to homeopathy, however many adherents (including the Queen of England) are advocates. The remedies may be providing a placebo benefit, or, may actually be labeled as homeopathic but contain measurable concentrations of drugs. In 2010, *Hyland's Teething Tablets* were recalled due to cases of belladonna toxicity. The amount of belladonna could be measured and was unsafe. It is tempting to use the term "homeopathic" on a label. It sounds nice, and if a manufacturer labels a product "homeopathic," they are permitted to make health claims, while natural products are not allowed by law to claim benefit for particular conditions. There have been other recent examples of products labeled as homeopathic which actually were not. Check the ingredients.

<u>Medical Foods: These are products that can also make health claims, since they are not FDA-approved drugs.</u> Medical foods are supposed to meet a nutritional need for a group that cannot be met with usual foods, such as specific formulations of enteral nutrition. A recent medical food that many pharmacists will have seen is a formulation of <u>folic acid</u> called *Deplin* that is being marketed for help in <u>treating depression</u>. The ad for this product states that "*Deplin* is a medical food containing L-methylfolate, the active form of the vitamin, folate. It is the only folate that can be taken up by the brain where it helps balance the chemical messengers that affect mood (serotonin, norepinephrine and dopamine)." It is less expensive to use over-the-counter folic acid supplements and there is no evidence that this supplement would provide more

VITAMINS	NAMES
Vitamin A	Retinol
Vitamin B1	Thiamine
Vitamin B12	Cobalamin
Vitamin B2	Riboflavin
Vitamin B3	Niacin
Vitamin B6	Pyridoxine
Vitamin B9	Folic Acid
Vitamin C	Ascorbic Acid

benefit, however the manufacturer can make this claim since it is a medical food. In a medical food, all ingredients must be Generally Recognized as Safe (G.R.A.S.) or be approved food additives. Most of the medical foods have Rx-only on the label and have NDC numbers.

Commonly Used Natural Products

CONDITION	TREATMENT
Anxiety	Valerian, lemon balm, glutamine, passion flower and hops (both as teas), chamomile tea, theanine and skullcap. Kava is used as a relaxant but can damage the liver and should not be recommended. Valerian may rarely be hepatotoxic (or some valerian products may have been contaminated with liver toxins); this is unclear at present. Passionflower is rated as "possibly effective" by the Natural Medicines Database. For most of the other agents the evidence is less robust but individual patients may get benefit from the various agents.
Sleep	Melatonin (also used for jet lag – carefully check doses for this use), valerian. Chamomile tea may help people relax. St. John's wort may help if the insomnia is due to depression (worry) but will lower levels of many other drugs. Kava is used but can damage the liver and should not be recommended.
ADHD	Fish oil supplements (which provide omega 3 fatty acids) with or without evening primrose oil (which provides omega-6 fatty acids) may be helpful in some patients.
Apthous Ulcers (canker sores)	Lysine
Cancer	Beta carotene, fish oil, black or green tea, garlic, soy, vitamins A and D Colon cancer: calcium Prostate cancer: lycopene (in cooked tomatoes)
Cholesterol	Fish oils (triglycerides), red yeast rice (monitor liver – may contain small amounts of an HMG CoA reductase inhibitor), plant sterols/stanols
Depression	St. John's wort, SAMe (do not use with MAO Is), fish oils, 5-HTP, tryptophan, glutamine, inositol (for OCD and panic disorder). Caution with induction and substrate drugs – see above.
Colds and Flu	Echinacea, elderberry, garlic, zinc, vitamin C. Caution for loss of smell (possibly permanent) with zinc nasal sprays and swabs.
Dementia/Memory	Ginkgo, huperzine A, vitamin E. Caution with ginkgo for increased bleeding risk.
Diabetes	Bitter melon, gymnema, chromium, alpha lipoic acid, cinnamon, acetyl-l-carnitine (neuropathy). Green tea may lower DM risk.
Energy/Weight Loss	Guarana, bitter orange; caution with bitter orange (similar to ephedra, CVD risk) and guarana (caffeine, caution with excessive intake.)
UTI	Cranberry. Caution on the risk of kidney stones with cranberry supplements.
Gastrointestinal Distress	Peppermint oil, chamomile tea
IBD	Cascara, senna (stimulant laxatives) for constipation. For diarrhea, psyllium (in *Metamucil* and many other formulations) or other "bulk-forming" fiber products can be useful. Peppermint (oil, sometimes teas) can be useful as an antispasmodic. Some use chamomile tea. The probiotic Lactobacillus or bifidobacterium infantis may help reduce abdominal pain, bloating, urgency, constipation or diarrhea in some patients. Antibiotics and probiotics are not taken together; separate the dosing by at least two hours. Fish oils (for the EPA and DHA, omega fatty acid components) are being used, although the evidence for benefit is contradictory. Indian frankincense gum resin taken TID may be beneficial for UC, based on preliminary studies. Comfrey is used for GI issues but can damage the liver and should not be recommended.

Commonly Used Natural Products Continued

CONDITION	TREATMENT
Probiotics	Lactobacillus, bifidobacterium infantis etc – check the efficacy of the individual probiotic for the condition – they vary. Separate probiotics from antibiotics or they will get destroyed by the drug.
Heart Health/Heart Failure	Coenzyme Q10, arginine (do not use with blood pressure meds – additive effect), fish oils, grape seed extract (grape seed extract used as a general health antioxidant and for atherosclerosis), garlic (mild decrease in blood pressure), hawthorne (caution – has additive effects with other drugs – can cause hypotension, dizziness with beta blockers, digoxin, calcium channel blockers, nitrates and PDE5-Is.)
Inflammation	Fish oils, willow bark (a salicylate)
Liver	Milk thistle
Menopausal Symptoms	Black cohosh (in popular menopause product Remifemin, generally safe, but reports of liver toxicity, some get GI upset), dong quai, red clover, evening primrose. Caution with dong quai and increased INR in patients using warfarin.
Migraine/Headache	Feverfew, willow bark, butterbur, guarana (a caffeine product), fish oils, magnesium, coenzyme Q10 and riboflavin. Combinations of these may be helpful.
Motion Sickness/Nausea	Ginger, peppermint
Osteoporosis	Soy, ipriflavone, calcium, vitamin D
Osteoarthritis	Glucosamine (may raise INR), Chondroitin, SAMe (do not use with MAO Is)
Prostate enlargement	Saw palmetto is used for BPH, but it is rated as "possibly ineffective" by The Natural Medicines Database. If men wish to try saw palmetto, they should be counseled to be seen first to rule out the possibility of prostate cancer and receive treatment, if needed. Pygeum is another natural product, and may be useful. Do not recommend a pygeum product unless it has been harvested ethically; ripping the bark off the trees to extract pygeum is not sustainable. Another natural product that may be useful is beta-sitosterol, which comes as supplements, in margarine substitutes, in African wild potato extract products, in pumpkin seed and in soy and red clover. Rye grass pollen is used, including commonly in Europe. (Lycopene is used for prostate cancer prevention, however there is not good evidence for taking supplements for this purpose.)
Skin	Aloe vera, Tea tree oil is used for a variety of skin conditions. It can be useful for treating acne. It may be helpful for onychomycosis symptoms (depending on the dose and application schedule), but is not useful in eradicating the infection in most patients. Tea tree oil may also be useful for athlete's foot symptoms if the 10% oil is used (not tea tree cream). Higher concentrations (25 or 50%) can cure the infection in up to half of patients, but are not as effective as the recommended antifungal agents. This efficacy data is from the Natural Medicines Database.

Vitamin Supplementation

People who consume an adequate diet do not require vitamin supplementation. However, many people eat poor diets. It is concerning to health care professionals that calcium and vitamin D intake remains insufficient for the majority of adults and children. Folic acid intake among women of child-bearing age can be insufficient. If thiamine (vitamin B1) is insufficient, this can cause Wernicke's encephalopathy. Symptoms of Wernicke's include ataxia, tremor and vision changes. A lack of vitamin B1 is common in alcoholism, and can be due to malabsorption, including from Crohn's, after obesity surgery, with advanced HIV and from a few other conditions. As the symptoms of Wernicke's fade, Korsakoff syndrome tends to develop (also called Korsakoff psychosis), which is permanent neurologic (mental) damage. Pharmacists are part of the solution to problems associated with vitamin deficiencies.

CALCIUM SUPPLEMENTATION

All prescription medicines for low bone density require adequate calcium and vitamin D supplementation taken concurrently (if dietary Intake is inadequate). Dietary intake of calcium should be assessed first, and supplements used if insufficient. Over half of the US population has low calcium and vitamin D intake. Adequate calcium intake is required throughout life, and is critically important in children (who can build bone stores), in pregnancy (when the fetus can deplete the mother's stores if intake is insufficient) and during the years around menopause, when bone loss is rapid. Vitamin D is required for calcium absorption, and low levels contribute to various health conditions, including autoimmune conditions and cancer. In 2010 there were news reports that calcium supplementation may increase heart attack risk; at present, recommend that patients use the recommended levels and use calcium with vitamin D – the increased risk was seen in patients who did not use vitamin D with calcium. Keep in mind that increased vitamin D intake will increase calcium absorption, and this may affect the amount of calcium required.

NIH's Recommended Adequate Intakes (AIs) for Calcium (2010)

AGE	MALE	FEMALE	PREGNANT	LACTATING
0-6 months	210 mg	210 mg		
7-12 months	270 mg	270 mg		
1-3 years	500 mg	500 mg		
4-8 years	800 mg	800 mg		
9-13 years	1,300 mg	1,300 mg		
14-18 years	1,300 mg	1,300 mg	1,300 mg	1,300 mg
19-50 years	1,000 mg	1,000 mg	1,000 mg	1,000 mg
50+ years	1,200 mg	1,200 mg		

Notes on calcium selection & absorption

- Calcium absorption is saturable; doses should be divided.

- Dietary calcium is generally not sufficient; most women need an additional 600-900 mg/day (2 to 3 dairy portions) to reach recommended levels.

- Calcium requires vitamin D for absorption (see below).

- Calcium citrate (*Citracal*, etc) has better absorption but is a larger pill to swallow and can be taken with or without food; usually tab has 315 mg calcium. It may be preferable with little or no stomach acid – such as with the use of H$_2$RAs and PPIs, which have been shown to increase fracture risk due to impaired calcium carbonate absorption (including dietary calcium.)

- Calcium carbonate (*Oscal, Tums*, etc) has acid-dependent absorption and should be taken with meals; usually tab is 500-600 mg.

- There is no known benefit of using more expensive formulations – recommend products made by reputable manufacturers, since lead may be present in untested products.

- Both forms come as chewables and in food products.

VITAMIN D SUPPLEMENTATION

The NIH's recommended intake for vitamin D for people up to age 70 years is 600 IU daily, and 71+ years is 800 IU daily. However, these levels are currently controversial and many endocrinologists are recommending a higher intake of 800-2000 IU daily. This is based on the recognition that low vitamin D levels is associated with a variety of health conditions – and the fact that many Americans have low vitamin D levels. A few years ago vitamin D levels were not routinely ordered; this has become commonplace.

The 50,000 unit vitamin D2 supplement (the green capsules) are used in renal disease or short-term in adults with deficiency to replenish stores. Cholecalciferol, or vitamin D3, is the preferred source, although vitamin D2 is often the type in supplements and will provide benefit. For information on vitamin D supplementation in renal disease, refer to the renal chapter.

FOLIC ACID

Any woman planning to conceive (and all women of child-bearing age) should be taking a folic acid supplement (400 - 800 mcg/daily, which is 0.4-0.8 mg/daily) to help prevent birth defects of the brain and spinal cord (neural tube defects). Folic acid needs to be taken at least one month before pregnancy and continued for the first 2-3 months of pregnancy. Once pregnant, the woman is likely taking a prescription prenatal vitamin and this is continued throughout since it also contains calcium (not enough, about 200 mg) and some iron. Folic acid is in many healthy foods, including fortified cereals (some of which are not healthy), dried beans, leafy green vegetables and orange juice. Multivitamins usually contain an amount in the recommended range. Prescription prenatal vitamins usually contain 1000 mcg, or 1 mg, of folic acid. The newer birth control pill *Beyaz* contains folate, however it less expensive to use a different birth control pill with a supplement. *Beyaz* contains the potassium-sparing progestin drospirenone, with ethinyl estradiol and folate.

VITAMIN E

It is unusual to have a vitamin E deficiency, since it is present in many foods. Vitamin E in foods is considered healthy, but excess intake in supplements is considered a health risk (particularly CVD risk); patients should not be exceeding 150 IU daily.

VITAMIN REQUIREMENTS FOR BABIES AND CHILDREN

Most children do not need vitamins, except as listed per the American Academy of Pediatrics:

- Exclusively breastfed infants or babies drinking less than 1 liter of baby formula need 400 IU of vitamin D daily (can use *Poly-Vi-Sol* or generic).

- Older children who do not drink at least 4 cups of Vitamin D fortified milk also need Vitamin D supplements.

IRON REQUIREMENTS FOR INFANTS & CHILDREN

0-4 months

- Supplemental iron not required.

4-6 months

- Formulas contain adequate iron; supplementation not required.

- Breast-fed babies need 1 mg/kg/day from 4-6 months old and until consuming iron-rich foods. At about 6 months most breast-fed babies get about half their calories from other foods.

6-12 months

- Need 11 mg/day of iron. Food sources are preferred; supplement as needed.

1-3 years old

- Need 7 mg/day of iron. Food sources are preferred; supplement as needed.

Adolescent girls

- At risk of anemia once they begin menstruating.

Iron-only supplements (generics available) – check bottle on iron drops because the iron mg/dropper ranges from 10-15 mg

- *Fer-In-Sol* Iron Supplement Drops

- *Feosol* Tablets and Caplets

Vitamin Supplements with Iron

- *Poly-Vi-Sol* Vitamin Drops With Iron: use if they need the vitamin D and iron

- Or others, such as: *Flintstones* Children's Chewable Multivitamin plus Iron, *Pokemon* Children's Multiple Vitamin with Iron, and store brands

DRUG INTERACTIONS

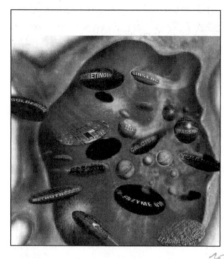

Background

CYP 450 enzymes are found in many cells, but are primarily located in the liver and intestine. The majority of drugs (75%) are metabolized by CYP 450 enzymes, and half of these are metabolized by CYP 450 3A4.

- Substrates are drugs that are metabolized by the CYP 450 enzymes.

- Inducers result in higher levels of enzymes, which ↓ levels of the substrate drugs.

- Inhibitors inactivate enzymes (causing less drug metabolism), and ↑ levels of the substrate drugs.

Note that the opposite will occur with "pro-drugs" – these are converted to the active form by the enzyme. Inhibitors will ↓ levels of the pro-drug (the drug cannot be converted to active form), and inducers will ↑ levels of the pro-drug.

P-glycoproteins (P-gp) are efflux transporters found in the gut and other organs. They pump drugs back into the gut (out of the bloodstream). If a drug is subject to efflux, and the transporter is inhibited by a different drug, the substrate drug concentration will increase. Drugs that are known to inhibit P-gp include cyclosporine, ketoconazole, itraconazole, lopinavir/ritonavir, ritonavir, indinavir/ritonavir, conivaptan, erythromycin, verapamil, quinidine and St. John's wort. Dabigatran *(Pradaxa)* and rivaroxaban *(Xarelto)* are P-gp substrates and will be subject to changes in concentration with P-gp inducers/inhibitors.

Inducers and Inhibitors included here are moderate or strong. The FDA characterizes strong inhibitors as drugs that cause ≥ 5-fold increase in the plasma AUC values or more than an 80% decrease in the substrate clearance. A moderate inhibitor is one that caused a ≥ 2 but < 5-fold increase.

QUICK STUDY TOOL
See more complete list of inducers and inhibitors below

PS PORCS (BIG INDUCERS)

Phenytoin

Smoking

Phenobarbital

Oxcarbazepine

Rifampin (and rifabutin, rifapentine)

Carbamazepine (and is an auto-inducer)

St. John's wort

G ♥ PACMAN (BIG INHIBITORS)

Grapefruit

♥

PIs Protease Inhibitors (don't miss ritonavir) but check all PIs since many are potent inhibitors

Azole antifungals, the agents that are used oral and IV: fluconazole, itraconazole, ketoconazole, posaconazole and voriconazole

C that's cimetidine, the H$_2$RA that is the most difficult to use due to DIs and androgen-blocking effects (that can cause gynecomastia – swollen, or painful breast tissue or impotence)

Macrolides (clarithromycin and erythromycin), not azithromycin, but DO include the related compound telithromycin

Amiodarone (and dronedarone)

Non-DHP CCBs diltiazem and verapamil

CYTOCHROME P 450 SUBSTRATES, INDUCERS, AND INHIBITORS

CLASS	SUBSTRATES	INDUCERS	INHIBITORS
3A4	alfentanil, alfuzosin, alprazolam, amiodarone, amlodipine, amprenavir, aprepitant, atazanavir, apomorphine, aripiprazole, atazanavir, atorvastatin, buprenorphine, buspirone, carbamazepine, citalopram, clarithromycin, dapsone, delavirdine, diazepam, diltiazem, dutasteride, efavirenz, eplerenone, erythromycin, escitalopram, esomeprazole, estrogens, felbamate, fentanyl, fosamprenavir, haloperidol, hydrocodone, indinavir, ketoconazole, lansoprazole, levonorgestrel, lidocaine, lopinavir, losartan, mirtazapine, modafinil, nateglinide, nelfinavir, nevirapine, nifedipine, omeprazole, ondansetron, oxycodone, progesterone, propoxyphene, quinidine, rabeprazole, ranolazine, repaglinide, ritonavir, rivaroxaban, saquinavir, sildenafil, simvastatin, sirolimus, tadalafil, tipranavir, tramadol, trazodone, vardenafil, venlafaxine, verapamil, (R)-warfarin, zolpidem	carbamazepine, oxcarbazepine, phenytoin, phenobarbital, primidone, rifabutin, rifampin, rifapentine, smoking, St. John's wort	amiodarone, amprenavir, aprepitant, atazanavir, cimetidine, clarithromycin, cyclosporine, delavirdine, diltiazem, efavirenz, erythromycin, fluconazole, fluvoxamine, fosamprenavir, grapefruit juice, haloperidol, indinavir, isoniazid, itraconazole, ketoconazole, lidocaine, metronidazole, nefazodone, nelfinavir, nevirapine, posaconazole, propofol, quinidine, ranolazine, ritonavir, saquinavir, sertraline, telithromycin, verapamil, voriconazole

Cytochrome P 450 Substrates, Inducers, and Inhibitors Continued

CLASS	SUBSTRATES	INDUCERS	INHIBITORS
1A2	alosetron, amitriptyline, clozapine, cyclobenzaprine, duloxetine, estradiol, methadone, mirtazapine, olanzapine, pimozide, propranolol, rasagiline, ropinirole, theophylline, (R)-warfarin	carbamazepine, estrogen, phenobarbital, phenytoin, primidone, rifampin, ritonavir, smoking, St. John's wort	cimetidine, ciprofloxacin, clarithromycin, erythromycin, fluvoxamine, gemfibrozil, isoniazid, ketoconazole, zileuton
2C8	amiodarone, pioglitazone, repaglinide, rosiglitazone	carbamazepine, phenobarbital, phenytoin, rifampin	atazanavir, gemfibrozil, irbesartan, ritonavir
2C9	carvedilol, celecoxib, diazepam, fluvastatin, phenytoin, ramelteon, (S)-warfarin	aprepitant, carbamazepine, phenobarbital, phenytoin, primidone, rifampin, rifapentine, St. John's wort	amiodarone, cimetidine, trimethoprim/ sulfamethoxazole, fluconazole, fluvoxamine, isoniazid, ketoconazole, metronidazole, voriconazole, warfarin, zafirlukast
2C19	clopidogrel, phenytoin, thioridazine, voriconazole	carbamazepine, phenobarbital, phenytoin, rifampin	cimetidine, esomeprazole, etravirine, efavirenz, fluoxetine, fluvoxamine, ketoconazole, modafinil, omeprazole, topiramate, voriconazole
2D6	amitriptyline, aripiprazole, atomoxetine, carvedilol, clozapine, codeine, desipramine, dextromethorphan, donepezil, doxepin, fentanyl, flecainide, haloperidol, hydrocodone, imipramine, lidocaine, meperidine, methadone, methamphetamine, mirtazapine, nortriptyline, oxycodone, propafenone, propoxyphene, propranolol, thioridazine, tramadol, trazodone, venlafaxine	carbamazepine, phenobarbital, phenytoin, primidone, rifampin, St. John's wort	amiodarone, cimetidine, darifenacin, duloxetine, fluoxetine, paroxetine, propafenone, quinidine, ritonavir, sertraline

Drugs with Significant Interactions – Watch For These

AMIODARONE

- A moderate inhibitor of 2C9, 2D6, and 3A4 and a substrate of 3A4 and 2C8 and a P-gp inhibitor.

- The following medications must have the doses ↓ 30-50% when starting amiodarone: digoxin, warfarin, quinidine and procainamide (note the serious problems if you don't decrease the dose, such as bleeding with warfarin from an INR or QT prolongation with the antiarrhythmics).

- Use lower doses of simvastatin, lovastatin and atorvastatin.

- Electrolyte abnormalities (K^+, Na^+, Ca^{2+}, Mg^{2+}, etc.) should be corrected before any antiarrhythmic therapy is initiated or the risk of arrhythmia is increased (true for all antiarrhythmics).

- Do not use grapefruit juice/products when using amiodarone.

AZOLE ANTIFUNGALS

All are 3A4 inhibitors (will ↑ concentration of 3A4 substrates). They also inhibit other CYP 450 enzymes; refer to above chart.

- Itraconazole and ketoconazole have pH-dependent absorption; ↑ pH causes ↓ absorption; avoid using with antacids, H_2RAs, PPIs.

- Voriconazole is notable for drug interactions (and dosing, and adverse effects).

- Voriconazole is metabolized by several CYP 450 enzymes (2C9, 2C19 and 3A4); the concentration of voriconazole can increase dangerously when given with drugs that inhibit voriconazole's metabolism or with small dose increases – it is 1st order, followed by Michaelis-Menten kinetics.

- Concurrent use of voriconazole and the following drugs are contraindicated: Alfuzosin, barbiturates, carbamazepine, cisapride, darunavir, dofetilide, ergot derivatives, lopinavir, nilotinib, pimozide, quinidine, ranolazine, rifampin, rifabutin, ritonavir, St. John's wort, thioridazine, etc.

COLCHICINE

- Colchicine should not be used with P-glycoprotein (P-gp) or strong 3A4 inhibitors, especially in patients with renal or hepatic impairment.

DIGOXIN

Digoxin is mostly renally cleared, and partially cleared hepatically. Decreased renal function requires a ↓ digoxin dose, or, if acute renal failure, the digoxin should be held.

- ↑ digoxin levels: amiodarone, quinidine, verapamil, erythromycin, clarithromycin, itraconazole, cyclosporine, propafenone, spironolactone, others – note that amiodarone (commonly) and verapamil are used in patients on digoxin. Caution: Amiodarone will cause levels of both digoxin and warfarin to increase. If started at the same time, lower doses are used. This is more of a concern when amiodarone is added to a stable dose of digoxin and warfarin – and the level increases.

- Hypokalemia (K+ < 3.5 mEq/mL) will ↑ digoxin levels. Potassium must be maintained between 3.5-5 mEq/mL.

- ↓ digoxin absorption with cholestyramine, colestipol and metoclopramide.

GRAPEFRUIT JUICE/FRUIT INTERACTIONS

Although the statin or CCB concentration may ↑ with grapefruit use, there are not many reports of clinical damage. However, it is best to counsel to avoid concurrent use. With other drugs, such as amiodarone, the interaction has more clinical relevance. This is not a gut interaction problem and separate administration times will not work. Avoid grapefruit products with:

- Lovastatin, simvastatin, atorvastatin

- Buspirone, amiodarone, carbamazepine, cyclosporine, tacrolimus, diazepam, triazolam, verapamil, nicardipine, felodipine, nisoldipine, nifedipine, telithromycin, voriconazole, etc.

LAMOTRIGINE & VALPROATE
- Increased risk severe rash, use caution and titrate slowly.

LITHIUM
100% renally cleared (excreted), but has important drug interactions with drugs that affect renal clearance, or cause toxicity.

- These will ↑ lithium levels: ↓ salt intake, NSAIDs, ACE Is, ARBs, dehydration (and caution with diuretics).

- These will ↓ lithium levels: salt intake, caffeine, theophylline.

- These will ↑ risk 5HT-syndrome if given with lithium: SSRIs, SNRIs, triptans, linezolid and other serotonergic drugs.

- ↑ neurotoxicity risk (ataxia, tremors, nausea) with verapamil, diltiazem, phenytoin and carbamazepine.

MONOAMINE OXIDASE INHIBITORS (MAO IS)
The non-selective MAO Is have drug interactions that can cause serotonin syndrome, hypertensive crisis, and potentially be fatal. Monoamines that would have reduced metabolism with monoamine oxidase inhibitors include dopamine, epinephrine, norepinephrine, serotonin (and tyramine, which is also a monoamine and thus the problem with foods rich in tyramine). This is mostly a risk with the antidepressants (which raise levels of the monoamines) and other agents that have a similar effect. There is some degree of risk with the Parkinson agents; refer to the chapter for specifics.

- DO NOT USE MAO Is with ephedrine and analogs (pseudoephedrine, etc.), buspirone, linezolid, lithium, meperidine, SSRIs, SNRIs, TCAs, tramadol, levodopa, mirtazapine, dextromethorphan, cyclobenzaprine (and other skeletal muscle relaxants), some of the triptans, St. John's wort, wellbutrin and some others.

- The non-selective MAO Is, the selegiline patch (at the two higher doses) and rasagiline should not be used with tyramine-rich foods, which include aged cheeses, air-dried meats, certain wines and beers and other foods which have been aged, fermented, pickled or smoked.

NSAIDS   renal
- All NSAIDs, including the selective agent celecoxib, raise blood pressure.

- The non-selective agents increase bleeding risk, including GI bleeding. The selective agent celecoxib has a reduced, but not eliminated, bleeding risk.

- All NSAIDs can cause renal toxicity and should be avoided with significant renal disease.

- NSAIDs cannot be used with lithium due to a risk of lithium toxicity.

- All NSAIDS, except ASA, have the risk of CV toxicity (causing MIs, etc.) COX-2 selectivity is pro-thrombotic and the selective agents have the highest risk. Celecoxib, at the present time, is considered to have the highest risk (except for the other COX-2 selective agents rofecoxib (*Vioxx*) and valdecoxib (*Bextra*), which have both been removed from the market due to MI/CVA risk.)

ORAL CONTRACEPTIVES (BIRTH CONTROL PILLS) AND SIMILAR CAUTION WITH RING AND PATCH

Decreases levels of OCs:

- Antibiotics (ampicillin, griseofulvin, sulfonamides, tetracycline, and rifampin – with rifampin need alternative method for 1 ½ months afterward, others use back-up while taking the antibiotic)

- Anticonvulsants (barbiturates, carbamazepine, phenytoin, and felbamate)

- St John's wort – do not use OC's concurrently

- Do not use with the following anti-retrovirals that increase OC metabolism, reducing the efficacy: atazanavir, lopinavir, nelfinavir, nevirapine, ritonavir

- Patients should not smoke; may ↓ efficacy and it is dangerous to smoke while using OC's.

OXYCONTIN AND OTHER OXYCODONE PRODUCTS (AND INCLUDE POSSIBLE RISK WITH HYDROCODONE, FENTANYL AND TRAMADOL)

- Increased opioid levels with 3A4 Inhibitors: ↑ side effects and risk of respiratory depression.

- Decreased opioid levels with 3A4 Inducers.

PD5-INHIBITORS- SILDENAFIL, TADALAFIL AND VARDENAFIL

- Contraindicated with nitrates due to severe hypotension.

- Use caution with alpha blockers, particularly with the non-selective agents (doxazosin, etc) that cause more dizziness and orthostatis. Start at lower dosing range and titrate slowly.

- These are 3A4 substrates; use lower doses with 3A4 inhibitors.

RIFAMPIN

Rifampin is a strong inducer of CYP 2C9, 2C19 and 3A4.

- Rifampin will ↓ warfarin (large decrease in INR).

- Will decrease effectiveness of oral contraceptives; cannot be used concurrently.

- Any other substrate of the above enzymes may be sub-therapeutic if given with rifampin.

STATINS

When the statin dose is increased, the risk is higher for muscle toxicity: muscle aches, soreness, or worse, including a rapid breakdown of muscle tissue called rhabdomyolysis. This can cause renal failure.

- For lovastatin, simvastatin and atorvastatin (these are the 3 statins with most of the drug interactions) - there is ↑ risk of muscle damage with amiodarone, dronedarone, cyclosporine, protease inhibitors, ketoconazole, grapefruit juice, diltiazem and other 3A4 inhibitors.

- Cannot use cyclosporine with pitavastatin.

- The safest choice with protease inhibitors is pravastatin, or low doses of atorvastatin or rosuvastatin.

  - With the combination of rosuvastatin and lopinavir/ ritonavir, the rosuvastatin dose should not exceed 10 mg.

  - Rosuvastatin cannot be used with indinavir or saquinavir.

  - Cyclosporine ↑ pravastatin and pitavastatin levels (Normally, pravastatin does not pose DI issues and is chosen when DI issues may be a concern.)

- Gemfibrozil and statins have an ↑ risk of muscle toxicity. The fenofibrates *(Tricor, Trilipix,* etc) with statins is a safer combination.

- Niacin and statins have ↑ risk muscle and liver toxicity. *Niaspan* can be used with lower doses of simvastatin and lovastatin if needed. Caution with any niacin and statin.

- Telithromycin with lovastatin, simvastatin or atorvastatin - hold these statins during telithromycin therapy due to an ↑ risk muscle damage.

TETRACYCLINE AND QUINOLONE ANTIBIOTICS

- These drugs chelate (complex) with aluminum, magnesium, calcium, iron and zinc leading to ↓ drug absorption. The administration time must be separated (2 hours before or 2 hours after, usually).

- This includes iron supplements, vitamins, antacids, dairy products, sucralfate and buffered aspirin and didanosine.

THEOPHYLLINE

Theophylline is metabolized by 1A2 and 3A4. It is first order kinetics, followed by Michaelis-Menten (saturable) kinetics (similar to phenytoin and voriconazole). This means that the concentration increases in a straight line initially and (suddenly) can become very high if a 1A2 or 3A4 inhibitor (for theophylline) is used at the same time, or if a dose increase is given. A small increase in dose can result in a large increase in the theophylline concentration.

- ↑ theophylline levels due to 1A2 inhibition: oral contraceptives, zafirlukast, zileuton, acyclovir, cimetidine, ciprofloxacin, ethinyl estradiol, fluvoxamine, isoniazid.

- ↑ theophylline levels due to 3A4 inhibition: amiodarone, azole antifungals, clarithromycin, cyclosporine, erythromycin, diltiazem, verapamil, lovastatin, simvastatin, atorvastatin, PI's, etc.

- ↑ theophylline levels, other mechanisms: allopurinol, erythromycin, propranolol, ephedrine, and possibly with other systemic bronchodilators (and possibly phenylephrine, pseudoephedrine).

- ↓ theophylline levels: carbamazepine, phenobarbital, phenytoin, primidone, rifampin, ritonavir, tobacco/marijuana smoking, St. John's wort, tipranavir/ritonavir, high protein diet, thyroid hormones (levothyroxine, etc.).

- Theophylline will ↓ lithium (theophylline ↑ renal excretion of lithium), and will ↓ zafirlukast.

Warfarin – Pharmacokinetic Drug Interactions

- Warfarin is a substrate of CYP 2C9 (major), 1A2 (minor) and 3A4 (minor) and an inhibitor of 2C9 (moderate). Avoid use with tamoxifen.

- 2C9 inducers - including phenobarbital, phenytoin, primidone, rifampin (large ↓ INR), and St. John's Wort - may ↓ INR.

- 2C9 inhibitors - including amiodarone, Bactrim, azole antifungals, macrolide antibiotics, and metronidazole - may ↑ INR. See drug interactions chapter.

- Check for 1A2 and 3A4 interactions; these occur, but usually have less of an effect on INR.

Warfarin – Pharmacodynamic Drug Interactions | NSAID, ginko, SSRI, SNRI

- The most common pharmacodynamic interaction is with NSAIDs, including aspirin and ibuprofen (but not selective agents such as celecoxib), and with antiplatelet agents. These interactions ↑ bleeding risk, but the INR will be in the usual range.

- Ginkgo biloba increases bleeding risk with no effect on the INR. Other natural products that can also pose a risk include bromelains, danshen, dong quai (this product may ↑ INR), vitamin E, evening primrose oil, high doses of fish oils, garlic, ginseng, glucosamine, grapefruit, policosanol, and willow bark.

- SSRIs and SNRIs, with the use of an anticoagulant, can increase bleeding risk without increasing the INR. Use extreme caution with these drugs in combination.

- Nutritional products, including drinks and supplements, can include vitamin K (e.g., green tea). Coenzyme Q10 may reduce the effectiveness of warfarin. Any additions of vitamin K will lower the INR. Check the product for vitamin K content. TPN mixtures usually contain vitamin K from the MVI component; the INR will be monitored. The MVI without vitamin K (MVI-12) may be used.

Additive Drug Interactions

These involve classes of drugs which may (or may not) pose a problem individually, but can become dangerous when used with other drugs that cause similar side effects.

BLEEDING RISK

Anticoagulants (warfarin, dabigatran, rivaroxaban, heparin and others) and antiplatelets (aspirin, dipyridamole, clopidogrel, prasugrel, ticagrelor) and other agents that increase bleeding risk have an additive effect: the more agents being used concurrently that increase bleeding risk, the higher the bleeding risk.

Caution: In some cases dual antiplatelets are recommended (such as clopidogrel and aspirin post-stent placement). In some high-risk cases (such as a patient on warfarin who had a stroke) there may even be use of an anticoagulant with an antiplatelet (such as warfarin plus aspirin). However, the use of this combination may be inadvertent; the cardiologist may have prescribed the warfarin (or other anticoagulant) and the patient is using the aspirin OTC on their own – or is using it based on an old recommendation.

Other agents that increase bleeding risk which should be avoided in patients on the above agents, or at higher bleeding risk for other reasons (such as having had a previous bleed): OTC or prescription NSAIDs, SSRIs and SNRIs, natural products, including ginkgo biloba (commonly used agent that inhibits platelet activating factor and must be stopped in advance of surgery), bromelains, danshen, dong quai (this product may increase the INR – the others listed in this paragraph generally do not raise INR), vitamin E, evening primrose oil, high doses of fish oils, garlic, ginseng, glucosamine, grapefruit, policosanol and willow bark.

- Anticoagulant and Antiplatelet Drug Interaction summary: dabigatran (*Pradaxa*) is neither a substrate, inducer or inhibitor of CYP 450 enzymes, rivaroxaban (*Xarelto)* is a substrate of CYP 450 3A4. Dabigatran (*Pradaxa*) and rivaroxaban (*Xarelto*) are P-gp substrates and will be subject to changes in concentration with P-gp inducers/inhibitors.

- Prasugrel (*Effient*) should not be used concurrently with rifampin. Clopidogrel (*Plavix*) is a pro-drug and is converted to active drug by the 2C19 enzyme; the effect of 2C19 inhibitors on this conversion is controversial at present (2C19 inhibitors include cimetidine, esomeprazole, etravirine, efavirenz, fluoxetine, fluvoxamine, ketoconazole, modafinil, omeprazole, topiramate and voriconazole); see anticoagulation section. The package insert for clopidogrel notes that persons who are poor metabolizers of 2C19 (they do not produce much of this enzyme) may have reduced effect from this drug (due to less conversion to active drug).

HYPERKALEMIA RISK

Potassium is renally cleared; severe renal disease causes hyperkalemia by itself. Potassium is cleared by dialysis.

- Additive potassium accumulation: ACE Is, ARBs, other K⁺-sparing agents, including amiloride, triamterene, eplerenone, spironolactone, salt substitutes (KCl), and the oral contraceptive pills *Yasmin*, *Natazia*, *Yaz*.

CNS DEPRESSION

CNS side effects are caused by drugs that enter the CNS (lipophilic) and primarily involve drugs that cause sedation (somnolence), dizziness, confusion (↓ cognitive function) and altered consciousness. CNS side effects can be activating (such as with the use of stimulants), but are primarily sedating.

- Additive CNS effects: alcohol, most pain medications (opioids, propoxyphene – this is off the US market, but it can come in from other places, NSAIDs), skeletal muscle relaxants, anticonvulsants, benzodiazepines, barbiturates, hypnotics, mirtazapine, trazodone, dronabinol, nabilone, propranolol, clonidine, and others.

QT PROLONGATION

The QT interval is measured from the beginning of the QRS complex to the end of the T wave. It reflects ventricular depolarization and repolarization. A prolonged QT interval is a risk factor for ventricular tachyarrhythmias (e.g. torsades de pointes) and sudden cardiac death.

Use the following QT-prolonging drugs with caution in patients with any arrhythmia risk (including those with existing arrhythmias, or if you see them on an antiarrhythmic). QT prolongation risk depends on the dose and duration. If a patient is using low dose amitriptyline for neuropathic pain, this should not be considered a particularly risky agent, although the risk may be additive with other agents.

Additive QT prolongation

- Any pre-existing cardiac condition (or history of arrhythmia).

- Class Ia and Class III antiarrhythmics (amiodarone, disopyramide, dronedarone, procainamide, quinidine, sotalol, and others).

- Antibiotics including quinolones (ciprofloxacin, levofloxacin, moxifloxacin, norfloxacin, gemifloxacin, and sparfloxacin), macrolides (azithromycin, erythromycin, clarithromycin and telithromycin), amantadine, foscarnet and others.

- Azole antifungals (fluconazole, itraconazole, ketoconazole, posiconazole and voriconazole).

- Anticancer agents (arsenic, dasatinib, lapatinib, nilotinib, sunitinib, tamoxifen).

- Protease inhibitors (saquinavir/ritonavir, atazanavir, lopinavir/ritonavir).

- Antidepressants including tricyclics (amitriptyline, nortriptyline, doxepin, desipramine, and others), and lower risk with SSRIs (citalopram, escitalopram, fluoxetine, paroxetine, sertraline) and SNRIs (venlafaxine and desvenlafaxine) and trazodone.

- Antiemetic agents including the 5-HT3 blockers (dolasetron, ondansetron, granisetron, palonosetron) and droperidol.

- Antipsychotics (chlorpromazine, thioridazine, pimozide, haloperidol, ziprasidone, risperidone, paliperidone, iloperidone, asenapine and lurasidone)

- Other agents: alfuzosin, apomorphine, chloroquine, galantamine, methadone and pentamidin

- Select Therapeutic Index Drugs

These drugs must stay within the safe range: too much can cause toxicity, and too little is sub-therapeutic.

DRUG	USUAL THERAPEUTIC RANGE
Carbamazepine	6-12 mcg/mL
Levothyroxine	FT4 normal range 0.8-1.7 mcg/dL TSH normal range 0.3 – 3.0µIU/mL
Lithium	0.6-1.2 mEq/L (can 1.5 mEq/L for acute symptoms)
Phenytoin	10-20 mcg/mL
Theophylline	5-15 mcg/mL
Digoxin	0.8-2.0 ng/mL
Procainamide NAPA	4-10 mcg/mL 15-25 mcg/mL
Valproic acid	50-100 mcg/mL
Warfarin	2-3 (INR) for most indications, use higher range (2.5-3.5) with thrombogenic valves and a few other indications

PRACTICE QUESTIONS

1. Drug A is a substrate of enzyme X. Drug B is an inducer of enzyme X. A patient has been using Drug A with good results. The patient has now started therapy with Drug B. What will happen to the concentration of Drug A?

    a. Increase
    b. Decrease
    c. Stay the Same
    d. There is not enough information given
    e. None of the above

2. Drug A is a substrate of enzyme X. Drug B is an inhibitor of enzyme X. A patient has been using Drug A with good results. The patient has now started therapy with Drug B. What will happen to the concentration of Drug A?

    a. Increase
    b. Decrease
    c. Stay the Same
    d. This is not enough information given
    e. None of the above

3. Drug A is a substrate of enzyme X. Drug A is also an inducer of enzyme Y. Drug B is a substrate of enzyme Y. Drug B is also an inhibitor of enzyme X. When these drugs are both administered, what will happen to the concentrations of Drug A and Drug B?

    a. Levels of both Drug A and Drug B will increase
    b. Levels of Drug A will increase and levels of Drug B will decrease
    c. Levels of Drug A will decrease and levels of Drug B will increase
    d. Levels of Drug A will increase and levels of Drug B will stay the same
    e. There is not enough information given.

4. A patient with heart failure is using many medications, including digoxin, warfarin and pravastatin. She is started on amiodarone therapy. Which statement is correct?

    a. The INR will increase; the warfarin dose will need to be reduced
    b. The digoxin will increase; the digoxin dose will need to be reduced
    c. The pravastatin level will increase; the pravastatin dose will need to be reduced
    d. A and B
    e. All of the above

5. A patient has been using warfarin for DVT treatment. She was hospitalized for afibrillation and started on amiodarone therapy. While hospitalized, she developed an infection and was prescribed trimethoprim/sulfamethoxazole and ketoconazole. Which of the following agents will increase the INR and could result in bleeding?

    a. Amiodarone
    b. Trimethoprim/sulfamethoxazole
    c. Ketoconazole
    d. A and B
    e. All of the above

6. The pharmacist is dispensing a prescription for ciprofloxacin. The only medication the patient is using is a daily multivitamin, which she takes with breakfast and an iron supplement, which she takes with dinner. She has yogurt or cheese every day with lunch. Which counseling statement is correct?

    a. She will need to separate the ciprofloxacin from the multivitamin
    b. She will need to separate the ciprofloxacin from the iron supplement
    c. She will need to separate the ciprofloxacin from the yogurt and cheese
    d. A and B
    e. All of the above

7. A patient is taking warfarin 5 mg once daily for DVT treatment. Which of the following medications will increase her bleeding risk, but leave the INR around the same range?

    a. Occasional Acetaminophen
    b. Ibuprofen 200 mg 1-2 tablets daily
    c. Celecoxib 200 mg once daily
    d. B and C only
    e. All of the above

8. Drug A is a substrate of 2C9 and a potent 3A4 inhibitor. Drug B is a substrate of 2D6 and 1A2 as well as a potent inhibitor of 2C19. Drug C is a substrate of 3A4 and a potent inhibitor of 2D6. If all three drugs were given together, what would the expected levels of each drug to do?

    a. Drug A levels would stay the same, Drug B levels would increase, Drug C levels would increase.
    b. Drug A levels would increase, Drug B levels would decrease, Drug C levels would increase.
    c. Drug A levels would decrease, Drug B levels would decrease, Drug C levels would increase.
    d. Drug A levels would increase, Drug B levels would stay the same, and Drug C levels would decrease.
    e. Drug A, B, and C levels would all increase.

9. A major drug interaction can occur with the use of grapefruit juice and which of the following medications?

    a. Atorvastatin and Amiodarone
    b. Celecoxib and Felodipine
    c. Lovastatin and Ranolazine
    d. Levetiracetam and Topiramate
    e. Duloxetine and Mirtazapine

10. A patient has an estimated creatinine clearance of 18 mL/min. Her potassium level is 4.8 mEq/L. The following drugs will increase her risk of hyperkalemia and should be used with extreme caution:

    a. Enalapril
    b. Valsartan
    c. Eplerenone
    d. A and B only
    e. All of the above

11. A patient is at risk for afibrillation; she has had this afibrillation in the past. The medical team has asked the pharmacist to check for drugs on her profile which can increase her risk of arrhythmia. The pharmacist should include the following medications:

    a. Fluconazole
    b. Erythromycin
    c. Ziprasidone
    d. B and C only
    e. All of the above

ANSWERS

1-b, 2-a, 3-b, 4-d, 5-e, 6-e, 7-b, 8-a, 9-a, 10-e, 11-e

RENAL DISEASE AND DOSING CONSIDERATIONS

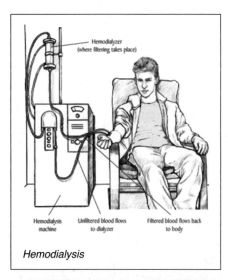

Hemodialyzer
(where filtering takes place)

Hemodialysis
machine

Unfiltered blood flows
to dialyzer

Filtered blood flows back
to body

Hemodialysis

GUIDELINES/REFERENCES

National Kidney Foundation. NKF/DOQI clinical practice guidelines for chronic kidney disease: evaluation, classification, and stratification. *Am J Kidney Dis.* 2002;39(2 suppl 1):S1–266.

Aronoff, GR. Drug Prescribing in Renal Failure: Dosing Guidelines for Adults. 4th Ed. Philadelphia, PA. American College of Physicians, 1999.

Lee, M. Basic Skills in Interpreting Laboratory Data. ASHP, 2009.

Johnson, C. Dialysis of Drugs, CKD Insights, LLC, 2010.

BACKGROUND

Chronic kidney disease (CKD) has increased from 10% to 13% in the U.S. over the past twenty years, due primarily to the increases in diabetes and hypertension. Awareness of CKD in the general population is low, including among patients who regularly see a physician. This is regrettable since CKD patients have a higher risk of cardiovascular disease morbidity and mortality, and risk progression to kidney failure. CKD is an important area for pharmacists, since many drugs require renal dose adjustment, and due to the treatment required for conditions related to CKD, including anemia, hyperphosphatemia, low vitamin D levels, bone metabolism problems and prevention and treatment of hyperkalemia.

A point worth mentioning:

Pharmacists should encourage patients to check, monitor and stay adherent with hypertension treatment. This is an asymptomatic condition with a high rate of nonadherence. Uncontrolled hypertension contributes to a high prevalence of young black males at dialysis centers, which is unfortunate. Any ethnicity can be at risk, but in this patient group there is a very high incidence of unrecognized or inadequately treated hypertension.

Dialysis

If the kidney disease progresses then dialysis will be required to eliminate wastes, electrolytes and water. The two primary types of dialysis are hemodialysis (HD), with a machine (usually at a dialysis center), and

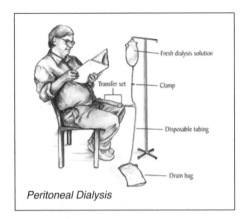

Peritoneal Dialysis

peritoneal dialysis (PD), which uses the peritoneal membrane on the abdomen to filter the blood.

In HD the blood is removed outside the body and into the dialyzer (dialysis machine) through a semi-permeable membrane. Solutes diffuse across the membrane and the cleansed blood goes back into the patient. This is a 3-4 hour process, done several times (usually three times) per week. Some patients get home HD, which is done more frequently with a portable device, often five days per week.

In PD a glucose solution is pumped into the peritoneal membrane, which acts as a semipermeable membrane. The solution is left in for a period of time, then drained. PD is done daily, usually by the patient at home. There are two types of PD: continuous ambulatory peritoneal dialysis (CAPD), which is done without a machine and automated peritoneal dialysis (ADP), in which the patient uses a machine in the home to do some of the dialysis.

FACTORS AFFECTING DRUG REMOVAL DURING DIALYSIS

When a patient is on dialysis the pharmacist needs to consider how much drug is lost to dialysis in order to obtain a reasonable dosing regimen and/or to schedule replacement dosing post-dialysis. These factors determine the dialyzability of drugs:

Molecular Size

In HD a fixed pore size determines the extent to which compounds can move through the membrane. Smaller molecules pass through more easily. In PD the pore size is larger and permits larger molecules to pass more easily through the membrane.

Protein Binding

In PD, with a larger membrane pore size, some (small percentage) of bound drugs may be lost, but in HD, with the smaller pore size, protein-binding prevents drug loss. The percentage of the drugs not bound to protein can be lost in HD, but this percentage is low with highly protein-bound drugs.

Volume of Distribution (VD)

If the VD is large (which means that much of the drug has gone into the tissues) there is a smaller concentration of drugs in the blood, and less will be lost to dialysis.

Water Solubility

The dialysis fluid, or dialysate, is aqueous and drugs with a high water solubility are dialyzed to a greater extent than highly lipid-soluble drugs (which concentrate in the tissues).

Plasma Clearance

If non-renal clearance mechanisms are large, the relative weight of renal clearance (which is replaced by dialysis) is low.

The Dialysis Membrane

The PD membrane (as it is part of the patient's body) cannot be altered, but the HD membrane types vary. Some newer membranes will affect drug loss differently. When using published references that indicate "percentage of drug lost" via different types of dialysis, the clinician must consider the type of membrane being used.

RENAL PHYSIOLOGY

The nephron is the functional unit of the kidney, or where the "work" takes place. There are about one million nephrons in each kidney. Blood is delivered into the glomerulus, a large filtering device at the entry point of each nephron that is located within the Bowman's capsule.

Glomerulus

Substances with a molecular weight below 40,000 daltons can pass through into the nephron filter. Larger substances cannot pass through this fine net and stay in the blood. If the filter is not damaged, albumin (which is large) stays in the blood. If the kidney filter is damaged some of the albumin passes into the urine. The level of albumin in the urine (micro or macroalbuminuria) can be used to gage the severity of renal damage in patients with nephropathy (nephron damage). This is discussed in the diabetes chapter.

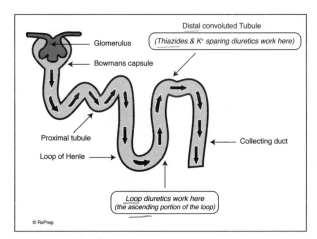

Most drugs are small enough to pass through the filter. Exceptions are large protein compounds and drugs that are bound (linked) to albumin.

Creatinine, a waste product of muscle metabolism, is also filtered through the glomerulus and in the proximal tubule. If the nephrons are damaged, the creatinine is not sent into the filtrate (urine) and the level of creatinine increases in the serum. We use the level of creatinine in the serum (by estimating the creatinine clearance, or CrCl) as an indirect method to estimate renal function (or the glomerular filtration rate, or GFR). It is not a fine measurement since the level of creatinine depends on the level of muscle mass (and metabolism) in the patient. In addition the creatinine does not increase during early stages of renal damage. For drug dosing purposes it is generally acceptable to use this estimation because drugs are not "dose adjusted" until the renal function has a significant degree of impairment, such as a creatinine clearance less than 60 mL/min (and in many drugs lower than this, or less than 25 or 30 mL/min).

There are more specific markers to estimate GFR, including inulin (which is a finer marker) and radioactive substances.

Blood urea nitrogen (BUN) measures the amount of nitrogen that comes from the waste product urea. The BUN increases with renal impairment, however it cannot be used independently to measure declines in renal function since other factors affect the BUN, including the level of hydration. In the calculations chapter there is a simple formula that can be used to ascertain if the patient is dehydrated, which would cause increases in both SCr and BUN. In actual practice the patient's signs and symptoms of dehydration including weakness, decreased urine output and tachycardia may be all that is required to assess hydration.

PROXIMAL TUBULE

A primary function of the nephron is to control the concentration of water and Na^+. The nephrons reabsorb what is needed (to go back into the circulation) and excrete the remainder as urine. This regulates the blood volume, and in turn, the blood pressure. "Proximal" means close to, and the proximal tubule is the closest part to the Bowman's capsule. Large amounts of water are reabsorbed here, along with Na^+ and Cl^+. The pH is regulated by exchange of hydrogen ions and bicarbonate ions. Water, Na^+ and Cl^+ absorption also continues further along the nephron.

LOOP OF HENLE

The loop of Henle has a descending limb and an ascending limb. As filtrate moves down the loop of Henle (the descending limb), water is reabsorbed, but sodium and chloride ions are not. This concentrates sodium and chloride in the lumen. The filtrate moves up the other side (the ascending limb) which is impermeable to water. Sodium and chloride

COMMON DRUGS (NOT ALL) THAT REQUIRE DOSAGE REDUCTIONS OR INCREASED DOSING INTERVALS WITH DECREASED RENAL FUNCTION

Some of these drugs would pose a DANGER if used at all in severe renal disease

Acyclovir

Allopurinol

Amantadine

Amphotericin

Aminoglycosides – increase dosing interval

Azole antifungals, including fluconazole, etc.

Antiarrhythmics (digoxin, ibutilide, procainamide, sotalol)

Beta-lactam antibiotics (most)

Bisphosphonates: do not use in severe disease

Chlorpropamide, glyburide – do not use, not preferred agents due to risk of drug accumulation

Cyclosporine

Famotidine, ranitidine

Gabapentin, pregabalin

Lithium: do not use in severe disease

LMWHs: enoxaparin

Meperidine

Metformin-has renal cut-offs, see diabetes chapter

Metoclopramide

Morphine and codeine: use lower starting dose

Nitrofurantoin: do not use in severe disease

NSAIDs – avoid with renal disease, higher risk ARF

Quinolone antibiotics (most), including ciprofloxacin and levofloxacin

Spironolactone, eplerenone – risk of hyperkalemia

Statins-most require dose adjustment

Tadalafil

Tramadol

Vancomycin

are reabsorbed but water is not. If antidiuretic hormone (ADH) is present water will pass through the walls of the duct. The more ADH present, the more water is passed back into the blood (anti-diuresis).

Loop diuretics inhibit the Na⁺-K⁺ pump in the ascending limb of the loop (the part that goes back up). About 25% of the sodium is reabsorbed here and inhibiting these pumps leads to a significant increase in the tubular concentration of sodium, and less water reabsorption. By blocking the pump the electrical gradient is altered and reabsorption of calcium decreases. Consequently, the long-term use of loop diuretics contributes to the development of osteoporosis.

DISTAL CONVOLUTED TUBULE

Distal means farthest away and the distal convoluted tubule is the farthest away from the entry point to the nephron. The distal tubule is also involved in regulating K^+, Na^+, Ca^{2+} and pH.

Thiazide diuretics inhibit the Na-Cl pump in the distal tubule. Only about 5% of the sodium is reabsorbed at this point, which makes thiazides weaker diuretics than loops. Thiazides also increase calcium absorption by affecting the calcium pump in the distal convoluted tubule. Consequently, the long-term use of thiazide diuretics has a protective effect on bone.

Collecting Duct

The collecting duct is a network of tubules and ducts that connect the nephrons to the ureter. Urine passes from the ureter into the bladder, and from there out of the body via the urethra. The collecting duct is involved with water and electrolyte balance and is affected by levels of ADH and aldosterone. Aldosterone also works in the distal tubule. The primary function of aldosterone is to increase Na^+ and water retention and to lower K^+. By blocking aldosterone (with spironolactone or eplerenone), potassium increases.

DRUGS AND RENAL CLEARANCE

Creatinine Clearance (CrCl) Estimation

$$\frac{140 - age}{72 \times Scr} \times wt \times 0.85$$

A normal range of serum creatinine is approximately 0.6 to 1.2 mg/dL. A creatinine above this range indicates that the kidneys are not functioning properly. However, the values can appear normal when renal function is compromised. This is especially true in the elderly because the production and excretion of creatinine declines with age. This concern increases in frail patients who are bed-bound and consequently have reduced muscle mass since creatinine is a break-down ("end") product of muscle metabolism.

In this text, for board exam purposes, we review how to use the Cockcroft-Gault equation in the calculations chapter since this is the most commonly used method of estimating renal functions used by clinical pharmacists. The Cockcroft-Gault formula may not be preferable in very young children, in end stage renal disease (ESRD) or when renal function is fluctuating rapidly.

Dehydration can cause both the serum creatinine (SCr) and the blood urea nitrogen (BUN) values to increase. Generally, a BUN:SCr ratio > 20 indicates dehydration. Correcting the dehydration will reduce both BUN and SCr, and can prevent or treat acute renal failure. Please refer to the Calculations chapter example that demonstrates a patient with elevated BUN and SCr due to dehydration.

CREATININE CLEARANCE VALUE AND DEGREE OF RENAL IMPAIRMENT

CRCL (ML/MIN)	INTERPRETATION
60-90	mild renal insufficiency
30-59	moderate renal insufficiency
15-29	severe renal insufficiency
< 15	kidney failure (or dialysis)

Depending on the extent of renal impairment, drug regimens may be altered by reducing the dose and/or extending the dosing interval to avoid accumulation and potential toxicity while maintaining clinically effective drug concentrations. If the dose is lowered, the concentrations will be more constant. If the interval is lengthened there is a lower risk of toxicities but the drug may become subtherapeutic towards the end of the dosing interval.

Impaired renal excretion – examples

Gabapentin (*Neurontin*), a drug commonly used for diabetic neuropathic pain (although it is not indicated for this condition and provides little benefit), causes primarily CNS side effects (dizziness, somnolence). Gabapentin is excreted renally. The kidneys have to be working well to excrete the drug, or the concentration of gabapentin in the body will increase. Gabapentin is "renally-dose adjusted" when the CrCl is < 60 mL/min. At this level, the dose is decreased by half since the kidneys are not able to eliminate the drug efficiently. If a person with a CrCl of 90 mL/min is using gabapentin 600 mg TID, the total daily dose will be 1,800 mg. At some later point, if the renal function has decreased to 45 mL/min, the person will experience excessive sedation and dizziness. In effect, the person is taking ~3,600 mg daily, or double the previous dose.

Metoclopramide (*Reglan*), a "do not use drug" in the elderly, is primarily used for nausea and poor GI motility, in the elderly. Metoclopramide is a dopamine-blocking agent and is renally cleared. In a patient with reduced renal clearance the typical dose of 10 mg QID (with meals and at bedtime) would be too high and the patient could present with "Parkinsonism," or movement difficulty due to dopamine blockade. (In elderly patients both reduced renal clearance and lower endogenous dopamine levels are likely.) The patient would certainly have increased CNS side effects (confusion, dizziness, etc.)

PROTEINURIA, BLOOD PRESSURE CONTROL, AND THE USE OF ACE IS AND ARBS

Proteinuria increases as renal disease advances. Once proteinuria has been identified, ACE Is or ARBs will be used, unless contraindicated. It is essential to control the blood pressure tightly. The goal blood pressure in kidney disease is < 130/80 mmHg. Glycemic control, if an issue, will also need to be tightly controlled to preserve kidney function.

ACE Is and ARBs help preserve renal function and reduce proteinuria, and provide cardio-vascular protection. These drugs inhibit the renin-angiotensin-aldosterone system (RAAS), causing efferent arteriolar dilation. This is described in some detail in the hypertension chapter.

Note that the use of ACE Is and ARBs can cause an acute decline in GFR during therapy initiation (most commonly occurring in patients with heart failure, or in those taking NSAIDs, which should not be used with renal disease.) Typically, the renal function will return to normal after several weeks of therapy but must be monitored during initiation. These are potassium-sparing agents and if the potassium increases (which will occur due to advanced renal disease as well) the ACE I or ARB may require a dose reduction or discontinuation.

ANEMIA AND BONE METABOLISM PROBLEMS IN ADVANCED RENAL DISEASE

Anemia of Chronic Kidney Disease

Erythropoietin is produced by the kidneys and stimulates production of reticulocytes in the bone marrow. As kidney function declines, the production of erythropoietin declines and anemia results. In addition, chronic kidney disease is a pro-inflammatory condition that can result in anemia of chronic disease. Nutritional deficiencies may be present that could require iron, folate or vitamin B12. Anemia identification and treatment is discussed in the anemia chapter.

Bone Metabolism Abnormalities

Patients with advanced kidney disease require screening for abnormalities associated with parathyroid hormone (PTH), phosphorus, calcium and vitamin D at regular intervals, according to the disease severity.

Bone metabolism abnormalities are initially caused by elevations in phosphorus, which is renally excreted.

To compensate for hyperphosphatemia, the parathyroid gland increases release of PTH. Vitamin D deficiency results when the elevated PTH is unable to sufficiently stimulate the hydroxylation of 25-OH vitamin D to its active form, resulting in a deficiency.

This is treated with dietary phosphate restriction, phosphate binders and vitamin D supplementation.

Treatment of Hyperphosphatemia

Initially, hyperphosphatemia treatment involves restricting dietary phosphorus, with monitoring. Eventually, phosphate binders may be required, primarily in patients on dialysis. There are three types of phosphate binders:

Aluminum-based (*AlternaGel,* others). They are effective, but aluminum is toxic to the nervous system and bone. They can only be used short-term and are not used much currently.

Calcium-based (primarily calcium acetate and carbonate). These are effective but do not bind phosphorus as well as aluminum. However, many renal patients are taking vitamin D (which raises calcium levels) and cannot tolerate additional calcium.

Aluminum-free, calcium-free binders are newer agents that are effective at controlling phosphorus. Because they do not contain aluminum or calcium, they do not cause problems with excess aluminum or calcium load. They are the most expensive.

Phosphate binders bind meal-time phosphate in the gut that is coming from the diet. If a dose is missed and the food is absorbed there is no point in taking it later or doubling up the next dose. Patients may be required to limit foods high in phosphate.

PHOSPHATE BINDERS

DRUG	DOSE	SIDE EFFECTS/MONITORING/CONTRAINDICATIONS
Aluminum-based		
Aluminum hydroxide (*AlternaGel, Amphojel,* others)	15-30 mL TID with meals	Constipation, poor taste, nausea Inexpensive, no effect on serum calcium, used short-term only
Calcium-based		
Calcium acetate (*PhosLo, Phoslyra,* others)	1,334 mg TID with meals	Constipation, nausea Can cause hypercalcemia, low gastric pH can reduce efficacy Provides calcium source, if needed
Calcium carbonate (*Tums,* store brands, others)	500 mg TID, with meals, chewable or not	Inexpensive, may contribute to hypercalcemia Provides calcium source, if needed

Phosphate Binders Continued

DRUG	DOSE	SIDE EFFECTS/MONITORING/CONTRAINDICATIONS
Aluminum-free, calcium-free		
Lanthanum carbonate (*Fosrenol*)	500 mg TID with meals, chewable – must chew thoroughly	Nausea
		Expensive, no effect on serum calcium, not affected by gastric pH
Sevelamer carbonate (*Renvela*)	800-1,600 mg TID with meals, tablets or powder (mix for suspension)	Nausea, constipation
		Expensive, no effect on serum calcium, affected by gastric pH, lowers LDL and total CH
Sevelamer hydrochloride (*Renagel*)	800-1,600 mg TID with meals	Nausea, constipation, risk acidosis, can lower fat-soluble vitamins (some may be told to take vitamin at other times)
		Expensive, no effect on serum calcium, affected by gastric pH, lowers LDL and total CH

TREATMENT OF VITAMIN D DEFICIENCY

Vitamin D deficiency is related to a host of conditions, including an increased risk of osteoporosis, fractures, poor immunity, psychiatric disorders and cardiovascular disease.

The term vitamin D refers to either vitamin D2 or vitamin D3. Vitamin D3, also known as cholecalciferol, is the active form of vitamin D. It is made in the skin or obtained in the diet from fatty fish. Vitamin D2, or ergocalciferol, is obtained from irradiated fungi, such as yeast. Vitamin D2 and vitamin D3 are used to supplement food products or are taken as supplements. Calcitriol (*Rocaltrol*) is a synthetic form of vitamin D3 that is often used in patients with advanced renal disease or on dialysis.

Vitamin D supplementation increases calcium absorption in the gut and decreases renal calcium excretion. It also increases the release of calcium from bone. This is done in conjunction with parathyroid hormone (PTH). Treatment of vitamin D deficiency can result in hypercalcemia or hyperphosphatemia. These values must be monitored during treatment. Further information on vitamin D is contained in the natural products and vitamins chapter, and the osteoporosis chapter.

TREATMENT OF HYPERKALEMIA

A normal potassium level is 3.5-5 mEq/L. Hyperkalemia, depending on the source, can be defined as a potassium level above 5.3 or above 5.5 mEq/L, although most clinicians are concerned with any level above 5 mEq/L.

Potassium is the most abundant intracellular cation and is essential for life. Humans obtain potassium through the diet from many foods, including meats, beans and fruits. Daily intake through the GI tract is about 1 mEq/kg/day. Any excess intake is excreted partially via the gut and primarily via the kidneys. Potassium excretion is increased by aldosterone, diuretics (strongly by loops, weakly by thiazides), by a high urine flow (via osmotic diuresis), and by negatively charged ions in the distal tubule (via bicarbonate).

Even if a person intakes a very rich potassium load the acute rise in potassium would be off-set by the release of insulin, which would cause potassium intake into the cells. Therefore, excessive intake is not normally a cause of hyperkalemia unless there is significant renal damage. Patients with renal insufficiency can become hyperkalemic, but the most common cause of hyperkalemia is decreased renal excretion due to renal failure.

This may be in combination with a high potassium intake or can be partially due to the use of drugs that interfere with potassium excretion. Drugs that raise potassium levels include potassium-sparing diuretics (including aldosterone blockers), ACE Is, ARBs, NSAIDs, the oral contraceptives that contain drospirenone (Yaz, etc.), cyclosporine, tacrolimus, heparin, pentamidine, trimethoprim/sulfamethoxazole, digoxin toxicity, potassium supplements and potassium present in IV fluids, including TPN.

Diabetes patients often have a diet high in sodium and low in potassium and are taking ACE Is or ARBs. They also have insulin deficiency, which reduces the ability to shift potassium into the cells. These factors make patients with diabetes at higher risk for hyperkalemia. Hospitalized patients, primarily due to the use of drugs, are at higher risk of hyperkalemia than outpatients. Rarely, acute hyperkalemia can be due to tumor lysis, rhabdomyolysis or succinylcholine administration.

A patient with elevated potassium, depending on the level, may be asymptomatic or symptomatic. Muscle weakness and bradycardia may be present. Fatal arrhythmia can develop. The risk for severe outcomes increases as the potassium level increases.

To Lower Potassium (↓ K⁺)

This does not lower potassium BUT an ECG may be needed to check for cardiotoxicity (monitor heart rhythm). If required, administer IV calcium to stabilize the cardiac tissue.

- Remove sources of potassium intake. This may require dietary changes.

- Enhance potassium uptake by the cells via:

  - Glucose (to stimulate insulin secretion – but not enough by itself).

  - Insulin, given with the glucose.

- If metabolic acidosis is present, administer sodium bicarbonate.

- Consider beta-agonists, such as nebulized albuterol.

  - Monitor for tachycardia, chest pain.

- Increase renal excretion with a loop diuretic, such as furosemide.

  - Monitor volume status.

- Another option to increase renal excretion is fluorohydrocortisone (Florinef), especially in a patient with hypoaldosteronism.

- Consider the use of the cation exchange resin sodium polystyrene sulfonate *(Kayexelate)*. This works within two hours and can decrease potassium by 2 mEq/L with a single enema. SPS is given orally or rectally. Rectal administration is preferred for high (emergency) treatment.

  - If using oral SPS, do NOT mix with sorbitol; in 2010 the FDA issued a warning against mixing the drug with sorbitol due to a risk of GI necrosis.

- Common side effects include ↓ appetite, nausea, vomiting, or constipation (less commonly diarrhea).

- Emergency dialysis can be used if the hyperkalemia could be fatal or for patients with renal failure; setting up dialysis takes time.

13

DRUG USE IN PREGNANCY

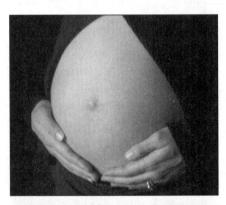

GUIDELINES (SELECTED)

CDC STD recommendations,
at www.cdc.gov

Department of Veteran Affairs, Department of Defense. VA/DoD clinical practice guideline for management of pregnancy. Washington (DC); 2009.

American College of Obstetricians and Gynecologists (ACOG) Practice Guidelines, various, available at www.guidelines.gov

FDA Pregnancy Categories

Pregnancy Category A

Controlled studies in animals and women have shown no risk in the 1st trimester, and possible fetal harm is remote.

Pregnancy Category B

Either animal studies have not demonstrated a fetal risk but there are no controlled studies in pregnant women, or animal studies have shown an adverse effect that was not confirmed in controlled studies in women in the 1st trimester.

Pregnancy Category C

No controlled studies in humans have been performed and animal studies have shown adverse events, or studies in humans and animals are not available; give only if potential benefit outweighs the risk.

Pregnancy Category D

Positive evidence of fetal risk is available, but the benefits may outweigh the risk if life-threatening or serious disease.

Pregnancy Category X

Studies in animals or humans show fetal abnormalities; use in pregnancy is contraindicated.

As a General Rule: Try to avoid all drugs if possible during 1st trimester (organogenesis) and use lifestyle recommendations first, to see if you can avoid the use of agents that may pose a risk.

ENCOURAGE ENROLLMENT IN THE PREGNANCY REGISTRIES

Pregnancy exposure registries exist for select disease states and for many individual drugs. They are designed to collect health information from women who take various drugs when they are pregnant and breastfeeding. Information is also collected on the newborn baby. This information is compared with women who have not taken medicine during pregnancy and the health of their babies.

The FDA pregnancy categories listed above do not always correctly define risk: consider that many drugs have had pregnancy categories changed recently in light of data that the drugs were not as safe as previously thought, including older drugs such as NSAIDs and SSRIs. Clinicians need real-life data on how the effect of these drugs; only with this information can we help parents make informed decisions. There are registries for drugs by condition (cancer, autoimmune conditions, HIV, epilepsy) and many other registries for individual drugs. Search for "pregnancy registries" at www.fda.gov.

COMMON TERATOGENS

If a case indicates hCG+, the patient is pregnant and teratogenic drugs should be discontinued, if possible. Well-known teratogens include alcohol, ACE Inhibitors, Angiotensin Receptor Blockers, carbamazepine, isotretinoin, lithium, NSAIDs, phenytoin, phenobarbital, topiramate, valproic acid, ribavirin, misoprostol, methotrexate, leflunomide, statins, dutasteride, finasteride, warfarin, lenalidomide and thalidomide. This list is far from complete; it represents large well-known drugs and classes only.

Many psychiatric drugs have risk in pregnancy. The drug's potential harm must be weighed against the risk of the condition not being treated adequately. In bipolar disorder, lithium and valproate are considered among the highest risk. In recent years, the use of sertraline and paroxetine (considered the riskiest SSRI; pregnancy category D) during pregnancy has become questionable, while bupropion is often the go-to drug during pregnancy. Specific drugs have more risk than others and guidelines include first-choice drugs for various psychiatric conditions.

FOLIC ACID IN WOMEN OF CHILD-BEARING AGE

Whenever a young woman enters the pharmacy, the pharmacist can ask if she consuming adequate folic acid (400-800 mcg daily, which is 0.4-0.8 mg/day), calcium (1,000 mg daily) and vitamin D (600 IU daily).

It is a safe and reasonable recommendation to women planning to conceive (and all women of child-bearing age, since many pregnancies are not planned) to take a folic acid supplement (at least one month prior to pregnancy) to help prevent birth defects of the brain and spinal cord (neural tube defects). Folic acid should be continued for the first 2-3 months of pregnancy. Folic acid is in many healthy foods, including fortified cereals (some of which are not healthy), dried beans, leafy green vegetables and orange juice. An OTC multivitamin that contains at least 400 mcg of folic acid can be recommended. Prescription prenatal vitamins *(PrimaCare ONE, Zenate*, others) usually contain 1,000 mcg, or 1 mg – this is an Rx dose of folic acid.

COMMON OTC-TREATABLE CONDITIONS IN PREGNANCY

Nausea/Vomiting

First, recommend eating smaller, more frequent meals, avoiding spicy or odorous foods, taking more frequent naps, and reducing stress, including working long hours. If this does not work recommend pyridoxine, which is vitamin B6. This is the 1st line recommendation by ACOG, with or without the antihistamine doxylamine *(Unisom)*. A natural product which may be helpful is ginger, in tea form, or cooked, do not recommend supplements. Dried, salted plums are used by certain ethnic groups.

GERD/Heartburn/Gas Pains

First recommend eating smaller, more frequent meals, avoiding foods that worsen GERD, and if symptoms occur while sleeping, recommend elevating the head of the bed and not eating three hours prior to sleep. If this does not work, calcium antacids are first-line, such as calcium carbonate in *Tums* or store brands. This is a good antacid choice since calcium intake is often deficient in pregnancy. Use caution with excessive use of antacids containing aluminum or calcium if renal disease is present *(Maalox, Mylanta*, etc.)

If gas is a concern, simethicone is considered safe *(Gas-X, Mylicon)* – and the *Mylicon* infant drops are considered safe for infants. H2 blockers *(Pepcid, Tagamet, Axid, Zantac* are all pregnancy category B); many doctors recommend OTC or Rx doses. PPIs are B's or C's.

Constipation

First recommend increasing fluid intake, increasing fiber in the diet, increasing physical activity, such as walking. If this does not work fiber is 1st-line and psyllium is pregnancy category B *(Metamucil*, store brands).

Cough/Cold/Allergies

The first-generation antihistamine doxylamine *(Unisom)* is pregnancy category B and is the usual first-line recommendation. Diphenhydramine is pregnancy category B (both of these antihistamines enter breast milk and neither are used during lactation). Decongestants (pseudoephedrine, phenylephrine, oxymetazoline), dextromethorphan and guaifenesin are pregnancy category C, but may be recommended by the physician.

Pain

Acetaminophen is pregnancy category B and is the analgesic and antipyretic drug-of-choice during pregnancy. Ibuprofen is pregnancy category D and naproxen is pregnancy category C; pharmacists should not recommend OTC NSAIDs in pregnancy. Caution for lactation: most opioids are excreted in breast milk. While this use may be acceptable in small amounts, the risk to the infant must be considered. Do not use codeine (in *Tylenol #3*, others), since rapid metabolizers of the CYP 450 2D6 enzyme will produce excessive amounts of morphine rapidly, which could be fatal to the infant.

SELECT CONDITIONS AND FIRST-LINE TREATMENT

DIT

Vaccine Use During Pregnancy

- Influenza vaccine (shot, inactivated): each fall, whether pregnant or not – this is recommended in all stages of pregnancy.

- No live vaccines [MMR, varicella (chickenpox), live influenza nasal, etc.] one month before and during pregnancy.

- Pregnant women > 20 weeks gestation should receive Tdap if they need a booster. If the woman has not been vaccinated or the history is unclear, a 3-dose series is needed (one with Tdap, the other two with Td only). If the woman delivers and has not received vaccination, she should receive it post-delivery. Vaccination protects the baby (and the mother) from pertussis (whooping cough).

- Other vaccines may be needed in unusual circumstances, such as a need for a tetanus update, or foreign travel; refer to CDC guidelines.

ANTIBIOTIC USE DURING PREGNANCY

Generally considered safe to use:

Penicillins (including amoxicillin and ampicillin, both B's) and cephalosporins, erythromycin and azithromycin (B's, but not clarithromycin, which is C)

Do not use during pregnancy: FQ, Tetra, Bactrim

Quinolones (due to cartilage damage) and tetracyclines (due to teeth discoloration)

Vaginal Fungal Infections

Use topical antifungals (creams, suppositories), at least 7 days.

Urinary Tract Infections

Beta lactams that cover the organism can be used, such as cephalexin (500 mg QID) or ampicillin. Nitrofurantoin 100 mg BID is used, but not in the last several weeks of pregnancy. Another option is fosfomycin (*Monurol*) 3 grams (1 packet, mixed with water) x 1. Sulfamethoxazole-trimethoprim (*Bactrim*) has been commonly used for UTIs in pregnancy; it is not clear if this is safe and is best avoided, if possible. The concern is over the use of agents that interfere with folic acid metabolism.

Chlamydia

Azithromycin 1 g x 1

Gonorrhea

Cephalosporin, or if contraindicated, azithromycin 2 g x 1

Bacterial Vaginosis

Clindamycin 300 mg BID or metronidazole (500 mg BID or 250 mg TID). Topical (vaginal) therapy for bacterial vaginosis is not recommended during pregnancy.

Vaginal Trichomoniasis

2 g metronidazole x 1 at any stage of pregnancy. Treatment may be deferred after 37 weeks.

ASTHMA IN PREGNANCY

- Inhaled corticosteroids are first-line controller therapy for persistent asthma during pregnancy.

- Budesonide is the preferred inhaled corticosteroid for use during pregnancy.

- Inhaled albuterol is recommended rescue therapy for pregnant women with asthma.

VENOUS THROMBOEMBOLISM/MECHANICAL VALVES

Heparin (UFH) or LMWH, convert to shorter half-life UFH during last month of pregnancy or if delivery appears imminent. Use pneumatic compression devices prior to delivery in women with thrombosis if they are getting a C-section. No warfarin during pregnancy (category X), the newer anticoagulants are category C and are not currently in the recommendations.

Hypothyroidism

Must test for and treat, with levothyroxine, which is pregnancy category A.

Hyperthyroidism

If treated, both drugs are pregnancy category D but may need to be used: propylthiouracil if trying to conceive and in 1st trimester, then switch to methimazole. Monitor for liver injury.

Anemia

Anemia due to iron deficiency can occur during pregnancy and will be treated with supplemental iron, in addition to prenatal vitamins (which contain some iron).

Do not use tobacco during pregnancy/encourage cessation: Smoking in pregnancy can cause adverse outcomes for the child, including spontaneous abortion, low birth weight and sudden infant death. If women smoke 5 or less cigarettes (occasional, "nervous" type smokers) they should be encouraged to quit with behavioral support. If they smoke more than 5 cigarettes daily, ACOG recommends bupropion (pregnancy category C), and other sources recommend nicotine replacement in pregnancy, however the efficacy is not as high in non-pregnant patients. All nicotine products are pregnancy category D except for the gum which is pregnancy category C.

Do not use alcohol during pregnancy/encourage cessation: No amount of alcohol is safe during pregnancy.

14

DRUG REFERENCES

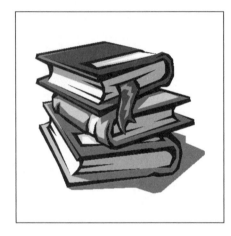

Drug Monographs

- Facts and Comparisons

- Lexi-Comp Clinical Online Databases

- Micromedex

- American Hospital Formulary Service Drug Information (AHFS) Drug Information

- Drug Information Handbook (Lacy's)

- Physician's Desk Reference (PDR) (Product Package Inserts, Vol I, and Patient Information, Vol II)

Bioequivalence

ORANGE BOOK

Can look up by active ingredient, proprietary name, applicant holder or applicant number. Published by the Food and Drug Administration (FDA) Center for Drug Evaluation and Research (CDER). Available at www.fda.gov/cder/ob

RATINGS

AA Products in conventional dosage forms not presenting bioequivalence problems.

AB Drugs that have been proven to meet the necessary bioequivalence requirements through in vivo and/or in vitro testing. AB is the most common designation. Drugs coded as AB are therapeutically equivalent and can be interchanged (brand to generic).

The FDA may not have compared each generic to each brand of the same drug. For example, the Orange Book lists *Cardizem SR*, *Cardizem CD*, *Dilacor XR*, and *Tiazac* under the heading for diltiazem. These are not bioequivalent to each other; however, some have generic equivalents. For example, *Cardizem SR* and the generic formulations are "AB1," *Dilacor XR* is "AB2,

The generic for *Cardizem CD* is "AB3." Products rated AB1 are bioequivalent to each other, products rated AB2 are bioequivalent to each other, and so forth.

The 2nd letter can also refer to the dosage form:

AN Solutions and powders for aerosolization

AO Injectable oil solutions; these are considered to be pharmaceutically and therapeutically equivalent only when the active ingredient, its concentration, and the type of oil used as a vehicle are all identical.

AP Injectable aqueous solutions

AT Topical products, including those for dermatologic, ophthalmic, otic, rectal, and vaginal administration formulated as solutions, creams, ointments, gels, lotions, pastes, sprays, and suppositories

DRUG PRICING

The Red Book

includes Average Wholesale Price (AWP) and the suggested retail price.

It is also useful to check if a drug is available: If a product is not listed in the Orange Book, it does not have an approved application (NDA or ANDA) with the FDA. [Note that DESI products (some of the pre-1962 drugs) are not listed in the Orange Book, since they do not have approved applications.] A manufacturer may have an approved drug with the FDA (and it will be listed in the Orange Book) but may not be marketing it at present which you could tell because it would not be listed in the Red Book.

Specific Drug References

REPORTING ADVERSE DRUG REACTIONS

- FDA's MedWatch Program (AERS, for drugs/devices) at http://www.fda.gov/medwatch/ or 1-800-FDA-1088 (1-800-332-1088).

- Vaccines: FDA's VAERS (see immunization section)

REPORTING MEDICAL ERRORS

In Hospital

- To the P&T Committee, at staff meetings (as defined by facility), to the Medication Safety Committee

In any setting

- ISMP's Medication Errors Reporting Program (MERP)

- FDA's MedWatch

- MedMARx program

IV STABILITY
- Trissel's Stability of Compounded Formulations (IV formulations)

- AHFS Drug Information

- Micromedex

COMPOUNDING AND MANUFACTURING
- Handbook on Extemporaneous Formulations

- International Journal of Pharmaceutical Compounding

- Stability of Compounded Formulations

- US Pharmacopoeia National Formulary (chapter on Pharmacy Compounding) (USP sets standards for quality, purity, identity, and strength of medicines, food ingredients and dietary supplements manufactured.)

- Allen's Compounded Formulations

- Remington: The Science and Practice of Pharmacy (chapter on Extemporaneous Prescription Compounding)

PEDIATRIC
- Harriet Lane Handbook

- Pediatric Dosage Handbook

- AHFS Drug Information

- Micromedex

FOREIGN DRUG IDENTIFICATION
- Martindales

- European Drug Index

- USP Dictionary of USAN and International Drug Names

- Drugs Available Abroad

- Micromedex

- International Drug Directory (Index Nominum)

NATURAL PRODUCTS

- Natural Medicines:Comprehensive Database
- US Pharmacopoeia
- PDR for Herbal Medicines
- The Complete German Commission E Monograph

PHARMACOTHERAPY DECISION MAKING OTC

- Handbook of Nonprescription Drugs (OTC)

PHARMACOTHERAPY DECISION MAKING OTC AND RX

- Pharmacotherapy: A Pathophysiologic Approach (DiPiro)
- Applied Therapeutics: The Clinical Use of Drugs (Koda-Kimble)
- Pharmacist's Letter
- Sanford Guide (for ID)
- Harrison's Principles of Internal Medicine
- Drugs of Choice from the Medical Letter
- Washington Manual of Medical Therapeutics
- The Merck Manual

PHARMACOLOGY/PHARMACEUTICS

- Goodman and Gilman's: The Pharmacological Basis of Therapeutics
- Merck Index
- Remington: The Science and Practice of Pharmacy
- Handbook of Pharmaceutical Excipients

PSYCHOLOGY

- DSM-IV (Diagnostic and Statistical Manual of Mental Disorders)

PREGNANCY AND LACTATION

- Briggs' Drugs in Pregnancy and Lactation
- Micromedex
- Breastfeeding: A Guide for the Medical Profession
- ACCP's Safety of Drugs in Pregnancy and Lactation

TABLET-CAPSULE ID

- Facts and Comparisons

- United States Pharmacopoeia Drug Information (USPDI)

- Physician's Desk Reference (PDR)

- Ident-A-Drug

- Micromedex

- Mosby's

Miscellaneous Drug References

LEGISLATIVE AND BUSINESS DEVELOPMENTS

- The Pink Sheet (for PhARMA news – the Pharmaceutical Research and Manufacturers Association of America), PhARMA news can be found the Wall Street Journal, NY Times & other news sources

- Pharmacist's Letter

- FDA Website

SELECT KEY GUIDELINES

- National Cholesterol Education Project Adult Treatment Panel (NCEP ATP 3), Cholesterol

- Joint National Commission (JNC) 7 and American Heart Association (AHA) Update, Hypertension

- American Diabetes Assoc (ADA) Clinical Practice Recommendations and American Association of Clinical Endocrinologists/American College of Endocrinology Consensus Statement (AACE), Diabetes

- CHEST guidelines for antithrombotic therapy

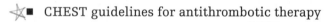

INN

- International Nonproprietary Names for Pharmaceutical Substances

NDC

- The National Drug Code (NDC) is the universal product identifier for human drugs.

DISPOSAL OF PRESCRIPTION DRUGS

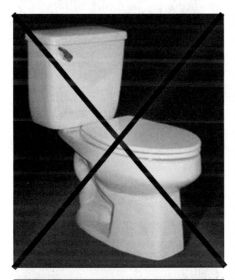

Proper Disposal of Prescription Drugs

Common prescription agents, including beta blockers and ACE Inhibitors, can be measured in fish in the Pacific basin. This region is not alone; drug concentrations in the ocean are an environmental disaster. It is important to realize that proper disposal is critical, but only part of the solution. The majority of drugs and drug metabolites end up in the oceans from the patient's urine and stool – the best way to reduce this exposure is to improve the health of the population to reduce the amount of drugs people are using. The federal prescription drug disposal guidelines recommend (in the absence of a "take-back" program – described below) mixing unwanted drugs (including controlled drugs) with unpalatable substances and placing them in a non-descript container before discarding in the trash unless the prescribing information specifically states the drug is to be flushed down the toilet or sink (see list of "okay to flush" drugs at the end of this section). The list of drugs that are acceptable to flush include only certain controlled drugs.

Some environmental experts disagree with the FDAs recommendations for flushing certain high-risk drugs and instead advise consumers to dispose of unwanted medications in their original prescription containers with any identifying information removed, and to not flush any medications, even if the patient information instructs otherwise. Note that the FDA is particularly concerned with the risk of the wrong person getting or taking the controlled drug – and subsequent harm.

Instruct patients: Do not flush prescription drugs down the toilet or drain unless the label or accompanying patient information specifically instructs you to do so.

To dispose of prescription drugs not labeled to be flushed, patients should be advised to take advantage of community drug take-back programs or other programs, such as household hazardous waste collection events, that collect drugs at a central location for proper disposal. <u>In 2010, the FDA started the first national "Take Back" day for unwanted drugs. Pharmacies have been involved, in all 50 states, in notifying patients where to take unused medications for destruction. These are annual events and have been very successful. The "Take Back" day in 2011 collected 498 tons of unused medications.</u>

The DEA's Take-Back events are a significant piece of the government's prescription drug abuse prevention strategy. Purging America's home medicine cabinets of unwanted or expired medications is one of four action items outlined in the strategy for reducing prescription drug abuse and diversion. The other action items include education of health care providers, patients, parents and youth; establishing prescription drug monitoring programs in all the states; and increased enforcement to address "doctor shopping" and pill mills.

PHARMACY INVOLVEMENT IN TAKING BACK UNWANTED DRUGS (THIS IS ONGOING, AND NOT "TAKE BACK DAYS" AS DESCRIBED ABOVE)

<u>In California and many other states, pharmacies, and other designated sites, have the ability to help patients dispose of unwanted prescription and over-the-counter drugs</u> – but <u>NOT controlled substances</u>, which must be returned only to law enforcement – without flushing them down the toilet or tossing them in the garbage. These are voluntary programs for community pharmacies.

The pharmacies can either:

- Use postage pre-paid envelopes so that consumers can return unwanted drugs to licensed waste disposal facilities, away from pharmacies where health care is provided, or

- Establish a collection bin for ongoing collection at pharmacies.

<u>Drugs should not be reviewed by staff</u> at a collection site (whether a pharmacy or community event) before being deposited into a secured collection bin. The patient or patient's agent should deposit the drugs themselves, thereby preventing staff from knowing what is being returned.

<u>Drugs that are collected should be separated from their containers</u> by patients or their agents before being placed in the collection bin, which reduces the disposal costs because the containers will not be part of the pharmaceutical waste.

Locking the "Take Back" Container

- There should be two separate locks on the secured collection bin: one key should be in the possession of the pharmacy, the other key in the possession of the licensed integrated waste hauler who will pick up what is now classified as "hazardous household waste."

- This dual lock ensures that the pharmacy cannot open the collection bin without the presence of the integrated waste hauler, and vice versa.

Some Pharmacies do not participate in Take Back Programs, but offer services for disposal by mail, including the common "TakeAway" mailers that are processed by companies, such as Sharps, Inc.

The "TakeAway" mailers are popular in many pharmacies and include return shipping and handling. They are for Rx (not controlled) and OTC drugs. At the receiving end the products are processed by law enforcement. Pharmacies can also have bins for medication drop off in the store. These services can also be used by pharmacies for their own medical waste, such as syringes during flu season.

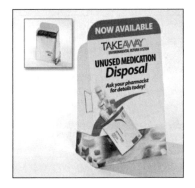 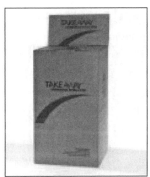 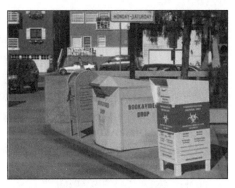

| Patient either gives TakeAway envelope to US postal service or UPS driver, or store – this picture is a display box that contains the mailing envelopes | Or, the patient drops off in the box of a pharmacy that has the container – neither option is for controlled drugs | Some communities have locked boxes for controlled drugs – if putting medicine into this container, the drug name must be visible (but not patient info) |

If the patient uses the mailer (rather than the drop-off box in a pharmacy) they put the medications into the brown mailing envelope, then put in the US mail or bring to a UPS store or driver. The return shipping is paid. Up to 4 ounces of liquids or gels can be put in a Ziploc bag into the envelope.

In the Absence of a Take Back Program or Access to Mailers, Instruct Patients to Follow Local Guidelines for Home Hazardous Waste (HHW) Collection.

Find the phone number of the local HHW collection site in the government section of the local white pages of the telephone directory. It is important for patients to know their local regulations. It may be that the locality requires drugs to be dropped off at certain sites, or be placed in the trash. If drugs are placed in the trash the following procedures should be followed:

Keep medicine in its original child-resistant container. Scratch or mark out the patient information on the label.

Place some water into solid medications, such as pills or capsules. Then add something nontoxic and unpalatable such as sawdust, kitty litter, charcoal, *Comet* or powdered spices (such as cayenne pepper).

Close and seal the container lids tightly with packing or duct tape. If discarding blister packs of unused medicines, <u>wrap in multiple layers of duct tape.</u>

Place medicine containers in durable <u>packaging that does not show what's inside</u> (such as a cardboard box).

Place in the trash close to garbage pickup time.

Syringe Disposal

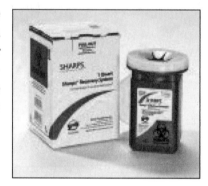

Improper management of discarded needles expose waste workers to potential needle stick injuries and infection risk when containers break open inside garbage trucks or needles are mistakenly sent to recycling facilities. Janitors, housekeepers and family members risk injury if loose sharps poke through plastic garbage bags. Used needles can transmit diseases, including HIV and hepatitis.

OPTIONS FOR SAFE SYRINGE DISPOSAL

Drop Box or Supervised Collection Sites

Sharps users can take their own sharps containers filled with used needles to appropriate collections sites: doctors' offices, hospitals, pharmacies, health departments, or fire stations. Services are free or have a nominal fee. Check for availability in your area.

Mail-Back Programs

Sharps users place their used sharps in special containers and return the container by mail to a collection site for proper disposal. Fees vary, depending on the size of the container. These are available in many pharmacies. Sharps, Inc. is a commonly used source for sharps mail-in containers, among others.

Syringe Exchange Programs (SEP)

Sharps users can exchange used needles for new needles. This is a proven method to decrease the transmission of blood-borne pathogens (HIV, hepatitis) by injection drug users. It is run by the North American Syringe Exchange Network at <u>www.nasen.org</u>.

At-Home Needle Destruction Devices

There are products patients use to destroy used needles at home. These devices sever, burn, or melt the needle. In general these are not recommended for places where others can be infected with a condition, because people can be pricked removing the needle. On the other hand, if the patient is in their own home and infection risk is low, this process reduces the cost of disposal because the plastic syringe can be disposed of in the trash if the needle has been removed. For example, this can be a cost-effective method for a patient injecting insulin several times daily.

Used Needle-Syringe Safety Tips

Disposable needles contaminated with drugs, chemicals or blood products should never be removed from their original syringes unless no other option is available. Throw the entire needle/syringe assembly (needle attached to the syringe) into the red plastic sharps container.

Never remove a needle by unscrewing it with your hands in a health care facility. At home, if infection risk is low, it may be possible to remove the needle by one of the devices described above.

Used disposable needles/sharps should be discarded immediately after use without recapping into a sharps container (a non-reusable plastic container that is puncture resistant, leak proof on the sides and bottom, properly labeled and closable).

Sharps containers should be easily accessible, replaced routinely, and not allowed to overfill. Never compress or "push down" on the contents of any sharps container.

If someone is stuck with a needle the patient should be seen by a health care provider immediately to assess infection risk and consider prophylactic therapy.

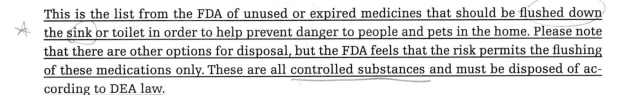

This is the list from the FDA of unused or expired medicines that should be flushed down the sink or toilet in order to help prevent danger to people and pets in the home. Please note that there are other options for disposal, but the FDA feels that the risk permits the flushing of these medications only. These are all controlled substances and must be disposed of according to DEA law.

DRUG	ACTIVE INGREDIENT
Actiq, oral transmucosal lozenge *	Fentanyl Citrate
Avinza, capsules (extended release)	Morphine Sulfate
Daytrana, transdermal patch system	Methylphenidate
Demerol, tablets *	Meperidine Hydrochloride
Demerol, oral solution *	Meperidine Hydrochloride
Diastat/Diastat AcuDial, rectal gel	Diazepam
Dilaudid, tablets *	Hydromorphone Hydrochloride
Dilaudid, oral liquid *	Hydromorphone Hydrochloride
Dolophine Hydrochloride, tablets *	Methadone Hydrochloride
Duragesic, patch (extended release) *	Fentanyl
Embeda, capsules (extended release)	Morphine Sulfate; Naltrexone Hydrochloride
Exalgo, tablets (extended release)	Hydromorphone Hydrochloride
Fentora, tablets (buccal)	Fentanyl Citrate
Kadian, capsules (extended release)	Morphine Sulfate
Methadone Hydrochloride, oral solution *	Methadone Hydrochloride
Methadose, tablets *	Methadone Hydrochloride
Morphine Sulfate, tablets (immediate release) *	Morphine Sulfate
Morphine Sulfate, oral solution *	Morphine Sulfate
MS Contin, tablets (extended release) *	Morphine Sulfate
Onsolis, soluble film (buccal)	Fentanyl Citrate
Opana, tablets (immediate release)	Oxymorphone Hydrochloride
Opana ER, tablets (extended release)	Oxymorphone Hydrochloride
Oramorph SR, tablets (sustained release)	Morphine Sulfate
Oxycontin, tablets (extended release) *	Oxycodone Hydrochloride
Percocet, tablets *	Acetaminophen; Oxycodone Hydrochloride
Percodan, tablets *	Aspirin; Oxycodone Hydrochloride
Xyrem, oral solution	Sodium Oxybate

These medicines have generic versions available or are only available in generic formulations.

Last revised March, 2010.

INFECTIOUS DISEASES

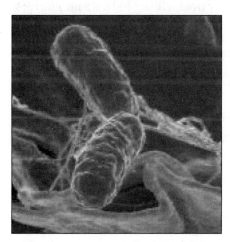

We gratefully acknowledge the assistance of Lee H. Nguyen, Pharm.D., BCPS, Infectious Diseases Pharmacist at St. Jude Medical Center and Assistant Professor at Loma Linda University, School of Pharmacy in preparing this section.

Background

An infectious disease is caused by one or more pathogenic viruses, bacteria, fungi, protozoa, parasites, and aberrant proteins known as prions. Transmission of disease can occur through various pathways including through physical contact with an infected individual, food, body fluids, contaminated objects, airborne inhalation or via vector-borne spread. Transmissible diseases, which occur through contact with an ill person or their secretions (or objects touched by them), are especially infective and are sometimes referred to as contagious diseases.

INFECTIOUS DISEASE PRINCIPALS

Bacterial organisms stain differently on a gram stain depending if they are gram positive or gram negative organisms. Gram positive (Gm+) organisms stain purple, or bluish in color, whereas gram negative (Gm-) organisms stain pink, or reddish in color. Empiric, broad-spectrum antibiotic treatment (that covers any possible organism) should be changed to directed antibiotic treatment as soon as possible (once gram stains, or preferably, specific cultures are available) in order to reduce the incidence of antibiotic resistance.

ANTIMICROBIAL STEWARDSHIP PROGRAMS (ASP)

- Antimicrobial stewardship has been defined as the optimal selection, dosage, and duration of antimicrobial treatment that results in the best clinical outcome for the treatment or prevention of infection, with minimal toxicity to the patient and minimal impact on subsequent resistance. It aims to promote the appropriate use of antimicrobials - the right drug, duration, dose, and route of administration. Promoting the appropriate use of antimicrobials is intended to improve clinical outcomes by reducing the emergence of resistance, limiting drug-related adverse events, and minimizing risk of unintentional consequences associated with antimicrobial use.

- Antimicrobial stewardship programs are typically a joint venture that contains infectious diseases physicians, infectious diseases pharmacist/s, and the pharmacy staff.

- Most programs contain an auditing component to determine the prescribing habits of physicians and an educational component to change poor prescribing habits and improve patient care.

- Other very common aspects of an ASP is to improve medication utilization through different means including 1) a restriction and/or pre-authorization policy, 2) intravenous-to-oral switch, and 3) de-escalation or streamlining.

- An antibiogram is a chart that contains the susceptibility patterns of select antibiotics and bacterial pathogens of a single institution or multiple institutions over a year's span. An example of an antibiogram is on the following page.

Common terms

- <u>Minimum inhibitory concentration (MIC)</u> – lowest drug concentration that prevents microbial growth in 24 hours.

- <u>Minimum bactericidal concentration (MBC)</u> – lowest drug concentration that reduces bacterial density by 99.9% in 24 hours.

- <u>Synergy</u> – effect of two or more agents produces a greater effect than each agent alone.

ANTIBIOGRAM *(JANUARY 1-DECEMBER 31 2009)*

	Acinotobacter baumenii	Citrobacter freundii	Citrobacter koseri	Enterobacter aeroenes	Enterobacter cloace	E. faecolis	E. faeccium	E. coli	Klebsiella pneumoniae	Morganella morganii	Proteus mirabilis	Providencai stuartii	Pseudomonas aeuginosas	Serratia marcescens	S. aureus
# isolates antibiotics	37	52	44	68	99	529	68	1,073	394	63	301	21	446	75	806
Amikacin	97	100	100	100	100			100	99	100	100	100	92	99	
Ampicillin	0	0	0	0	3	100	16	43	0	0	62	0		0	
Amp/sulbactam	69	0	84	0	6			43	0	0	62	0		0	
Cefazolin	0	0	86	0	1			87	94	0	86	0		0	41
Cefepime	57	100	100	99	94			98	97	98	98	100	92	100	
Ceftriaxone	0	79	89	82	81			97	96	95	96	100		99	
Ceftazidime	46	79	86	79	80			97	95	95	94	95	92	97	
Ciprofloxacin**	59	81	86	94	87			68	95	84	57	33	78	95	
Clyndamycin*															81*
Gentamicin	73	87	100	100	95			88	97	81	83	0	85	99	
Imipenen	84	100	100	100	100			100	100		100	95	90	100	
Oxacillin															41
Pennicillin G						99	15								6
Pip/tazobactan	62	90	93	85	86			98	98	92	99	100	93	99	
Tetracucline															95
Tobramycin	81	96	100	100	96			90	97	92	84	0	94	93	
TMP/Sulfa	54	73	86	100	85			71	90	68	65	71		99	99
Vancomycin						99	28								100

* may not reflect inducible MLS resistance

** can be used to predict susceptibility to moxifloxacin except Pseudomonas

Factors to consider when selecting a drug regimen

- Site of infection

- Severity of disease

- Patient characteristics (age, renal function, liver function, allergies, pregnancy status, etc.)

- Spectrum of activity of the drug

- Etiology of infection

Monitoring for therapeutic effectiveness

- Fever curve

- WBC count

- Radiographic findings

- Pain/inflammation

- Elevated markers of inflammation

- Reduction in signs and symptoms

Lack of therapeutic effectiveness

- Misdiagnosis

- Improper drug regimen

- Inappropriate choice of agent(s) selected

- Drug resistance

SAMPLE CULTURE AND SENSITIVITY REPORT

- Urine culture

- Organism 1: *Pseudomonas aeruginosa*

- Organism 2: *Morganella morganii*

DRUG	ORGANISM 1	ORGANISM 2
Ampicillin	-	R
Ampicillin/sulbactam	-	R
Cefazolin	-	R
Cefoxitin	-	R
Ceftazidime	S	S
Ceftriaxone	-	S
Ciprofloxacin	S	R
Ertapenem	-	S
Gentamicin	S	R
Imipenem	S	-
Levofloxacin	S	R
Meropenem	S	-
Nitrofurantoin	-	R
Piperacillin/tazobactam	S	-
Tobramycin	S	R
Trimethoprim/sulfamethoxazole	-	R

S = susceptible; I = intermediately susceptible; R = resistant

When deciding upon an antibiotic regimen, consider the following:

- If an infection is present or not – the urine culture report above does not determine presence of infection or not. A urinary analysis and/or clinical signs and symptoms should be the determinant whether an infection is present.

- Drug allergies and antibiotic use history.

- Location of infection. Hepatically cleared antimicrobials may not get appreciable drug concentrations in the urine.

- Drug regimen: ideally a single antimicrobial would be best for most infections (certain infections may require more than one drug for treatment).

  - Other co-infections should also be taken into account. This could easily justify the use of more than one antibiotic.

- Absence of susceptibility results – ["S", "I", or "R"] does not constitute resistance. It represents information not given. This is typically due to either the FDA or Clinical and Laboratory Standards Institute (CLSI) suppression rules where a preferred antibiotic therapy is available and non-preferred (i.e. broader therapy) is suppressed.

- To effectively treat the urinary tract infection listed above, it is best to pick the narrowest spectrum antibiotic as possible to limit the spread of resistance.

  - The narrowest spectrum antibiotic that can treat both infections would most likely be ceftazidime.

ANTIBACTERIAL AGENTS

Aminoglycosides (AMGs)

AMGs interfere with bacterial protein synthesis by binding to 30S and 50S ribosomal subunits resulting in a defective bacterial cell membrane. AMGs exhibit concentration dependent kill and they have a post antibiotic effect (PAE). The PAE is defined as the continued suppression of bacterial growth when antibiotic levels are below the MIC of the organism.

DRUG	NOTES	SIDE EFFECTS/CONTRAINDICATIONS/MONITORING
Gentamicin, Tobramycin, Amikacin	Mainly active against (Gm -) bacteria (e.g. *Pseudomonas*), used for synergy in treating (Gm +) cocci (e.g. *Staphylococcus/Enterococcus endocarditis*) Tobramycin comes in an inhaled formulation, ***TOBI***, used in CF (with a PARI-LC PLUS nebulizer) Amikacin – has broadest activity Dose on IBW, unless total body weight (TBW) is less Use AdjBW if TBW > 30% of IBW (morbidly obese)	**BLACK BOX WARNINGS** AMGs may cause neurotoxicity (vertigo, ataxia) and nephrotoxicity **SIDE EFFECTS** Nephrotoxicity and ototoxicity. Use with caution in patients with impaired renal function, in the elderly, and those on other nephro toxic drugs (amphotericin B, cisplatin, NSAIDs, vancomycin, contrast dyes, cyclosporine and others) **MONITORING** Renal function, hearing tests, and peak and trough levels if using traditional dosing or a random level with extended interval dosing Pregnancy Category D May ↑ levels of neuromuscular blocking agents

DOSING OF AMGs

DOSING TYPE	DOSE	FREQUENCY			
Traditional dosing (AKA conventional)	Gent/tobra: 1 - 2 mg/kg/dose Amikacin: 5 - 7.5 mg/kg/dose	CrCl > 60 mL/min	CrCl 40-60 mL/min	CrCl 20-40 mL/min	CrCl < 20 mL/min
		Q8H	Q12H	Q24H	Give loading dose, monitor levels
		Take trough level right before next dose, take a peak level ½ hour after the end of drug infusion			
Extended Interval dosing	Gent/tobra: 4-7 mg/kg Amikacin: 15-20 mg/kg	Draw random level within 6-16 hours post dose; determine frequency based on nomogram (example of nomogram on next page). Extended Interval dosing is less nephrotoxic and more cost-effective.			

TRADITIONAL DOSING DRUG CONCENTRATIONS

DRUG	PEAK (MCG/ML)	TROUGH (MCG/ML)
Gentamicin	5 - 10	< 2
Tobramycin	5 - 10	< 2
Amikacin	20 - 30	< 5

Organism specific peak goals are typically 8-10 times the MIC of the bacteria causing the infection. (J. Infect. Dis. 155:93–99.)

Example of Extended Interval Dosing Nomogram

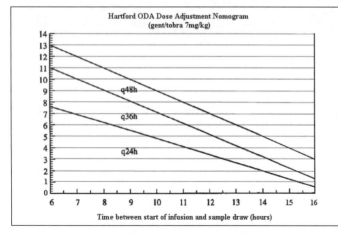

Antimicrob Agents Chemother. 1995 Mar;39(3):650-5

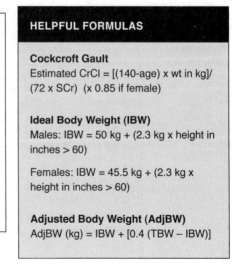

HELPFUL FORMULAS

Cockcroft Gault
Estimated CrCl = [(140-age) x wt in kg]/ (72 x SCr) (x 0.85 if female)

Ideal Body Weight (IBW)
Males: IBW = 50 kg + (2.3 kg x height in inches > 60)

Females: IBW = 45.5 kg + (2.3 kg x height in inches > 60)

Adjusted Body Weight (AdjBW)
AdjBW (kg) = IBW + [0.4 (TBW – IBW)]

Penicillins (PCNs)

Penicillins are beta-lactams that <u>inhibit bacterial cell wall synthesis</u> by binding to one or more penicillin-binding proteins (PBP's), which in turn prevents the final transpeptidation step of peptidoglycan synthesis in bacterial cell walls. Penicillins exhibit <u>time dependent kill</u>.

SELECT PENICILLINS

DRUG	NOTES	SIDE EFFECTS/CONTRAINDICATIONS/ MONITORING
Amoxicillin *(Amoxil, Moxatag)* + clavulanate *(Augmentin)* Ampicillin *(Principen)* Ampicillin + sulbactam *(Unasyn)* Penicillin *(Pen VK)* Piperacillin + tazobactam *(Zosyn)* Ticarcillin + clavulanic acid *(Timentin)*	Mainly active against (Gm +) cocci (*Staph* and *Strep*) and some (Gm -) bacilli. No atypical coverage Amoxicillin – DOC in acute otitis media, *H pylori* regimen, pregnancy, prophylaxis for endocarditis Agents combined with a beta-lactamase inhibitor have a broader spectrum of activity and are very popular in hospitals for treating many types of infections Reduce dose in renal impairment except for nafcillin, oxacillin, dicloxacillin, and cloxacillin Can be used for empiric coverage when combined with beta-lactamase inhibitor	**SIDE EFFECTS** Allergic reactions (including anaphylaxis), rash, pruritus, GI upset, diarrhea, seizures with accumulation, interstitial nephritis, colitis, agranulocytosis, ↑ LFT's **MONITORING** Renal function, signs of anaphylaxis with 1st dose Do not use in PCN-allergic patients Pregnancy Category B Test Interactions: can cause false (+) urinary glucose test as well as a false (+) galactomannan test for aspergillosis *Augmentin oral susp* must be refrigerated, *Amoxil oral susp* may be refrigerated to improve taste, but is stable for 14 days at room temperature Take *Moxatag* within 1 hour of finishing a meal Take *Pen VK* on an empty stomach. *Pen VK susp* should be refrigerated after reconstitution

PENICILLIN DRUG INTERACTIONS

- Uricosuric agents (e.g. probenecid, allopurinol) can ↑ levels of PCNs by interfering with renal excretion.

- May ↓ effectiveness of oral contraceptives – check package insert for individual drug.

Cephalosporins

Cephalosporins are beta-lactams that <u>inhibit bacterial cell wall synthesis</u> by binding to one or more penicillin-binding proteins (PBP's), which in turn prevents the final transpeptidation step of peptidoglycan synthesis in bacterial cell walls. Cephalosporins exhibit <u>time dependent kill</u>. Spectrum of activity is dependent upon the generation of cephalosporin (see chart below).

DRUG	DOSING	SIDE EFFECTS/ CONTRAINDICATIONS/MONITORING
1st Generation [Better (Gm +) activity than (Gm -) activity]		**SIDE EFFECTS** Allergic reactions (anaphylaxis), rash, GI upset, diarrhea, seizures with accumulation, colitis, ↑ LFTs
Cefadroxil *(Duricef-N/A)*	500-1,000 mg Q12H (PO)	
Cefazolin *(Ancef, Kefzol)*	250-2,000 mg Q8H (IV)	**MONITORING** Renal function, signs of anaphylaxis with 1st dose
Cephalexin *(Keflex)*	250-500 mg Q6H (PO)	
2nd Generation [Better (Gm -) activity compared to 1st generation with similar (Gm +) activity]		Cross sensitivity (< 10%) with PCN allergy – DO NOT USE in patients who have a PCN allergy
Cefaclor *(Raniclor)*	250-500 mg Q8H (PO)	Pregnancy Category B
Cefotetan *(Cefotan-N/A)*	1-2 grams Q12H (IV)	Test Interactions – positive direct Coomb's test, false positive urinary glucose test
Cefoxitin *(Mefoxin)*	1-2 grams Q6-8H (IV)	Reduce dose in renal impairment except cefoperazone and ceftriaxone
Cefprozil *(Cefzil- N/A)*	250-500 mg Q12-24H (PO)	
Cefuroxime *(Ceftin, Zinacef)*	250-1,500 mg Q8H (PO/IV)	Cephalosporins that contain the N-methylthiotetrazole (NMTT or 1-MTT) side chain can lead to risk of hypoprothrombinemia (bleeding) and a disulfiram-like reaction with alcohol ingestion. These agents are cefamandole, cefmetazole, cefoperazone, cefotetan
Cefamandole *(Mandol – N/A)*		
Loracarbef *(Lorabid-N/A)*		
3rd Generation [Better (Gm -) activity compared to 2nd generation and less *Staphylococcal* (Gm +) activity compared to 2nd generation but better *Streptococcal* activity]		
Cefdinir *(Omnicef)*	300 mg Q12H or 600 mg daily (PO)	
Cefditoren *(Spectracef)*	200-400 mg Q12H (PO)	
Cefixime *(Suprax)*	400 mg divided every 12-24H (PO)	
Cefoperazone *(Cefobid)*	1,000-2,000 mg Q12H (IV)	
Cefotaxime *(Claforan)*	1-2 grams Q8-12H (IV/IM)	
Cefpodoxime *(Vantin)*	200-400 mg Q12H (PO)	
Ceftazidime *(Fortaz, Tazicef)*	1,000–2,000 mg Q8-12H (IV)	
Ceftibuten *(Cedax)*	400 mg daily (PO)	
Ceftriaxone *(Rocephin)*	1-2 grams Q12-24H (IV/IM)	
4th Generation [Best (Gm -) activity and (Gm +) activity similar to 1st generation]		
Cefepime *(Maxipime)*	1-2 grams Q8-12H (IV)	
5th generation **[Best (Gm +) activity; covers MRSA, some (Gm -) similar to ceftriaxone]**		
Ceftaroline fosamil *(Teflaro)*	600 mg Q12H (IV)	

DIT

CEPHALOSPORIN DRUG INTERACTIONS

- Uricosuric agents (e.g. probenecid, allopurinol) can ↑ levels of cephalosporins by interfering with renal excretion.

- Cephalosporins with the NMTT side chain may cause disulfiram-like reaction with ingestion of ethanol and can ↑ INR.

- May ↓ effectiveness of oral contraceptives – check package insert for individual drug.

Carbapenems

Carbapenems are beta-lactams that inhibit bacterial cell wall synthesis by binding to one or more penicillin-binding proteins (PBP's), which in turn prevents the final transpeptidation step of peptidoglycan synthesis in bacterial cell walls. Carbapenems exhibit time dependent kill.

DRUG	DOSING	SIDE EFFECTS/CONTRAINDICATIONS/ MONITORING
Imipenem/Cilastatin (Primaxin)	250 -1,000 mg IV Q6H	Active against most (Gm +), (Gm -), and anaerobic pathogens. No atypical coverage. **SIDE EFFECTS** Diarrhea, rash, and seizures with higher doses and in patients with impaired renal function (mainly imipenem)
Meropenem (Merrem)	500 - 2,000 mg IV/IM Q8H	**MONITORING** Renal function, signs of anaphylaxis with 1st dose Pregnancy Category B (except imipenem, C) Imipenem is combined with cilastatin to prevent its degradation by renal tubular dehydropeptidase Reduce dose in renal impairment
Ertapenem (Invanz)	1,000 mg IV/IM daily Ertapenem is not active against *Pseudomonas* or *Acinetobacter*	DO NOT USE in patients with PCN allergy, cross-reactivity is approximately 50%
Doripenem (Doribax)	500 mg IV Q8H	

CARBAPENEM DRUG INTERACTIONS

- Uricosuric agents (e.g. probenecid, allopurinol) can ↑ levels of carbapenems by interfering with renal excretion. Carbapenems can ↓ serum concentrations of valproic acid leading to a loss of seizure control. Avoid concomitant use of imipenem with ganciclovir due to the compounded increased risk of seizures.

- Use with caution in patients at risk for seizures.

Fluoroquinolones (FQ)

Fluoroquinolones inhibits bacterial DNA topoisomerase IV and inhibits DNA gyrase (topoisomerase II). This prevents supercoiling of DNA and promotes breakage of double-stranded DNA. Fluoroquinolones exhibit concentration dependent killing.

DRUG	DOSING	SIDE EFFECTS/CONTRAINDICATIONS/MONITORING
Ofloxacin *(Floxin)*	Ciprofloxacin dosing 250-750 mg PO or 200-400 IV CrCl > 50 mL/min: Q8-12H	Extensive activity against (Gm -), (Gm +), and average to excellent atypical coverage (levofloxacin, moxifloxacin, & gemifloxacin – excellent atypical coverage)
Norfloxacin *(Noroxin)*	CrCl 30-50 mL/min: Q12H CrCl < 30 mL/min: Q18-24H Levofloxacin dosing (IV/PO)	**BLACK BOX WARNING** Tendon inflammation and/or rupture (most often in Achilles tendon) – risk with concurrent corticosteroid use, organ transplant patients, and patients > 60 years of age
Ciprofloxacin (Cipro, Cipro XR, *Proquin XR*, *Ciloxan* ophthalmic, *Cetraxal, Ciprodex* Otic)	CrCl > 50 mL/min: 500 mg daily CrCl 20-49 mL/min: 500 mg, then 250 mg daily CrCl < 20 mL/min: 500 mg, then 250 mg Q48h	**SIDE EFFECTS** Photosensitivity, hypo (mostly) and hyperglycemia, arthropathy in children, crystalluria, potential for seizures, Q-T prolongation – caution using with agents that prolong Q-T interval and Class Ia and Class III antiarrhythmics - GI upset, nausea, vomiting, diarrhea, headache, rash
Levofloxacin (Levaquin, *Iquix* and *Quixin* ophthalmic)	Moxifloxacin dosing (IV/PO) 400 mg Q24H	Pregnancy Category C – may cause cartilage damage in immature animals (benefit must outweigh risk) *Cipro Oral Susp* should not be given through a NG or other feeding tube (the oil based suspension binds to the tubing). Also, need to shake vigorous for 15 seconds each
Gatifloxacin *(Zymar ophthalmic)*		time before use and do not chew the microcapsules. Can crush immediate release tablet, mix with water and give via NG tube. Hold tube feedings at least 1 hour before and 2 hours after dose
Moxifloxacin (Avelox, Vigamox ophthalmic)		*Proquin XR* should be given with a main meal of the day, evening meal is preferred. Never crush, split, or chew *Proquin XR* Dose adjust in renal impairment except for moxifloxacin These agents can be used in PCN-allergic patients
Gemifloxacin *(Factive)*		

QUINOLONE DRUG INTERACTIONS

- Antacids, didanosine, sucralfate, bile acid resins, magnesium, aluminum, calcium, iron, zinc, multivitamins or any product containing multivalent cations can chelate and inhibit absorption of FQ (separate the FQ by 2 hours before or 4-6 hours after above listed drugs; *Proquin XR* is given 4 hours before or 2 hours after).

- Can ↑ the levels of warfarin, sulfonylureas and QT-prolonging drugs (moxifloxacin prolongs the QTc interval the most).

- Probenecid and NSAIDs can ↑ FQ levels.

- Ciprofloxacin is a potent 1A2 inhibitor and a weak 3A4 inhibitor.

Macrolides

Macrolides bind to the 50S ribosomal subunit, resulting in inhibition of RNA-dependent protein synthesis.

DRUG	DOSING	SIDE EFFECTS/CONTRAINDICATIONS/MONITORING
Azithromycin *(Zithromax, Z-Pak, Zmax, Azasite ophthalmic)*	500 mg on day 1, then 250 mg days 2-5 -or- 500 mg daily x 3 days -or- Gonorrhea: 2 g x 1 <u>Do not refrigerate azithromycin oral susp *(Zmax)*</u> Better (Gm -) coverage compared to erythromycin	Activity against (Gm +), some (Gm -), and good atypical coverage **SIDE EFFECTS** GI upset (diarrhea, abdominal pain/cramping especially with erythromycin), liver dysfunction, Q-T prolongation Pregnancy Category B/C (clarithromycin) *Azasite* – viscous solution for ophthalmic use. Store at room temp once dispensed (cold makes solution more viscous) These agents can be used in PCN-allergic patients Azithromycin - use caution when CrCl < 10 mL/min ER suspension (*Zmax*) is not bioequivalent with *Zithromax*
Clarithromycin *(Biaxin, Biaxin XL)* better (Gm+) coverage	250-500 mg BID or 1 gm daily <u>Take *Biaxin XL* with food. Do not refrigerate *Biaxin oral susp.*</u>	ER suspension (*Zmax*) must be consumed within 2 hours of reconstitution on an EMPTY stomach.
Erythromycin *(E.E.S., Ery-tab)*	E.E.S.: 400 mg QID Erythromycin base/stearate: 250-500 mg PO QID <u>Must refrigerate erythromycin ethylsuccinate (E.E.S.) oral granule suspension.</u> <u>Erythromycin powder suspension stable at room temperature x 14 d</u>	L M C

MACROLIDE DRUG INTERACTIONS

- Erythromycin and clarithromycin are major 3A4 inhibitors whereas azithromycin is a minor 3A4 inhibitor. See drug interactions chapter for a more complete list.

- Do not concurrently use agents that can prolong the Q-T interval with erythromycin or clarithromycin.

Tetracyclines

Tetracyclines inhibit bacterial protein synthesis by reversible binding to 30S ribosomal sub-unit.

DRUG	DOSING	SIDE EFFECTS/CONTRAINDICATIONS/MONITORING
Doxycycline (*Vibramycin, Vibra-Tab, Oracea, **Doryx**, others*)	100 mg Q12H Take *Oracea* on an empty stomach (1 hr before or 2 hrs after meals). Take other forms with food to ↓ GI irritation	Activity against atypicals, spirochetes, Rickettsial diseases, anthrax, syphilis, acne, etc. A viable option for the treatment of MRSA in mild skin infections and VRE in urinary tract infections **SIDE EFFECTS** GI upset, photosensitivity, rash, colitis, tooth discoloration (in children), exfoliative dermatitis and fixed drug eruption
Minocycline (*Minocin, Dynacin, **Solodyn***)	50-100 mg Q12-24H	**CONTRAINDICATIONS** Children ≤ 8 years of age, pregnancy (Preg Category D - retards bone growth and skeletal development) Take with 8 oz water to minimize GI irritation. Remain upright for 30 minutes. Do not adjust dose of doxycycline in renal impairment
Tetracycline (*Sumycin*)	250-500 mg Q6H	

TETRACYCLINE DRUG INTERACTIONS

- Tetracycline absorption is impaired by antacids containing magnesium, aluminum, or calcium or medications that contains divalent cations such as iron-containing preparations, sucralfate, bile acid resins, or bismuth subsalicylate – separate doses (take 1-2 hours before or 4 hours after).

- May ↑ INR in patients taking warfarin

- Can ↓ effectiveness of oral contraceptives (check package insert).

- Many anticonvulsants ↓ level of tetracyclines. Avoid concomitant use with retinoic acid derivatives due to the risk of pseudotumor cerebri.

Sulfonamides

Sulfamethoxazole (SMZ) interferes with bacterial folic acid synthesis via inhibition of di-hydrofolic acid formation from para-aminobenzoic acid and trimethoprim (TMP) inhibits dihydrofolic acid reduction to tetrahydrofolate resulting in inhibition of enzymes of the folic acid pathway

DRUG	DOSING	SIDE EFFECTS/CONTRAINDICATIONS/MONITORING
Sulfamethoxazole and trimethoprim *(**Bactrim, Septra**, others)* Single Strength (SS) = 400 mg SMZ/80 mg TMP Double Strength (DS) = 800 mg SMZ/160 mg TMP (Always a 5:1 ratio)	<u>Adult UTI</u>: 1 DS tab BID x 3 days <u>Adult bronchitis</u>: 1 DS tab x 14 days <u>PCP prophylaxis</u>: 1 DS or SS tab daily Children UTI/AOM: urinary tract infections or acute otitis media is 40 mg/kg SMZ and 8 mg/kg TMP, divided BID x 10 days Other doses exist as well	Activity against (Gm +) and some (Gm -); no atypical and no anaerobic coverage **SIDE EFFECTS** GI upset (nausea, vomiting, diarrhea), skin reactions (rash, urticaria, SJS, TENS), crystalluria (take with 8 oz of water), photosensitivity **CONTRAINDICATIONS** Sulfa allergy, pregnancy (at term), anemia due to folate deficiency, marked renal or hepatic disease Pregnancy Category C/D (at term) *Bactrim IV* – store at room temp, short stability (~6 hrs; however, the more concentrated the solution, the shorter the stability), <u>dilute with D5W</u>. Protect from light. *Bactrim susp* should be stored at room temp and protected from light.

SULFONAMIDE DRUG INTERACTIONS

- Sulfonamides are moderate inhibitors of 2C8/9, <u>caution with concurrent use of warfarin</u>. See drug interactions chapter for more 2C8/9 substrates.

- May ↑ levels of sulfonylureas, phenytoin, dofetilide, azathioprine, methotrexate and others.

- Levels of SMZ/TMP may be ↓ by 2C8/9 inducers and the therapeutic effects may be diminished by the use of leucovorin/levoleucovorin.

Other Agents

DRUG	MOA	SIDE EFFECTS/CONTRAINDICATIONS/MONITORING

Agents to treat (Gm+)s

DRUG	MOA	SIDE EFFECTS/CONTRAINDICATIONS/MONITORING
Vancomycin *(Vancocin)* <u>Vancomycin PO (oral) is used to treat *C. difficile* (not IV)</u>- 125-500 mg QID for severe *C. diff* infections or recurrent infections <u>DOC: MRSA infections – 15 mg/kg Q8-12H IV</u> <u>Infuse IV at a concentration not to exceed 5 mg/mL</u>	Inhibits bacterial cell wall synthesis by blocking glycopeptides polymerization by binding to D-alanyl-D-alanine portion Time dependent kill	**SIDE EFFECTS** <u>Nephrotoxicity, ototoxicity, red man syndrome (maculopapular rash from too rapid of an infusion rate), hypotension, flushing</u>, neutropenia. Infuse slowly to reduce risk of red man syndrome (30 min for each 500 mg of drug given) Caution with the use of other nephrotoxic or ototoxic drugs (AMGs, cisplatin, others) **MONITORING** <u>Troughs (15-20 mcg/mL – pneumonia, endocarditis, osteomyelitis, meningitis, bacteremia and 10-15 mcg/mL for other infections) and renal function. Dose adjust in renal impairment</u> <u>Consider alternative agent when MIC of organism ≥ 2 mcg/mL</u>

Other Agents Continued

DRUG	MOA	SIDE EFFECTS/CONTRAINDICATIONS/MONITORING
Linezolid *(Zyvox)* 400-600 mg Q12H PO/IV	Oxazolidinone class – binds to bacterial 23S ribosomal RNA of the 50S subunit inhibiting bacterial translation and protein synthesis Treats (Gm +)s, including MRSA, VRE *faecium* and *faecalis*	**SIDE EFFECTS** Myelosuppression (duration related-typically > 14 days), headache (up to 11%), diarrhea, ↑ pancreatic enzymes A weak MAO inhibitor – avoid tyramine containing foods (wine and fermented foods), serotonergic and adrenergic drugs Do not dose adjust in renal impairment Store oral suspension at room temp
Quinupristin and dalfopristin ***(Synercid)*** 7.5 mg/kg IV Q8-12H	Streptogramin class – binds to different sites on the 50S bacterial ribosomal subunit inhibiting protein synthesis Treats MRSA, VRE *faecium* (not *E. faecalis*)	**SIDE EFFECTS** Hyperbilirubinemia (up to 35%), phlebitis (40%), inflammation, edema and pain at infusion site (13-44%), arthralgias and myalgias (up to 47%) Do not dose adjust in renal impairment Must be in a volume of 250 mL or greater (D5W only) to be given peripherally
Daptomycin *(Cubicin)* 4-6 mg/kg IV daily	Cyclic lipopeptide class – binds to cell membrane components causing rapid depolarization, inhibiting all intracellular replication processes including protein synthesis Concentration dependent kill Treats MRSA, VRE *faecium* and *faecalis*	**SIDE EFFECTS** > 10% diarrhea/constipation, vomiting, anemia. Also can cause peripheral edema, chest pain, hypo- and hyperkalemia, ↑ CPK and myopathy. **MONITORING** CPK level weekly (more frequently if on a statin) Frequency adjustment in renal impairment (Q24H to Q48H) DO NOT USE to treat pneumonias as it is inactivated by surfactant FDA alert 2010 - May ↑ risk of eosinophilic pneumonia Compatible with NS (not D5W)
Telavancin (*Vibativ*) 10 mg/kg IV daily	Lipoglycopeptide derivative of vancomycin – inhibits bacterial cell wall synthesis Active against MRSA, not VRE strains	**BLACK BOX WARNING** Fetal risk, obtain pregnancy test prior to starting therapy **SIDE EFFECTS** Taste disturbance (33%), nausea, vomiting (20%), foamy urine (13%), renal dysfunction, QT prolongation, red man syndrome **MONITORING** Renal function, pregnancy status Can ↑ PT, INR, aPTT, ACT, Xa Pregnancy Category C Reduce dose in renal impairment
Aztreonam *(Azactam IV,* *Cayston*- inhaled for CF) 500-2,000 mg IV Q8-12H	Monobactam that inhibits bacterial cell wall synthesis by binding to PCPs Covers *Pseudomonas* and many other gram negatives	**SIDE EFFECTS** Rash, diarrhea, nausea, vomiting Used in PCN-allergic patients. Reduce dose in renal impairment

Other Agents Continued

DRUG	MOA	SIDE EFFECTS/CONTRAINDICATIONS/MONITORING

Broad Spectrum Agents

Chloramphenicol Rarely used due to side effects (dose: max 4 g/day)	Reversibly binds to 50S ribosomal subunit of susceptible organisms inhibiting protein synthesis Activity against (Gm +)s, (Gm -)s, anaerobes, and atypicals	**BLACK BOX WARNING** Serious and fatal blood dyscrasias (aplastic anemia, thrombocytopenia) – must monitor CBC **SIDE EFFECTS** Myelosuppression (pancytopenia), gray syndrome (circulatory collapse, acidosis, coma, death) **MONITORING** CBC, liver and renal function Do not dose adjust in renal impairment
Telithromycin *(Ketek)* 800 mg PO daily	Ketolide class - inhibits bacterial protein synthesis by binding to 2 sites on the 50S ribosomal subunit Activity against (Gm +)s, (Gm -)s, some anaerobes, and atypicals	**BLACK BOX WARNING** Do not use in myasthenia gravis, causes respiratory failure **SIDE EFFECTS** Diarrhea, headache, nausea, vomiting **CONTRAINDICATIONS** Allergy to macrolides, or history of hepatitis or jaundice from macrolides Warnings include acute hepatic failure (can be fatal), QT prolongation, visual disturbances, loss of consciousness, and colitis **MONITORING** LFTs and visual acuity Pregnancy Category C Reduce dose in renal impairment
Tigecycline *(Tygacil)* **Derivative of minocycline** 100 mg IV x 1 dose, then 50 mg IV Q12H on day two	Glycylcyclines class – binds to 30S ribosomal subunit inhibiting protein synthesis Activity against (Gm +)s including MRSA, VRE *faecium* and *faecalis*, (Gm -)s, anaerobes, and atypical No activity against *Pseudomonas, Proteus, Providencia* species	**SIDE EFFECTS** Nausea and vomiting (20%), diarrhea, ↑ LFTs, photosensitivity, not to be used in children ≤ 8 years of age Pregnancy Category D Do not reduce dose in renal impairment FDA alert - risk of death when used to treat serious infections (e.g. ventilator-associated pneumonia)

Other Agents

| **Clindamycin *(Cleocin)***
150-450 mg PO 3-4 times/day

600-900 mg IV Q8H | Reversibly binds to the 50S ribosomal subunit and inhibits bacterial protein synthesis

Activity against most (Gm +)s (not *Enterococcus*) and anaerobes | **BLACK BOX WARNING**
Can cause severe and possibly fatal colitis

SIDE EFFECTS
Nausea, vomiting, diarrhea, rash, urticaria, antibiotic-associated diarrhea including pseudomembranous colitis

Pregnancy Category B

Do not dose adjust in renal impairment |

Other Agents Continued

DRUG	MOA	SIDE EFFECTS/CONTRAINDICATIONS/MONITORING
Metronidazole *(Flagyl, Metrogel* topical) 250-500 mg Q6-8H (IV, PO) Use 500 mg TID for 10-14 days for *C.diff* – mild-to-moderate infections	Causes a loss of helical DNA structure and inhibits protein synthesis Activity against anaerobes and protozoal infections DOC for bacterial vaginosis, trichomoniasis, giardiasis, amoebiasis and pseudomembranous colitis	**SIDE EFFECTS** GI upset, metallic taste, furry tongue, glossitis, darkened urine, disulfiram-like reaction with alcohol (no ethanol 24-48 hrs post last dose), peripheral neuropathy Immediate release can be taken without regard to food Take extended release tablets on empty stomach Pregnancy Category B (CI in 1st trimester) No dose adjustment in mild-moderate renal impairment, adjust when CrCl < 10 mL/min
Tinidazole *(Tindamax)* 2,000 mg PO x 1, up to 5 days	Activity against protozoa and bacterial vaginosis organisms	**SIDE EFFECTS** Metallic/bitter taste, nausea, vomiting, GI discomfort, anorexia, darkened urine, rash, peripheral neuropathy and disulfiram-like reaction with alcohol Take with food to minimize GI effects No dose adjustment in renal impairment
Rifaximin *(Xifaxan)* **Derivative of rifampin** 200 mg TID x 3 days	Used for treatment of traveler's diarrhea caused by non-invasive *E. coli*	Not systemically absorbed (< 0.4%) Also used to treat hepatic encephalopathy (550 mg PO BID) It can be taken with or without of food
Fosfomycin *(Monurol)* 3 grams in 3-4 oz of water x 1	Bacterial cell wall inhibitor Single dose used to treat uncomplicated UTI due to *E. coli* and *E. faecalis*	Major side effect is diarrhea Pregnancy Category B
Nitrofurantoin *(Macrodantin, MacroBID)* **Macrodantin 50-100 mg PO 4 times/day** **MacroBID 100 mg PO BID**	Bacterial cell wall inhibitor Used for UTI due to *E. coli, S. aureus, Enterococcus, Klebsiella* and *Enterobacter*	Contraindicated in patients with renal impairment (CrCl < 60 mL/min) and pregnancy at term Can cause pulmonary toxicity long term Pregnancy Category B (at term, Category D) Take with food to enhance absorption
Fidaxomicin *(Dificid)* 200 mg PO BID x 10 days	RNA synthesis inhibitor Used for *Clostridium difficile* associated diarrhea	Major side effect is nausea and vomiting Not effective for systemic infections. Absorption is minimal and concentrates in the bowel. Pregnancy Category B This medication can be taken without regards to food

SELECT DRUG INTERACTIONS FOR ABOVE AGENTS

- Vancomycin ↑ toxicity with other nephro- and ototoxic drugs (e.g. AMGs, amphotericin).

- Linezolid is a weak monoamine oxidase inhibitor: Avoid tyramine containing foods and alcohol. AVOID serotonergic agents (e.g. TCAs, MAO-Is, SSRIs, SNRIs) as they may cause serotonin syndrome. Avoid amphetamines, meperidine, dextromethorphan and others. Adrenergic agents may cause hypertensive crisis. Avoid products containing caffeine, tyrosine, tryptophan, or phenylalanine.

- Quinupristin/dalfopristin is a weak 3A4 inhibitor; can ↑ levels of CCBs, cyclosporine and HMG-CoA reducatase inhibitors.

- Daptomycin – There is an additive risk of rhabdomyolysis when used in conjunction with HMG-CoA reductase inhibitors.

- Telavancin is a minor 3A4/5 inhibitor. Additive QTc prolongation effects when used with antiarrhythmics or other medications that increase the QT interval.

- Telithromycin is a potent 3A4 inhibitor and can ↑ levels of many agents (azoles, CCBs, digoxin, simvastatin, lovastatin, atorvastatin, midazolam, triazolam, cyclosporine, warfarin). Can have additive effects with the class Ia and class III antiarrhythmics and other drugs, which prolong the QT interval. See drug interactions chapter for more details on 3A4 drug interactions.

- Tigecycline may ↑ INR if patient is also on warfarin (non-P450 interactions).

- Metronidazole and tinidazole cannot be used with alcohol and can increase the INR if used with warfarin. Both agents are 3A4 substrates.

Organism Classification

- Remembering the different types of bacterial genus and species names can be difficult. Knowing where the infection is located will be the largest clue on the type of bacteria causing the infection. Most types of infections discussed later in this chapter will discuss likely pathogens. In general, being able to identify a bacteria as gram positive or gram negative will markedly increase the likelihood of determining the correct antimicrobial agent to treat any infection.

- Gram-positive bacteria consists mainly of the following species: *Staphylococcus, Streptococcus, Enterococcus, Clostridium*, and *Listeria*.

- In general, gram-negative or atypical bacteria are simply NOT *Staphylococcus, Streptococcus, Enterococcus, Clostridium*, and *Listeria*.

- A more comprehensive list of bacteria can be found below.

CLASSIFICATION	ORGANISMS	
Gram Positive Cocci	*Enterococcus (VRE)*	*Staphylococcus saprophyticus*
	Peptostreptococcus sp.	*Streptococcus agalactiae (Grp. B)*
	Staphylococcus aureus (MSSA/MRSA)	*Streptococcus bovis (Grp. D)*
	Staphylococcus epidermidis (MSSE/MRSE)	*Streptococcus pneumoniae (DRSP)*
	Viridans group streptococcus	*Streptococcus pyogenes (Grp. A)*
Gram Positive Rods	*Propionibacterium acnes*	*Corynebacterium jeikeium*
	Bacillus anthracis	*Listeria monocytogenes*
	Clostridium difficile	*Nocardia asteroids (branched)*
	Clostridium perfringens	*Actinomyces israelii (branched)*
	Corynebacterium diphtheriae	
Gram Negative Cocci	*Neisseria gonorrhoeae*	*Neisseria meningitidis*
	Neisseria gonorrhoeae (PRNG)	
Spirochetes	*Borrelia burgdorferi*	*Leptospira interrogans*
	Borrelia recurrentis	*Treponema pallidum*
Atypicals	*Chlamydia/Chlamydophilia*	*Mycoplasma pneumoniae*
	Mycoplasma hominis	*Ureaplasma urealyticum*
Gram Negative Coccobacillary	*Acinetobacter sp.*	*Francisella tularensis*
	Bartonella henselae	*Moraxella catarrhalis*
	Bordetella pertussis	*Pasteurella multocida*
	Family rickettsiaceae	
Gram Negative Rods	*Aeromonas hydrophila*	*Helicobacter pylori (curved rod)*
	Alcaligenes xylosoxidans	*Klebsiella pneumoniae*
	Bacteroides fragilis	*Legionella pneumophilia*
	Brucella sp.	*Morganella morganii*
	Burkholderia cepacia	*Prevotella melaninogenica*
	Campylobacter jejuni (curved rod)	*Proteus mirabilis*
	Citrobacter diversus	*Proteus sp.*
	Citrobacter freundii	*Providencia sp.*
	Eikenella corrodens	*Pseudomonas aeruginosa*
	Enterobacter cloacae	*Salmonella sp.*
	Enterobacter aerogenes	*Samonella typhi*
	Escherichia coli	*Serratia sp.*
	Flavobacteriae	*Shigella sp.*
	Fusobacteriae	*Stenotrophomonas maltophilia*
	Gardnerella vaginalis	*Vibrio cholerae (curved rod)*
	Haemophilus ducreyi	*Yersinia enterocolitica*
	Haemophilus influenzae	*Yersinia pestis*

(Bartlett. Johns Hopkins Antibiotic Guide: Diagnosis & Treatment of Infectious Diseases 2nd Ed. 2010)

Peri-Operative Antibiotic Prophylaxis

- Short course of antibiotic administered before there is clinical evidence of infection

- Treatment usually begins within 1 hour before the surgical incision and continues for no longer than 24 hours post surgery, except some surgeries (e.g., 48 hours post cardiac surgery)

- In general, first or second generation cephalosporins (e.g. cefazolin/cefuroxime) are the drugs of choice for most procedures. In penicillin-allergic patients, a suitable alternative is vancomycin (given within 2 hrs prior to surgical incision).

- Surgeries that involve parts of the bowel or put patients at risk of an anaerobic infection will commonly use an antibiotic such as cefotetan.

SURGICAL PROCEDURE	RECOMMENDED ANTIBIOTICS	IF BETA-LACTAM ALLERGY
CABG, other cardiac or vascular surgeries	Cefazolin, Cefuroxime or Vancomycin	Vancomycin or Clindamycin
Hip/Knee Arthroplasty	Cefazolin, Cefuroxime or Vancomycin	Vancomycin or Clindamycin
Colon (colorectal)	Cefotetan, Cefoxitin, Ampicillin/ Sulbactam or Ertapenem OR Cefazolin or Cefuroxime + Metronidazole	Clindamycin + Aminoglycoside or Clindamycin + Quinolone or Clindamycin + Aztreonam OR Metronidazole + Aminoglycoside or Metronidazole + Quinolone
Hysterectomy	Cefotetan, Cefazolin, Cefoxitin, Cefuroxime or Ampicillin/Sulbactam	Clindamycin + Aminoglycoside or Clindamycin + Quinolone or Clindamycin + Aztreonam OR Metronidazole + Aminoglycoside or Metronidazole + Quinolone

Skin and Soft-Tissue Infections (SSTIs)

INFECTION	ADULT TREATMENT OPTIONS	COMMENTS

Empiric oral therapy options for purulent* cellulitis

| Outpatient SSTI | Clindamycin 300-450 mg TID OR TMP-SMX 1 to 2 DS tabs BID OR Doxycycline 100 mg BID OR Minocycline 200 mg X 1, then 100 mg BID OR Linezolid 600 mg BID Duration of therapy = 5 to 10 days | Primary treatment for cutaneous abscess is incision and drainage (I & D) Use antibiotics for severe infections, rapid progression, systemic illness, etc. For recurrent SSTIs, consider nasal decolonization with mupirocin BID for 5 to 10 days and/or topical body decolonization with chlorhexidine for 5 to 14 days or dilute bleach baths twice weekly for 3 months *If nonpurulent, treat with beta-lactam (e.g. cephalexin) |

Skin and Soft-Tissue Infections (SSTIs) Continued

INFECTION	ADULT TREATMENT OPTIONS	COMMENTS

Empiric therapy options for complicated SSTIs (pending culture results)

Inpatient SSTI	Vancomycin IV OR Linezolid 600 mg IV/PO BID OR Daptomycin 4 mg/kg/dose once daily OR Telavancin 10 mg/kg/dose once daily OR Clindamycin 600 mg IV/PO TID; Duration of therapy = 7 to 14 days	MRSA risk high compared to outpatient

Urinary Tract Infection (UTI)

- UTIs are typically more common in females than males

- An uncomplicated UTI is not associated with structural or neurologic abnormalities that may interfere with the normal flow of urine. A complicated UTI generally results from an obstruction or abnormality (e.g. congenital abnormality of urinary tract, a stone, indwelling catheter) or neurologic deficit (neurogenic bladder; spinal cord injury patient) that interferes with the normal flow of urine.

- Typical signs and symptoms of lower urinary tract infections (cystitis) are dysuria, urgency, frequency, burning, nocturia, suprapubic heaviness, and/or hematuria (fever is uncommon).

- Typical signs and symptoms of upper urinary tract infections (pyelonephritis) are flank pain, abdominal pain, fever, nausea, vomiting, costovertebral angle pain, and malaise.

UTI TREATMENT GUIDELINES

DIAGNOSIS	PATHOGENS	DRUGS OF CHOICE/ GUIDELINES	COMMENTS
Acute uncomplicated cystitis in females	E. coli, S. saprophyticus, Enterococcus	If < 20% local E. coli resistant to SMX/TMP and no allergy to sulfa; use SMX/TMP DS tab BID x 3 days If ≥ 20% local E. coli resistant to SMX/TMP or sulfa allergy; Use 3 day regimen of: Cipro 250 mg BID or Cipro ER 500 mg daily or Levofloxacin 250 mg daily OR nitrofurantoin 100 mg BID x 5 d OR fosfomycin x 1 (3 g in 4 oz water)	May add phenazopyridine 200 mg PO TID x 2 days to the regimen to relieve symptoms Usually empirically treated as an outpatient Prophylaxis: ≥ 3 episodes in 1 yr; use 1 SMX/TMP SS daily, macrodantin 50 mg PO daily, or 1 SMX/TMP DS post coitus If no response on 3-day course, culture and treat for 2 weeks Do NOT recommend moxi (does not reach high levels in the urine) or gemifloxacin (poor to limited activity vs. normal UTI pathogens) Treat pregnant women for 7 days

UTI Treatment Guidelines Continued

DIAGNOSIS	PATHOGENS	DRUGS OF CHOICE/ GUIDELINES	COMMENTS
Acute uncomplicated pyelonephritis	*E. coli, Enterococci, P. mirabilis, K. pneumoniae, P. aeruginosa*	<u>Moderately ill : outpatient tx (PO):</u> FQ PO x 5-7 d for unknown FQ resistance or resistance < 10% Cipro 500 mg PO BID or Cipro ER 1,000 mg daily; Levo 750 mg daily; Oflox 400 mg BID FQ-resistance; consider amox/clav, cefdinir, cefaclor, or cefpodoxime <u>Severe - hospitalized tx (IV):</u> FQ, AMP + Gent, Pip/Tazo, or ceftriaxone x 10-14 days	Most require hospitalization Need urinalysis, urine and blood cultures
Complicated UTI	*E.coli, Klebsiella, Enterobacter, Serratia, Pseudomonas, Enterococcus, Staph species*	AMP + Gent or Pip/Tazo or Ticar/ clav, ceftriaxone or cefotaxime +/- FQ Or If ESBL producers are present: Doripenem or Imipenem or Meropenem x 2 weeks	Need urinalysis, urine and blood cultures May be due to obstruction, catheterization – remove or change catheter if possible Treat for 7 days if there is prompt symptom relief Treat for 10-14 days with delayed response regardless of catheterization or not

(Clinical Infectious Diseases 2011;52;e103–e120; Clinical Infectious Diseases 2010; 50:625-663; Postgrad Med. 2010;122;:7-15.)

Additional Notes

- Longer term therapy needed for acute uncomplicated UTIs in men, pregnancy, elderly, people with diabetes, and children.

- <u>Must treat pregnant women (for 7 days).</u> If not, can lead to premature birth or pyelonephritis. <u>In pregnant women, avoid quinolones (cartilage toxicity and arthropathies) and TCNs (teratogenic). SMX/TMP can cause hyperbilirubinemia and kernicterus in 3rd trimester (Pregnancy Category D near term); otherwise, category C).</u> See drug use in pregnancy section.

Phenazopyridine

- Phenazopyridine *(Azo, Uristat, Pyridium)* is an azo dye and urinary analgesic.

- Dose = 200 mg TID (Rx), 100 mg TID (OTC)

- <u>Take with or following food to minimize stomach upset.</u>

- <u>Do not use longer than two days because it may mask worsening symptoms.</u>

- <u>May cause red-orange coloring of the urine and other body fluids. Contact lenses and clothes can be stained.</u>

- Can cause hemolytic anemia in patients with G6PD deficiency

- CrCl < 50 mL/min: avoid use

TRAVELER'S DIARRHEA

- Prevention is not routinely recommended.

- Treatment – recommend an antibiotic + loperamide. Do not use loperamide if patient has a fever or blood in the stool.

- Main etiologies are *E. coli, Shigella, Salmonella,* or *Campylobacter.*

- If diarrhea persists > 7 days (especially in immunocompromised patients), consider parasites as a possible cause *(Giardia, Cryptosporidium)*

(Bartlett. Johns Hopkins Antibiotic Guide: Diagnosis & Treatment of Infectious Diseases 2nd Ed. 2010; Dis Mon. 2006 Jul;52(7):289-302.)

CLOSTIDIUM DIFFICILE ASSOCIATED-DIARRHEA

- Discontinue offending agent as soon as possible.

- <u>Mild-to-moderate infections</u>, use metronidazole 500 mg PO TID x 10-14 days. Do not use after treating a 2nd episode due to the risk of neurotoxicity.

- <u>Severe infections</u>, use vancomycin 125 mg PO QID x 10-14 days.

TRAVELER'S DIARRHEA TREATMENT

Drug Therapy

Cipro 500 mg PO BID x 3 days or

TMP/SMX DS PO BID x 7-10 days or

Ofloxacin 300 mg BID x 3 days or

Levofloxacin 500 mg daily x 1-3 days or

Rifaxamin 200 mg TID x 3 days or

Metronidazole 250-750 mg TID x 7-10 days or

Tinidazole 2 gm PO x1, may repeat daily for a total of 3 days or

Nitazoxanide 500 mg PO BID x 3 days or

Azithromycin 1,000 mg x 1 or 500 mg daily x 1-3 days – drug of choice for pregnancy and children

PLUS

Loperamide 4 mg x 1, then 2 mg after each loose stool – max 16 mg/d

---

- <u>Severe, complicated infections</u>, use vancomycin 500 mg PO QID ± metronidazole 500 mg IV Q8H. Consider vancomycin per rectum if ileus is present (500 mg in 100 mL NS PR Q6H). Consider fidaxomicin instead of vancomycin for patients at high risk of recurrence (such as patients receiving chemotherapy or immunosuppressed patients). Fidaxomicin's place in *C. difficile* therapy has not been fully established. In clinical trials, fidaxomicin was as efficacious as vancomycin oral therapy, but with lower recurrence rates. Fidaxomicin is effective in mild to severe *C. difficile* infections.

- Treat all first recurrences with the same agent that was used previously, unless the recurrence infection has increased in severity.

- For 3rd episode of any severity, use vancomycin taper therapy. Start 125 mg PO QID for 2 weeks, BID for 1 week, and then 3 times per week for 2-8 weeks.

- Avoid antimotility agents due to the risk of toxic megacolon. Probiotics are not beneficial with initial *C. difficile* infections, but may have some utility in patients with persistent recurrence.

- Wash hands with soap and water to prevent transmission. Alcohol sanitizers do NOT kill *C. difficile* spores.

BRONCHITIS

- Acute bronchitis is almost always self-limiting and many cases (~50%) are viral. If bacterial, common etiologies are *Mycoplasma pneumonia, Strep pneumonia, H. influenza, Moraxella catarrhalis,* and others.

- Treatment is generally symptomatic and supportive – fluids to prevent dehydration, antipyretics for fever, cough suppressants, vaporizers to thin secretions, etc.

- Signs and symptoms of acute bronchitis include cough persisting > 5 days to weeks, sore throat, coryza, malaise, headache, possible fever, bilateral rales, purulent sputum in ~50% of patients.

(J Am Geriatr Soc. 2010;58;570-9, MMWR Recomm Rep. 2005 Dec 9;54(RR-14):1-16, others)

BRONCHITIS NOTES & TREATMENT

Acute Bronchitis – expect cough to last 2 weeks
Usually viral – antibiotics not indicated. Recommend antitussive ± inhaled bronchodilators

Persistent Cough/Pertussis (whooping cough) – 10-20% adults with cough > 14 days have pertussis
Azithromycin 500 mg x 1, then 250 mg daily 2-5 days or

Erythromycin estolate 500 mg QID x 14 days or

SMX/TMP DS 1 tab BID x 14 days or

Clarithromycin 500 mg BID or 1 gm ER daily x 7 days

Acute Bacterial Exacerbation of Chronic Bronchitis (ABECB)
Mild-to-moderate disease

- No antibiotic treatment or if used, choose: amoxicillin, doxycycline, SMX/TMP, or cephalosporin

Severe disease

- Inhaled anti-cholinergic bronchodilator plus oral corticosteroid, taper over 2 weeks.

- Role of antibiotic therapy debated even for severe disease. If used, choose: amoxicillin/clavulanic acid, or azithromycin, or clarithromycin, or cephalosporin, or FQ (moxi, gemi, or levo). Treat or 3-10 days or longer if needed.

COMMUNITY-ACQUIRED PNEUMONIA (CAP)

- Patients with CAP are empirically treated until the infectious organism is known (cultures and sensitivities are available).

Guidelines adapted from the Infectious Diseases Society of America/American Thoracic Society Consensus Guidelines on the Management of CAP in Adults. (Clin Infect Dis 2007;44 suppl 2:S27-72)

MOST COMMON ETIOLOGIES OF CAP

PATIENT TYPE	ETIOLOGY
Outpatient	Streptococcus pneumonia
	Mycoplasma pneumonia *Moraxella k.*
	Haemophilus influenzae
	Chlamydophila pneumonia
	Respiratory viruses

Most Common Etiologies of CAP Continued

PATIENT TYPE	ETIOLOGY
Inpatient (non-ICU)	*Streptococcus pneumonia*
	Mycoplasma pneumonia
	Chlamydophila pneumonia
	Haemophilus influenzae
	Legionella sp.
	Aspiration
	Respiratory viruses
Inpatient (ICU)	*Streptococcus pneumonia*
	Staphylococcus aureus
	Legionella sp.
	Gram-negative bacilli
	Haemophilus influenzae

RECOMMENDED EMPIRICAL ANTIBIOTIC COVERAGE FOR CAP

Outpatient Treatment

Previously healthy and no use of antimicrobials within the past 3 months:

- Macrolide* (azithromycin, clarithromycin, erythromycin) OR

- Doxycycline

At risk for drug-resistant S. pneumonia (age > 65 y/o, comorbidities – such as HF, DM, cancer, renal/liver dysfunction – and use of antibiotics within past 3 months):

- A respiratory fluoroquinolone (moxifloxacin, gemifloxacin,or levofloxacin [750mg]) OR

- Beta-lactam (amox, amox/clav, cefpodoxime, cefuroxime) PLUS a macrolide (azithromycin, clarithromycin, erythromycin)

Inpatient (non-ICU)

- Respiratory fluoroquinolone (moxifloxacin, gemifloxacin, or levofloxacin) – IV or PO OR

- Beta-lactam (ceftriaxone, cefotaxime, ampicillin-sulbactam) PLUS Macrolide (azithromycin, clarithromycin, erythromycin)

Inpatient (ICU) - IV therapy preferred

- Beta-lactam (ceftriaxone, cefotaxime, ampicillin-sulbactam) PLUS Azithromycin or an IV fluoroquinolone (levofloxacin, moxifloxacin)

If *Pseudomonas* is a consideration, use drugs that cover *Pseudomonas* (antipseudomonal beta-lactam + antipseudomonal FQ or AMG)

If CA-MRSA is a consideration, add vancomycin or linezolid

* preferred

ORAL ANTIBIOTICS FOR COMMUNITY ACQUIRED PNEUMONIA (CAP)

DRUG	USUAL ADULT DOSE

Cephalosporins

Cefpodoxime (*Vantin*)	200 mg Q12H
Cefuroxime (*Ceftin*)	500 mg Q12H

Macrolides

Azithromycin (*Zithromax*)	500 mg x 1, then 250 mg daily (days 2-5)
Clarithromycin (*Biaxin*)	250-500 mg Q12H
(*Biaxin XL*)	1,000 mg daily
Erythromycin base (*E-mycin*)	250-500 mg Q6H

Fluoroquinolones

Gemifloxacin (*Factive*)	320 mg daily
Levofloxacin (*Levaquin*)	750 mg daily
Moxifloxacin (*Avelox*)	400 mg daily

Tetracyclines

Doxycycline (*Vibramycin*)	100 mg Q12H

Penicillins

Amoxicillin (*Amoxil*)	1 g Q8H
Amoxicillin/clavulanate (*Augmentin XR*)	2 g Q12H

HOSPITAL ACQUIRED PNEUMONIA (HAP)/VENTILATOR ASSOCIATED PNEUMONIA (VAP)

- Treatment regimens for nosocomial pneumonias vary by institution based on the frequency of pathogens seen and the susceptibility profile. Many hospitals generate an antibiogram, which describes overall sensitivities seen with the different pathogens to aid in proper antibiotic selection (see example at the front of the chapter).

- One key factor is the prevention of hospital-acquired pneumonia – elevate head of bed by 30 degrees, wean off ventilator quickly, remove naso-gastric (NG) tube, and discontinue use of stress ulcer prophylaxis medication if not needed.

MOST COMMON ETIOLOGIES OF HAP/VAP

PATIENT TYPE	ETIOLOGY
Acquired infection	Streptococcus pneumoniae
≥ 5 days after hospitalization	Haemophilus influenzae
	Enteric gram-negative bacteria (such as E. coli, Klebsiella pneumoniae)
	Pseudomonas aeruginosa
	Methicillin-resistant Staphylococcus aureus (MRSA)
	Acinetobacter species
	ESBL Klebsiella pneumoniae

Am J Respir Crit Care Med Vol 171. pp 388–416, 200

- Hospital acquired pneumonia that occurs < 5 days after admission are caused by pathogens similar to that of CAP except for fact that the incidence of enteric gram-negative bacteria is more prevalent.

DRUGS TO TREAT HAP/VAP	
Primary Regimens Piperacillin-tazobactam 4.5 gm IV Q6H or Ceftriaxone 1-2 gm IV Q24H or Ampicillin-sulbactam 3 gm IV Q6H or Ertapenem 1 gm IV Q24H PLUS If suspect Legionella or bioterrorism, add or replace therapy with a respiratory FQ (levofloxacin or moxifloxacin)	**If suspect *P. aeruginosa*, empirically start 2 antipseudomonal drugs to ↑ likelihood that at least one agent will be active** Choose an anti-pseudomonal beta-lactam PLUS Anti-pseudomonal FQ (ciprofloxacin or levofloxacin) OR Aminoglycoside (e.g. tobramycin) If MRSA is suspected, add vancomycin or linezolid

Am J Respir Crit Care Med Vol 171. pp 388–416, 200

USEFUL LISTS

Agents used for skin and skin structures infections caused by Community-Associated Methicillin-Resistant *Staphylococcus aureus* (CA-MRSA)
TMP-SMX *(Bactrim* DS) 10-15 g/kg/day in 2 or 3 divided doses

Doxycycline 100 mg PO/IV Q12H

Minocycline 100 mg PO/IV Q12H

Clindamycin 600 mg PO/IV Q8H*

Linezolid 600 mg PO/IV Q12H

Daptomycin 4 mg/kg IV daily

Tigecycline 100 mg IV x 1, then 50 mg IV Q12H

Ceftaroline 600 mg IV Q12H

Vancomycin 10-15 mg/kg IV Q12H

Telavancin 10 mg/kg IV daily

Agents used to treat Nosocomial-Associated Methicillin-Resistant *Staphylococcus aureus*
Vancomycin (If VISA, then use agents listed below or consider agents below if MIC ≥ 2)

Linezolid

Quinupristin-dalfopristin

Daptomycin (not for pneumonia)

Ceftaroline

Telavancin

Tigecycline

Rifampin (combination therapy, e.g. prosthetic infections)

Agents used to treat *VRE. faecalis*
PenG

Ampicillin

Linezolid

Daptomycin

Tigecycline

Doxycycline (for urinary isolates when susceptible)

Agents used to treat *VRE. faecium*
Pen G (when susceptible – typically resistant)

Ampicillin (when susceptible – typically resistant)

Linezolid

Quinupristin-dalfopristin

Daptomycin

Tigecycline

Doxycycline (for urinary isolates when susceptible)

Agents used to treat *Pseudomonas aeruginosa*
Imipenem

Meropenem

Doripenem

Cefepime

Ceftazidime

Ciprofloxacin

Levofloxacin

Aztreonam

Ticarcillin/Clavulanic acid

Piperiacillin/Tazobactam

Colistimethate (colistin)

Amikacin

Tobramycin

Gentamicin

Before using clindamycin, an induction test (D test) should be performed on isolates sensitive to clindamycin but resistant to erythromycin – look for a flattened zone between the disks → this signifies that inducible clindamycin resistance is present. Also, never use FQs regardless of susceptibility profile

Sexually Transmitted Infections (STIs)

INFECTION	DOC	DOSING	ALTERNATIVES/NOTES
Syphilis - caused by *Treponema pallidum*, a spirochete Early (primary, secondary, or latent < 1 year duration)	Penicillin G benzathine	2.4 MU IM x 1	Doxycycline 100 mg PO BID x 2 weeks If patient is pregnant and PCN-allergic, desensitize and treat with PCN
Syphilis - Late (> 1 year's duration, cardiovascular, gummas, late-latent, or unknown duration)	Penicillin G benzathine	2.4 MU IM weekly x 3 wks	Doxycycline 100 mg PO BID x 4 weeks If patient is pregnant and PCN-allergic, desensitize and treat with PCN
Neurosyphilis (including ocular syphilis)	Penicillin G (aqueous)	3-4 MU IV Q4H x 10-14 days	Penicillin G procaine 2.4 MU IM daily + probenecid 500 mg PO QID x 10-14 days
Congenital syphilis	Penicillin G (aqueous)	50,000 units/kg IV Q12H x 7 days, then Q8H for 10 days total	Penicillin G procaine 50,000 units/kg IM daily x 10 days
Gonorrhea – caused by *Neisseria gonorrhea*, a (Gm -) diplococcus Urethral, cervical, rectal, pharyngeal	Ceftriaxone *(Rocephin)* or Cefixime *(Suprax)* or Cefpodoxime *(Vantin)*	250 mg IM x 1 400 mg PO x 1 400 mg PO x 1	Should also treat patients for chlamydia infection if not ruled out Azithromycin 2 g PO x 1 – effective for both gonorrhea and chlamydia but poorly tolerated (GI effects) and more expensive *Ceftriaxone is most effective for pharyngeal infections Alternative options: Cefoxitin 2,000 mg IM x 1 PLUS probenecid Or Cefotaxime 500 mg x 1

INFECTION	DOC	DOSING	ALTERNATIVES/NOTES
Chlamydial Infection – caused by *Chlamydia trachomatis*, intracellular obligate parasite	Azithromycin	1 g PO x 1	Doxycycline 100 mg PO BID x 7 days or Erythromycin 500 mg PO QID x 7 days
Bacterial Vaginosis – caused by many different organisms	Metronidazole or	500 mg PO BID x 7 days	Clindamycin 300 mg PO BID x 7 days or or Clindamycin ovules 100 mg intravaginally at bedtime x 3 days or Tinidazole 2 g PO daily x 2 days or Tinidazole 1 g PO daily x 5 days
	Clindamycin 2% cream	5 g intravaginally at bedtime x 7 days	
	Metronidazole 0.75% gel	5 g intravaginally daily x 5 days	
Trichomoniasis – caused by *Trichomonas vaginalis*, a flagellated protozoan	Metronidazole	2 g PO x 1	Metronidazole 500 mg PO BID x 7 days
	Tinidazole	2 g PO x 1	

CDC. MMWR Recomm Rep. 2010;59(RR-12):1-110.

All sexual partners must also be treated concurrently to prevent re-infection

HERPES SIMPLEX VIRUS (HSV)

- HSV-1 is most commonly associated with oropharyngeal disease, and HSV-2 is associated more closely with genital disease. However, each virus is capable of causing infections clinically indistinguishable in both anatomic areas.

- Genital herpes is a chronic, life-long viral infection. 1 in 6 people in the U.S. have herpes.

- Clinical manifestations of first episodes of genital herpes usually begin within 2-14 days post exposure but up to 50% of patients are asymptomatic. First episode symptoms can include flu-like symptoms, fever, headache, malaise, myalgias, and development of pustular or ulcerative lesions on external genitalia. Lesions usually begin as papules or vesicles that rapidly spread and clusters of lesions form, crust, and re-epithelialize. Lesions are described as painful. Itching, dysuria, and vaginal or urethral discharge are common symptoms.

- Recurrent infections are not associated with systemic manifestations. Symptoms are localized to the genital area, milder, and of shorter duration. Patients typically experience a prodrome prior to symptoms. Must start treatment during prodrome or within 1 day of lesion onset for patient to experience benefit.

- Suppressive therapy reduces the frequency of genital herpes recurrences by 70-80% among patients who have frequent recurrences (e.g. > 6 recurrences/yr) and many report no symptomatic outbreaks.

- Acyclovir *(Zovirax)* is usually the cheapest regimen. Valacyclovir *(Valtrex)* is a prodrug of acyclovir that results in higher concentrations than with oral acyclovir. If resistant to acyclovir, patient will obviously be resistant to valacyclovir. Famciclovir *(Famvir)* is a prodrug of penciclovir. Strains resistant to acyclovir are generally resistant to famciclovir.

GENITAL HERPES

DRUG	DOSING	SIDE EFFECTS
Primary (initial episode)		**Side Effects** Acyclovir: malaise, headache, nausea, vomiting, diarrhea, [Thrombotic Thrombocytopenic Purpura and Hemolytic Uremic Syndrome (TTP/HUS), renal failure – both rare]
Acyclovir *(Zovirax)* or	400 mg PO TID x 7-10 days	
Valacyclovir *(Valtrex)* or	1 g PO BID x 7-10 days	Valacyclovir: ↑ LFTs, headache, GI upset, neutropenia [Thrombotic Thrombocytopenic Purpura and Hemolytic Uremic Syndrome (TTP/HUS), renal failure – both rare]
Famciclovir *(Famvir)*	250 mg PO TID x 7-10 days	
For severe cases, use acyclovir 5-10 mg/kg IV Q8H x 2-7 days**		Dose adjust these agents in renal impairment
If acyclovir-resistant HSV, use Foscarnet	40 mg/kg IV Q8H until clinical resolution. Most cases take ~7 days	**IV treatment maybe be cut short for clinical improvement and PO (oral) therapy initiated for a treatment duration of at least 10 days
Recurrent episodes		
Acyclovir or	800 mg PO TID x 2 days	
Acyclovir or	800 mg PO BID x 5 days	
Acyclovir or	400 mg PO TID x 5 days	
Valacyclovir or	500 mg PO BID x 3 days	
Valacyclovir or	1 g PO daily x 5 days	
Famciclovir or	1 g BID x 1 day	
Famciclovir or	125 mg PO BID x 5 days	
Chronic suppression (daily)		
Acyclovir or	400 mg PO BID	
Valacyclovir or	500-1,000 mg PO daily	
Famciclovir	250 mg PO BID	

CDC. MMWR Recomm Rep. 2010;59(RR-12):1-110. Bartlett. Johns Hopkins Antibiotic Guide: Diagnosis & Treatment of Infectious Diseases 2nd Ed. 2010

TUBERCULOSIS

- Tuberculosis is caused by *Mycobacterium tuberculosis* (aerobic, non-spore forming bacillus). It is transmitted by aerosolized droplets (via sneezing, coughing, talking, etc.) and is highly contagious. There are strains resistant to multiple drugs (MDR-TB) including INH and rifampin and these strains are on the rise.

- Diagnosed by tuberculin skin test (TST), same as PPD. Look for induration (raised area) within 48-72 hours after injection. Also, can do a sputum smear, culture, and PCR for AFB.

- 2 categories of TB; latent and active disease. Latent disease is treated with INH 300 mg PO daily for 9 months (or 15 mg/kg given 2 x/wk). Alternatively, rifampin 600 mg PO daily for 4 months can be used. Previous recommendations of rifampin 600 mg PO + pyrazinamide for 2 months has been withdrawn and not recommended by the CDC secondary to hepatotoxicity.

SYMPTOMS OF ACTIVE TB
Coughing (may be productive)
Fatigue
Night sweats
Infiltrates on chest x-rays (cavitary lesions)
Anorexia/weight loss (unintentional)
Pleuritic chest pain
Hemoptysis
Fever

Tuberculosis Drug Regimen

CONDITION	MEDICATIONS	DURATION OF THERAPY
Take all 4 drugs for 8 weeks (by 8 wks, cultures and sensitivities are available). Then, if sensitive, take isoniazid + rifampin for the next 18 weeks	Isoniazid + Rifampin + Pyrazinamide + Ethambutol	26 weeks
If resistance to INH	Rifampin + Pyrazinamide + Ethambutol ± FQ	6 months
If resistance to RIF	Isoniazid + Ethambutol + FQ + (Pyrazinamide x 2 months)	12-18 months
If MDR-TB (defined as resistant to at least 2 drugs including INH and RIF)	FQ + Pyrazinamide + Ethambutol + aminoglycoside (streptomycin/amikacin/ kanamycin) +/- alternative agent	18-24 months

CDC. MMWR Recomm Rep. 2003;52(RR-11):1-77. Am J Respir Crit Care Med. 2003;15;167;603-62.

Alternative anti-TB agents include cycloserine, ethionamide, clarithromycin, ampicillin/ clav., linezolid, streptomycin (used instead of ethambutol).

- Use Directly Observed Therapy (DOT) regimen, if possible. DOT regimens are dosed 2 or 3 times per week instead of daily.

- Patients with active TB should be in isolated, single negative pressure rooms!! Essential.

- Recommended to add pyridoxine (vitamin B6) 25-50 mg PO daily to INH regimens to ↓ risk of neuropathy.

- Rifabutin can be used instead of rifampin in cases of unacceptable drug-drug interactions with rifampin.

DRUG	MOA	DOSING	SIDE EFFECTS/CONTRAINDICATIONS/MONITORING
Isoniazid (INH)	Inhibits cell wall synthesis of susceptible isolates	5 mg/kg (max 300 mg) daily or 15 mg/kg (max 900 mg) 2-3x/wk Take 1 hour before or 2 hours after a meal on an empty stomach Store oral solution at room temp.	**BLACK BOX WARNING** Severe (and fatal) hepatitis may occur; usually within first 3 months of treatment **SIDE EFFECTS** ↑ LFTs, hepatitis, peripheral neuropathy, lupus-like syndrome, abdominal pain, nausea, agranulocytosis, rash, hypersensitivity reactions **CONTRAINDICATIONS** Active liver disease, previous adverse reaction to INH Monitoring: LFTs periodically
Rifampin *(Rifadin)*	Inhibits RNA synthesis, by blocking RNA transcription, in susceptible isolates	10 mg/kg (max 600 mg) daily or 2-3x/wk Take 1 hour before or 2 hours after a meal on an empty stomach	**SIDE EFFECTS** Flu-like syndrome, rash, pruritus, hepatotoxicity, nausea, vomiting, diarrhea, abdominal pain, hyperbilirubinemia, leukopenia, thrombocytopenia, renal failure, ↑ uric acid, orange-red discoloration of body secretions (stain contact lens) **MONITORING** LFTs, CBC, mental status, sputum culture, chest X-ray
Ethambutol *(Myambutol)*	Suppresses mycobacteria replication by interfering with RNA synthesis	15-25 mg/kg (max 1,600 mg) daily or 25-30 mg/kg (max 2.5 grams) 3x/wk or 50 mg/kg (max 4 grams) 2x/wk Take without regards to meals	**SIDE EFFECTS** Optic neuritis, ↓ visual acuity, scotoma and/or color blindness (usually reversible); rash, hyperuricemia, headache, confusion, hallucinations, nausea, vomiting, abdominal pain **MONITORING** Routine vision tests (monthly) Dose adjust in renal impairment
Pyrazinamide	Converts to pyrazinoic acid in susceptible strains of *Mycobacterium* which ↓ pH	15-30 mg/kg (max 2 grams) daily; 50 mg/kg given 2-3x/wk	**SIDE EFFECTS** Hepatotoxicity, malaise, nausea, vomiting, GI upset, arthralgias, myalgias, rash, hyperuricemia and others **CONTRAINDICATIONS** Acute gout, severe hepatic damage Dose adjust in renal impairment
Streptomycin	Binds to 30S ribosomal subunit and inhibits bacterial protein synthesis	20-40 mg/kg (max 1 gram) daily or 20 mg/kg (max 1.5 grams) 2-3x/wk	**BLACK BOX WARNING** Neurotoxicity, nephrotoxicity, and neuromuscular blockade and respiratory paralysis IV form can cause ototoxicity

Tuberculosis Agents Drug Interactions

- INH - Major 3A4 and 2C19 inhibitor, and moderate 2D6 inhibitor. Avoid concomitant use with alfuzosin, eplerenone, nilotinib, nisoldipine, ranolazine, salmeterol, silodosin, thioridazine, alcohol. Can ↑ levels of phenytoin, carbamazepine, and benzodiazepines; avoid tyramine and histamine containing foods. ↑ dietary intake of folic acid, niacin, and magnesium while taking INH.

- Rifampin – Potent <u>inducer</u> of 1A2, 2C8, 2C9, 2C19 and 3A4. Avoid concomitant use with protease inhibitors, mycophenalate, nilotinib, ranolazine, voriconazole and alcohol. Can ↓ levels of warfarin, antiretroviral agents, corticosteroids, quinidine, benzodiazepines, oral contraceptives, methadone, sulfonylureas, calcium channel blockers, digoxin, cyclosporine, amiodarone, and 100+ others.

- Pyrazinamide – Can ↑ rifampin and ↓ cyclosporine; can cause fatal hepatotoxicity with rifampin; monitor liver function tests, uric acid, etc.

- Streptomycin – ↑ effect with neuromuscular blocking agents; ↑ nephrotoxicity with amphotericin B, cisplatin, loop diuretics, NSAIDS and vancomycin.

ACUTE OTITIS MEDIA (AOM)

Guidelines: American Academy of Pediatrics and American Academy of Family Physicians. Diagnosis and management of acute otitis media for children 2 months to 12 years of age. (Am Fam Physician. 2004 Jun 1;69(11):2713-5.; Pediatrics. 2004 May;113(5):1451-65.)

- Most common infection for which children in the United States receive antibiotic treatment.

- Signs of infection include rapid onset, middle ear effusion and signs and symptoms of middle-ear inflammation plus fever, tugging or rubbing ears, crying.

- <u>Many of the infections are viral (i.e. antibiotics will not work)</u>.

- <u>Observation without antibiotics may be an option – depending on age, diagnostic certainty, and illness severity. The "observation" period is 48-72 hours and used to assess clinical improvement without antibiotics.</u> However, it is recommended that <u>children < 6 months are given antibiotics (even with an uncertain diagnosis)</u>. Children 6 mos - 2 years should be given antibiotics if severe illness or with certain diagnosis. <u>Once children are ≥ 2 years, give antibiotics if severe illness. Otherwise, can observe.</u>

- <u>Treat the pain with acetaminophen or ibuprofen. Can use topical benzocaine *(Auralgan, Americaine Otic)* in children > 5 years of age.</u>

- Primary treatment is high-dose <u>amoxicillin (90 mg/kg/day)</u> divided Q12H or Q8H. The higher dose will cover most *S. pneumoniae*. It is also safe and cheap.

- More severe cases or in cases where amoxicillin does not work, <u>the next step is high-dose amoxicillin/clavulanate *(Augmentin)* (90mg/kg/d of amoxicillin component). Can also use cefdinir, cefpodoxime, cefprozil, or cefuroxime.</u>

- <u>Patients who had anaphylaxis from penicillin can get azithromycin, clarithromycin, erythromycin-sulfisoxazole, trimethoprim-sulfamethoxazole or clindamycin.</u>

- Recommended to treat children < 2 years of age or those with severe disease for 10 days; ≥ 2 years of age with mild to moderate disease for 5-7 days.

- Ceftriaxone (50 mg/kg) can be given IM/IV x 3 days for those who cannot tolerate oral medication (e.g. vomiting). All the others are oral.

Select drugs for AOM

DRUG	DOSING
Amoxicillin *(Amoxil)*	90 mg/kg/day in 2 divided doses
Amoxicillin/clavulanate *(Augmentin)*	90 mg/kg/day of amoxicillin and 6.4 mg/kg/day of clavulanate in 2 divided doses *Augmentin ES*-600 is a powder. Each 5 mL contains 600 mg amoxicillin and 42.9 mg clavulanic acid.
Azithromycin *(Zithromax)*	10 mg/kg/day on day 1, then 5 mg/kg/day once daily on days 2-5
Clarithromycin *(Biaxin)*	15 mg/kg/day in 2 divided doses
Erythromycin-sulfisoxazole *(Pediazole)*	40-50 mg/kg/day of erythromycin in 3 or 4 divided doses (not to exceed 2 gm of erythromycin/6 gm sulfisoxazole per day)
Sulfamethoxazole-trimethoprim *(Bactrim, Septra)*	6-10 mg/kg/day of trimethoprim in 2 divided doses
Ceftriaxone *(Rocephin)*	50 mg/kg IM/IV x 3 days (max 1,000 mg per day)

- *Prevnar 13,* the Pneumococcal Conjugate Vaccine (PCV) which contains 13 serotypes is now given to all children 2-23 months. Children receive four doses of PCV13 intramuscularly at age 2, 4, 6, and 12 to 15 months old. *(Pneumovax* is the adult polyvalent vaccine which contains 23 serotypes.)

- ACIP also recommends the *Pneumovax* vaccine for children aged > 24 months who are at increased risk for pneumococcal disease (e.g., children with sickle cell hemoglobinopathies, HIV, and other immunocompromising or chronic medical conditions).

- *Prevnar 13* is primarily for preventing pneumococcal meningitis and pneumonia, but also reduces otitis media.

INFECTIVE ENDOCARDITIS (IE)

- The incidence of infective endocarditis is relatively rare in comparison to other infections such as UTI or pneumonia with less than 15,000 cases per year.

- IE is commonly determined by the Modified Duke Criteria and treatment is based on the American Heart Association guidelines.(Circulation. 2005;111:e394-e433)

Infective Endocarditis Treatment

NATIVE VALVE	PRIMARY DRUG REGIMEN
Infective endocarditis – empiric treatment Methicillin-Sensitive *Staphylococcus aureus*	Nafcillin or oxacillin 2 gm IV Q4H x 6 weeks (native valve) +/- Gentamicin 1 mg/kg IM/IV Q8H x 3-5 days Prosthetic valve: extend gentamicin therapy for 2 weeks PCN allergic patients or MRSA: replace beta-lactam with vancomycin 15 mg/kg Q12H x 6 weeks

NATIVE VALVE	PRIMARY DRUG REGIMEN
Infective endocarditis due to *Viridans Strep, S. bovis* (Pen G MIC ≤ 0.12 mcg/mL) If higher MICs (> 0.12 - ≤ 0.5 mcg/mL), need to treat with higher doses of Pen G (24 MU) and for longer durations (4 weeks) + gentamicin (2 weeks).	Pen G 12-18 MU IV divided Q4H + gentamicin 1 mg/kg IV Q8H x 2 weeks or Pen G 12-18 MU IV divided Q4H or ceftriaxone 2 gm IV daily x 4 weeks
Infective endocarditis due to *Entercocci* – sensitive to PCN, gentamicin, vancomycin	Pen G 18-30 MU IV divided Q4H x 4-6 weeks Or Ampicillin 12 gm/day IV divided Q4H x 4-6 weeks PLUS Gentamicin 1 mg/kg IV Q8H x 4-6 weeks
Infective endocarditis due to *Entercocci* – resistant to gentamicin	Pen G 24 MU IV divided Q4H x 4-6 weeks or Ampicillin 12 gm/day IV divided Q4H x 4-6 weeks PLUS Streptomycin 7.5 mg/kg IV/IM Q12H x 4-6 weeks
Infective endocarditis due to *Entercocci* – resistant to Pen G/ampicillin	Vancomycin 15 mg/kg IV Q12H x 6 weeks PLUS Gentamicin 1 mg/kg IV Q8H x 6 weeks
Infective endocarditis due to *Entercocci* – resistant to PCN, vancomycin, gentamicin *E. faecium species*	Linezolid 600 mg PO/IV Q12H x ≥ 8 weeks or Quinupristin/dalfopristin 22.5 mg/kg per day divided in 3 doses x ≥ 8 weeks

Notes

- When gentamicin is used for synergy, do not need peak levels to exceed 4 mcg/mL (~3 mcg/mL is sufficient), and trough levels should be < 1 mcg/mL.

- Do not use extended interval dosing for AMG when dosing for endocarditis.

Endocarditis Prevention

INFECTIVE ENDOCARDITIS PROPHYLAXIS	
Cardiac Conditions Associated With the Highest Risk of Adverse Outcome From Endocarditis for Which Prophylaxis With Dental Procedures Is Recommended (2007 AHA Guidelines)	
Prosthetic cardiac valve(s)	Repaired CHD with residual defects at the site or adjacent to the site of a prosthetic patch or prosthetic device
Previous IE	
Congenital heart disease (CHD)	Cardiac transplantation recipients who develop cardiac valvulopathy
Unrepaired cyanotic CHD, including palliative shunts and conduits	Mitral Valve Prolapse with regurgitation and/or thickened valve leaflets
Completely repaired congenital heart defect with prosthetic material or device, whether placed by surgery or by catheter intervention, during the first six months after the procedure	Hypertropic Cardiomyopathy
	Acquired Valvular Dysfunction
	Non-cardiac reason – Total joint replacement in the last 2 years

Regimen: Single dose 30 to 60 min before procedure

AGENT	ADULTS	CHILDREN
Oral		
Amoxicillin	2 g	50 mg/kg
Unable to take oral medication		
Ampicillin OR	2 g IM/IV	50 mg/kg IM/IV
Cefazolin or ceftriaxone	1 g IM/IV	50 mg/kg IM/IV
Allergic to penicillins		
Cephalexin or cefadroxil[e] OR	2 g	50 mg/kg
Clindamycin OR	600 mg	20 mg/kg
Azithromycin or clarithromycin	500 mg	15 mg/kg
Allergic to penicillins and unable to take oral medication		
Cefazolin or Ceftriaxone OR	1 g IM/IV	50 mg/kg IM/IV
Clindamycin	600 mg IM/IV	20 mg/kg IM/IV

[e]*Cephalosporins should not be used in an individual with a history of anaphylaxis, angioedema, or urticaria with penicillins or ampicillin.*

MENINGITIS

- Classic signs and symptoms include fever, nuchal rigidity, and altered mental status (classic triad), chills, vomiting, photophobia, and severe headache. In children, may also see bulging fontanelles, apneas, and convulsions. (Clin Infect Dis. 2004;39:1267-84; N Engl J Med. 2006;354;44-53)

- A lumbar puncture (LP) is mandatory for all suspected bacterial meningitis. The LP will help differentiate viral from bacterial meningitis as well as culture and sensitivities.

- Gram stain is both rapid and sensitive for diagnosis of bacterial meningitis; however, the sensitivity decreases in patients who received prior antibiotic therapy.

- Antibiotic dosages must be maximized to optimize penetration of the CNS.

- The most likely organisms causing bacterial meningitis are *S. pneumonia*, *N. meningitidis*, *H. influenza* and *L. monocytogenes*.

TREATMENT	NOTES

Acute Bacterial Meningitis – Empiric Therapy

Cefotaxime 2 gm IV Q4-6H or	Give dexamethasone 15-20 min prior to or concomitantly with 1st dose of antibiotic
Ceftriaxone 2 gm IV Q12H or	
Meropenem 2 gm IV Q8H (alternative to 3rd gen. ceph)	Need high doses of vancomycin to penetrate CSF
PLUS	Add ampicillin 2 gm IV Q4H if age < 1 month or > 50 years, have impaired cellular immunity, if suspect *Listeria*
Dexamethasone 0.15 mg/kg IV Q6H x 2-4 days PLUS	
Vancomycin 30-45 mg/kg per day in divided doses	

For severe PCN allergy

Chloramphenicol 4,000-6,000 mg per day in 4 doses	Chloramphenicol and vancomycin will provide adequate coverage for *Neisseria* and *Streptococcus pneumoniae*. SMX/TMP can be added for suspected *Listeria*.
PLUS Vancomycin 30-45 mg/kg per day in divided doses	
+/- SMX/TMP 5 mg/kg IV Q6H	

(Eur J Neurol. 2008;15;649-59; Bartlett. Johns Hopkins Antibiotic Guide: Diagnosis & Treatment of Infectious Diseases 2nd Ed. 2010)

RICKETTSIAL DISEASES

Rickettsia species are carried by many ticks, fleas, and lice.

DISEASE	TREATMENT
Rocky Mountain Spotted Fever	Doxycycline 100 mg PO/IV BID x 7 days
Lyme Disease	Doxycycline 100 mg PO BID or amoxicillin 500 mg PO TID x 14-21 days
Typhus	Doxycycline 100 mg PO/IV BID x 7 days
Ehrlichiosis	Doxycycline 100 mg PO/IV BID x 7-14 days
Tularemia	Gentamicin or tobramycin 5 mg/kg/d divided Q8H IV x 7-14 days

Clin Infect Dis. 2006;43;1089-134.

SYSTEMIC FUNGAL INFECTIONS

BACKGROUND

- Certain types of fungi (including yeasts such as *Candida)* are normally present on body surfaces or in the intestine. They do not normally cause serious fungal infections unless the immune system is weakened, or compromised, by drugs or diseases.

- However, candidemia is the 4th most common nosocomial blood stream infection in the U.S. with mortality rates up to 30%. (Curr Med Res Opin. 2009;25;1732-40)

- Some fungi reproduce by spreading microscopic spores. These spores are often present in the air, where they can be inhaled or come into contact with the skin; therefore, causing lung and skin infections.

- Some fungal organisms include *Aspergillus spp., Blastomycosis spp., Candida spp., Crytococcosis spp., Coccidioidomycosis spp., Histoplasmosis spp.* and others.

- *Candida* infections can be generally treated with fluconazole. However, there are fluconazole-resistant species of *Candida* such as *C. krusei* and while other species require higher doses of fluconazole to be effective such as *C. glabrata* but resistance to fluconazole is also present in this species. (Clinical Infectious Diseases 2009; 48:503–35)

PHARMACOLOGIC TREATMENTS

Amphotericin B binds to ergosterol altering cell membrane permeability in susceptible fungi and causing cell death.

DIFFERENT FORMULATIONS	SIDE EFFECTS/NOTES
Amphotericin B desoxycholate (conventional) - *(Amphocin)*	Hypokalemia, hypomagnesemia, nephrotoxicity, hypotension , tachypnea, fever, chills, headache, malaise, rigors, nausea, vomiting, normochromic, normocytic anemia and others
	Compatible with D5W
	Amphotericin B deoxycholate – most nephrotoxic
	AmBisome - most expensive – can cause back/chest pain with 1st dose
	Infusion-related reactions = *Amphotec* > Ampho B deoxycholate > ***Abelcet*** > ***AmBisome***
Lipid formulations Amphotericin B Lipid Complex *(Abelcet)*	**Pre-medicate for infusion-related reactions (including fever, chills, hypotension, nausea, etc.). Give 30-60 minutes prior to infusion:** Acetaminophen or NSAID
Liposomal Amphotericin B *(AmBisome)*	Diphenhydramine 25 mg IV and/or hydrocortisone 50-100 mg IV Meperidine 25-50 mg IV for reducing the duration of rigors
Amphotericin B cholesteryl sulfate complex *(Amphotec)*	Saline boluses (500-1,000 mL) to reduce the nephrotoxicity

Clin Infect Dis. 1998;27;603-18.

Amphotericin B Drug Interactions

- Risk of nephrotoxicity with Ampho B will be ↑ when used with other nephrotoxic agents such as cyclosporine, AMGs, flucytosine, cisplatin and others. Nephrotoxic effects are additive. May enhance digoxin toxicity due to hypokalemia.

- Use caution with any agent that ↓ potassium and magnesium since amphotericin decreases both of these.

Flucytosine (Ancobon, 5-FC) penetrates fungal cells and is converted to fluorouracil which competes with uracil, interfering with fungal RNA and protein synthesis.

CAUTIONS	SIDE EFFECTS/DRUG INTERACTIONS
Causes bone marrow suppression	Dose-related bone marrow suppression, many CNS effects, hypoglycemia, hypokalemia, pancytopenia, aplastic anemia, hepatitis, ↑ bilirubin, ↑ SCr, ↑ BUN and others
Avoid use as monotherapy due to rapid resistance	↑ effect with concurrent Ampho B. May be used for synergy with Ampho B for certain fungal infections (*Cryptococcus* spp.)

Azole Antifungals decrease ergosterol synthesis and inhibit cell membrane formation

DRUG	DOSING	SIDE EFFECTS/CONTRAINDICATIONS/MONITORING
Itraconazole *(Sporanox)*	200- 400 mg daily-BID PO	**SIDE EFFECTS** Nausea, vomiting, diarrhea, abdominal pain, rash/pruritus, ↑ LFTs, hypertriglyceridemia, hypokalemia, HTN, edema Itraconazole - due to differences in bioavailability, oral capsules and oral solution CAN NOT be used interchangeably Capsule form has low bioavailability on an empty stomach; take with food and requires gastric acidity for absorption Oral solution is more bioavailable than capsules; take on an empty stomach With ketoconazole shampoo, ↑ hair loss and altered hair texture **CONTRAINDICATIONS** **Itraconazole Black Box Warning** Heart failure (HF) or history of heart failure – capsules should not be administered for the treatment of onychomycosis in patients with HF
Fluconazole *(Diflucan)*	100-400 mg daily PO/IV IV/PO 1:1	Concurrent administration with cisapride, dofetilide, pimozide, and quinidine. Hypersensitivity to azoles **Fluconazole Black Box Warning** Hypersensitivity to azoles Concomitant use with cisapride **Ketoconazole Black Box Warning** Concurrent administration with cisapride due to fatal ventricular arrhythmias
Ketoconazole *(Nizoral, Kuric, Xolegel*, others)*	200-400 mg PO daily	Has been associated with hepatotoxicity, some fatal Hypersensitivity to azoles

Azole Antifungals decrease ergosterol synthesis and inhibit cell membrane formation Continued

DRUG	DOSING	SIDE EFFECTS/CONTRAINDICATIONS/MONITORING
Voriconazole *(VFEND)*	PO: 100-300 mg Q12H IV: 6 mg/kg Q12H x 2 doses, then 4 mg/kg Q12H Take 1 hr before or 1 hr after meals (empty stomach)	**SIDE EFFECTS** Visual changes (~20% - dose related - blurred vision, photophobia, altered color perception, altered visual acuity), ↑ SCr, hallucinations, photosensitivity, others as above Correct K^+, Ca^{2+}, and Mg^{2+} prior to initiating therapy **CONTRAINDICATIONS** Hypersensitivity to azoles Contraindicated with many 3A4 substrates (rifampin, rifabutin, ergot alkaloids, long acting barbiturates, carbamazepine, pimozide, quinidine, cisapride, efavirenz, St. John's wort) **MONITORING** LFTs, electrolytes, visual function Caution driving at night due to vision changes. Avoid direct sunlight. In patients with CrCl < 50 mL/min, the IV vehicle, SBECD (sulfobutyl ether beta-cyclodextrin), may accumulate. Therefore, it is recommended to use oral dosing after the initial IV loading doses More active against *Aspergillus spp, C. glabrata, C. krusei,* and *Fusarium spp* compared to intraconazole/fluconazole
Posaconazole *(Noxafil)*	40 mg/mL suspension in a 4 oz. bottle packaged with dosing spoon; shake well before use Must be taken with a full meal	**SIDE EFFECTS** Diarrhea, nausea, vomiting, headache, ↑ LFTs, rash, QT-prolongation, hypokalemia Correct K^+, Ca^{2+}, and Mg^{2+} prior to initiating therapy **CONTRAINDICATIONS** Hypersensitivity to azoles Concurrent administration with ergot alkaloids, pimozide, cisapride, quinidine, or sirolimus **MONITORING** LFTs, renal function, electrolytes, visual function

AZOLE ANTIFUNGALS DRUG INTERACTIONS

- All are 3A4 inhibitors (will ↑ concentration of 3A4 substrates). Itraconazole is an inhibitor of 3A4 (major). Ketoconazole inhibits 1A2 (strong), 2C9 (strong), 2C19 (moderate), 2D6 (moderate), 3A4 (strong). Fluconazole is an inhibitor of 2C9 (strong), 2C19 (strong), and 3A4 (moderate). Voriconazole is an inhibitor of 3A4 (strong), 2C9 (moderate) and posaconazole is a strong inhibitor of 3A4.

- Itraconazole and ketoconazole have pH-dependent absorption; ↑ pH causes ↓ absorption; avoid using with antacids, H_2RAs, PPIs.

- Voriconazole is notable for being the drug of choice for *Aspergillus* infections and for drug interactions (and dosing and adverse effects – visual changes).

- Voriconazole is metabolized by several CYP 450 enzymes (2C9, 2C19 and 3A4); the concentration of voriconazole <u>can increase dangerously when given with drugs that inhibit voriconazole's metabolism or with small dose increases – it is 1st order, followed by Michaelis-Menten kinetics.</u>

- <u>Concurrent use of voriconazole and the following drugs are contraindicated:</u> alfuzosin, barbiturates, carbamazepine, cisapride, darunavir, dofetilide, ergot derivatives, lopinavir, nilotinib, pimozide, quinidine, ranolazine, rifampin, rifabutin, ritonavir, St. John's wort, thioridazine, and others.

Echinocandins inhibit synthesis of β(1,3)-D-glucan, an essential component of the fungal cell wall

DRUG	DOSING	SIDE EFFECTS/CONTRAINDICATIONS/MONITORING
Caspofungin *(Cancidas)*	LD: 70 mg IV on day 1, then 50 mg daily Do not mix with dextrose-containing solutions Increase dose to 70 mg IV daily when used in combination with rifampin or other strong enzyme inducers	**SIDE EFFECTS** ↑ LFTs, hypotension, peripheral edema, tachycardia, headache, fever, rash, nausea, vomiting, hypokalemia, ↓ Hgb/Hct, ↑ SCr, etc. Rare: Histamine-mediated symptoms (rash, pruritus, facial swelling, flushing, hypotension) have occurred; anaphylaxis Caution use with cyclosporine due to hepatotoxicity; Caution in hepatic impairment **MONITORING** LFTs
Micafungin *(Mycamine)*	Candidemia 100 mg IV daily Esophageal candidiasis: 150 mg IV daily over 60 minutes	**SIDE EFFECTS** ↑ LFTs, fever, headache, nausea, vomiting, diarrhea, hypomagnesemia, hypokalemia, bone marrow suppression Rare: Histamine-mediated symptoms (rash, pruritus, facial swelling, flushing, hypotension) have occurred; anaphylaxis **MONITORING** LFTs Minor 3A4 interactions
Anidulafungin *(Eraxis)*	Esophageal candidiasis: 100 mg IV on day 1, then 50 mg daily Candidemia: 200 mg IV on day 1, then 100 mg IV daily	**SIDE EFFECTS** ↑ LFTs, diarrhea, hypokalemia Rare: Histamine-mediated symptoms (rash, pruritus, facial swelling, flushing, hypotension) have occurred; anaphylaxis **MONITORING** LFTs All 3 agents are given once daily and do not require dose adjustment in renal impairment. Very little drug interactions

TREATMENT GUIDELINES FOR VARIOUS FUNGAL ORGANISMS

ORGANISM	DISEASE	TREATMENT
Aspergillus spp	Invasive pulmonary disease	Voriconazole 6 mg/kg IV Q12H on day 1, then 4 mg/kg IV Q12H (or 200 mg PO Q12H) **ALTERNATIVE THERAPIES** Liposomal ampho B: 3-5 mg/kg/d IV OR Ampho B lipid complex: 2.5-5 mg/kg/d IV OR Caspofungin: 70 mg IV on day 1, then 50 mg IV daily OR Micafungin 100-150 mg IV daily OR Posaconazole 200 mg PO QID, then 400 mg BID, once stable OR Itraconazole tablets 600 mg PO daily x 3 days, then 400 mg/day
Candida albicans	Bloodstream infection	Clinically stable and not infected with *C. glabrata* or *C. krusei* Fluconazole 800 mg x 1, then 400 mg daily IV/PO OR Caspofungin 70 mg IV on day 1, then 50 mg IV daily OR Micafungin 100 mg IV daily OR Anidulafungin 200 mg IV x 1, then 100 mg IV daily <u>Treatment duration: 2 weeks after the last positive blood culture</u>
Oral candidiasis	Thrush	**NON-AIDS PATIENT** Clotrimazole troches 10 mg PO 5 times/day OR Nystatin suspension or 1-2 pastilles 4 times/day OR Fluconazole 100-200 mg PO daily OR **AIDS PATIENT** Fluconazole 100-200 mg PO daily OR Itraconazole oral solution 200 mg PO daily OR Posaconazole 100 mg BID x 1 day, then 100 mg daily OR Echinocandins OR Ampho B 0.3 mg/kg IV daily <u>Treatment duration: 7-14 days</u>
Esophageal candidiasis		Fluconazole 200-400 mg/day IV/PO OR Itraconazole oral solution 200 mg PO daily OR Voriconazole 200 mg IV/PO Q12H OR Posaconazole 400 mg PO BID x 3 days, then 400 mg PO daily (refractory cases) OR Caspofungin 50 mg IV daily OR Micafungin 150 mg IV daily OR Anidulafungin 100 mg IV day 1, then 50 mg daily OR Ampho B 0.3-0.7 mg/kg daily <u>Treatment duration: 14-21 days</u>

SUPERFICIAL FUNGAL INFECTIONS AND TREATMENT

- Superficial mycotic infections of the skin are referred to as dermatophytoses.

- Risk factors for development of an infection include prolonged exposure to sweaty clothes, failure to bathe regularly, many skin folds, sedentariness, and confinement to bed.

- Diagnosis based on patient history, physical exam, and direct microscopic exam of a specimen after addition of potassium hydroxide (KOH).

- General approach to treatment is to keep the infected area dry and clean and limiting exposure to the infected reservoir.

- Topical agents are considered first-line therapy for infections of the skin.

- Oral therapy is preferred when the infection is extensive or severe or when treating tinea capitis (involves scalp/hair follicles) or onychomycosis.

Superficial Fungal Infections: see Skin (Derm) section

VAGINAL CANDIDA INFECTIONS

Background

- About 75% women will have at least one episode

- 40-45% will have 2 or more episodes

- < 5% will have recurrent episodes

Causative Agents

- *Candida albicans*

- Predisposing factors: broad-spectrum antibiotics, oral contraceptives (high estrogen), poorly controlled diabetes, pregnancy, chronic use of steroids, obesity

Signs & Symptoms

- Intense pruritus, thick, curd-like vaginal discharge, soreness, vulvar pain, swelling and irritation (discharge may or not be present, but itching is universal)

Diagnosis

- Based on signs and symptoms; confirmed by a wet preparation of vaginal secretions using a 10% potassium hydroxide (KOH) solution showing budding yeast and pseudohyphae

Pharmacologic Treatment

- Topical azole agents are typically used and usually do not cause systemic side effects (just local side effects such as burning or irritation). They are all equally effective (except nystatin is less effective) and have > 80% cure rates.

- Only topical azole therapies, applied for 7 days, are recommended in pregnant women.

- Severe infection and pregnant: prefer 7-day regimen.

- Recurrent infection (> 4 episodes/yr): 7-14 day regimen.

- Not usually acquired through sexual contact, thus not necessary to treat partner unless developing recurrent infection.

- Check case first for diabetes or HIV – these patients should see the physician for treatment. An infection could mean the disease is uncontrolled.

- Do not recommend self-treatment until after a first infection has been diagnosed by the primary care provider.

Topical agents

- Butoconazole *(Femstat-3, Gynazole-1)* 2% cream 5 g intravaginally x 3 d or intravaginally x 1

- Clotrimazole *(Gyne-Lotrimin-7, Mycelex-7)* 1% cream 5 g intravaginally x 7 days

- Clotrimazole 100 mg vaginal tab daily x 7 days or 2 tabs daily x 3 days

- Clotrimazole 500 mg vaginal tab x 1

- Miconazole *(Monistat-7)* 2% cream 5 g intravaginally x 7 days

- Miconazole *(Monistat-3, Monistat-7)* - 200 mg vaginal supp daily x 3 days or 100 mg daily x 7 days

- Miconazole *(Monistat-1)* 1,200 mg vaginal supp. x 1

- Nystatin *(Mycostatin)* 100,000 unit vaginal tab daily x 14 days

- Tioconazole *(Vagistat-1)* 6.5% oint 5 g intravaginally x 1

- Terconazole *(Terazol)* 0.4% cream 5 g intravaginally x 7 days or 0.8% cream x 3 days

- Terconazole *(Zazole)* 80 mg vaginal supp daily x 3 days

- Fluconazole *(Diflucan)* 150 mg PO x 1 – only oral formulation

PATIENT COUNSELING

- Insert applicator, suppository, or tab at night before bed. Complete entire course of treatment.

- Use protective pad if desired

- The creams and suppositories are oil-based medications that can weaken latex condoms and diaphragms; avoid sexual intercourse

- If you get your menstrual cycle during treatment, continue the treatment, otherwise a woman can wait until her menstrual cycle is over before starting treatment if she desires (this is not necessary)

- Medical care is warranted if symptoms persist/recur within 2 months after using an OTC product

Counseling That Applies to All Antibiotics

- Antibiotics only treat bacterial infections. They do not treat viral infections (e.g., the common cold).

- Skipping doses or not completing the full course of therapy may decrease the effectiveness of treatment, cause the infection to return, and increase the likelihood that this medicine will not work for you in the future.

- If your symptoms worsen, contact your doctor.

- All beta lactams (and most other antibiotics) can cause rash. If the rash looks serious, the patient should be seen right away. Beta lactams can cause severe skin rashes in rare cases.

- If using a suspension, all need shaking and most (but not clarithromycin, clindamycin, voriconazole, others) should be refrigerated.

- Measure liquid doses carefully using a measuring device/syringe. These should be dispensed with the medicine if the patient does not have one already. Tell the patient not to use a household spoon because they may not get the correct dose.

- For all antibiotics, especially clindamycin and drugs with broad-spectrum coverage, instruct the patient to report symptoms of a C. *diff* infection, including watery diarrhea several times a day with (possibly) mild abdominal cramping. This can occur during treatment, or weeks after the antibiotic treatment has finished. If present, the doctor should be contacted right away. Patients should be instructed not to self-treat this condition with anti-diarrhea medicine. Taking yogurt with active cultures, or certain probiotics, can help reduce the incidence, but should be taken at a time separate from the antibiotic.

SPECIFIC COUNSELING POINTS FOR COMMON AGENTS

Acyclovir *(Zovirax)* – Antiviral

- This medicine works best when taken at the first sign of an outbreak within the first day.

- The most common side effect (less than 3%) is nausea. Headache can also occur.

- Take this medication by mouth with or without food, usually 2 to 5 times daily, as directed. The intervals should be evenly spaced.

- Drink plenty of fluids while taking this medication.

- For the cream, side effects including dry/cracked lips, burning, stinging, or flaky skin may occur. If any of these effects persist or worsen, tell your doctor or pharmacist promptly.

Amoxicillin products

- Take this medication by mouth with a meal or snack, usually every 8 or 12 hours, or as directed by your doctor.

- If you develop a rash, especially one that looks serious, you should be seen right away. This medicine can rarely cause serious skin rashes.

- The suspensions should be refrigerated (especially important for *Augmentin*).

Azithromycin *(Zithromax)*

- The most common side effect (less than 1%) is nausea or abdominal discomfort.

- Common dosing is two 250 mg tablets on day 1, followed by one 250 mg tablets on days 2-5.

- The tablets and immediate release oral suspension can be taken with or without food; extended release suspension should be taken on an empty stomach (1 hour before, 2 hours after a meal). The suspension does not require refrigeration.

Clarithromycin *(Biaxin)*

- Common side effects (2-3%) include diarrhea, abdominal pain, nausea or abnormal (metallic) taste.

- The tablets and oral suspension are taken with or without food and can be taken with milk.

- *Biaxin XL* tablets should be taken with food.

- The liquid suspension is not refrigerated.

- There are interactions with this drug and other medicines. Please discuss with your pharmacist to make sure this will not pose a problem.

Ciprofloxacin *(Cipro)*

- Common side effects (1-3%) include nausea, diarrhea or rash. You may feel dizzy or lightheaded. Rarely, seizures can occur, especially in those with seizure disorders. (Quinolones should be avoided with a seizure history.)

- This medicine can make your skin more sensitive to the sun, and you can burn more easily. Use sunscreen and protective clothing, and try to avoid staying in the sun.

- This medicine can rarely cause a serious problem called tendon rupture or swelling of the tendon (tendinitis). If you notice, pain, swelling and inflammation of the tendons on the back of the ankle (Achilles), shoulder, hand or other sites, stop the medicine and be seen right away. This is uncommon, but occurs more frequently in people over 60, and in patients who have had transplants and use steroid medicine, such as prednisone.

- This is not a first choice medicine in patients under 18 years of age due to a risk of bone and joint problems. However, it is used occasionally on a short-term basis for certain conditions.

- Do not use this medicine if you take a different medicine called tizanidine *(Zanaflex)*. Please tell your pharmacist about all medicines you are using, since this medicine can interact with many others.

Levofloxacin *(Levaquin)*

- Same for ciprofloxacin (above). Levofloxacin is taken once daily (ciprofloxacin is BID or daily).

- The tablets can be taken with or without food. The suspension is taken 1 hour before or 2 hours after eating. Maintain adequate hydration to prevent crystalluria.

- If you use warfarin, your INR may increase. Your doctor should check your INR more frequently, and you should watch for symptoms of bleeding.

- If you use blood sugar-lowering medicines, your blood sugar may get unusually low. Be careful to check your sugar level frequently and treat low blood sugar if it occurs.

- If you have kidney disease, you will need to use a lower dose. Your doctor or pharmacist will make sure the dose is correct.

- This medicine should be taken 2 hours before, or 4-6 hours after taking antacids, vitamins, magnesium, calcium, iron or zinc supplements, dairy products, bismuth subsalicylate or the medicines sucralfate *(Carafate)* or didanosine *(Videx)*.

- Drink plenty of fluids while using this medicine.

Doxycycline *(Doryx*, others)

- Common side effects include stomach upset, mild diarrhea, nausea, headache, or vomiting.

- This medicine can make your skin more sensitive to the sun, and you can burn more easily. Use sunscreen and protective clothing, and try to avoid staying in the sun.

- Drink plenty of fluids while using this medicine.

- This medicine should be taken 2 hours before, or 4-6 hours after taking antacids, vitamins, magnesium, calcium, iron or zinc supplements, dairy products, bismuth subsalicylate or the medicines sucralfate *(Carafate)* or didanosine *(Videx)*.

- Tell your doctor immediately if any of these unlikely but serious side effects occur: stomach pain, yellowing of the eyes/skin, vision changes, mental/mood changes.

Erythromycin *(EES)*   يعمل

- Typical dosing is 400 mg erythromycin ethylsuccinate every 6 hours.

- Chew the tablet thoroughly before swallowing. You may take this medication with or without food.

- Nausea commonly occurs with the use of erythromycin, especially when taken on an empty stomach. To reduce this side effect, take with food or milk.

- Common side effects are nausea, abdominal pain and cramping, and diarrhea.

- The liquid suspension combination with sulfisoxazole *(Pediazole)* is refrigerated.

- There are many interactions with this drug and other medicines. Please discuss with your pharmacist to make sure this will not pose a problem.

Fluconazole *(Diflucan)* [all true for ketoconazole *(Nizoral)* and itraconazole *(Sporanox)* as well, except the single dosing]

- Common side effects (5-16%) are headache, nausea and abdominal pain.

- Commonly given as one 150 mg tablet for a vaginal fungal infection. If taken longer, counsel on possible hepatotoxicity or serious skin rash issues.

- Contact your doctor right away if you are passing brown or dark-colored urine, have pale stools, feel more tired than usual or if your skin and whites of your eyes become yellow. These may be signs of liver damage.

- If you develop a rash, especially one that looks serious, you should be seen right away. This medicine can rarely cause serious skin rashes.

- If you have kidney disease, you will need to use a lower dose. Your doctor or pharmacist will make sure the dose is correct.

- This medicine can increase the levels of many other medicines. Please discuss with your pharmacist to make sure this will not pose a problem.

- Ketoconazole and Itraconazole (except dosing): same as above, and do not use with antacids (two hour separation) and stop the use of PPIs or H_2RAs while using this medicine. These other medicines will reduce the amount of the anti-fungal medicine that gets absorbed.

Clindamycin *(Cleocin)*

- Common side effects include diarrhea (> 10%), abdominal pain, nausea, abnormal taste.

- This medication can cause a serious intestinal condition called *Clostridium difficile*-associated diarrhea, or pseudomembranous colitis. If this develops, you will have watery diarrhea, several times or more daily, with possible cramping and bloody stool. If this happens, tell your doctor immediately. This could occur even after you have finished the medicine. You will need to be treated for this condition. Do not self-treat it with anti-diarrheal medication.

- Take by mouth with or without food, 3-4 times a day.

- Take with a full glass of water.

- The liquid suspension is not refrigerated.

Metronidazole *(Flagyl)*

- Generally taken 250-500 mg three to four times daily.

- Common side effects are nausea (12%), and occasional headache and loss of appetite.

- Do not use any alcohol products while using this medicine, and for at least 1-2 days afterward.

- Take with food or water or milk to help prevent stomach upset.

Oseltamivir *(Tamiflu)* – antiviral (in the immunizations section)

- Treatment should begin within 2 days of onset of influenza symptoms.

- Adult treatment dose is 75 mg twice daily for 5 days. Prophylaxis is once daily for 10 days.

- Children (1-12 years) are dosed from 30-75 mg BID for treatment, based on weight, for 5 days. Prophylaxis is once daily for 10 days.

- Common side effects are nausea and vomiting. Take with or without food. There is less chance of stomach upset if you take it with a light snack, milk, or a meal.

- Please let your doctor know if you have received the nasally administered influenza virus vaccine during the past two weeks. (Risk that drug may inhibit replication of the live virus vaccine).

- This medicine can occasionally cause a severe rash. If you develop a rash, stop taking the medicine and contact your doctor.

- People with the flu, particularly children and adolescents, may be at an increased risk of self injury and confusion shortly after taking this medicine and should be closely monitored for signs of unusual behavior. Contact the doctor immediately if the patient shows any signs of unusual behavior.

- Vaccination is considered the first line of defense against influenza; this medicine does not replace an annual (fall) influenza vaccine.

Nitrofurantoin *(Macrodantin, Macrobid)*

- Take this medication with food, as direct by your doctor. Swallow the medication whole.

- Do not use magnesium trisilicate-containing antacids while taking this medication. These antacids can bind with nitrofurantoin, preventing its full absorption into your system.

- Antibiotics work best when the amount of medicine in your body is kept at a constant level. Therefore, take this drug at evenly spaced intervals.

- Continue to take this medication until the full prescribed amount is finished, even if symptoms disappear after a few days. Stopping the medication too early may allow bacteria to continue to grow, which may result in a return of the infection.

- Side effects including nausea and headache may occur. If any of these effects persist or worsen, notify your doctor or pharmacist promptly.

- This medication may cause your urine to turn dark yellow or brown in color. This is usually a harmless, temporary effect and will disappear when the medication is stopped. However, dark brown urine can also be a sign of rare side effects (liver problems or anemia). Therefore, seek immediate medical attention if you notice dark urine along with any of the following symptoms: persistent nausea/vomiting, stomach/abdominal pain, yellowing eyes/skin, tiredness, fast/pounding heartbeat.

- Tell your doctor immediately if any of these rare but very serious side effects occur: eye pain, vision changes, mental/mood changes, persistent/severe headaches, new signs of infection (e.g., fever, persistent sore throat), easy bruising/bleeding.

- This medication may rarely cause very serious (possibly fatal) lung problems. Lung problems may occur within the first month of treatment or after long-term use of nitrofurantoin (generally for 6 months or longer). Seek immediate medical attention if you develop symptoms of lung problems, including: persistent cough, chest pain, shortness of breath/ trouble breathing, joint/muscle pain, bluish/purplish skin.

- This medication may rarely cause a severe intestinal condition (*Clostridium difficile*-associated diarrhea) due to a resistant bacteria. This condition may occur during treatment or even weeks to months after treatment has stopped. Do not use anti-diarrhea products or narcotic pain medications if you have the following symptoms because these products may make them worse. Tell your doctor immediately if you develop: persistent diarrhea, abdominal or stomach pain/cramping, blood/mucus in your stool.

Sulfamethoxazole and Trimethoprim *(Bactrim, Septra)*

- Do not use if you have an allergy to sulfa medicines.

- Common side effects are nausea and rash.

- Take with a full glass of water to prevent crystalluria.

- If stomach upset occurs, take with food or milk.

- The suspension does not need to be refrigerated.

- This medicine can make your skin more sensitive to the sun, and you can burn more easily. Use sunscreen and protective clothing, and try to avoid staying in the sun.

- If you develop a rash, especially one that looks serious, you should be seen right away. This medicine can rarely cause serious skin rashes.

- Shake the suspension prior to use. The suspension should be kept at room temperature.

Terbinafine *(Lamisil)*

- Terbinafine is used to treat certain types of fungal infections (e.g. fingernail or toenail). It works by stopping the growth of fungus.

- Take this medication by mouth with or without food, usually once a day. Dosage and length of treatment depend on the location of the fungus and the response to treatment.

- It may take several months after you finish treatment to see the full benefit of this drug. It takes time for your new healthy nails to grow out and replace the infected ones.

- Continue to take this medication until the full prescribed amount is finished. Stopping the medication too early may allow the fungus to continue to grow, which may result in a return of the infection.

- Side effects such as diarrhea, stomach upset, or temporary change or loss of taste may occur. If any of these effects persist or worsen, tell your doctor or pharmacist.

- Tell your doctor immediately if any of these rare, but serious side effects occur: new signs of infection (fever, chills, etc.) or vision changes.

- This drug has rarely caused very serious (and fatal) liver disease. Tell your doctor immediately if you develop symptoms of liver disease including persistent nausea, loss of appetite, severe stomach/abdominal pain, dark urine, yellowing of eyes/skin, or pale stools.

Valacyclovir *(Valtrex)* – for herpes simplex

- *Valtrex* used daily with the following safer sex practices can lower the chances of passing genital herpes to your partner.

  - Do not have sexual contact with your partner when you have any symptom or outbreak of genital herpes.

  - Use a condom made of latex or polyurethane whenever you have sexual contact.

- *Valtrex* does not cure herpes infections (cold sores, chickenpox, shingles, or genital herpes)

- Do not stop or change your treatment without talking to your healthcare provider.

- Can be taken with or without food.

- Start treatment as soon as possible after your symptoms start. *Valtrex* may not help you if you start treatment too late.

- If you miss a dose, take it as soon as you remember and then take your next dose at its regular time. However, if it is almost time for your next dose, do not take the missed dose. Wait and take the next dose at the regular time.

- Kidney failure and nervous system problems are not common, but can be serious in some patients taking *Valtrex*. Nervous system problems include aggressive behavior, unsteady movement, shaky movements, confusion, speech problems, hallucinations (seeing or hearing things that are really not there), seizures, and coma. Kidney failure and nervous system problems have happened in patients who already have kidney disease and in elderly patients whose kidneys do not work well due to age. Always tell your healthcare provider if you have kidney problems before taking *Valtrex*. Call your doctor right away if you develop any of these symptoms.

- Common side effects in adults include headache, nausea, stomach pain, vomiting, and dizziness. These side effects usually are mild and do not cause patients to stop taking *Valtrex*.

- Store caplets at room temperature.

- Store suspension in a refrigerator. Discard after 28 days.

Voriconazole *(VFEND)*

- Common side effects include eyesight changes, rash, vomiting, nausea, diarrhea, headache, chills, and fever.

- Avoid night driving because this medicine may cause vision problems like blurry vision. If you have any change in your eyesight, avoid all driving or using dangerous machinery.

- Avoid sunlight. Your skin may burn more easily. Your eyes may hurt in bright sunlight.

- Discuss with the pharmacist if you have trouble digesting dairy products, lactose, or regular table sugar. The tablets contain lactose (milk sugar). The liquid contains sucrose (table sugar).

- Take this medication by mouth, at least 1 hour before or 1 hour after meals, usually every 12 hours or as directed. ☆ BID w/o meal

- There are many interactions with this drug and other medicines. Please discuss with your pharmacist to make sure this will not pose a problem.

- Do not use if you are pregnant, if you could become pregnant, or if you are breastfeeding.

- Contact your doctor right away if you are passing brown or dark-colored urine, feel more tired than usual or if your skin and whites of your eyes become yellow. These may be signs of liver damage.

- You will need to be seen by a doctor quickly if you develop any signs of a rash or have difficulty breathing.

Practice Case

MJ is a 43 year old female who presents to the doctor with fever, runny nose, congestion, productive cough, and body aches. She tells you that she has been feeling this way for the past 36 hours and she needs to get better to return to work. She noticed a lot of people coughing on the bus she takes to work and figures that were she picked it up.

CATEGORY	
PMH	Depression
	GERD
Vitals	BP 164/81 HR 114 RR 24 Temp 102.3
Current medications	Fluoxetine 20 mg PO daily
	Ranitidine 150 mg PO BID
	Tums PRN
Labs	K⁺ 3.5 mEq/L, SCr 1.1 mg/dL
Allergies	Sulfa (major hives, extreme rash)

QUESTIONS

CAP

1. The doctor confirms by culture that MJ has community-acquired pneumonia. What is the most appropriate therapy for MJ?

    a. *Zithromax* 500 mg PO x 1, then 250 mg PO daily (days 2-5)
    b. *Avelox* 400 mg IV daily x 5-7 days
    c. *Levaquin* 500 mg PO x 1, then 250 mg PO daily x 5-7 days
    d. *Ceftin* 500 mg PO Q12H x 5-7 days
    e. *Bactrim* 1 DS tab PO Q12H x 5-7 days

CAP

2. MJ has accidentally lost the prescription and she cannot afford another office visit. She decides to tough it out and goes back to work. Two days later, MJ is admitted to the hospital due to worsening symptoms. What is the best agent(s) to treat her community-acquired pneumonia?

    a. Ciprofloxacin 500 mg PO daily
    b. Ceftriaxone 1 gram IV daily
    c. Ceftriaxone 1 gram IV daily + azithromycin 500 mg IV daily
    d. Vancomycin 1 gram IV Q12H + imipenem 500 mg Q6H
    e. Gemifloxacin 320 mg PO daily + clarithromycin 500 mg PO Q12H

3. While in the hospital, MJ develops a *Pseudomonal* infection in her lungs as well. Which of the following antibiotics would be an appropriate choice for coverage of *Pseudomonas*?   carbapenem

    a. Ampicillin
    b. *Cubicin*   Daptomycin
    c. *Invanz*   Ertapenem (no p. a. coverage)
    d. *Doribax*   doripenem
    e. *Tygacil*

4. MJ's condition is not improving. She was placed on vancomycin a few days ago and now she has developed vancomycin-resistance *Enterococcus faecium*. The medical team puts her on linezolid. Which of the following statements is TRUE regarding linezolid?

    a. It is in a new class called cyclic lipopeptides
    b. It is a weak MAO inhibitor and should be avoided with serotonergic agents.
    c. It is a combination product consisting of quinupristin and dalfopristin.
    d. It needs to be dose adjusted in patients with renal impairment.
    e. It is not effective for treating infections in the lung.

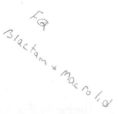

5. MJ has now been in the hospital for a month. She is still febrile, has an increased WBC count, and remains unable to wean from the ventilator. She has been on most intravenous antibacterial agents. The team decided to re-culture her and now they find *C. albicans* in the blood. They tried treating with itraconazole with no improvement. The team decides to treat with anidulafungin. Which of the following is correct regarding anidulafungin?

   a. This medication should be taken with meals for best absorption.
   b. This medication can cause an increase in liver transaminases.
   c. This medication is not effective for the treatment of candidemia.
   d. This medication needs to be dose adjusted in renal impairment.
   e. The brand name is *Epistaxis*.

6. MJ has turned the corner and was discharged to home a few weeks later. After about 3-4 months, she returns to the doctor complaining of intense burning on urination, dysuria, and frequency of bathroom visits. The doctor confirms that she has a urinary tract infection caused by *E. coli*, which is sensitive to everything. Which of the following is the best choice to treat MJ's UTI?

   a. *Bactrim* SS 1 tab PO BID x 3 days
   b. *Bactrim* DS 1 tab PO BID x 3 days
   c. Nitrofurantoin 100 mg PO BID x 3 days
   d. Nitrofurantoin 100 mg PO BID x 5 days
   e. Phenazopyridine 200 mg TID x 2 days

7. Which of the following statements regarding the intravenous formulation of *Bactrim* is/are correct?

   a. *Bactrim* IV should be protected from light.
   b. *Bactrim* IV should be refrigerated.
   c. *Bactrim* IV is compatible with NS.
   d. A and B.
   e. A and C.

8. You are working in the ER when an intern comes to you and asks how to treat the patient in room 4 who has a gonorrheal STD infection. What is the best recommendation to treat this patient?

   a. Levofloxacin 750 mg PO x 1
   b. Doxycycline 100 mg PO BID x 7 days
   c. Benzathine penicillin G 2.4 million units IM x 1
   d. Metronidazole 2 grams PO x 1
   e. Ceftriaxone 250 mg IM x 1 + azithromycin 1 gram PO x 1

9. The intern is back. This time to ask you about herpes simplex virus and *Valtrex*. Which of the following statements are TRUE regarding *Valtrex*?

   a. *Valtrex* is a prodrug of acyclovir and can be used as suppressive therapy in patients with herpes simplex virus.
   b. *Valtrex* is a prodrug of penciclovir and should not be used as suppressive therapy in patients with herpes simplex virus.
   c. *Valtrex* should only be used for herpes zoster virus.
   d. *Valtrex* needs to be taken with a fatty meal for best absorption.
   e. *Valtrex* is contraindicated in patients with a CrCl < 30 mL/min.

10. Tommy is taking isoniazid (INH) as part of his tuberculosis treatment. Which of the following is/are TRUE regarding INH?

   a. INH should be taken 1 hour before or 2 hours after a meal on an empty stomach.
   b. INH is a potent enzyme inducer.
   c. INH is contraindicated in acute gout
   d. A and B
   e. A, B, and C

11. Which of the following medications will prevent peripheral neuropathies in patients taking isoniazid?

   a. Pyrazinamide
   b. Pyridoxine
   c. Pyridium
   d. Pyridostigmine
   e. Pyrimethamine

12. A patient taking amphotericin B is at risk for which electrolyte abnormalities?

    a. Hypocalcemia and hypomagnesemia
    b. Hyponatremia and hypokalemia
    c. Hypernatremia and hyperkalemia
    d. Hypokalemia and hypernatremia
    e. Hypokalemia and hypomagnesemia

13. A patient comes into your clinic. She is 5 months pregnancy and has a UTI. She is allergic to penicillin. Which of the following regimens would be the best choice for her?

    a. *Bactrim* 1 DS tab BID x 3 days
    b. *Cipro ER* 500 mg PO daily x 7 days.
    c. Nitrofurantoin 100 mg PO BID x 7 days
    d. Cefpodoxime 100 mg PO Q12H x 7 days
    e. Do not treat since she is pregnant.

14. Which of the following statements is/are TRUE regarding *VFEND*?

    a. *VFEND* can cause visual changes and patients should be instructed not to operate heavy machinery while taking the medication.
    b. *VFEND* must be taken on an empty stomach.
    c. *VFEND* oral tablets should not be used in patients with poor renal function.
    d. A and B
    e. A, B, and C

15. Which of the following antibiotics do NOT require dose adjustment in renal impairment?

    a. Gentamicin
    b. Clarithromycin
    c. Cefixime
    d. Tigecycline
    e. Daptomycin

16. Which of the following antibiotics should be refrigerated?

    a. *Cipro*   FQ
    b. *Keflex*   ceph
    c. *Levaquin*   FQ
    d. *Septra*
    e. *Zithromax*   azithromycin

Aug
Erythro

ANSWERS

1-a, 2-c, 3-d, 4-b, 5-b, 6-d, 7-a, 8-e, 9-a, 10-a, 11-b, 12-e, 13-c, 14-d, 15-d, 16-b

IMMUNIZATION

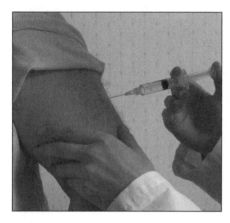

We gratefully acknowledge the assistance of Jerry Prentice, BS Pharmacy, Pharmacist Consultant, RxPrep, Inc., in preparing this section.

Background

Immunizations in the United States over the past century are one of the greatest public health achievements. Since vaccines are medications, pharmacists should review immunization history with patients. Vaccines prevent patients from acquiring serious or potentially fatal diseases. Many formerly prevalent childhood diseases (diphtheria, measles, meningitis, polio, tetanus) are rare because many children are vaccinated to prevent the illness, and others are protected by herd immunity (people around them are protected – thus they are less likely to catch the illness). If immunization rates drop, vaccine-preventable diseases may once again become common threats, as the pertussis cases in recent years demonstrate.

GUIDELINES/REFERENCES

Immunization recommendations are written by the CDC Advisory Committee on Immunization Practices (ACIP) and the Committee on Infectious Diseases of the American Academy of Pediatrics (AAP). The pediatric and adult schedules are updated annually and published in January. Since the ACIP meets several times throughout the year to review new information, updates are published in Morbidity and Mortality Weekly Report (MMWR). Updated immunization schedules are available at www.cdc.gov.

The CDC's Pink Book, *Epidemiology and Prevention of Vaccine-Preventable Disease* is published every 2 years and is available at www.cdc.gov.

Helpful resources for immunizing pharmacists are available on the following three websites:

- www.pharmacist.com/imz (American Pharmacists Association)

- www.cdc.gov/vaccines (Centers for Disease Control and Prevention/Vaccines and Immunizations)

- www.immunize.org (Immunization Action Coalition)

Read through the background information before reviewing the individual vaccines. Immunization is currently taught in most pharmacy schools and has become standard pharmacy practice in many settings, especially in the community pharmacy. Principles of immunization should be well understood.

As stated above, the CDC Advisory Committee on Immunization Practices (ACIP) develops written recommendations for the routine administration of vaccines to children and adults in the civilian population. The Immunization Action Coalition's website has useful information for clinicians, such as vaccine records and clinic tools.

SAFETY CONCERNS

Some parents withhold vaccines due to the risk of autism, a debilitating illness. There is no evidence that vaccines cause autism. Some had thought the risk may have come from thimerosal, a mercury-containing preservative. Thimerosal has been removed from most childhood vaccines, which is beneficial, since mercury can accumulate and is a known neurotoxin. Others thought the risk was due to providing multiple vaccines concurrently at an early age. Although the rates of autism have not decreased among communities with a high rate of abstaining from vaccinations, the concern of a possible link between autism and vaccines remains strong among some parents. This will likely continue to be an issue until the causes of autism are better understood. Promoting vaccination requires open communication and education.

Usually, vaccine side effects are minor and include mild fever and soreness or swelling at the injection site. Some vaccines cause headache, loss of appetite and dizziness – but these quickly dissipate. Very rarely (and mostly in children who have limited vaccine experience) anaphylaxis can occur. Anyone giving vaccines must screen for previous reactions and be prepared to treat a severe reaction. Some vaccines have specific contraindications to use, such as a true egg allergy with the influenza vaccines. Give the most up-to-date version of the Vaccine Information Statement (VIS) BEFORE EACH vaccine is administered. The VIS standardized forms describes the risk and benefit of the vaccines, purpose of the vaccine, who should receive it and who should not, and what the patient can expect for both mild and serious adverse effects. VISs are created by the CDC and updated versions are available on the CDC and IAC websites.

PHARMACIST'S ROLE IN IMMUNIZATION

Pharmacists in the community setting have contributed to increased immunization rates, particularly in providing influenza, pneumococcal, pertussis (in Tdap)and herpes zoster (shingles) vaccinations. We have been expanding this role – to include more vaccines and management of immunization clinics in health care settings. Some of our colleagues have set-up travel clinics and advise and administer vaccines for foreign travel.

PRINCIPLES OF IMMUNITY

Immunity is the ability of the human body to tolerate the presence of material indigenous to the body ("self"), and to eliminate foreign ("nonself") material. This discriminatory ability provides protection from infectious disease, since most microbes are identified as foreign by the immune system. Immunity to a microbe is usually indicated by the presence of antibody to that organism. There are two basic mechanisms for acquiring immunity, active and passive.

ACTIVE AND PASSIVE IMMUNITY

Active immunity is protection that is produced by the person's own immune system. This type of immunity is usually permanent. One way to acquire active immunity is to survive infection. Another way to produce active immunity is by vaccination. Passive immunity is protection by products produced by an animal or human and transferred to another human, usually by injection. This protection wanes with time, usually within a few weeks or months. The most common form of passive immunity is the antibodies an infant receives from the mother. Many types of blood products contain antibody, including intravenous immune globulin and plasma products.

LIVE ATTENUATED AND INACTIVATED VACCINES

Live attenuated vaccines (weakened) are produced by modifying a disease-producing ("wild") virus or bacterium in a laboratory; they retain the ability to replicate (grow) and produce immunity, but usually do not cause illness. Live vaccine administration to immune compromised patients may be contraindicated since uncontrolled replication of the pathogen could take place. Live attenuated vaccines produce a strong immune response – since the body's response to the vaccine is similar to actual disease.

Inactivated vaccines can be composed of either whole viruses or bacteria, or fractions of either. Antibody titers against inactivated antigens diminish with time. As a result, some inactivated vaccines may require periodic supplemental doses to increase, or "boost" antibody titers.

General rule

The more similar a vaccine is to the disease-causing form of the organism, the better the immune response to the vaccine.

TIMING AND SPACING OF VACCINES

The presence of circulating antibody to a vaccine antigen may reduce or completely eliminate the immune response to the vaccine. The amount of interference produced by circulating antibody generally depends on the type of vaccine administered and the amount of antibody.

Inactivated antigens are generally not affected by circulating antibody, so they can be administered before, after, or at the same time as the antibody. Live vaccines, however, must replicate in order to cause an immune response and antibody against injected live vaccine antigen may interfere with replication. If the live vaccine is given first, it is necessary to wait at least 2 weeks (i.e., an incubation period) before giving the antibody.

The necessary interval between an antibody-containing blood product and MMR

ANTIBODY AND MEASLES- AND VARICELLA-CONTAINING* VACCINES	
Product Given First	**Action**
Vaccine	Wait 2 weeks before giving antibody
Antibody	Wait 3 months or longer before giving vaccine
*Except zoster vaccine	

or varicella-containing vaccine (except zoster vaccine – this is not affected by circulating antibody) is always 3 months and up to 11 months. The product and dose administered of the blood product is used to determine the time interval. Consult "The Pink Book" to determine the specific recommended interval. During vaginal childbirth maternal antibodies are passed from the mother to the baby and may reduce the live vaccine response in the baby. This is why live vaccines are withheld until the child is 12 months. Inactivated vaccines are started at birth.

Simultaneous administration of antibody (in the form of immune globulin) and vaccine is recommended for postexposure prophylaxis of certain diseases, such as hepatitis B, rabies and tetanus.

SIMULTANEOUS ADMINISTRATION

Simultaneous administration on the same day of the most widely used live and inactivated vaccines does not result in decreased antibody responses or increased rates of adverse reactions. Simultaneous administration of all vaccines for which a child is eligible is very important in childhood vaccination programs because it increases the probability that a child will be fully immunized at the appropriate age.

According to the ACIP, there are no contraindications to simultaneous administration of any of the vaccines currently available in the United States and EVERY EFFORT SHOULD BE MADE TO PROVIDING ALL NECESSARY VACCINATIONS AT ONE VISIT.

NON-SIMULTANEOUS ADMINISTRATION OF DIFFERENT VACCINES

In some situations, vaccines that could be given at the same visit are not. If live parenteral (injected) vaccines (MMR, MMRV, varicella, zoster, and yellow fever) and live intranasal or intra-dermal influenza vaccine (LAIV) are not administered at the same visit, they should be separated by at least 4 weeks.

INTERVALS OF DOSES BETWEEN VACCINES GIVEN IN SERIES

Increasing the interval between doses of a multidose vaccine does not diminish the effectiveness of the vaccine after completion of all doses. It may, however, delay more complete protection. Decreasing the interval between doses of a multidose vaccine may interfere with antibody response and protection. Following a high risk exposure, a shorter interval may be used. In that situation either revaccinate after the recommended interval or check antibody titers.

INTERVAL FOR ADMINISTRATION OF LIVE VACCINES AND TB TEST

The skin test with purified protein derivative (PPD) of tuberculin and live vaccines can be administered on the same day and is the preferred method to avoid a false negative response to the skin test. When a live vaccine has been given recently but not on the same day as the live vaccine, wait 4 weeks before giving the TB test in order to avoid a false negative TB test result. False negative TB test results delay treatment of tuberculosis infection and are a significant risk to the patient and to public health. If the TB test was given recently but not on the same day as the live vaccine, then wait 48-72 hours for the TB test results are determined before administering the live vaccine.

VACCINE SIDE EFFECTS OR ADVERSE REACTIONS

Vaccine adverse reactions fall into three general categories: local, systemic, and allergic. Local reactions are generally the least severe and most frequent. Allergic reactions are the most severe and least frequent.

The most common type of adverse reactions are local reactions, such as pain, swelling and redness at the site of injection. Local reactions may occur with up to 80% of vaccine doses, depending on the type of vaccine. Local reactions are most common with inactivated vaccines, particularly those, such as DTaP, that contain an adjuvant. Local adverse reactions generally occur within a few hours of the injection and are usually mild and self-limited. On rare occasions, local reactions may be very exaggerated or severe.

Systemic adverse reactions are more generalized events and include fever, malaise, myalgias (muscle pain), headache, loss of appetite, and others. These symptoms are common and non-specific; they may occur in vaccinated persons because of the vaccine or may be caused by something unrelated to the vaccine, like a concurrent viral infection, stress, or excessive alcohol consumption. Systemic adverse reactions following live vaccines are usually mild, and occur 7–21 days after the vaccine was given (i.e., after an incubation period of the vaccine virus). Intranasal LAIV is cold adapted, meaning it can replicate in the cooler temperatures of upper airways (nose and throat) but not in the higher temperatures of the lower airways and the lungs. Mild cold-like symptoms such as a runny nose may occur.

A third type of vaccine adverse reaction is a severe (anaphylactic) allergic reaction. The allergic reaction may be caused by the vaccine antigen itself or some other component of the vaccine, such as cell culture material, stabilizer, preservative, or antibiotic used to inhibit bacterial growth. Severe allergic reactions may be life-threatening. Fortunately, they are rare, occurring at a rate of less than one in half a million doses. The risk of an allergic reaction can be minimized by good screening prior to vaccination. A severe (anaphylactic) allergic reaction following a dose of vaccine will almost always contraindicate a subsequent dose of that vaccine. Anaphylactic allergies are those that are mediated by IgE, occur within minutes or hours of receiving the vaccine, and require medical attention. Examples of symptoms and signs typical of anaphylactic reactions are generalized urticaria (hives), swelling of the mouth and throat, difficulty breathing, wheezing, abdominal cramping, hypotension, or shock. Immunizations should never be administered if epinephrine is not available.

Providers should report a clinically significant adverse event to the Vaccine Adverse Event Reporting System (VAERS) even if they are unsure whether a vaccine caused the event.

All providers who administer vaccines must have an emergency protocol and supplies to treat anaphylaxis. If symptoms are generalized, activate the emergency medical system (EMS; e.g., call 911) and notify the on-call physician. This should be done by a second person, while the primary health care provider assesses the airway, breathing, circulation, and level of consciousness of the patient.

- Administer aqueous epinephrine 1:1000 dilution intramuscularly, 0.01mg per kg of body weight per dose, up to a 0.5 mg maximum per dose.* If EpiPens are stocked, at least three adult EpiPens (0.30 mg) should be available. If the patient is taking a beta blocker they may need a higher dose or more frequent doses of epinephrine.

- In addition, for systemic anaphylaxis, administer diphenhydramine either orally or by injection.

- Monitor the patient closely until EMS arrives. Perform cardiopulmonary resuscitation (CPR), if necessary, and maintain airway. Keep patient in supine position (flat on back) unless he or she is having breathing difficulty. If breathing is difficult, patient's head may be elevated, provided blood pressure is adequate to prevent loss of consciousness. If blood pressure is low, elevate legs. Monitor blood pressure and pulse every 5 minutes.

- If EMS has not arrived and symptoms are still present, repeat dose of epinephrine. If EMS has not arrived and symptoms are still present, repeat dose of epinephrine, if needed.

- Record all vital signs, medications administered to the patient, including the time, dosage, response, and the name of the medical personnel who administered the medication, and other relevant clinical information.

- Notify the patient's primary care physician.

- Report reaction to VAERS (Vaccine Adverse Event Reporting System).

CONTRAINDICATIONS AND PRECAUTIONS

Contraindications and precautions to vaccination generally dictate circumstances when vaccines will not be given. Most contraindications and precautions are temporary, and the vaccine can be given at a later time.

A contraindication is a condition in a recipient that greatly increases the chance of a serious adverse reaction. It is a condition in the recipient of the vaccine, not with the vaccine per se. For instance, administering influenza vaccine to a person with a true anaphylactic allergy to egg could cause serious illness or death in the recipient. In general, vaccines should not be administered when a contraindication condition is present.

Two conditions are temporary contraindications to vaccination with live vaccines: pregnancy and immunosuppression. Two conditions are temporary precautions to vaccination: moderate or severe acute illness (all vaccines), and recent receipt of an antibody-containing blood product. The latter precaution applies only to MMR and varicella-containing (except zoster) vaccines.

Immunosuppression

Live vaccines can cause severe or fatal reactions in persons with immunosuppression due to uncontrolled replication of the vaccine virus or reduced vaccine efficacy. Live vaccines should not be administered to severely immuno-suppressed persons for this reason. Certain drugs may cause immunosuppression. For instance, anyone receiving cancer treatment with alkylating agents or antimetabolites, or radiation therapy should not be given live vaccines. Live vaccines can be given after chemotherapy has been discontinued for at least 3 months. Persons receiving large doses of corticosteroids should not receive live vaccines. This includes persons receiving 20 milligrams or more of prednisone daily or 2 or more milligrams of prednisone per kilogram of body weight per day for 14 days or longer. Persons infected with human immunodeficiency virus (HIV) may have no symptoms, or they may be severely immunosuppressed. Live vaccines are only contraindicated for HIV patients with CD4 T lymphocyte counts < 200 cells/microliter. In general, the same vaccination recommendations apply as with other types of immunosuppression. Live-virus vaccines are usually contraindicated, but the disease may indicate the need for certain inactivated vaccines like pneumococcal.

IMMUNOSUPPRESSION
Corticosteroids
■ 20 mg or more per day of prednisone*
■ 2 mg/kg or more per day of prednisone
■ NOT intra-articular injections, metered-dose inhalers, topical, alternate day or short course for less than 14 days
For 14 days or longer

INVALID CONTRAINDICATIONS TO VACCINATION

Review the table for invalid contraindications to vaccination. Note that mild illness, such as a cold, or patients receiving antibiotics can receive vaccinations.

VACCINATIONS DURING PREGNANCY

The common vaccination administered by pharmacists to women who are pregnant is the influenza vaccine. This is indicated in all trimesters of pregnancy. The live vaccine (*FluMist*) cannot be used in pregnant women. Pregnant women > 20 weeks gestation should receive Tdap if they need a booster. If the woman has not been vaccinated or the history is unclear, a 3-dose series is needed (one with Tdap, the other two with Td only). If the woman delivers and has not

INVALID CONTRAINDICATIONS TO VACCINATION	
■ Mild acute illness (slight fever, mild diarrhea)	■ Breastfeeding
■ Antimicrobial therapy (exceptions are certain antiviral medications and oral typhoid vaccine)	■ Preterm birth
	■ Allergy to products not present in vaccine or allergy that is not anaphylactic
■ Local skin reactions (mild/moderate)	
■ Bird feather allergies	■ Family history of adverse events
■ Recent infectious disease exposure	■ Tuberculin skin test (see above for timing and spacing with live vaccines only)
■ Penicillin allergy	
■ Disease exposure or convalescence	■ Multiple vaccines
■ Pregnant or immunosuppressive person in the household	

VACCINATION OF PREGNANT WOMEN

- Live vaccines should not be administered to women 1 month before or during pregnancy

- In general, inactivated vaccines may be administered to pregnant women for whom they are indicated

- HPV vaccine should be deferred during pregnancy

- Pregnant women should receive the influenza shot (in season) and Tdap, if needed.

received vaccination, she should receive it post-delivery. Vaccination protects the baby (and the mother) from pertussis (whooping cough).

ALLERGIES TO VACCINE COMPONENTS

Anaphylaxis to a previous dose of the vaccine is a contraindication to the vaccine in the future. Influenza and yellow fever vaccines are the only vaccines that are contraindicated for people who have a history of a severe (anaphylactic) allergy to eggs. Allergy to eggs is no longer considered a contraindication for giving MMR vaccine. Several vaccines are not absolute contraindications but caution is advised if the patient has a history of Guillian-Barré syndrome (tetanus containing vaccines, influenza, MCV). Both varicella vaccines (*Zostavax* and *Varivax*) and MMR should not be given to anyone with a true gelatin or neomycin allergy. Inactivated poliovirus vaccine (IPV) is contraindicated with streptomycin, polymyxin B and neomycin allergies. Check for contraindications for any vaccine in the CDC's Guide to Vaccine Contraindications and Precautions or by using the vaccine's package insert.

SCREENING PRIOR TO VACCINE ADMINISTRATION

Use screening form to rule out specific contraindications to the vaccine:

1. Are you sick today?

2. Do you have allergies to medications, food, a vaccine component, or latex?

3. Have you ever had a serious reaction after receiving a vaccination?

4. Do you have a long-term health problem with heart disease, lung disease, asthma, kidney disease, metabolic disease (e.g., diabetes), anemia, or other blood disorder?

5. Do you have cancer, leukemia, AIDS, or any other immune system problem?

6. Do you take cortisone, prednisone, other steroids, or anticancer drugs, or have you had radiation treatments?

7. Have you had a seizure or a brain or other nervous system problem?

8. During the past year, have you received a transfusion of blood or blood products, or been given immune (gamma) globulin or an antiviral drug?

9. For women: Are you pregnant or is there a chance you could become pregnant during the next month?

10. Have you received any vaccinations in the past 4 weeks?

IMMUNIZATION REGISTRIES

Immunization registries are computerized information systems that collect vaccination histories and help ensure correct and timely immunizations, especially for children. They are useful for healthcare providers who use the registries to obtain patient's history, produce vaccine records, manage vaccine inventories, among other benefits. It helps the community at-large to identify groups who are not receiving vaccines in order to target outreach efforts. Some systems are able to notify parents if vaccines are needed.

Registries in one state or area may not be compatible with other registries, and information may have to be manually transferred from between registries. Also, to protect personal information in registries, this information cannot be directly retrieved by individuals.

DRUG	ADMINISTER TO	STORAGE/ ADMINISTRATION
Diphtheria Toxoid-, Tetanus Toxoid- and acellular Pertussis-Containing Vaccines		
DTaP: *DAPTACEL, Infanrix, Tripedia* DTaP-IPV: *KINRIX* DTaP-HepB-IPV: *Pediarix* DTaP-IPV/Hib: *Pentacel*	DTaP series given to children.	Store in the refrigerator. Do not freeze. Shake the prefilled syringe or vial before use. IM.
Haemophilus influenzae type b-Containing Vaccines		
Hib: *ActHIB, Hiberix, PedvaxHIB* Hib-HepB: *Comvax* DTaP-IPV/Hib: *Pentacel*	Hib: Given to children. Sometimes in adults if HIV+, splenectomy, sickle cell disease, leukemia, or if they have not previously received Hib vaccine.	Store in the refrigerator. Do not freeze. Shake the prefilled syringe or vial before use. IM.
Hepatitis-Containing Vaccines		
HepA: *Havrix, Vaqta* **HepB: *Engerix-B, Recombivax HB*** **HepA-HepB: *Twinrix*** DTaP-HepB-IPV: *Pediarix* Hib-HepB: *Comvax*	Hep A and B given to children. Hep A in adults for men who have sex with men, IV drug abusers, chronic disease, travelers to countries with high Hep A incidence. Hep B Health care workers (required by OSHA), men who have sex with men, anyone who has sex with multiple partners, IV drug users, ESRD, chronic liver disease. Hep B is 3-dose series: 2nd dose 1 month after 1st, 3rd dose at least 2 months after 2nd and at least 4 months after 1st. If combined Hep A/Hep B vaccine (*Twinrix*) is used, administer 3 doses at 0, 1, and 6 months; alternatively, a 4-dose *Twinrix* schedule, administered on days 0, 7, and 21 to 30, followed by a booster dose at month 12.	Store in refrigerator. Do not freeze. Shake the vial or prefilled syringe before use. IM. HepA: Older than 18 years inject 1mL intramuscularly. HepB: Brands not same dose. Inject correct dose/volume for each brand shortly after preparing.

Immunization Registries Continued

DRUG	ADMINISTER TO	STORAGE/ ADMINISTRATION

Human Papillomavirus Vaccines

DRUG	ADMINISTER TO	STORAGE/ ADMINISTRATION
HPV2: *Cervarix* **HPV4:** *Gardasil* Either vaccine recommended for females.	HPV vaccination for females HPV vaccine is indicated for females age 9-26 years. ACIP recommends the 3 dose series between the age of 11-12 years, with catch-up vaccination age 13-26 years. Vaccination can begin at age 9 years and ideally prior to sexual activity. Males 9-26 to reduce their likelihood of genital warts. Requires 3 doses. The 2nd dose is 1–2 months after the 1st and the 3rd 6 months after the 1st.	Store in the refrigerator. Do not freeze. Protect from light. Shake the prefilled syringe or vial before use. IM, deltoid preferred.

Influenza Vaccines

DRUG	ADMINISTER TO	STORAGE/ ADMINISTRATION
LAIV: *FluMist* **TIV:** *Afluria, Agriflu, Fluarix, FluLaval, Fluvirin, Fluzone, Fluzone High-Dose, Fluzone Intradermal* **High-dose** *(Fluzone)* licensed in 2010 for adults aged ≥ 65, trivalent like others but contains 60 mcg of each strain vs 15 mcg in others. ***Fluzone Intradermal*** uses smaller needle (30 gauge, 1.5 mm vs 22 to 25 gauge, 15.8-38.1 mm). Smaller needle, no more pain but more redness, swelling, itching. Preg B (other influenza shots are Preg C)	ACIP recommends flu vaccine for ALL people 6 months and older each year. The 1st year children get two shots, otherwise it is one shot/each fall. Can get nasal spray age 2-49 years. Healthy, nonpregnant adults aged 2-49 years, without high-risk medical conditions can receive either live attenuated influenza vaccine (LAIV:*FluMist*) or trivalent inactivated vaccine (TIV: IM or *Intradermal*). Flu vaccine for 2011-12 contains the same strains as the previous years. Immunity declines and patients who got vaccine last year should be revaccinated. 3 Strains A/California/7/2009-like (2009 H1N1) A/Perth/16/2009-like (H3N2) B/Brisbane/60/2008-like (B/Victoria lineage)	All influenza vaccines are stored in the refrigerator. Do not freeze. LAIV Intranasal TIV: intramuscular & intradermal injections Do not give if true egg allergy.

Measles, Mumps and Rubella-Containing Vaccine

DRUG	ADMINISTER TO	STORAGE/ ADMINISTRATION
MMR: *M-M-RII* MMRV: *ProQuad*	Given to children. Adults born before 1957 generally are considered immune to measles and mumps. Health care providers born before 1957 must prove immunity or receive 2 doses MMR vaccine at least 4 weeks apart. Live vaccine, not in pregnancy.	MMR: Refrigerator or freezer MMRV: Freezer only due to varicella component. Always store diluents in refrigerator. Protect from light. SC.

Meningococcal Vaccines

DRUG	ADMINISTER TO	STORAGE/ ADMINISTRATION
MCV4: *Menactra, Menveo* MPSV4: *Menomune* Adults usually 1 dose but 2 doses for HIV+, asplenia, complement component deficiencies	Vaccinate: 11-12 year old adolescents 13-18 year old if previously unvaccinated 2-55 years old if in high risk, such as: College freshman in dormitories, asplenia, military service, immunodeficiencies, travelers to high-risk countries like the meningitis belt in sub Saharan Africa, lab workers with N. meningitidis exposure.	Refrigerate. Protect from light. MCV is IM, MPSV is SC.

Immunization Registries Continued

DRUG	ADMINISTER TO	STORAGE/ ADMINISTRATION

Pneumococcal Vaccines

PCV13: *Prevnar 13* (**Pneumococcal conjugate**) PPSV23: *Pneumovax 23* (**Pneumococcal polysaccharide**) Minimum ages: 6 weeks for PCV (*Prevnar 13*) 2 years for PPSV(*Pneumovax 23*). Polysaccharide does not invoke immunity in patients < 2 years old. Only conjugate invokes immunity in < 2 years old. *Prevnar* had 7 serotypes previously; current vaccine has 13. If start series with PCV7, finish with PCV13.	*Prevnar* (conjugate) 4 dose series to children at 2 months, 4 months, 6 months and 12-15 months. **Pneumovax** (polysaccharide) > 2 years old with chronic disease, 19-64 years if smoke or asthma, 2-64 years with chronic illness. **Revaccinate:** ■ All adults with 1 dose age > 65 years, give 2nd dose if 1st dose was 5 years earlier and < 65 years old. ■ Age 2-64 years if high risk of death from pneumococcal disease give 2nd dose 5 years after initial dose (sickle cell, immune compromised, asplenia).	**All Pneumococcal Vaccines Storage** Store in refrigerator. Do not freeze. **Conjugate (PCV7 & PCV13)** Shake the vial or prefilled syringe prior to use. IM. **Polysaccharide (PPSV23)** Shake the vial or prefilled syringe prior to use. IM or SC.

Poliovirus-Containing Vaccine

IPV: IPOL 49 DTaP-HepB-IPV: *Pediarix* DTaP-IPV: *KINRIX* DTaP-IPV/Hib: *Pentacel*	Vaccine series to ALL children.	**Inactivated Poliomyelitis Vaccines (IPV)** Store in the refrigerator. Do not freeze. Shake the prefilled syringe or vial before use. IM or SC.

Rotavirus Vaccines

RV1: *Rotarix* RV5: *RotaTeq*	Vaccine series to ALL children.	Oral suspensions. (other oral vaccine is *Vivotif Berna* (typhoid) capsules that must be refrigerated)

Tetanus Toxoid Vaccine

TT: *Tetanus Toxoid*		

Tetanus Toxoid- and diphtheria toxoid-Containing Vaccines

Td: *DECAVAC* DT: *Diphtheria and Tetanus Toxoid*	May be used in wound prophylaxis.	IM

Immunization Registries Continued

DRUG	ADMINISTER TO	STORAGE/ ADMINISTRATION
Tdap: *Adacel, Boostrix* See above for DTaP series, indicated for children 6 weeks to 6 years of age. Single Tdap dose for age 7 years to 10 years who were not fully vaccinated with DTaP series (missed dose in series). Tdap is the one time booster age 11 years to 64 years with no previous record of Tdap, then one dose of Td every 10 years. Read recommendations to right to help reduce pertussis infections which have been epidemic in recent years.	Administer a one-time dose of Tdap to adults aged < 65 years who have not received Tdap previously or for whom vaccine status is unknown to replace one of the 10-year Td boosters, and as soon as feasible to all 1) postpartum women, 2) close contacts of infants younger than age 12 months (e.g., grandparents and child-care providers), and 3) health-care personnel with direct patient contact. Adults aged 65 years and older who have not previously received Tdap and who have close contact with an infant aged less than 12 months also should be vaccinated. Other adults aged 65 years and older may receive Tdap. Tdap can be administered regardless of interval since the most recent tetanus or diphtheria-containing vaccine in order to administer the pertussis component since adults often infect children with pertussis. Pregnant women > 20 weeks gestation should receive Tdap if they need a booster. If the woman has not been vaccinated or the history is unclear, a 3-dose series is needed (one with Tdap, the other 2 with Td only). If the woman delivers and has not received vaccination, she should receive it post-delivery. Vaccination protects the baby (and the mother) from pertussis (whooping cough).	All tetanus, diphtheria, and pertussis containing vaccines: Store in the refrigerator. Do not freeze. Shake the prefilled syringe or vial before use. IM.

Varicella containing vaccines

DRUG	ADMINISTER TO	STORAGE/ ADMINISTRATION
VAR: *Varivax* **(chickenpox)** **ZOS:** *Zostavax* **(herpes zoster/shingles)** MMRV: *ProQuad*	Children get varicella at 12 months & again at 4 yrs. All adults without evidence of immunity to varicella should receive 2 doses of varicella vaccine. Varicella vaccines are live vaccines, not in pregnancy. Herpes zoster vaccination (potency 14 times greater than varicella in order to elicit needed immune response) May 2011 the FDA licensed zoster vaccine for adults 50 years of age and older. *Zostavax* is indicated for prevention of shingles and not for treatment of active case. Also reduces complications such as severity of postherpatic neuralgia following infections. Vaccinate even if history of zoster infection since you can get it again.	SC Freeze Vaccine Varicella-containing vaccines have 2 components: vaccine & diluent. Store vaccine in Freezer & protect from light (keep in original container). Store diluent in refrigerator or room temp. LIVE vaccines: do not give if immuno-compromised, pregnant or if pregnancy is expected within 4 weeks. Do not give if hypersensitivity to gelatin or neomycin. SC vaccines, reconstituted; reconstitute immediately upon removal from freezer and inject within 30 minutes or discard. Inject adults in fatty tissue at triceps.

VACCINE STORAGE/NAME & MISC REVIEW INFORMATION THAT IS GOOD TO KNOW.

- If the wrong vaccine is chosen the patient is not covered for the intended disease.

- Review the brand name/components for vaccines that can be confused, including combos.

- If the vaccine is not stored properly it may not be active and, again, the patient may not be protected. Use vaccines quickly if removed from refrigerator/if reconstituted. Short stability.

VACCINE	NOTES
DT, Td, DTaP, DTAP combos w/other vaccines (all), TDaP	Refrigerate
Hib, Hib combos	
HPV	
Polio, IPV, SC or IM	
Influenza, all	
MMR (reconstituted, SC)	
Pneumococcal vaccines, *Pneumovax* is SC or IM	
Rotavirus vaccines (*Rotarix*), (*RotaTeq*)	
Meningococcal, combos *Menactra, Menveo, Menomune* (this one is 56+ ages only)	Refrigerate, all reconstituted
Typhoid vaccine, live oral (*Vivotif*)	Refrigerate (capsules) – if vaccines are not stored properly the vaccine is wasted and this one is tricky because it is capsules.
MMR w/varicella (*ProQuad*)	Freezer, prior to reconstitution
Varicella (chickenpox) (*Varivax*)	Diluent kept at room temp or refrigerate – not frozen.
(herpes	If not used within 30 minutes, discard.
zoster/shingles (*Zostavax*)	Note these are all SC vaccines (including *ProQuad*, which also contains MMR which is also SC.
IPV, Pneumococcal polysaccharide (*Pneumovax*)	IPV and *Pneumovax* are SC or IM.
Rabies Vaccine	Rabies vaccine only in high-risk exposure, otherwise vaccine + rabies immune globulin (RIG) post-exposure.
Yellow Fever	Yellow fever is SC.

Tips

- OHSA does not require gloves when giving vaccines, unless likely to come into exposure with bodily fluids. However, most wear gloves. If using gloves they must be changed between each patient.

- The CDC does NOT recommend using acetaminophen before or at vaccination as it may decrease the immune response. It can be used to treat pain and fever after vaccination.

- Never mix vaccines in the same syringe yourself – they have to come mixed.

- Do not aspirate. If this occurs, withdraw the needle, discard, and start over. This is an expensive waste so try not to aspirate. (this is when you see a flash of blood come up into the syringe)

- All vaccines can be given simultaneously. If a vaccine is missed, then any 2 live vaccines not given at the same time must be given at least 4 weeks apart.

- You can vaccinate through a tattoo.

Storage

Store refrigerated vaccines immediately upon arrival. Stand alone units are preferred but household combination units with separate exterior doors and thermostats can be used. <u>Dormitory-style refrigerators should not be used</u>. Keep a calibrated thermometer in the refrigerator and freezer. Post "Do Not Unplug" signs next electrical outlets and "Do Not Stop Power" signs near circuit breakers to maintain a consistent power source. <u>Store vaccines on the shelves away from the walls</u>. <u>Vaccines should never be stored in the door of the freezer or refrigerator</u>. The temperature there is not stable. Read and document refrigerator and freezer temperatures at least <u>twice each workday</u>: in the morning and before the end of the workday. <u>Keep temperature logs for at least 3 years</u>. Rotate stock so vaccine and diluent <u>with the shortest expiration date is used first. Place vaccine with the longest expiration date behind the vaccine that will expire the soonest.</u>

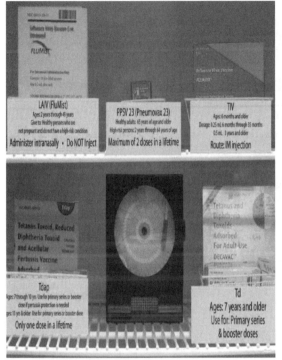

Staff can easily confuse the vaccines within the storage unit. Use labels & separate containers.

Store refrigerated vaccines between 35°F and 46°F (2°C and 8°C). Store frozen vaccines between -58°F and +5°F (-50°C and -15°C).

ADMINISTRATION

See the chart at the end of this chapter for injection technique. In adults intramuscular <u>(IM) injections are given in the deltoid muscle</u> at the central and thickest portion above the level of the armpit and below the acromion. <u>Adults require a 1" syringe</u> (or 5/8" for a person less than 130 lbs & or 1½" needle for women greater than 200 lbs or men greater than 260 pounds. Use a 22-25 gauge. (The higher the gauge, the thinner the needle.)

<u>Subcutaneous (SC) vaccinations are given in the fatty tissue above the triceps with a 5/8", 23-25 gauge syringe.</u> The vaccines pharmacists administer in the community setting that are SC are <u>varicella and zoster (shingles)</u> and <u>pneumococcal polysaccharide vaccine (PPSV23, Pneumovax) can be given either SC or IM.</u>

INFLUENZA (THE FLU)

<u>Influenza is the most common vaccine preventable illness in the U.S.</u>

Make sure patients know:

- The influenza shot cannot cause the flu. They may get a sore arm, or mild systemic reactions that go away.

- The only patients who can use the nasal mist vaccine are healthy (no chronic disease) non-pregnant females and males from age 2 to 49 years. This is a live vaccine; the others are inactivated injections.

- Everyone 6 months and older should get vaccinated annually – patients at highest risk will get vaccinated first if there is a vaccine shortage; check the CDC vaccination website if a shortage is present.

- Pregnant women are at risk for severe disease & should be vaccinated – in all trimesters.

- If someone has not gotten the shot early in the fall and it is still influenza season they should get vaccinated.

Influenza A and B are the two types of influenza viruses that cause epidemic human disease. Influenza A viruses are further categorized into subtypes on the basis of two surface antigens: hemagglutinin and neuraminidase. Immunity to the surface antigens, particularly the hemagglutinin, reduces the likelihood of infection and severity of disease if infection occurs. Frequent development of antigenic variants through antigenic drift is the virologic basis for seasonal epidemics and the reason for the usual incorporation of one or more new strains in each year's influenza vaccine, which is made as a trivalent vaccine. More dramatic antigenic changes, or shifts, occur less frequently and can result in the emergence of a novel influenza virus with the potential to cause a pandemic.

The virus spreads from person to person, primarily through respiratory droplet transmission (e.g., when an infected person coughs or sneezes in close proximity to an uninfected person). If someone sneezes in their hands and touches something it is possible to spread illness.

Uncomplicated influenza illness is characterized by the abrupt onset of these symptoms: fever, myalgia, headache, malaise, nonproductive cough, sore throat, and rhinitis. Among children, otitis media, nausea, and vomiting also are commonly reported with influenza illness.

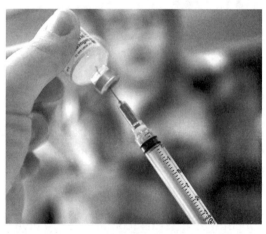

Influenza (inactivated) injection – annually, each fall

Uncomplicated influenza illness typically resolves after 3-7 days for the majority of persons, although cough and malaise can persist for more than 2 weeks. However, among certain persons, influenza can exacerbate underlying medical conditions (e.g., pulmonary or cardiac disease), leading to secondary bacterial pneumonia or primary influenza viral pneumonia, or occur as part of a co-infection with other viral or bacterial pathogens.

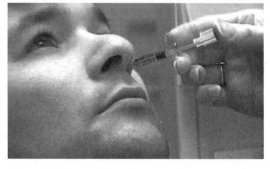

*Influenza – live nasal vaccine, annually,
each fall, if healthy, ages 2-49*

ANTIVIRAL TREATMENT OF PATIENTS WITH INFLUENZA

- Check to see if there is *Tamiflu*-resistant flu in the area prior to solo treatment with oseltamivir: if present, use zanamivir or oseltamivir plus rimantidine or amantadine.

- For most cases stick with starting neuraminidase inhibitors within 48 hours of illness onset.

- Vaccinate if they haven't been vaccinated and are willing.

NEURAMINIDASE INHIBITORS

Inhibits the neuraminidase enzyme which affects the release of viral particles, thereby reducing the amount of virus in the body

DRUG	DOSING	SIDE EFFECTS/MONITORING/ CONTRAINDICATIONS
Oseltamivir (*Tamiflu*)	START within 48 hours of symptoms Treatment: 75 mg BID X 5 d Prevention: 75 mg daily x 10 d 30, 45, 75 mg capsules 300 mg/25 ml suspension – Children dosed by weight ↓ dose with ↓ renal function	Aches and pains, rhinorrhea, dyspepsia and upper respiratory tract infections Rare side effects of sudden confusion, delirium, hallucinations, unusual behavior, or self-injury; more often in children.
Zanamivir (*Relenza*)	Treatment: 10 mg (two 5-mg inhalations) twice daily Prevention: 10 mg (two 5-mg inhalations) once daily	Rare side effects of sudden confusion, delirium, hallucinations, unusual behavior, or self-injury; more often in children. The inhaler can't be used by very young children: prophylaxis 5+, treatment 7+. Bronchospasm risk: Do not use if asthma/COPD/any breathing problem. Tell patient to stop if wheezing or breathing problems.

OTHER ANTIVIRALS	DOSING	SIDE EFFECTS/MONITORING/ CONTRAINDICATIONS
Rimantidine (*Flumadine*) – for Influenza A Amantadine (*Symmetrel*) can be used instead but has higher incidence adverse effects (↑ insomnia, dizziness, etc.)	Treatment/Prevention: 100 mg BID	Nausea, vomiting, diarrhea, loss of appetite, stomach pain, dry mouth, insomnia, dizziness, headache Rare: euphoria, hallucinations, higher if overdosed; caution to ↓ dose with ↓ renal function

How to Administer IM and SC Vaccine Injections to Adults

Intramuscular (IM) Injections

Administer these vaccines via IM route:

Tetanus, diphtheria (Td), or with pertussis (Tdap); hepatitis A; hepatitis B; human papillomavirus (HPV); trivalent inactivated influenza (TIV); and quadrivalent meningococcal conjugate (MCV4). Administer polio (IPV) and pneumococcal polysaccharide vaccine (PPSV23) either IM or SC.

Injection site:

Give in the central and thickest portion of the deltoid—above the level of the armpit and below the acromion (see the diagram).

Needle size:

22–25 gauge, 1–1½" needle *(see note at right)*

Needle insertion:

- Use a needle long enough to reach deep into the muscle.
- Insert the needle at a 90° angle to the skin with a quick thrust.
- Separate two injections given in the same deltoid muscle by a minimum of 1".

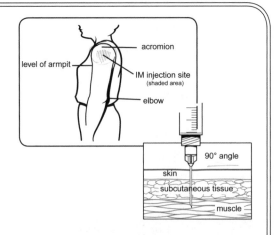

Note: A ⅝" needle is sufficient in adults weighing <130 lbs (<60 kg); a 1" needle is sufficient in adults weighing 130–152 lbs (60–70 kg); a 1–1½" needle is recommended in women weighing 152–200 lbs (70–90 kg) and men weighing 152–260 lbs (70–118 kg); a 1½" needle is recommended in women weighing >200 lbs (>90 kg) or men weighing >260 lbs (>118 kg). A ⅝" (16mm) needle may be used only if the skin is stretched tight, the subcutaneous tissue is not bunched, and injection is made at a 90-degree angle.

Subcutaneous (SC) Injections

Administer these vaccines via SC route:

MMR, varicella, meningococcal polysaccharide (MPSV4), and zoster (shingles). Administer polio (IPV) and pneumococcal polysaccharide vaccine (PPSV23) either SC or IM.

Injection site:

Give in fatty tissue over the triceps (see the diagram).

Needle size:

23–25 gauge, 5/8" needle

Needle insertion:

- Pinch up on the tissue to prevent injection into the muscle. Insert the needle at a 45° angle to the skin.
- Separate two injections given in the same area of fatty tissue by a minimum of 1".

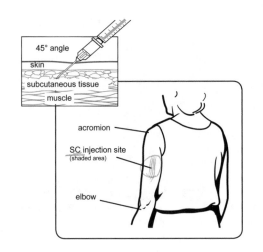

Adapted by the Immunization Action Coalition, courtesy of the Minnesota Department of Health

Technical content reviewed by the Centers for Disease Control and Prevention, November 2010.

www.immunize.org/catg.d/p2020A.pdf Item #P2020A (11/10)

Immunization Action Coalition • 1573 Selby Ave. • St. Paul, MN 55104 • (651) 647-9009 • www.immunize.org • www.vaccineinformation.org

HUMAN IMMUNODEFICIENCY VIRUS (HIV)

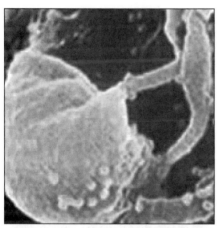

We gratefully acknowledge the assistance of Jim Scott, PharmD, M.Ed, FCCP, Western University of Health Sciences College of Pharmacy in preparing this section.

Background

1981 marked the year when case reports from Los Angeles and San Francisco first identified what is now known as Acquired Immunodeficiency Syndrome (AIDS). The causative agent, human immunodeficiency virus (HIV), is a RNA retrovirus and was discovered several years later. This virus attacks the immune system, mainly the CD4+ T cells, causing a progressive decrease in the CD4+ T cell count. Once CD4+ cell counts fall below a critical level, the person becomes more susceptible to opportunistic infections due to the loss of cell-mediated immunity. CD4+ counts are commonly used to assess the severity of the disease and to determine whether a person should start antiretroviral therapy. HIV viral loads are also measured. The viral load quantifies the degree of viremia by measuring the amount of HIV RNA in the blood and is used to assess disease progression and possible drug resistance.

GUIDELINES

Panel on Antiretroviral Guidelines for Adults and Adolescents. Guidelines for the Use of Antiretroviral Agents in HIV-1 Infected Adults and Adolescents. Department of Health and Human Services. October 14, 2011; 1-167. Available at http://www.aidsinfo.nih.gov/ContentFiles/AdultandAdolescentGL.pdf. Accessed October 15, 2011.

HIV can be spread through blood, semen, vaginal fluid, pre-ejaculate, breast milk and amniotic fluid. Transmission of the virus mainly occurs via unsafe sex, needles contaminated with bodily fluids, breast milk, and from infected mothers to their babies at birth.

Antiviral medications can limit or significantly slow down the destruction of the immune system, improve the health of people living with HIV, and likely reduce their ability to transmit the disease. Untreated early HIV infection is also associated with many diseases including cardiovascular disease, kidney disease, liver disease, and various types of cancer.

500 – 1500

Pharmacologic Treatment

- Treatment for HIV requires combination therapy known as antiretroviral therapy (ART). Previously, the term highly active antiretroviral therapy (HAART) was used, but was simplified to ART because all recommended regimens are highly active. A diagram of the HIV replication cycle is included at the end of the chapter. Understanding the steps involved in viral replication will assist you in determining where each drug class works.

- ART should be initiated in *all* patients with a history of an AIDS-defining illness or with CD4 counts < 350 cells/mm³. ART is also recommended for patients with CD4 counts between 350 and 500 cells/mm³. Treatment for patients with CD4 counts > 500 cells/mm³ is considered optional.

- ART should also be initiated, regardless of CD4 count, in patients with the following conditions: pregnancy, HIV-associated nephropathy, and hepatitis B virus co-infection when treatment of HBV is indicated.

- Plasma HIV-1 RNA levels should be monitored frequently when treatment is initiated or changed for virologic failure. Baseline genotypic testing for resistance should be performed in *all* treatment-naïve patients regardless of whether therapy will be started and be *considered* for all patients experiencing a suboptimal response to therapy (a minimum HIV RNA viral load of 1,000 copies/mL is preferred for an accurate resistance assay). Genotypic testing for patients on therapy should be completed before or within 4 weeks of discontinuing ART.

- Monitoring includes HIV RNA viral load and CD4 cell counts plus many other lab values.

- ↑ in viral load and ↓ in CD4 counts may indicate development of drug resistance and the need for susceptibility testing.

Antiretroviral Therapy Guidelines in Treatment-Naïve Patients with HIV-1 Infection

CLINICAL CONDITION AND/OR CD4 COUNT	RECOMMENDATION
History of AIDS-defining illness or with CD4 count < 350 cells/mm³	Initiate *ART*
CD4 counts between 350-500 cells/mm³	Recommend *ART*
Pregnant women	Initiate *ART* (regardless of CD4 count)
Persons with HIV-associated nephropathy	Initiate *ART* (regardless of CD4 count)
Persons co-infected with hepatitis B virus (HBV) when HBV treatment is indicated (Treatment with fully suppressive antiviral drugs active against both HIV and HBV is recommended).	Initiate *ART* (regardless of CD4 count)
The treatment guidelines panel were split 50-50 with regards to patients with CD4 count > 500 cells/mm³ who do not meet any of the specific conditions listed above	Consider *ART*

Patients initiating ART should be counseled on medication risks and benefits and committed to medication adherence and lifelong treatment.

Antiretroviral Regimens Recommended for Treatment-Naïve HIV Patients

Initiate ART with one of the following combination regimens:

- NNRTI + 2 NRTIs; or

- PI (preferably boosted with ritonavir) + 2 NRTIs; or

- INSTI + 2 NRTIs

Selection of a regimen should be individualized based on virologic efficacy, toxicity, pill burden, dosing frequency, drug-drug interaction potential, resistance testing results, and co-morbid conditions. The regimens in each category are listed in alphabetical order.

REGIMEN	COMMENTS

Preferred Regimens

REGIMEN	COMMENTS
NNRTI-BASED REGIMEN Efavirenz/tenofovir/emtricitabine	Efavirenz should not be used during the 1st trimester of pregnancy or in women trying to conceive or not using 2 forms of effective and consistent contraception (Pregnancy Category D).
PI-BASED REGIMENS Atazanavir + ritonavir + tenofovir/emtricitabine Darunavir + ritonavir + tenofovir/emtricitabine	Omeprazole is contraindicated in atazanavir treatment-experienced patients; give omeprazole dose 12 hours before atazanavir dose in treatment-naïve patients, maximum omeprazole dose is 20 mg daily (or PPI equivalent dose). Atazanavir absorption and levels decrease at higher gastric pH.
INSTI-BASED REGIMEN Raltegravir + tenofovir/emtricitabine	Tenofovir should be used with caution in patients with renal insufficiency.
PREFERRED REGIMEN FOR PREGNANT WOMEN Lopinavir + ritonavir + zidovudine/lamivudine	Do not use once daily dosing of lopinavir/ritonavir in pregnant women. Always use twice daily dosing.

Alternative Regimens

REGIMEN	COMMENTS
NNRTI-BASED REGIMENS Efavirenz + abacavir/lamivudine Rilpivirine/tenofovir/emtricitabine Rilpivirine + abacavir/lamivudine	Use rilpivirine with caution in patients with pretreatment HIV RNA > 100,000 copies/mL Use of proton pump inhibitors is contraindicated with rilpivirine
PI-BASED REGIMENS Atazanavir + ritonavir + abacavir/lamivudine Darunavir + ritonavir + abacavir/lamivudine Fosamprenavir + ritonavir + either [abacavir/lamivudine or tenofovir/emtricitabine] Lopinavir + ritonavir + either [abacavir/lamivudine or tenofovir/emtricitabine]	Once daily lopinavir/ritonavir is not recommended in pregnant women. **Abacavir:** should not be used in patients who test positive for HLA-B*5701 use with caution in patients with high risk of cardiovascular disease or with pre-treatment HIV-RNA > 100,000 copies/mL.
INSTI-BASED REGIMEN Raltegravir + abacavir/lamivudine	

Adopted from www.aidsinfo.nih.gov on 10/15/11

Drug Resistance Testing

Drug resistance testing is used to determine viral strains and assist in determining drug selection. Two types of drug resistance testing are currently available, genotypic and phenotypic. Both types have pros and cons associated with them, and which test is chosen is usually based on the preference of the medical provider. Genotypic testing is preferred over phenotypic testing in guiding treatment decisions in ART naïve patients, suboptimal response to ART, virologic failure and pregnant women. Phenotypic tests are used in addition to a genotype test when multiple drug resistant mutations are known or suspected, especially with protease inhibitors. Genotypic testing is available for all current ART drug classes except CCR5 inhibitors. A trofile assay (explained below) is used to select patients for CCR5 inhibitor therapy. Drug resistance testing is recommended for persons with HIV infection in the following situations:

- When they enter into care regardless of whether treatment will be initiated or deferred. If treatment is deferred, then a genotype should be repeated later, prior to initiating ART.

- To assist in the selection of active drugs when changing ART in patients with virologic failure and HIV RNA levels > 1,000 copies/mL.

- When managing suboptimal viral load reductions, or a rebounding viral load that was previously suppressed.

- All pregnant women prior to therapy, and for those entering pregnancy with detectable viral loads while on therapy.

Nucleoside/tide Reverse Transcriptase Inhibitors (NRTIs)

NRTIs work by binding to the catalytic site of reverse transcriptase, interfering with HIV viral RNA-dependent DNA polymerase and resulting in inhibition of viral replication.

DRUG	DOSING	SIDE EFFECTS/CONTRAINDICATIONS/MONITORING
Entire Class		**BLACK BOX WARNING** Lactic acidosis and severe hepatomegaly with steatosis, sometimes fatal, have occurred especially with stavudine, didanosine and zidovudine. Increased risk in females and in obesity Mortality up to 50% in some case series.
Abacavir *(Ziagen)* + lamivudine *(Epzicom)* + lamivudine and zidovudine *(Trizivir)*	300 mg BID or 600 mg daily 1 tab daily (for *Epzicom*) 1 tab BID (for *Trizivir*)	**BLACK BOX WARNING** Serious, possibly fatal, hypersensitivity reaction – look for fever, skin rash, respiratory symptoms (dyspnea, cough) and/or GI symptoms (nausea, abdominal pain). Reversed when drug is discontinued. Must screen for the HLA-B*5701 allele prior to starting therapy– if positive, ↑ risk for hypersensitivity reaction; do not use. Record as abacavir allergy in patient record. **SIDE EFFECTS** Headache, nausea, ↑ LFTs, rash, GI upset, ↑ triglycerides **MONITORING** CBC, CPK, LFTs, triglycerides, amylase

Nucleoside/tide Reverse Transcriptase Inhibitors (NRTIs) Continued

DRUG	DOSING	SIDE EFFECTS/CONTRAINDICATIONS/MONITORING
Didanosine *(Videx, Videx EC)*	≥ 60 kg: 400 mg daily < 60 kg: 250 mg daily *Videx EC* - Take on an empty stomach (1 hour before or 2 hours after a meal); swallow whole; store in tightly closed bottles at room temp. ↓ dose when CrCl< 60 mL/min	**BLACK BOX WARNINGS** Pancreatitis (sometimes fatal) – dose related **SIDE EFFECTS** Peripheral neuropathy (~20%), nausea and vomiting, ↑ amylase (16%), diarrhea (20%), abdominal pain (10%), ↑ LFTs/steatosis, retinal changes and optic neuritis (rare), myocardial infarction., diabetes mellitus/insulin resistance, SJS/TEN **CONTRAINDICATIONS** Concurrent use with allopurinol or ribavirin **MONITORING** Dilated retinal exam every 6-12 months; CBC, electrolytes, uric acid, SCr, LFTs, bilirubin, albumin, amylase and lipase (↑ with pancreatitis) New reports of portal HTN from liver complications Avoid didanosine and stavudine combo due to ↑ risk of hepatic failure. In pregnant women, additional risk of lactic acidosis
Emtricitabine (Emtriva) **+ tenofovir *(Truvada)*** **+ efavirenz and tenofovir *(Atripla)***	Cap: 200 mg daily Soln: 240 mg daily (stable for 3 months at room temp) ↓ dose when CrCl < 50 mL/min One tab daily (for *Truvada* and *Atripla)* Take *Atripla* on an empty stomach, preferably at bedtime	Recommended for initial ART **BLACK BOX WARNING** May exacerbate Hep B once drug is discontinued or HBV resistance may develop. **SIDE EFFECTS** Hyperpigmentation usually of the palms and/or soles (primarily among non-whites) but can include lip, tongue, arms, and nails; rash, insomnia, N/V/D, ↑ CPK **MONITORING** LFTs, CPK
Lamivudine *(Epivir)* + zidovudine *(Combivir)* + abacavir *(Epzicom)* + abacavir and zidovudine *(Trizivir)*	150 mg BID or 300 mg daily ↓ dose when CrCl < 50 mL/min Caution solution in diabetic patients 1 tab daily (for *Epzicom)* 1 tab BID (for *Trizivir)*	**Black Box Warnings (2)** Do not use *Epivir-HBV* for treatment of HIV May exacerbate Hep B once drug is discontinued or HBV resistance may develop. **SIDE EFFECTS** Headache, fatigue, N/V/D, neutropenia, peripheral neuropathy, ↑ LFTs, pancreatitis (rare) **MONITORING** LFTs, amylase, bilirubin, CBC, signs and symptoms of pancreatitis

Nucleoside/tide Reverse Transcriptase Inhibitors (NRTIs) Continued

DRUG	DOSING	SIDE EFFECTS/CONTRAINDICATIONS/MONITORING
Stavudine *(Zerit)*	≥ 60 kg: 40 mg Q12h < 60 kg: 30 mg Q12h ↓ dose when CrCl < 50 mL/min	**BLACK BOX WARNING** Pancreatitis (sometimes fatal) seen in combo with didanosine **SIDE EFFECTS** Hyperbilirubinemia, ↑ LFT's, peripheral neuropathy (can be reversible), headache, rash, N/V/D, lipoatrophy (more with efavirenz than boosted PI) **CONTRAINDICATIONS** Do not combine with zidovudine (antagonistic – decreased efficacy of both drugs) **MONITORING** LFTs, renal function, bilirubin, signs and symptoms of peripheral neuropathy
Zidovudine *(Retrovir)* + lamivudine *(Combivir)* + abacavir and lamivudine *(Trizivir)*	300 mg BID ↓ dose when CrCl < 15 mL/min 1 tab BID (for *Combivir* and *Trizivir*)	**BLACK BOX WARNINGS (2)** Associated with bone marrow suppression/hematologic toxicities (severe anemia requiring transfusions) and/or pancytopenia, especially in advanced HIV Prolonged use has been associated with myopathy and myositis **SIDE EFFECTS** Nausea, vomiting, anorexia, headache, ↑ LFTs, hyperpigmentation of skin/nails, muscle pain, lipoatrophy (more with efavirenz than boosted PI), diabetes mellitus/insulin resistance, dyslipidemia (↑ LDL, ↑ TG) **CONTRAINDICATIONS** Do not combine with stavudine (antagonistic – decreased efficacy of both drugs) **MONITORING** SCr at baseline, CBC, LFTs, mean corpuscular volume (MCV), CPK
Tenofovir *(Viread)* + emtricitabine *(Truvada)* + emtricitabine and efavirenz *(Atripla)*	300 mg daily ↓ dose when CrCl < 50 mL/min 1 tab daily (for *Truvada* and *Atripla*) Take *Atripla* on an empty stomach, preferably at bedtime	**BLACK BOX WARNING** May exacerbate Hep B once drug is discontinued or HBV resistance may develop. **SIDE EFFECTS** Fanconi syndrome, renal insufficiency, osteomalacia and ↓ bone density, diarrhea, abdominal pain, rash, ↑ CPK **MONITORING** CBC, CPK, LFTs, renal function, phosphorus, bone density (long term) Recommended for initial ART

NUCLEOSIDE/TIDE REVERSE TRANSCRIPTASE INHIBITOR DRUG INTERACTIONS

NRTIs do not undergo hepatic transformations via the CYP metabolic pathway, therefore, they have fewer significant drug interactions compared to PIs and NNRTIs. Some NRTIs have other routes of hepatic metabolism with reported drug interactions.

- Ribavirin may ↑ levels of all NRTIs (combo ↑ risk lactic acidosis).

- Abacavir: Levels of abacavir may be ↓ by PIs.

- Didanosine: Levels of didanosine may be ↑ by allopurinol and stavudine and ↓ by PIs. Avoid combining with hydroxyurea due to increased didanosine intracellular drug levels and toxicities.

- Emtricitabine: Avoid use with lamivudine.

- Lamivudine: Avoid use with emtricitabine. SMX/TMP may ↑ lamivudine levels.

- Stavudine: Avoid use with zidovudine (combo may ↓ levels of both drugs). Levels of didanosine may be ↑ by stavudine.

- Tenofovir: Levels of tenofovir may be ↑ by PIs and tenofovir may ↓ levels of PIs.

- Zidovudine: Avoid use with stavudine (combo may ↓ levels of both drugs). Combining with ganciclovir produces ↑ bone marrow suppression. Clarithromycin, divalproex, fluconazole, interferons, and valproic acid may ↑ levels of zidovudine.

Non-Nucleoside Reverse Transcriptase Inhibitors (NNRTIs)

NNRTIs work by binding to reverse transcriptase and blocking the RNA-dependent and DNA-dependent DNA polymerase activities including HIV-1 replication

DRUG	DOSING	SIDE EFFECTS/CONTRAINDICATIONS/MONITORING
Entire Class		**SIDE EFFECTS** Rash (SJS/TEN) sometimes severe (most common with nevirapine), ↑ LFTs, GI upset, ↓ bone mineral density when combined with NRTIs Many drug interactions
Delavirdine (*Rescriptor*)	400 mg TID Patients with achlorhydria should take with acidic beverage; separate dose from antacids by 1 hour	**SIDE EFFECTS** Rash, GI upset, headache, ↑ LFTs **CONTRAINDICATIONS** Concurrent use of alprazolam, ergot alkaloids, midazolam, pimozide, rifampin and triazolam
Efavirenz *(Sustiva)* **+ emtricitabine and tenofovir** *(Atripla)*	600 mg daily Take on an empty stomach, preferably at bedtime	**SIDE EFFECTS** CNS (impaired concentration, drowsiness, vivid dreams) and psychiatric symptoms (depression, mania, suicide), rash, ↑ triglycerides, ↑ LDL, ↑ HDL, and GI upset **CONTRAINDICATIONS** Concurrent use of atazanavir, ergot alkaloids, midazolam, pimozide, triazolam, and voriconazole, ranolazine, St John's Wort **MONITORING** LFTs and triglycerides Pregnancy Category D – not to be used in pregnant women (particularly the 1st trimester) Recommended for initial ART

Non-Nucleoside Reverse Transcriptase Inhibitors (NNRTIs) Continued

DRUG	DOSING	SIDE EFFECTS/CONTRAINDICATIONS/MONITORING
Etravirine (*Intelence*)	200 mg BID after meals	**SIDE EFFECTS** Rash, peripheral neuropathy, nausea, HTN
Nevirapine (*Viramune, Viramune XR*)	200 mg daily x 14 d; then 200 mg BID (*Viramune*) or 400 mg daily (*Viramune XR*) Need 14 day lead-in period	**BLACK BOX WARNINGS (2)** Severe hepatotoxic reactions may occur (liver failure, death); risk is greatest in the first 6 weeks and with female gender. Severe, life-threatening skin reactions (SJS, TENS, etc.) have occurred; intensive monitoring is required in the first 18 weeks of therapy. Stop drug if rash is severe or if there is a fever. **SIDE EFFECTS** Rash, ↑ LFTs, GI upset **CONTRAINDICATIONS** Moderate-to-severe hepatic impairment, post-exposure prophylaxis regimens **MONITORING** LFTs (every 2 weeks for first month, then monthly for 3 months, then quarterly), signs of drug rash Do not initiate therapy in women with CD4+ counts > 250 cells/mm^3 and in men with CD4+ counts > 400 cells/mm^3
Rilpivirine (*Edurant*) + emtricitabine and tenofovir (*Complera*)	25 mg daily with a meal 1 tab daily with a meal (*Complera*) Keep in original container to protect from light	**SIDE EFFECTS** Depressive disorders, insomnia, headache and rash **CONTRAINDICATIONS** Co-administration with drugs that lower levels of rilpivirine, such as 3A4 inducers and PPIs [PPIs are contraindicated (CI), H$_2$RAs give 12 hours before or 4 hours after rilpivirine, antacids give 2 hours before or 4 hours after rilpivirine]. Phenobarbarbital, carbamazepine, phenytoin, rifabutin and rifampin are CI with rilpivirine. More than a single dose of dexamethasone is CI with rilpivirine. **MONITORING** Signs and symptoms of mood changes and body rash Higher rates of failure have been seen in patients with HIV-RNA levels > 100,000 at treatment initiation.

Non-Nucleoside Reverse Transcriptase Inhibitor (NNRTI) Drug Interactions

All NNRTIs and PIs are metabolized in the liver via the CYP 450 system. All NNRTIs are 3A4 substrates and may also be an inducer (neviripine and etravirine), inhibitor (delavirdine) or both inducer and inhibitor (efavirenz). Etravirine is also a substrate of 2C9 and 2C19. NNRTIs have many drug interactions.

- Delavirdine: Strong inhibitor of 2C9, 2C19, 2D6 (weak) and 3A4 and major 3A4 substrate. Avoid concurrent use with alfuzosin, alprazolam, clopidogrel, dronedarone, dutasteride, eletriptin (within 72 hours of use), ergot alkaloids, eplerenone, fosamprenavir, H_2RAs, PPIs, midazolam, nilotinib, pimozide, ranolazine, rifampin, rivaroxaban, silodosin, St. John's wort, tamoxifen, tamsulosin, and triazolam.

- Efavirenz: Moderate inhibitor of 2C9, 2C19 and 3A4 and strong inducer of 3A4 and a major substrate of 3A4. Avoid use with atazanavir, clopidogrel, dronedarone, ergot derivatives, midazolam, nilotinib, pimozide, ranolazine, St. John's wort, triazolam and voriconazole.

- Etravirine: Inhibitor of 2C9, 2C19, and p-glycoprotein and inducer of 3A4 and substrate of 3A4, 2C9, and 2C19.

- Nevirapine: Strong 3A4 inducer and major 3A4 substrate. Watch for strong 3A4 inhibitors.

- Rilpivirine: Contraindicated with strong 3A4 inducers (carbamazepine, oxcarbazepine, phenobarbital, phenytoin, rifampin, rifabutin, St. John's wort) and proton pump inhibitors.

Protease Inhibitors (PIs)

PI work by inhibiting HIV-1 protease and rendering the enzyme incapable of cleaving the Gag-Pol polyprotein, resulting in the production of immature, noninfectious virions.

DRUG	DOSING	SIDE EFFECTS/CONTRAINDICATIONS/MONITORING
PI Class		**SIDE EFFECTS** Hyperglycemia
		Lipodystrophy; loss of subcutaneous fat in face, buttocks, arms and legs
		Lipohypertrophy; fat accumulation in various areas of the body (buffalo hump in the upper back, ↑ abdominal obesity, ↑ breast size in females and males). Observed with PIs although causal relationship not established (may be HIV infection and not ART)
		Dyslipidemia; Ritonavir boosted PIs may ↑ TG, ↑ LDL, ↑ HDL
		↑ amylase
		Hepatitis and hepatic decompensation (highest with tipranavir), ↑ LFTs, ↑ bilirubin
		Immune reconstitution syndrome
		Bleeding in patients with hemophilia
		Hypersensitivity reactions (rare)
		↓ bone mineral density when combined with NRTIs
		Associated with MI and stroke
		Gastrointestinal intolerance (N/V/D)
		MONITORING Glucose, LFTs, cholesterol, triglycerides, bilirubin

Protease Inhibitors (PIs) Continued

DRUG	DOSING	SIDE EFFECTS/CONTRAINDICATIONS/MONITORING
Atazanavir *(Reyataz)*	300 mg + 100 mg ritonavir daily 400 mg daily if therapy-naïve and unable to tolerate ritonavir Take with food (better absorption)	**SIDE EFFECTS** (in addition to the class side effects above) May prolong the PR interval, ↑ CPK, indirect hyperbilirubinemia (which can result in uncomplicated jaundice) Rash including SJS/TEN cases have been reported Can cause nephrolithiasis/urolithiasis;(stone, crystal formation). May reduce risk if drink at least 48 oz (1.5 L) of water daily Note that atazanavir +/- ritonovir does NOT alter insulin sensitivity **MONITORING** ECG in at-risk patients Treatment naive patients can take dose simultaneously with, or at least 10 hours after H2 blockers; can take dose 12 hours after a PPI. Max 80 mg famotidine/day, 20 mg omeprazole/day, or equivalent. PPIs are not recommended in non-boosted atazanavir. Recommended for initial ART
Darunavir *(Prezista)*	Treatment naïve: 800 mg + 100 mg ritonavir daily Treatment-experienced: 600 mg + 100 mg ritonavir BID Take with food. Swallow whole.	Use caution in patients with a sulfa allergy. Rash including SJS/TEN cases have been reported Must be given with ritonavir Recommended for initial ART
Fosamprenavir *(Lexiva)*	Treatment naïve: 1,400 mg + 100-200 mg ritonavir daily or 700 mg + 100 mg ritonavir BID Treatment-experienced: 700 mg + 100 mg ritonavir BID	Use caution in patients with a sulfa allergy Rash including SJS/TEN cases have been reported Nephrolithiasis
Indinavir *(Crixivan)*	800 mg every 8 hours without ritonavir 800 mg BID with 100-200 mg ritonavir BID or 400 mg + 400 mg ritonavir BID Take without food (unless co-administered with ritonavir), 1 hour before or 2 hours after a meal with water.	**SIDE EFFECTS** ↑ SCr, dysuria: hydronephrosis or renal atrophy Can cause nephrolithiasis/urolithiasis;(stone, crystal formation). May reduce risk if drink at least 48 oz (1.5 L) of water daily Indirect hyperbilirubinemia (which can result in uncomplicated jaundice) SJS/TEN cases have been reported Must dispense in the original container with the desiccant to protect from moisture
Nelfinavir *(Viracept)*	750 mg TID or 1,250 mg BID Take with food	**SIDE EFFECTS** Diarrhea (~17%) Oral powder contains phenylalanine, caution in patients with phenylketonuria. Mixed oral powder is stable for 6 hrs under refrigeration.

Protease Inhibitors (PIs) Continued

DRUG	DOSING	SIDE EFFECTS/CONTRAINDICATIONS/MONITORING
Ritonavir *(Norvir)* .	600 mg BID 100-400 mg/d – booster dose Take with food.	**BLACK BOX WARNING** May interact with many medications, resulting in potentially serious and/or life-threatening adverse events **SIDE EFFECTS** ↑ CPK, ↑ uric acid, can cause prolongation of the PR interval Note that side effects are less significant when lower dose ritonavir is used as a boosting agent for other PIs **MONITORING** CPK and uric acid levels Oral solution contains 43% ethanol by volume; also has unpleasant taste – can mix with chocolate milk. Store at room temp (capsules good for 30 days at room temp) Recommended for initial ART
Lopinavir + Ritonavir *(Kaletra)*	Treatment naïve: 800 mg lopinavir/200 mg ritonavir daily or 400/100 mg BID Treatment-experienced: 400/100 mg BID Solution: Take with food.	**SIDE EFFECTS** Can cause pancreatitis, sometimes fatal Can cause prolongation of PR interval SJS/TEN cases have been reported Insulin resistance/diabetes mellitus Tablet must be swallowed whole
Saquinavir *(Invirase)*	1,000 mg + ritonavir 100 mg BID Take within 2 hours of a full meal	**SIDE EFFECTS** Ritonavir-boosted saquinavir can prolong the PR and QT intervals on ECG. The degree of QT prolongation is greater than that seen with some other boosted PIs. Use caution in patients at risk of these ECG abnormalities. ECG prior to initiating and during therapy Contraindicated with trazadone
Tipranavir *(Aptivus)*	500 mg + ritonavir 200 mg BID	**BLACK BOX WARNINGS (2)** May cause hepatitis (including fatal) and/or exacerbate pre-existing hepatic dysfunction when taken with ritonavir. (CI with Child-Pugh B or C) Rare reports of fatal and nonfatal intracranial hemorrhage. Risks include CNS lesions, trauma, surgery, hypertension, alcohol abuse, coagulopathy, anti-coagulant or anti-platelet agents including vitamin E. Use caution in patients with a sulfa allergy. Caps: Refrigerate unopened bottles; once opened, stable at room temp up to 60 days. Solution: Contains vitamin E (additional vitamin E supplements are not recommended). Store at room temp and use within 60 days.

PROTEASE INHIBITOR (PI) DRUG INTERACTIONS

All NNRTIs and PIs are metabolized in the liver via the CYP 450 system. All PIs are 3A4 substrates. Most PIs are strong 3A4 inhibitors including all PI regimens in the treatment guidelines. Ritonovir is a potent 3A4 inhibitor used at low doses to increase ("boost") the level of other PIs. Tipranavir is a strong 3A4 inducer that is always boosted with ritonivir in clinical practice. The combined PI regimen of tipranivir/ritonivir results in inhibiting 3A4. PIs have many drug interactions.

- Avoid concomitant use with alfuzosin, amiodarone, conivaptan, dronedarone, eplerenone, ergot derivatives, lovastatin, midazolam, nilotinib, nisoldipine, PDE-5 inhibitors, phenobarbital, phenytoin, pimozide, quinidine, ranolazine, rifampin, rivaroxaban, salmeterol, silodosin for PAH, simvastatin, St. John's wort, tamsulosin, triazolam, and voriconazole.

- PIs can alter the INR (↑ or ↓) in patients taking warfarin; the INR should be closely monitored.

- When combining PI regimens with statins, avoid lovastatin, pitavastatin and simvastatin due to increased statin levels and risk of rhabdomyolysis.

- PIs decrease the levels of bupropion, paroxetine and sertraline levels. PIs increase the levels of trazodone and many tricyclic antidepressants. Titrate anti-depressant doses based upon clinical response.

- Trazodone with saquinavir/ritonavir is CI.

- PPIs are not recommended in PI-experienced patients.

Fusion Inhibitors

Fusion inhibitors block the attachment (or fusion) of the HIV-1 virus with the CD4 cells by blocking the conformational change in gp41 required for membrane fusion and entry into CD4 cells. They are also known as cell entry inhibitors.

DRUG	DOSING	SIDE EFFECTS/CONTRAINDICATIONS/MONITORING
Enfuvirtide (Fuzeon)	90 mg SC BID	**SIDE EFFECTS** Local injection site reactions in almost 100% of patients (pain, erythema, induration, nodules and cysts, pruritus, ecchymosis); ↑ risk of bacterial pneumonia Hypersensitivity reactions have been reported (rash, fever, N/V, hypotension). Re-challenge is not recommended Reconstituted solution should be refrigerated and used within 24 hours

CCR5 Antagonist

CCR5 inhibitors bind to the CCR5 co-receptor on the CD4 cells and prevent the conformational change required for HIV cell entry.

DRUG	DOSING	SIDE EFFECTS/CONTRAINDICATIONS/MONITORING
Maraviroc (Selzentry)	300 mg BID (150 mg – 600 mg BID if taking 3A4 inhibitors and/or inducers) Take without regard to meals	**BLACK BOX WARNING** Possible drug-induced <u>hepatotoxicity</u> with allergic type features **SIDE EFFECTS** Upper respiratory tract infections, fever, <u>rash (including SJS)</u>, cough, abdominal pain, dizziness, orthostatic/postural hypotension (especially in renal impairment). If postural hypotension develops, reduce the dose **CONTRAINDICATIONS** Patients with severe renal impairment (CrCl < 30 mL/min) who are taking potent 3A4 inhibitors or inducers <u>Prior to starting therapy, patients must undergo a screening test (Trofile) to determine the tropism of their HIV since this agent will not work for patients with CXCR4-tropic disease or dual/mixed tropic HIV disease</u>

CCR5 INHIBITOR DRUG INTERACTIONS

Maraviroc is a P-glycoprotein and major 3A4 substrate. Maraviroc concentrations can be significantly increased in the presence of strong 3A4 inhibitors and reduced with 3A4 inducers. Dose adjust maraviroc when combined with these agents: ritonavir and other PIs (except tipranavir/ritonavir), efavirenz or rifampin. Use of St. John's wort is not recommended with maraviroc.

Integrase Inhibitors

Integrase inhibitors block the integrase enzyme needed for viral DNA to enter into the host nucleus.

DRUG	DOSING	SIDE EFFECTS/CONTRAINDICATIONS/MONITORING
Raltegravir (Isentress)	400 mg BID Take without regard to meals	**SIDE EFFECTS** Nausea, diarrhea, headache, pyrexia, <u>hypertension</u>, ↑ cholesterol (↑ LDL, ↑ TGs), ↑ <u>glucose</u>, ↑ LFTs, ↑ CPK ; muscle weakness/myopathy and rha<u>bdomy</u>olysis **MONITORING** Lipid panel <u>Recommended for initial ART</u>

INTEGRASE INHIBITOR DRUG INTERACTIONS

Raltegravir: Metabolized by the UGT1A1-mediated glucuronidation pathway. Rifampin, a strong inducer of UGT1A1, will ↓ levels of raltegravir. When given concurrently with rifampin, use raltegravir 800 mg BID. Avoid St. John's wort. PPIs can ↑ levels of raltegravir.

Recommendations for Post-Exposure Prophylaxis (PEP) Following Occupational Percutaneous Injuries

EXPOSURE TYPE	WELL-CONTROLLED HIV	POORLY-CONTROLLED HIV	HIV STATUS OF SOURCE PATIENT
Less severe (solid needle or superficial injury)	Recommend 2-drug PEP	Recommend 3-drug PEP	If unknown, but high risk, consider 2 drug prophylaxis. If known negative or unknown but low risk, no PEP is needed
More severe (large-bore hollow needle, deep puncture, visible blood on device, needle in source patient's artery or vein)	Recommend 3-drug PEP	Recommend 3-drug PEP	If unknown, but high risk, consider 2 drug prophylaxis. If known negative or unknown but low risk, no PEP is needed

PREFERRED OPTIONS FOR TWO-DRUG REGIMENS

- Zidovudine + lamivudine

- Tenofovir + emtricitabine

- Tenofovir + lamivudine

- Zidovudine + emtricitabine

PREFERRED THIRD DRUG OF THREE-DRUG REGIMEN:

- Lopinavir/ritonavir

Patients receiving PEP should complete a full 4-week regimen and the regimen should be started as soon as possible.

Strategies to Improve Adherence to Antiretroviral Therapy

STRATEGIES	EXAMPLES
Utilize a multidisciplinary team approach Provide an accessible, trusting healthcare team	Nurses, social workers, pharmacists, and medications managers
Establish a trusting relationship with the patient	
Establish readiness to start ART	
Identify potential barriers to adherence prior to starting ART	Psychosocial issues Active substance abuse or at high risk for relapse Low literacy level Busy daily schedule and/or travel away from home Lack of disclosure of HIV diagnosis Skepticism about ART Lack of prescription drug coverage
Provide resources for the patient	Referrals for mental health and/or substance abuse treatment Resources to obtain prescription drug coverage Pillboxes, reminder tools
Involve the patient in ARV regimen selection	For each option, review potential side effects, dosing frequency, pill burden, storage requirements, food requirements, and consequences of nonadherence
Assess adherence at every clinic visit	Simple checklist patient can complete in the waiting room Assessment also by other members of the healthcare team Ask the patient open-ended questions (e.g., In the last three days, please tell me how you took your medicines?)
Identify the type of nonadherence	Failure to fill the prescription(s) Failure to take the right dose(s) at the right time(s) Nonadherence to food requirements
Identify reasons for nonadherence	Adverse effects from medications Complexity of regimen – pill burden, dosing frequency, etc. Difficulty swallowing large pills Forgetfulness Failure to understand dosing instructions Inadequate understanding of drug resistance and its relationship to adherence Pill fatigue Reassess other potential barriers listed above
Assess and simplify regimen, if possible	

Adopted from www.aidsinfo.nih.gov on 10/15/11

Prophylaxis to Prevent First Episode of Opportunistic Infections in Patients with HIV

PATHOGEN	INDICATION	DOC
Pneumocystis Carinii (PCP)	CD4+ count < 200 cells/mL or oropharyngeal candidiasis	TMP-SMZ 1 DS tab PO daily OR TMP-SMZ 1 SS tab PO daily
Toxoplasma gondii	Toxoplasma IgG positive patients with CD4+ count < 100 cells/ mL	TMP-SMZ 1 DS tab PO daily
Mycobacterium avium complex (MAC)	CD4+ count < 50 cells/mL (after ruling out active MAC infection)	Azithromycin 1,200 mg PO every week OR Clarithromycin 500 mg PO BID
Mycobacterium tuberculosis	Tuberculin skin test (TST) reaction ≥ 5mm OR prior positive TST result without adequate treatment OR contact with person with active TB regardless of TST result	Isoniazid 300 mg PO + pyridoxine 50 mg PO daily x 9 months OR Isoniazid 900 mg PO twice weekly + pyridoxine 50 mg PO daily x 9 months.

Source: www.aidsinfo.nih.gov, accessed 10/15/11

Patient Counseling

ALL HIV MEDICATIONS

- This medication is not a cure for HIV and it does not prevent the spread of HIV to others through sexual contact or blood contamination (such as sharing used needles).

- It is very important to continue taking this medication (and other HIV medications) exactly as prescribed by your doctor. Do not skip any doses. Do not stop taking it (or other HIV medicines) even for a short time unless directed to do so by your doctor. Skipping or stopping your medication without approval from your doctor may cause the amount of virus to increase and make the infection more difficult to treat (resistant). Refill your medication before you run out.

NRTIs PATIENT COUNSELING

- Dizziness, nausea, vomiting, diarrhea, headache, or trouble sleeping may occur. If any of these effects persist or worsen, tell your doctor or pharmacist promptly.

- Rarely, this medication can cause severe (sometimes fatal) liver problems and a certain metabolic problem (lactic acidosis). Tell your doctor immediately if you develop symptoms of liver problems (such as persistent nausea, vomiting, stomach/abdominal pain, pale stools, dark urine, yellowing eyes/skin, unusual tiredness), or of a build-up of acid in your blood (such as stomach discomfort, nausea, vomiting, fast/difficult breathing, drowsiness, muscle pain, weakness, cold skin). These serious side effects may occur more often in women and obese patients.

- If you have hepatitis B infection, your hepatitis symptoms may get worse or become very serious if you stop taking this medication. Talk with your doctor before stopping this medication. Your doctor will monitor liver tests for several months after you stop this medication. Tell your doctor immediately if you develop symptoms of worsening liver problems.

For Emtricitabine, add:

- Rarely, this medication can cause darkening skin color on the palms of hands and on the soles of feet. Notify your doctor if this is problematic to you.

For Tenofovir, add:

- Tell your doctor immediately if any of these rare but serious side effects occur: signs of kidney problems such as a change in the amount of urine, unusual thirst, muscle cramps/weakness, bone pain, or easily broken bones.

EFAVIRENZ

- Take this medication by mouth on an empty stomach, without food, usually once daily at bedtime or as directed by your doctor. Swallow this medication with water. Taking efavirenz with food increases the blood level of this medication, which may increase your risk of certain side effects.

- Efavirenz can cause side effects that may impair your thinking or reactions. Be careful if you drive or do anything that requires you to be awake and alert.

- Avoid drinking alcohol. It can increase some of the side effects of efavirenz.

- Dizziness, trouble sleeping, drowsiness, unusual dreams, and trouble concentrating may frequently occur. These side effects may begin 1-2 days after starting this medication and usually go away in 2-4 weeks. They are also reduced by taking efavirenz on an empty stomach at bedtime.

- Tiredness, headache, nausea, vomiting, and diarrhea may also occur. If any of these effects persist or worsen, tell your doctor or pharmacist promptly.

- Infrequently, serious psychiatric symptoms may occur during efavirenz treatment, although it is unclear if they are caused by efavirenz. These effects may be seen especially in people who have mental/mood conditions. Tell your doctor immediately if any of these unlikely but serious side effects occur: mental/mood changes (such as depression, rare thoughts of suicide, nervousness, angry behavior, hallucinations).

- Tell your doctor immediately if any of these rare but serious side effects occur: signs of liver problems (such as persistent nausea/vomiting, stomach/abdominal pain, severe tiredness, yellowing eyes/skin, dark urine).

- Efavirenz can commonly cause a rash that is usually not serious. A rash may occur in the first 2 weeks after starting treatment and if it is not serious, it will usually resolve in 4 weeks. However, you may not be able to tell it apart from a rare rash that could be a sign of a severe reaction. Therefore, seek immediate medical attention if you develop any rash.

- Efavirenz can speed up or slow down the removal of many other medications from your body, which may affect how they work. Examples of affected drugs include some drugs for anxiety/sleep (such as alprazolam, midazolam, triazolam), azole antifungals (such as itraconazole, ketoconazole, voriconazole), calcium channel blockers (such as diltiazem, verapamil), cisapride, ergot drugs (such as ergotamine), macrolide antibiotics (such as clarithromycin), methadone, pimozide, rifabutin, sertraline, some cholesterol-lowering statins (such as atorvastatin, pravastatin, simvastatin), warfarin, among others.

- This medication may decrease the effectiveness of hormonal birth control such as pills, patch, or ring. This could cause pregnancy. However, to reduce the risk of spreading HIV to others, always use barrier protections during all sexual activity.

- This medication can cause harm to an unborn baby. Do not use efavirenz without your doctor's consent if you are pregnant. Use two forms of birth control, including a barrier form (such as a condom or diaphragm with spermicide gel) while you are taking efavirenz, and for at least 12 weeks after your treatment ends. Tell your doctor if you become pregnant during treatment.

PI PATIENT COUNSELING

- Diarrhea, nausea, vomiting, heartburn, stomach pain, loss of appetite, headache, dizziness, tiredness, weakness, or changes in taste may occur. If any of these effects persist or worsen, tell your doctor or pharmacist promptly.

- A mild rash (redness and itching) may occur within the first few weeks after the medicine is started and usually goes away within 2 weeks with no change in treatment.

- If a severe rash develops with symptoms of fever, body or muscle aches, mouth sores, shortness of breath, or swelling of the face, contact your doctor immediately.

- Tell your doctor immediately if any of these unlikely but serious side effects occur: persistent nausea/vomiting, stomach/abdominal pain, dark urine, yellowing eyes/skin, mental/mood changes (such as depression, anxiety), joint pain, muscle weakness/cramps/aches, increased urination (especially at night), or increased thirst.

- Before using this medication, tell your doctor or pharmacist your medical history, especially of: diabetes, heart problems (coronary artery disease, heart attack), hemophilia, high cholesterol/triglycerides, gout/high uric acid in the blood, liver problems (such as hepatitis B, hepatitis C) and/or pancreatitis.

- If you have diabetes, this product may increase your blood sugar levels. Check your blood sugar levels regularly as directed by your doctor. Tell your doctor immediately if you have symptoms of high blood sugar, such as increased thirst, increased urination, confusion, drowsiness, flushing, rapid breathing, or fruity breath odor. Your doctor may need to adjust your diabetes medication.

- Changes in body fat may occur while you are taking this medication (such as increased fat in the upper back and stomach areas, decreased fat in the arms and legs). The cause and long-term effects of these changes are unknown. Discuss the risks and benefits of treatment with your doctor, as well as the possible use of exercise to reduce this side effect.

- If you are taking HIV medications for the first time, you may experience symptoms of an old infection. This may happen as your immune system begins to work better. Contact your doctor immediately if you notice any of the following symptoms: new cough, trouble breathing, fever, new vision problems, new headaches, new skin problems.

- This medication interacts with many medications. Your doctor or pharmacist may already be aware of any possible drug interactions and may be monitoring you for them. Do not start, stop or change the dosage of any medicine before checking with your doctor or pharmacist first.

For Atazanavir, add: *not w̄ PPI*

- If you are taking antacids or a buffered form of didanosine (e.g., chewable/dispersible buffered tablets), take atazanavir 2 hours before or 1 hour after these medicines.

- Also, other acid-lowering medications for indigestion, heartburn, or ulcers (e.g., prescription or over-the-counter medications such as famotidine, omeprazole) may prevent your HIV drugs from working. Ask your doctor or pharmacist how to use these medications safely

- Seek immediate medical attention if any of these rare but serious side effects occur: symptoms of a heart attack (such as chest/jaw/left arm pain, shortness of breath, unusual sweating), change in heart rhythm, dizziness, lightheadedness, severe nausea or vomiting, severe stomach pain, extreme weakness (especially in arms and legs), trouble breathing, signs of a kidney stone (e.g., pain in side/back/abdomen, painful urination, blood in the urine).

For Atazanavir, add:

- Liquid ritonavir can be mixed with chocolate milk or a nutrition drink such as *Ensure*. Drink the mixture within 1 hour after mixing.

- Store ritonavir capsules in the refrigerator or at room temperature, away from heat or moisture. If you store the capsules at room temperature you must use them within 30 days.

- Store ritonavir liquid at room temperature with the cap tightly closed. Do not refrigerate.

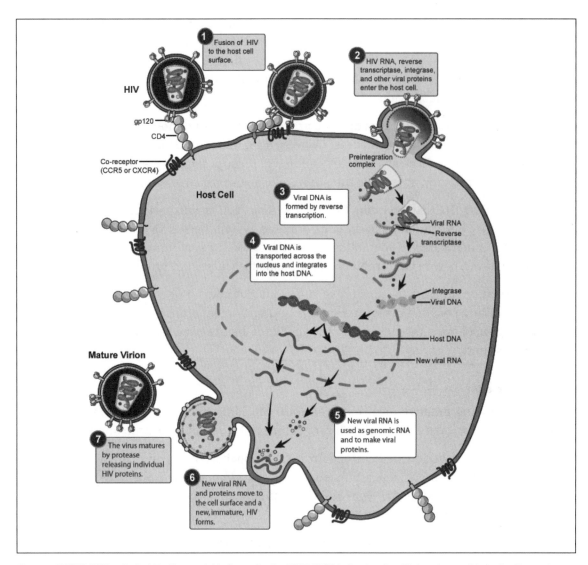

Source: DHHS-NIH website http://www.niaid.nih.gov/topics/HIVAIDS/Understanding/Biology/pages/hivreplicationcycle.aspx

HIV REPLICATION CYCLE

Steps in the HIV Replication Cycle

1. Fusion of the HIV cell to the host cell surface.

2. HIV RNA, reverse transcriptase, integrase, and other viral proteins enter the host cell.

3. Viral DNA is formed by reverse transcription.

4. Viral DNA is transported across the nucleus and integrates into the host DNA.

5. New viral RNA is used as genomic RNA and to make viral proteins.

6. New viral RNA and proteins move to cell surface and a new, immature, HIV virus forms.

7. The virus matures by protease releasing individual HIV proteins.

Credit: NIAID

HEPATITIS AND LIVER DISEASE

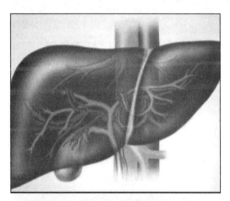

GUIDELINES

An Update on Treatment of Genotype 1 Chronic Hepatitis C Virus Infection: 2011 Practice Guidelines by the American Association for the Study of Liver Diseases. Hepatology 2011;55:1433-1444. Available at www.aasld.org

Chronic Hepatitis B: Update 2009: Practice Guidelines by the American Association for the Study of Liver Diseases. Hepatology 2009;50:661-699. Available at www.aasld.org

Background

The term hepatitis means inflammation of the liver. There are many possible causes of hepatitis, including viral hepatitis and liver inflammation due to drugs, including alcohol.

Symptoms of Liver Disease

Symptoms can include nausea, loss of appetite, vomiting, diarrhea, malaise, abdominal pain in the upper right quadrant, yellowed skin and yellowed whites of the eyes (jaundice), darkened urine and/or lightened color (white or clay-colored) stool, which indicates a severe liver condition, caused by increased bilirubin in the blood. This occurs when red blood cells are being broken down faster than the liver is able to process them.

OBJECTIVE CRITERIA

Alanine aminotransferase (ALT) and asparatate aminotransferase (AST) are liver enzymes. The ALT normal range is 7-55 units per liter (units/L), and the AST normal range is 10-40 units/L. In general, the higher the values, the worse the liver disease. Clinical signs of liver disease, in addition to ↑ ALT and ↑ AST, include ↓ albumin (protein produced by the liver; normal range 3.5-5.5 g/dL), ↑ alkaline phosphatase (Alk Phos), and ↑ total bilirubin (Tbili).

NATURAL PRODUCT

Milk thistle, an extract derived from a member of the daisy family, is often used by patients with liver disease. Most studies show benefit, and milk thistle may help protect liver cells through a variety of mechanisms, including antioxidant and anti-inflammatory properties.

However, the study designs were not rigorous enough to make definitive statements regarding its benefit. Milk thistle does not seem harmful and is well-tolerated. A possible side effect is mild diarrhea.

DRUGS THAT CAN CAUSE LIVER DAMAGE

If a drug is damaging the liver, the primary treatment (in most cases) is to STOP THE DRUG. Many drugs that are hepatotoxic are discontinued when the liver enzymes are 3 times the upper limit of normal (> 150 ALT or AST).

DRUGS THAT CAN CAUSE LIVER DAMAGE

Below are some common drugs in which patients should monitor for symptoms of liver disease. Also, tell patients (with some of these such as statins, niacin, etc) that they may require blood tests done to check on their liver.

Acetaminophen (acute, high doses)	Felbamate	Mitomycin	Anabolic steroids, testosterone, estrogen
Acarbose	Febuxostat	Nefazodone	Tacrine
Adriamycin	Fenofibrate	Niacins	Tamoxifen
Amiodarone	Flutamide	Nitrofurantoin	Terbinafine
Atomoxetine	Gemfibrozil	NSAIDs: many	Tizanidine
Azathioprine	Gold	Pentamidine	Tolcapone
Azole antifungals	Griseofulvin	Phenobarbital	Valproic acid
Bosentan	HIV drugs: many	Phenytoin	Thionamides (PTU, Methimazole)
TNF-blockers and other biologics	Hydralazine	Pioglitazone, Rosiglitazone	Zileuton
Bicalutamide	Imatinib and other "ibs"	Pyrazinamide	Zafirlukast
Carbamazepine	Interferons	Quinidine	and the natural products comfrey and kava – these should be considered dangerous due to potential liver damage.
Dronedarone	Isoniazid	Ribavirin	
Erythromycin	Isotretinoin	Rifampin	
Ethambutol	Methotrexate	Statins	
	Methyldopa		

Viral Hepatitis

Viruses that damage the liver include hepatitis A through E (most cases of viral hepatitis are caused by hepatitis A, B and C), along with herpes, CMV, Epstein-Barr virus, and adenoviruses.

Hepatitis A causes an acute, self-limiting illness and does not lead to chronic infection. Transmission is primarily via the fecal-oral route and is most likely to occur through travel to countries with high rates of hepatitis A, over-crowded areas and through ingestion of contaminated food or drinks. The hepatitis A vaccine *(Havrix, Vaqta)* is given to children beginning at one year of age (2 shots are required), and to older persons if risk factors are present: homosexual (male-male intercourse), prostitution, IVDA, if someone lives in or travels to areas with high prevalence, if liver disease is present, if receiving blood products, or if working with HIV-A infected animals. Treatment of hepatitis A is supportive and no antiviral agents are needed. Immunoglobulin (IgG) can be given for post-exposure prophylaxis.

Hepatitis B virus (HBV) causes acute illness and leads to chronic infection, cirrhosis (scarring) of the liver, liver cancer, liver failure, and death. Transmission requires contact with infectious blood, semen, or other body fluids by having sex with an infected person, sharing contaminated needles to inject drugs, or from an infected mother to her newborn (perinatal transmission). The vaccination schedule for adults and children is typically three IM injections, the second and third administered 1 and 6 months after the first, respectively (using *Engerix-B*). *Recombivax H* is given in a two dose schedule for ages 11-15 years. *Twinrix* has also been approved as a four dose accelerated schedule. Many antivirals (NRTIs) and interferons are used for chronic therapy of HBV. Patient status, viral load, severity of disease, and resistance patterns are all considered when deciding on an appropriate therapeutic regimen.

> 6 months

 Hepatitis C virus (HCV) can cause acute disease, but more commonly is silent until chronic disease emerges, with consequences similar to hepatitis B. Transmission is the same (requires body fluid transfer) but is most commonly transmitted in the United States via intravenous drug use. Vaccines are available for hepatitis A and B; however, there is no vaccine currently for hepatitis C prevention. There are 3 different genotypes for hepatitis C; genotype 1 which requires 48 weeks of treatment and is the most difficult to treat, and genotype 2 and 3 which require 24 weeks of treatment.

TREATMENT

The primary treatment for hepatitis B and C viruses are interferons. Interferons are naturally-produced cytokines that stimulate an immune response and can prevent the virus from replicating and infecting surrounding cells. The common agents include non-pegylated and pegylated interferons, such as interferon-α-2a *(Pegasys* or *PEG-Intron)*. The pegylated forms have polyethylene glycol added to the interferon via pegylation, which enhances the drug's half-life. This reduces dosing frequency from three-times weekly to once weekly.

Different antivirals are used in combination with interferons. Ribavirin *(Rebetol, Copegus)* is used for hepatitis C infections (and for RSV). Ribavirin is not used alone for hepatitis C, but when used in combination with an interferon, the response rate is doubled. Protease inhibitors can be used with ribavirin and interferon therapy for hepatitis C genotype 1 virus. For hepatitis B infections, there are several other antivirals (NRTIs) that can be used.

Interferons

Interferons have antiviral, antiproliferative, and immunomodulatory effects. They inhibit cell growth, alter cellular differentiation, alter surface antigen expression, interfere with oncogene expression, and augment cytotoxicity of lymphocytes for target cells.

DRUG	DOSING	SIDE EFFECTS/CONTRAINDICATIONS/MONITORING
Interferon-α-2b (*Intron A*) – for HBV, HCV, many cancers Pegylated interferon–α-2b (*PegIntron*) – for HCV Pegylated interferon–α-2a (*Pegasys*) – for HBV and HCV Interferon Alfacon-1 (*Infergen*) – for HCV Combo product: Interferon-α-2b and ribavirin (*Rebetron*) Other interferons are used for Multiple Sclerosis – the side effects are the same and all require Med Guides: -Interferon-β-1b (*Betaseron*) -Interferon-β–1a, liquid form (*Rebif*) -Interferon-β-1a, lyophilized (*Avonex*) Med Guides must be dispensed with each new prescription and refill.	HCV dosing example: *Intron A* 3 million units SC 3 times weekly Pegylated formulations are given once weekly + ribavirin (different doses depending on interferon type used) Treatment duration for ribavirin depends on the genotype (which determines disease severity) As in the example above, interferons are often given with ribavirin (*Rebetol, Copegus*)	**BLACK BOX WARNING** May cause or aggravate fatal or life-threatening autoimmune disorders, psychiatric symptoms (including depression and/or suicidal behavior), ischemic disease and/or infection. STOP THE DRUG if this happens. **SIDE EFFECTS** Interferons can cause many adverse effects. Flu-like syndrome 1-2 hrs after administration (fever, chills, malaise, tachycardia, arthralgia, myalgia, diaphoresis – can last 24 hrs (can pre-treat with APAP, antihistamine). **Bone Marrow Suppression** Neutropenia, thrombocytopenia and anemia **CNS** Fever, headache, chills and fatigue (~50%), headache, insomnia, blurry vision, depression, anxiety, psychosis **Pulmonary** Dyspnea, pulmonary infiltrates, pneumonitis **Endocrine/Metabolic** Hypothyroidism (~4%), hyperthyroidism (~1%), ↑BG, pancreatitis, hypertriglyceridemia **Muscle-Joint Pain** Myalgias, arthralgias, joint pain, back pain **Cardiovascular** Chest pain, arrhythmias, hypotension, syncope, murmurs, palpitations, edema **Eye** Decreased vision, optic neuritis, retinal hemorrhages **GI** Dry mouth, anorexia, cough, nausea **Dermatologic** Alopecia, skin lesions, rash **CONTRAINDICATIONS** Autoimmune hepatitis **MONITORING** Chest X-ray, ECG, CBC, LFTs, SCr, electrolytes, triglycerides, thyroid function tests, weight, and eye exam High increases in liver enzymes are expected. Withhold treatment when ANC< 500/mm³ or platelets < 25,000/mm³

INTERFERON COUNSELING

Injection Technique for Interferon Injections

- Keep the pre-filled syringes in refrigerator (never frozen). Avoid exposure to direct sunlight. Patients get 4 prefilled syringes/pack (or vials with empty syringes – in this case, they will reconstitute).

- Like insulin and other protein injectables, always instruct patient to check for discoloration and expiration date. Warm by gently rolling in hand; do not shake.

- Attach needle to pre-filled syringes. If drawing up from a vial, the instruction is similar to insulin vials.

- Interferons are injected in the abdomen (but not if patient is too thin), the top of the thigh, or the outer surface of the upper arm; rotate sites. (This is different than *Lovenox*, which is injected into the abdomen, and insulin, in which you have several possible SC sites – although the abdomen is preferred.)

- Interferons should not be injected IV; avoid areas where you can see veins. When you inject, pull the plunger of the syringe back very slightly and see if you get blood in the syringe. If you see blood in the syringe, do not inject.

- Gently tap the area you are going to inject into with your fingers, clean with alcohol, let alcohol dry 10 seconds.

- Tap syringe to push bubbles to top, inject out the bubbles (by pressing slightly). Make sure the edge of the stopper is at the correct dose. Patients may have to discard excess medicine, depending on the dose.

- Pinch a fold of skin and inject at 45- to 90-degree angle. Insert needle as far as it will go and press plunger. Press the needle into the safety (orange cover) to prevent needlestick injuries. If the patient is using syringes they fill from a vial, they should also have an orange safety cover. Due to the risk of contracting hepatitis, only syringes with safety tops are used.

- You will likely experience flu-like symptoms after injection; these can be reduced by taking acetaminophen and an antihistamine. *≥1-2 hrs after*

Tell your doctor if any of the following occurs:

- you become pregnant or your female partner becomes pregnant

- new or worsening mental health problems such as thoughts about hurting or killing yourself or others

- decreased vision

- trouble breathing or chest pain

- severe stomach or lower back pain

- bloody diarrhea or bloody bowel movements

- high fever

- easy bruising or bleeding

Ribavirin

Ribavirin is an antiviral agent that inhibits replication of RNA & DNA viruses. <u>It is indicated for hepatitis C virus (HCV) in combination with interferon alfa-2a/2b.</u>

DRUG	DOSING	SIDE EFFECTS/CONTRAINDICATIONS/MONITORING
Ribavirin *(Rebetol, Ribasphere, RibaPak, Copegus, Virazole)* 200 mg caps, 40 mg/mL soln, and 20 mg/mL for nebulization	Med Guides must be dispensed with each new prescription and refill. Dose varies based on indication, patient weight and genotype (which determines severity). In Hep C infections, stop ribavirin if there has not been an early viral response (EVR) by week 12. Take with food (better tolerated). <u>Not recommended in patients with CrCl < 50 mL/min</u>	**BLACK BOX WARNINGS (4)** <u>Significant teratogenic effects</u> Monotherapy not effective for HCV Hemolytic anemia (primary toxicity of oral therapy mostly occurring within 1-2 weeks of therapy) Caution with inhalation formulation in patients on a ventilator (precipitation of drug may interfere with ventilation) **SIDE EFFECTS** Hemolytic anemia - primary toxicity. Can worsen cardiac disease and lead to MIs. Do not use with unstable cardiac disease. Can also cause pancytopenia, GI upset, hyperuricemia, hyperbilirubinemia and others. **CONTRAINDICATIONS** Pregnancy, women of childbearing age who will not use contraception reliably, male partners of pregnant women, hemoglobinopathies **MONITORING** CBC, electrolytes, uric acid, bilirubin, and LFTs which are measured at baseline, then at weeks 1, 2, 4, 6, 8 and then every 4 weeks. Monitor TSH every 12 weeks. <u>Highly teratogenic; Pregnancy Category X</u> Can stay in body for as long as 6 months. <u>Avoid pregnancy in female patients and female partners of male patients.</u> Extreme care must be taken to avoid pregnancy during therapy and for 6 months after completion of treatment in both female patients and in female partners of male patients. At least <u>two reliable forms of effective contraception must be utilized during treatment and during the 6-month post-treatment follow-up period.</u>

RIBAVIRIN DRUG INTERACTIONS

- Do not use with didanosine due to cases of fatal hepatic failure, peripheral neuropathy and pancreatitis.

- Ribavirin may ↑ levels of nucleoside reverse transcriptase inhibitors.

RIBAVIRIN COUNSELING

- Ribavirin can cause <u>birth defects</u> or death of an unborn child. If you are pregnant or your sexual partner is pregnant, do not use. If you could become pregnant, you must not become pregnant during therapy and for <u>6 months after you have stopped therapy.</u> During this time, you must use 2 forms of birth control, and you must have pregnancy tests that show that you are not pregnant.

- Female sexual partners of male patients being treated must not become pregnant during treatment and for 6 months after treatment has stopped. Therefore, you must use 2 forms of birth control during this time.

- If you or a female sexual partner becomes pregnant, you should tell your health care provider. There is a Ribavirin Pregnancy Registry that collects information about pregnancy outcomes in female patients and female partners of male patients exposed to ribavirin. You or your doctor should contact the Registry at 1-800-593-2214. All information is confidential.

- If using the oral solution, wash the measuring cup or spoon to avoid swallowing of the medicine by someone other than the person to whom it was prescribed.

- This medicine can cause a dangerous drop in your red blood cell count, called anemia. Your doctor should check your red blood cell count before you start therapy and often during the first 4 weeks of therapy. Your red blood cell count may be checked more often if you have any heart or breathing problems.

- Do not take ribavirin alone to treat hepatitis C infection. Ribavirin is used in combination with interferon for treating hepatitis C infection.

Protease Inhibitors For Hepatitis C Only

These agents are NS3/4A protease inhibitors indicated for the treatment of chronic hepatitis C genotype 1 infection. They are direct-acting antiviral agents (DAA) that are used in combination with peginterferon alfa and ribavirin in adult patients.

DRUG	DOSING	SIDE EFFECTS/CONTRAINDICATIONS/MONITORING
Boceprevir (*Victrelis*)	800 mg 3 times/day (every 7-9 hours) with food (a meal or light snack) starting on week 5 of peginterferon alfa plus ribavirin for 24-44 weeks With compensated cirrhosis – treat for 44 weeks Without cirrhosis – treat for 24 to 44 weeks	**SIDE EFFECTS** Fatigue, anemia (requiring ESA use), neutropenia, taste distortion (dysgeusia), nausea, headache **CONTRAINDICATIONS** Due to co-administration with ribavirin, pregnancy (use of 2 non-hormonal contraceptives and negative pregnancy test before use and monthly is required) and men whose female partner is pregnant. Concurrent administration of drugs dependent on 3A4 for clearance where ↑ concentrations result in serious or life-threatening events and concurrent use of 3A4 inducers **MONITORING** CBC (to monitor anemia and neutropenia) at baseline and every 4 weeks, HCV-RNA levels, electrolytes Never reduce the dose or interrupt therapy as treatment failure may result. Never use as monotherapy; must always be combined with peginterferon and ribavirin.

Protease Inhibitors For Hepatitis C Only Continued

DRUG	DOSING	SIDE EFFECTS/CONTRAINDICATIONS/MONITORING
Telaprevir (*Incivek*)	750 mg 3 times/day (every 7-9 hours) with food (containing ~20 grams of fat) plus peginterferon alfa plus ribavirin for 12 weeks	**SIDE EFFECTS** Serious skin rash (discontinue all treatment if progressive or severe), fatigue, itching, taste distortion (dysgeusia), anemia, nausea, diarrhea **CONTRAINDICATIONS** Due to co-administration with ribavirin, pregnancy (use of 2 non-hormonal contraceptives and negative pregnancy test before use and monthly is required) and men whose female partner is pregnant. Concurrent administration of drugs dependent on 3A4 for clearance where ↑ concentrations result in serious or life-threatening events and concurrent use of 3A4 inducers **MONITORING** CBC (to monitor anemia) at baseline and every 4 weeks, HCV-RNA levels, electrolytes, bilirubin, uric acid Never reduce the dose or interrupt therapy as treatment failure may result. Never use as monotherapy; must always be combined with peginterferon and ribavirin.

PROTEASE INHIBITOR DRUG INTERACTIONS

Boceprevir and telaprevir are 3A4 inhibitors (strong) and 3A4 substrates as well as p-glycoprotein inhibitors. Major 3A4 inhibitors and inducers are contraindicated with the use of these agents. There are many drug interactions.

Nucleoside Reverse Transcriptase Inhibitors for Hepatitis B (HBV) Only

These agents inhibit HBV replication by inhibiting HBV polymerase resulting in DNA chain termination.

DRUG	DOSING	SIDE EFFECTS/CONTRAINDICATIONS/MONITORING
Entire Class ↓ in CrCl < 50 mL/min		**BLACK BOX WARNINGS (2)** Lactic acidosis and severe hepatomegaly with steatosis, which may be fatal Exacerbations of hepatitis B may occur upon discontinuation, monitor closely **SIDE EFFECTS** Headache, fatigue, nausea, vomiting, diarrhea, abdominal pain, ↑ LFTs, ↑ bilirubin, rash **MONITORING** LFTs, bilirubin, CBC, renal function, HBV DNA, signs and symptoms of HBV relapse/exacerbation upon discontinuation

Nucleoside reverse transcriptase inhibitors for Hepatitis B (HBV) Only Continued

DRUG	DOSING	SIDE EFFECTS/CONTRAINDICATIONS/MONITORING
Lamivudine *(Epivir HBV)*	100 mg PO daily 150 mg BID if co-infected with HIV	**BLACK BOX WARNINGS (3)** Do not use *Epivir HBV* for treatment of HIV **SIDE EFFECTS** Peripheral neuropathy, neutropenia, rare pancreatitis
Adefovir *(Hepsera)*	10 mg PO daily	**BLACK BOX WARNINGS (4)** May cause HIV resistance in patients with unrecognized or untreated HIV infection Use caution in patients with renal impairment or those at risk of renal toxicity **SIDE EFFECTS** Nephrotoxicity
Tenofovir *(Viread)*	300 mg PO daily	**SIDE EFFECTS** Fanconi syndrome, renal insufficiency, osteomalacia and ↓ bone density
Entecavir *(Baraclude)* Used for some cases of lamivudine-resistant HBV	Nucleoside-treatment naïve: 0.5 mg PO daily Lamivudine-resistant: 1 mg PO daily Take on empty stomach	**BLACK BOX WARNINGS (3)** May cause HIV resistance in patients with unrecognized or untreated HIV infection **SIDE EFFECTS** Peripheral edema, pyrexia, ascites Food reduces AUC by 20%; take on an empty stomach (2 hrs before or after a meal)
Telbivudine *(Tyzeka)*	600 mg PO daily	**SIDE EFFECTS** Myopathy, myalgia, peripheral neuropathy (interrupt therapy if suspected), ↑ CPK **MONITORING** CPK

NUCLEOSIDE REVERSE TRANSCRIPTASE INHIBITOR DRUG INTERACTIONS

- Ribavirin may ↑ levels of all NRTIs

- Lamivudine: SMX/TMP and ribavirin may ↑ lamivudine levels; do not use with emtricitabine

- Adefovir: Caution with other medications that are renally cleared or those which can reduce renal clearance

- Tenofovir: Levels of tenofovir may ↑ with the use of PIs, while tenofovir may ↓ the level of PIs

- Telbivudine: Caution with other medications that are renally cleared or those which can reduce renal clearance

NUCLEOSIDE REVERSE TRANSCRIPTASE INHIBITOR COUNSELING

- *EPIVIR-HBV* Tablets and Oral Solution are not exchangeable with *Epivir* tablets and solution (which have higher doses).

- Entecavir: Food reduces AUC by 20%; take on an empty stomach (take 2 hrs before or after a meal).

- Lactic Acidosis: Some people (rarely) have developed a serious condition called lactic acidosis (a buildup of an acid in the blood). Lactic acidosis is a medical emergency and must be treated in the hospital. Be seen right away if you feel very weak or tired, have unusual muscle pain, have trouble breathing, have stomach pain with nausea and vomiting, and feel dizzy or light-headed.

- Lamivudine - Pancreatitis: Some people (rarely) have developed pancreatitis, which is a medical emergency and must be treated in the hospital. Be seen right away if you have upper abdominal pain that radiates to your back, or abdominal pain that feels worse after eating with or without nausea or vomiting.

PRACTICE CASE

PATIENT PROFILE

Patient Name	Patrick Mally
Address	18 Santa Rosa
Age 44	**Sex** Male **Race** White **Height** 5'11" **Weight** 140 lbs.
Allergies	None known

DIAGNOSES

Hepatitis C

Depression

Anxiety

Insomnia

MEDICATIONS

Date	No.	Prescriber	Drug & Strength	Quantity	Sig	Refills
7/12/09	64538	Kroner	Ribivarin 200 mg	150	2AM, 3 PM	
7/12/09	64537	Kroner	Intron A 18 MU multidose #2	2	3 MU TIW	3
5/11/09	56825	Beebee	Citalopram 40 mg	30	1 TID	3
5/11/09	56826	Beebee	Zolpidem 10 mg	30	1 PO QHS	3

LAB/DIAGNOSTIC TESTS

Test	Normal Value	Results Date 7/10/09	Date	Date
Protein, T	6.2-8.3 g/dL			
Albumin	3.6-5.1 g/dL			
Alk Phos	33-115 u/L			
AST	10-35 u/L	90 u/L		
ALT	6-40 u/L	180 u/L		
CH, T	125-200 g/dL			
TG	<150 g/dL			
HDL	g/dL			
LDL	g/dL			
GLU	65-99 mg/dL			
Na	135-146 mEq/L			
K	3.5-5.3 mEq/L			
Cl	98-110 mEq/L			
C02	21-33 mmHg			
BUN	7-25 mg/dL	14		
Creatinine	0.6-1.2 mg/dL	0.9		
Calcium	8.6-10.2 mg/dL			
WBC	4-11 cells/mm³			
RBC	3.8-5.1 mL/mm³			
Hemoglobin	Male: 13.8- 17.2 g/dL Female: 12.1-15.1 g/dL			
Hematocrit	Male: 40.7-50.3% Female: 36.1- 44.3%			
MCHC	32-36 g/dL			
MCV	80-100 µm			
Platelet count	140-400 x 10³/mm³			

ADDITIONAL INFORMATION

Date	Notes
7/12/09	Recent diagnosis Hepatitis C infection. HIV negative. Patient states previous IVDA; none currently. Smokes 1 PPD; occasional alcohol. Counseled to discontinue alcohol. Nurse to instruct on injection technique & safe needle disposal. Return to clinic 4 weeks. Significant anxiety. Case mgmt to ensure safe needle storage, patient support.

Questions

1. The patient is receiving interferon therapy. Which of the following adverse effects will most likely occur in this patient?

   a. Worsening of anxiety and depression
   b. Hypertension
   c. High triglycerides
   d. Weight gain
   e. All of the above

2. The patient should be counseled that he will likely experience the following side effects post-injection of interferon therapy:

   a. Myalgia
   b. Fever
   c. Chills
   d. Diaphoresis
   e. All of the above

3. The patient is receiving ribavirin therapy. He is in a sexual relationship with a female partner. Which of the following statements is correct?

   a. No precautions are required since she is not using ribavirin.
   b. Female sexual partners of male patients being treated must not become pregnant during treatment and for 6 months after treatment has stopped. Therefore, use 2 forms of birth control are required during this time.
   c. Female sexual partners of male patients being treated must not become pregnant during treatment and for 1 year after treatment has stopped. Therefore, 2 forms of birth control are required during this time.
   d. If she becomes pregnant, she should notify the Center for Disease Control.
   e. If she becomes pregnant, the baby will be fine, however the mom will develop anemia.

4. The patient requires counseling for ribavirin therapy. Which is the most serious, potential adverse reaction of this drug?

   a. Hemolytic anemia
   b. Hemorrhagic cystitis
   c. Pancreatitis
   d. Agranulocytosis
   e. Gastrointestinal hemorrhage

5. The patient is requesting information on a natural product that might help protect his liver from further damage. Which product might be helpful?

   a. Ginkgo biloba
   b. Hawthorn
   c. St. John's wort
   d. Milk thistle
   e. Saw palmetto

6. Which of the following drugs are best avoided in this patient?

   a. Atorvastatin
   b. Nevirapine
   c. Isoniazid
   d. Felbamate
   e. All of the above

Questions 7 - 11 do not apply to the case

7. A pharmacist is reviewing a hepatic panel to assess improvement after interferon-ribavirin therapy. Which of the following lab values would indicate improvement?

   a. ↑ AST
   b. ↑ ALT
   c. ↑ albumin
   d. ↑ total bilirubin
   e. ↑ alkaline phosphatase

8. Which of the following serious adverse drug reactions may occur with the use of interferon therapy?

   a. Bone marrow suppression, including neutropenia
   b. Arrhythmias
   c. Progressive multifocal leukoencephalopathy
   d. A and B
   e. All of the above

9. What is the rationale behind adding polyethylene glycol to interferons?

   a. Reduce incidence of bone marrow suppression
   b. Decrease administration time
   c. Decrease administration frequency
   d. Reduce ischemic complications
   e. All of the above

10. Which of the following medications can lead to renal insufficiency and osteomalacia?

    a. Telaprevir
    b. Tenofovir
    c. Boceprevir
    d. Lamivudine
    e. Entecavir

11. Which of the following statements is correct regarding syringes for interferon self-injection?

    a. Safety tips are required to prevent accidental needle-stick injuries
    b. The syringes should be at least 1-inch long
    c. This medication cannot be self-injected
    d. A and B
    e. None of the above

ANSWERS

1-a, 2-e, 3-b, 4-a, 5-d, 6-e, 7-c, 8-d, 9-c, 10-b, 11-a

20

DIABETES

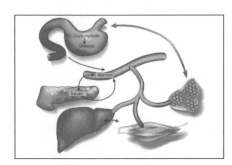

Guidelines

American Diabetes Association (ADA). Diabetes Care 2011;34:Supplement 1. Update to the 2009 guidelines.

American Association of Clinical Endocrinologists (AACE)/American College of Endocrinology Consensus Panel on Type 2 Diabetes Mellitus: An Algorithm for Glycemic Control. Endocrine Practice 2009;15:540-559.

Background

Diabetes is characterized by high blood glucose, or hyperglycemia. Glucose is the body's main source of energy. High blood glucose indicates that the glucose cannot get into the cell or cannot be properly stored. Insulin moves glucose into muscle and other tissue cells. Either there is a complete lack of insulin which occurs in type 1 diabetes, or there is a combination of insulin resistance and decreased insulin production as in type 2 diabetes. Hyperglycemia leads to micro- and macro-vascular health complications.

TYPE 1 DIABETES

Type 1 diabetes is an autoimmune disease. The patient's antibodies destroy the pancreatic beta cells which produce insulin. There is no correlation with obesity. Family history is less of a risk factor than with type 2 diabetes. Patients may present (initially) with diabetic ketoacidosis (DKA), which is a life-threatening condition. This disease usually presents in younger, thinner patients.

TYPE 2 DIABETES

This is the most common type of diabetes. While genetic risk is important, the primary cause of type 2 diabetes is lifestyle. When a person's weight increases and they have a low level of physical activity and poor nutritional intake, they are more at risk. Some lifestyle factors can be altered to reduce the risk of disease. Risk factors for type 2 diabetes include:

- Family history

- Ethnicity (African-Americans, Asians, Hispanics, Native Americans, Pacific Islanders)

- Overweight (BMI ≥ 25 kg/m²)

- Pre-diabetes

- A history of gestational diabetes mellitus (GDM, or diabetes of pregnancy)

- Poor diet and low physical activity level

Drug-induced Hyperglycemia

Corticosteroids and protease inhibitors are the most likely culprits to raise blood glucose levels. The drug may be required, in which case the resultant hyperglycemia would need to be treated. Niacin can raise blood glucose (modestly), but it is also a useful agent in many patients with diabetes. Thiazide diuretics were used in higher doses in the past, with resultant hyperglycemia. HCTZ 25 mg daily, the typical dose, may raise blood glucose, but it would be a slight increase. The atypical antipsychotics, with some worse than others, can raise blood glucose (and blood pressure and lipids). Olanzapine (*Zyprexa*) may be the worst offender. Other drugs that can raise blood glucose include diazoxide (*Proglycem*, a drug used rarely for hypoglycemia), pentamidine (*Nebupent*, for PCP prophylaxis or treatment), beta-agonists, phenytoin, cyclosporine, and tacrolimus.

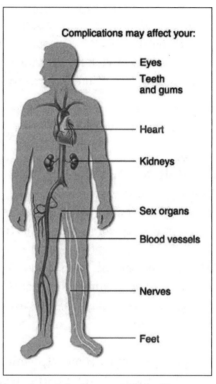

Complications may affect your: Eyes, Teeth and gums, Heart, Kidneys, Sex organs, Blood vessels, Nerves, Feet

CLINICAL SIGNS AND SYMPTOMS

Hyperglycemia, polyuria, polyphagia, polydipsia (the 3 Ps) and weight loss are usually present in type 1 patients.

Type 2 patients have hyperglycemia, but may not have the 3 Ps. Hyperglycemia can cause fatigue, recurring infections (vaginal fungal infections) and blurred vision.

CATEGORIES OF RISK FOR DIABETES (PRE-DIABETES)
- Fasting plasma glucose (FPG) 100-125 mg/dL, or
- A 75 g oral glucose tolerance test (OGTT) between 140-199 mg/dL
- HbA1C 5.7-6.4%

CRITERIA FOR THE DIAGNOSIS OF DIABETES
- Signs and symptoms of diabetes (polyuria, polydipsia and unexplained weight loss) AND a random plasma glucose ≥ 200 mg/dL, or

- FPG ≥ 126 mg/dL, or

- 2-hr plasma glucose of ≥ 200 mg/dL during a 75 g oral glucose tolerance test (OGTT), or

- HbA1C ≥ 6.5%

LONG-TERM COMPLICATIONS

Long-term complications of diabetes are classified as micro-vascular (involving small vessels) and macrovascular (involving large vessels).

- Microvascular complications include retinopathy (this is the most common microvascular complication), nephropathy (which can lead to renal dysfunction and ESRD), peripheral neuropathy (which can lead to loss of sensation in the peripheral nerves and put the patient at risk for foot ulcers and amputation) and autonomic neuropathy (including erectile dysfunction and gastroparesis).

- Macrovascular disease, or large vessel disease, includes coronary artery disease (MI, HF, HTN), cerebrovascular disease (stroke, TIA), and/or peripheral artery disease (PAD).

Diabetic Ketoacidosis (DKA)

DKA can occur when there is not enough insulin and the body breaks down fat to make energy. The breakdown of fats causes the concentration of ketones in the blood to increase. DKA can lead to coma, and if not treated quickly, can result in death.

DKA may be the initial presentation of type 1 diabetes, or can be due to a person stopping insulin therapy (running out, cutting the dose due to weight gain, etc.) Acute illness such as infection, pancreatitis, myocardial infarction and stroke can precipitate DKA. Symptoms develop rapidly.

- DKA Symptoms: Hyperglycemia, polyuria, polyphagia, polydipsia, blurred vision, metabolic acidosis (fruity breath, dyspnea) and dehydration (dry mouth, excessive thirst, poor skin turgor, fatigue).

- DKA Lab Abnormalities: Glucose > 300 mg/dL, ketones present in urine and blood, pH < 7.2, bicarb < 15 mEq/L, WBC 15-40 cells/mm³ ↑ K

- DKA Treatment: Treatment involves giving IV fluids and insulin → closely monitoring and replacing electrolytes. This typically involves using NS, followed by ½ NS, and correcting potassium to bring the level > 3.5 mEq/L.

  ❏ Potassium, even if high initially, should be expected to drop as insulin is administered. It may be necessary to replace potassium as the insulin drives the potassium into the cells (intracellular).

  ❏ It may be required to administer an anticoagulant to prevent DVT – the hospitalized patient should be considered at high risk for clotting.

TREATMENT GOALS

While a meter tests the blood glucose (BG) at that given moment, the hemoglobin A1C (or A1C) measures the average blood glucose level over the past few months. The A1C is measured quarterly if not controlled, and semiannually if controlled. The American Diabetes Association (ADA) goal for A1C is < 7%, and states that < 6% may be better, especially for type 1 patients. The American Association of Clinical Endocrinologists (AACE) guidelines have an A1C goal of < 6.5%.

A1C (%)	eAG (mg/dL)
5	97
6	126
7	154
8	183
9	212
10	240
11	269
12	298

The eAG (estimated Average Glucose) is a newer test that is becoming more popular. It may be easier for patients to understand because the value is like a blood glucose number they are used to seeing when they measure their BG. The eAG is a 3-month blood glucose average. The goal eAG is < 154 mg/dL.

The preprandial blood glucose (taken before eating) should stay between 70-130 mg/dL and the postprandial BG (1-2 hours after eating) should be < 180 mg/dL. (ADA).

LDL cholesterol should be < 100 mg/dL in patients without overt CVD. In patients with overt CVD, a LDL goal of < 70 mg/dL is an option. Triglycerides should be < 150 mg/dL. HDL should be > 40 mg/dL in men and > 50 mg/dL in women.

Blood pressure should be < 130/80 mmHg. ACE Is or ARBs should be chosen for initial treatment to help reduce the development of nephropathy. The only time an ARB is indicated over an ACE I is when a type 2 patient has hypertension, macroalbuminuria and chronic renal insufficiency, defined as a SCr > 1.5. If patient is still not at BP goal with ACE-I or ARB therapy, a thiazide diuretic should be added (if CrCl > 30 mL/min) or a loop diuretic (if CrCl < 30 mL/min).

An annual urine test for albumin is required. Any protein in the urine indicates renal disease and requires strict blood glucose and blood pressure control. Microalbuminemia is defined as 30-300 mg. Macroalbuminemia is a urine protein level > 300 mg and indicates worsening renal disease.

The feet should be examined daily by the patient or caregiver, every visit to the physician, and annually by a podiatrist. Wear clean, dry socks, comfortable shoes, cut toe-nails straight across (do not curve), dry well between toes. Keep all body skin hydrated and moisturize to avoid dry, cracked skin. Keep BG and BP controlled!

An initial dilated retinal exam is recommended to check for retinopathy. Eye exams are recommended annually, but may be done less frequently (every 2-3 years) if past eye exam(s) were normal.

All patients with diabetes should get the fall influenza immunization, and a pneumococcal vaccine once (repeat if > 65 years old or if it was longer than 5 years since 1st immunization).

Consider aspirin therapy for primary prevention in those with ↑ CV risk (10-year risk > 10%). This includes men > 50 years of age and women > 60 years of age with at least one additional major risk factor (e.g. family history of CVD, HTN, smoking, dyslipidemia, or albuminuria). The dose of ASA should be 75-162 mg daily (usually 81 mg EC) if there is no contraindication (ASA allergy, bleeding tendency, a recent GI bleed, or active hepatic disease). If the patient has an aspirin allergy, clopidogrel 75 mg daily can be used as an alternative.

DIAGNOSIS OF TYPE 2 DIABETES

Counsel patients regarding lifestyle modification (weight loss, exercise)
(expected decrease in A1c 1-2%) [well-validated*]

and

Initiate metformin [**Glucophage**, others] 500 mg once or twice daily, titrate to 850 mg to 1,000 mg twice daily (expected decrease in A1c 1-2%) [well-validated*]

↓

(A1c 7% or greater three months later)

Add sulfonylurea, not glyburide or chlorpropamide (expected decrease in A1c 1- 2%) [well validated*]

or

Add basal insulin (bedtime intermediate-acting insulin or bedtime or morning long-acting insulin) (expected decrease in A1c 1.5%) [well-validated*]

or

Add pioglitazone [*Actos*], NOT rosiglitazone [*Avandia*] (expected decrease in A1c 0.5-1.4%) [less well-validated]

or

Add exenatide [*Byetta*] (expected decrease in A1c 0.5-1%) [insufficient clinical use to be confident regarding safety, less-well-validated]

↓

(A1c 7% or greater three months later)

In those receiving metformin and basal insulin or sulfonylurea, change to metformin plus intensive or basal insulin, respectively [well-validated*]

or

In those receiving metformin plus pioglitazone, add sulfonylurea or change to metformin plus basal insulin [less well-validated]

or

In those receiving metformin plus exenatide, change to metformin plus pioglitazone and sulfonylurea or metformin plus basal insulin [less well-validated]

↓

(A1c 7% or greater three months later)

In patients not yet receiving metformin plus insulin, change to metformin plus basal insulin [well- validated*]

or

In those receiving metformin plus basal insulin, intensify insulin and continue to adjust [well-validated*]

- Well-validated therapies are those which are the best established, most effective, and cost effective therapies. These therapies are the preferred route of therapy for most patients with type 2 diabetes.

- When insulin is added, insulin secretagogues such as sulfonylureas or the meglitinides (repaglinide, nateglinide) should be discontinued.

- Consider insulin as initial therapy (with lifestyle modification) in patients with fasting glucose greater than 250 mg/dL or A1C > 10% or those with ketouria or symptoms of hyperglycemia.

- The algorithm does not include pramlintide [*Symlin*], alpha-glucosidase inhibitors [*Precose, Glyset*], glinides [*Prandin, Starlix*], or sitagliptin [*Januvia*] because of their lower or equivalent overall glucose-lowering effectiveness compared with other agents and/or limited clinical data or relative expense. However, these agents may be appropriate for certain patients. This algorithm also does not include liraglutide (*Victoza*) or saxagliptin (*Onglyza*) which were not available at the time of writing this consensus statement.

ADA Treatment Guidelines for TYPE 2 Diabetes

The AACE guidelines agree with the ADA in recommending metformin as initial therapy (unless insulin is required or the patient cannot use metformin) – but they differ in 2nd line treatment options. The ADA prefers the older drugs (sulfonylureas) and the AACE prefers to avoid these due to risk of hypoglycemia and weight gain. AACE recommends metformin first. Pioglitazone, incretin mimetics (such as exenatide), and DPP-4 inhibitors are favored as second line therapies. The AACE treatment algorithm recommends evaluating the initial A1C and, based on the value, initiating single, double or triple drug therapy. Note that the AACE treatment plan may be cost-prohibitive for the patient.

Biguanide

Metformin works primarily by ↓ hepatic glucose output (the liver releases less glucose into the bloodstream). Metformin also decreases intestinal absorption of glucose and improves insulin sensitivity.

DRUG	DOSING	SIDE EFFECTS/CONTRAINDICATIONS/MONITORING
Metformin (*Glucophage, Glucophage XR, Fortamet, Glumetza*) **Immediate release: 500, 850, 1,000 mg** **Extended release 500, 750, 1,000 mg** *Riomet liquid* (500 mg/5 mL) + glipizide (*Metaglip*) **+ glyburide (*Glucovance*)** **+ pioglitazone (*Actoplus Met*)** + rosiglitazone (*Avandamet*) **+ sitagliptin (*Janumet*)** + saxagliptin (*Kombiglyze XR*) + repaglinide (*PrandiMet*)	Start IR 500 mg daily-BID or 850 mg daily Start ER 500-1,000 mg with dinner. Titrate to 2 g daily, although higher doses are sometimes used. ↓ A1C 1-2% The ADA treatment guidelines state that metformin should be used as first-line therapy, unless A1C > 10% or FBG > 250 mg/dL. The ER formulations may appear in the stool.	**SIDE EFFECTS** Diarrhea, or loose stools, occurs in up to 20% of patients, but it often goes away. Possible abdominal discomfort. WEIGHT NEUTRAL, NO HYPOGLYCEMIA. **Renal** Contraindicated with SCr ≥ 1.5 mg/dL (males) or ≥ 1.4 mg/dL (females) or CrCl < 60 mL/min. Adequate renal function should be confirmed if the patient is > 80 years old. **Lactic acidosis (Black Box Warning)** Rare, but can be fatal. More common if patient has renal impairment and cardiac disease. Counsel for symptoms. **Caution in heart failure** If heart failure is acute or worsening, it is best to hold the metformin. The patient may experience hypoperfusion, which can lead to hypoxia and acute renal failure. **CONTRAINDICATIONS** Metformin should be stopped in any case of hypoxia, such as decompensated heart failure, respiratory failure or sepsis. Hold prior to use of IV contrast dye and wait 48 hours after the procedure. Check for normal renal function. **MONITORING** FBG, HbA1C

METFORMIN DRUG INTERACTIONS

- Alcohol can increase risk for lactic acidosis, especially with renal impairment and advanced heart disease.

- Iodinated contrast dye increases risk of lactic acidosis – hold x 48 hrs and recheck renal function prior to restarting metformin.

- Metformin ↓ folate and vitamin B-12 absorption: this can lead to neuropathic damage. Consider vitamin supplement.

METFORMIN COUNSELING

- Some people have developed a very rare, life-threatening condition called lactic acidosis while taking metformin. Get emergency medical help if you have any of these symptoms of lactic acidosis: weakness, increasing sleepiness, slow heart rate, cold feeling, muscle pain, shortness of breath, stomach pain, feeling light-headed, and fainting.

- If you need to have any type of X-ray or CT scan using a dye that is injected into your vein, you may need to temporarily stop taking metformin. Be sure the physician knows ahead of time that you are using metformin.

- Take metformin twice daily with your morning and evening meals (daily with evening meal if ER).

- Do not crush, chew, or break an extended-release tablet. Swallow the pill whole. It is specially made to release medicine slowly in the body. Breaking the pill would cause too much of the drug to be released at one time.

- Diarrhea and abdominal discomfort may occur; it often goes away. If the immediate dose is used, it should be given twice daily with meals. The stomach upset may be worse if taken on an empty stomach. You may find relief with the extended release formulation which is taken with dinner.

- If using *Glumetza*, you may see a shell of the medicine in the stool. This is not a problem; the medicine has been absorbed. If using *Fortamet*, you may see what looks like a lumpy tablet in the stool. This is not a problem; the medicine has been absorbed.

Sulfonylureas

Sulfonylureas work by stimulating insulin secretion from the pancreatic beta cells. <u>Do not use with meglitinides due to similar MOA.</u>

DRUG	DOSING	SIDE EFFECTS/CONTRAINDICATIONS/MONITORING
Acetohexamide (*Dymelor – N/A*) **Chlorpropamide (*Diabinese*)** Tolazamide (*Tolinase – N/A*) Tolbutamide (*Orinase – N/A*)	↓ A1C 1-2% Older agents no longer routinely used; ADA guidelines state not to use chlorpropamide due to long duration and risk hypoglycemia.	**SIDE EFFECTS** <u>Hypoglycemia</u>, weight gain ↓ efficacy after long-term use **Renal** ADA guidelines recommend against use of chlorpropamide and glyburide. Both can cause long-lasting hypoglycemia. Glyburide has a partially active metabolite that is renally cleared; it accumulates with renal dysfunction and is not recommended in patients with a CrCl < 50 mL/min. Micronized glyburide has better absorption than glyburide; 3 mg micronized glyburide = 5 mg of glyburide
Glipizide (*Glucotrol, Glucotrol XL*) + metformin (*Metaglip*)	IR 2.5-10 mg BID XL 2.5-10 mg daily, max 20 mg daily	
Glimepiride (*Amaryl*) + pioglitazone (*Duetact*) + rosiglitazone (*Avandaryl*)	2-4 mg, max 8 mg daily	**MONITORING** FBG, HbA1C
Glyburide (*Diabeta, Micronase*) Micronized glyburide (*Glynase PresTab*) + metformin (*Glucovance*)	1.25-5 mg daily *Glynase PresTab:* 1.5-12 mg daily	

SULFONYLUREA DRUG INTERACTIONS

- Primary interaction is with insulin because both can cause hypoglycemia.

- Use caution with drugs that can cause hypoglycemia: alcohol, azole antifungals (fluconazole, voriconazole), penicillamine, pentamidine, quinine, quinolones, pramlintide and sulfamethoxazole-trimethoprim.

SULFONYLUREA COUNSELING

- Do not crush, chew, or break an extended-release tablet. Swallow the pill whole. It is specially made to release medicine slowly in the body. Breaking the pill would cause too much of the drug to be released at one time.

- If dosed once daily, take before breakfast. If dosed twice daily, take before breakfast and dinner.

- This medicine can cause low blood sugar. Be able to recognize the symptoms of low blood sugar including shakiness, irritability, hunger, headache, confusion, drowsiness, weakness, dizziness, sweating, and fast heartbeat. Very low blood sugar can cause seizures (convulsions), fainting, or coma. Always keep a source of sugar available in case you have symptoms of low blood sugar.

Meglitinides

Meglitinides work by stimulating insulin secretion from the pancreatic beta cells. Do not use with sulfonylureas due to similar MOA.

DRUG	DOSING	SIDE EFFECTS/CONTRAINDICATIONS/MONITORING
Repaglinide (*Prandin*) + metformin (*PrandiMet*)	0.5 mg TID if A1C < 8%, 1-2 mg TID if A1C ≥ 8% Take 15-30 minutes before meals	↓ A1C 0.5-1.5%; used for ↓ postprandial BG Nateglinide is slightly less effective than repaglinide **SIDE EFFECTS** Hypoglycemia Weight neutral – benefit over sulfonylureas **MONITORING** FBG, HbA1C
Nateglinide (*Starlix*)	60 mg TID if near goal A1C, otherwise 120 mg TID. Take 15-30 minutes before meals	

MEGLITINIDES DRUG INTERACTIONS

- Primary interaction is with insulin because both can cause hypoglycemia.

- Gemfibrozil increases *Prandin* concentrations and can ↓ BG: recommend fenofibrate instead.

- Use caution with drugs that can cause hypoglycemia: alcohol, azole antifungals (fluconazole, voriconazole), penicillamine, pentamidine, quinine, quinolones, pramlintide and sulfamethoxazole-trimethoprim.

MEGLITINIDES COUNSELING

- Take 15-30 minutes prior to meals. If you forget to take a dose until after eating, skip that dose and take only your next regularly scheduled dose, before a meal.

- If you plan to skip a meal, skip the dose for that meal. (Some patients will be told to increase dose if they eat significantly more food at a meal).

- This medicine can cause low blood sugar. Be able to recognize the symptoms of low blood sugar including shakiness, irritability, hunger, headache, confusion, drowsiness, weakness, dizziness, sweating, and fast heartbeat. Very low blood sugar can cause seizures (convulsions), fainting, or coma. Always keep a source of sugar available in case you have symptoms of low blood sugar.

Thiazolidinediones (TZDs)

Thiazolidinediones are peroxisome proliferator-activated receptor gamma (γ) agonists causing $\uparrow$ peripheral insulin sensitivity ($\uparrow$ insulin entry into muscle cells; insulin sensitizers).

DRUG	DOSING	SIDE EFFECTS/MONITORING/CONTRAINDICATIONS
Pioglitazone (*Actos*) + metformin (*Actoplus Met,* *Actoplus Met XR*) + glimepiride (*Duetact*)	$\downarrow$ A1C 0.5-1.4% 15-45 mg daily	**BLACK BOX WARNING** May cause or exacerbate heart failure in some patients **SIDE EFFECTS** Peripheral edema, weight gain, macular edema, CHF, fracture risk, pioglitazone has $\uparrow$ risk of bladder cancer when used beyond 1 year **Hepatic** Discontinue when ALT > 3x normal or signs and symptoms of hepatitis–monitor liver enzymes before start of therapy and periodically thereafter.
Rosiglitazone (*Avandia*) + metformin (*Avandamet*) + glimepiride (*Avandaryl*)	2-8 mg daily Not in any guidelines. Restricted use (2011) due to CVD risk. Patients must be enrolled in the Avandia-Rosiglitazone Medicines Access Program - REMS program.	**Cardiovascular Risk** Use caution in CHF, can cause fluid retention, peripheral edema, HF decompensation – contraindicated in NYHA 3 or 4. Rosiglitazone can increase the risk of MI (Black Box Warning). Pioglitazone is better for lipids: rosiglitazone LDL (both HDL) **CONTRAINDICATIONS** NYHA Class 3 and 4 heart failure. Do not use pioglitazone in patients with active bladder cancer. **MONITORING** LFTs, FBG, HbA1C, and signs and symptoms of heart failure

GLITAZONE COUNSELING

- May take several weeks for the drug to lower blood sugar; monitor your levels carefully.

- Take once daily, with or without food.

- Contact your doctor right away if you are passing dark-colored urine, have pale stools, feel more tired than usual or if your skin and/or whites of your eyes become yellow. These may be signs of liver damage.

■ This drug can cause water retention and can cause your ankles to swell. You may develop trouble breathing. If this happens, inform your doctor right away.

Alpha-Glucosidase Inhibitors

These agents inhibit alpha-glucosidase in the intestines and alpha-amylase in the pancreas resulting in delayed absorption of glucose. They also inhibit metabolism of sucrose to glucose and fructose.

DRUG	DOSING	SIDE EFFECTS/CONTRAINDICATIONS/MONITORING
Acarbose (Precose)	↓ A1C 0.5-0.8%; used to ↓ postprandial BG Both acarbose and miglitol are started at 25 mg with the first bite of each main meal; ↑ by 25 mg every 1-2 months, max 300 mg/d, divided.	**SIDE EFFECTS** GI effects [flatulence, diarrhea, abdominal pain (all > 20%)] – so titrate slowly. Good: ↑ HDL, ↓ TGs and ↓ total cholesterol Weight neutral **CONTRAINDICATIONS** Irritable bowel syndrome (IBS); colonic ulceration, intestinal obstruction – do not use with any significant GI disease **MONITORING** Postprandial BG, HbA1C, SCr, and LFTs with acarbose Acarbose can rarely ↑ liver enzymes; check LFTs every 3 months during 1st year
Miglitol (Glyset)		

ALPHA-GLUCOSIDASE INHIBITOR COUNSELING

■ Take with a full glass of water with your first bite of food; the medicine needs to be in the stomach with your food. If you plan to skip a meal, you do not need to take the meal-time dose.

■ This medicine will cause flatulence (gas) and diarrhea, but this usually goes away with time. The dose may be increased as you get over these side effects.

■ These agents, by themselves, do not cause low blood sugar. If you get low blood sugar after taking acarbose or miglitol, you cannot treat it with sucrose (present in fruit juice) or with table sugar or candy. If you are using this agent with a drug that causes low blood sugar (such as insulin, a sulfonylurea or a meglitinide), you will need to purchase glucose tablets or gel to have on-hand to treat any hypoglycemia.

■ This medicine can improve your cholesterol levels. And, they do not cause any weight gain.

DPP4-Inhibitors

DPP-4 inhibitors prevent the enzyme DPP-4 from breaking down incretin hormones, glucagon-like peptide-1(GLP-1) and glucose-dependent insulinotropic polypeptide (GIP). These hormones help to regulate blood glucose levels by increasing insulin release from the pancreatic beta cells and decreasing glucagon secretion from pancreatic alpha cells. A reduction in glucagon results in decreased hepatic glucose production. These are *incretin enhancers*.

DRUG	DOSING	SIDE EFFECTS/CONTRAINDICATIONS/MONITORING
Sitagliptin (*Januvia*) **+ metformin (*Janumet*)** + simvastatin (*Juvisync*)	100 mg daily (can start 50 mg) 25 mg with CrCl < 30 mL/min, including dialysis.	↓ A1C 0.5-0.8%, ↓ (primarily) postprandial BG **SIDE EFFECTS** Nasopharyngitis, upper respiratory tract infections, peripheral edema, rash and hypoglycemia. Rarely can cause acute pancreatitis Weight neutral
Saxagliptin (*Onglyza*) + metformin (*Kombiglyze XR*)	5 mg daily 2.5 mg if CrCl < 50 mL/min or with strong CYP 3A4 inhibitors *Kombiglyze XR* is given daily with evening meal	**MONITORING** FBG, HbA1C, renal function
Linagliptin (*Tradjenta*)	5 mg daily No renal dose adjustment	

DPP-4 INHIBITOR DRUG INTERACTIONS

- Saxagliptin (*Onglyza*): Use the lower 2.5 mg dose with strong CYP 3A4 inhibitors including ketoconazole, atazanavir, clarithromycin, indinavir, itraconazole, nefazodone, nelfinavir, ritonavir, saquinavir and telithromycin.

- Linagliptin *(Tradjenta)* is a 3A4 and P-glycoprotein substrate. Linagliptin levels are decreased by strong inducers (carbamazepine, efavirenz, phenytoin, rifampin, St. John's wort).

DPP-4 INHIBITOR COUNSELING

- Take once daily in the morning, with or without food.

- If you have trouble breathing, or any kind of rash, see the doctor at once.

- Counsel patients to be seen right away if they develop symptoms of pancreatitis, which include severe stomach pain that does not go away, with or without vomiting. The pain can radiate from the abdomen through to the back.

Glucagon-Like Peptide-1 (GLP-1) Agonists

These agents are analogs of glucagon-like peptide-1 (GLP-1) which ↑ insulin secretion, ↓ glucagon secretion, slow gastric emptying, improve satiety, and may result in weight loss. These are *incretin mimetics*.

DRUG	DOSING	SIDE EFFECTS/CONTRAINDICATIONS/MONITORING
Exenatide *(Byetta)* 5 mcg and 10 mcg pens A synthetic version of exendin, a substance found in Gila monster saliva	Start at 5 mcg SC BID for 1 month; then 10 mcg SC BID Should be given within 60 minutes (usually 30) before the morning and evening meal Abdomen is preferred SC injection site, but can use thigh or upper arm. Count to 5 before withdrawing syringe Can be stored at room temperature for up to 30 days	↓ A1C 0.5-1%, primarily ↓ postprandial BG **SIDE EFFECTS** Nausea (primary side effect), vomiting, diarrhea, anti-exenatide antibodies, hypoglycemia, weight loss – different for all patients, usually ~5 pounds. Can cause pancreatitis **Pancreatitis** Pancreatitis (fatal and non-fatal) can occur, but occurs most commonly in patients with risk factors. Do not use in patients with history of pancreatitis, gallstones, alcoholism, or high triglycerides. This is in the required MedGuide. May cause thyroid neoplasms **Renal** Use caution with moderate impairment, avoid in severe impairment (CrCl < 30 mL/min) **MONITORING** FBG, HbA1C, renal function
	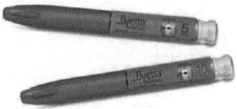	
Liraglutide (*Victoza*)	0.6, 1.2, or 1.8 mg SC daily - available in prefilled pens Start with 0.6 mg SC daily x 1 wk, then 1.2 mg SC daily x 1 wk. Can ↑ to 1.8 mg SC daily, if needed. Given without regard to meals Can be stored at room temperature for up to 30 days	↓ A1C 0.5-1.1% Can be used as mono- or combination therapy only in type 2 diabetes **Black Box Warning** Thyroid C-cell carcinomas seen in rats and mice – unknown if this could happen in humans. Contraindicated in patients with a personal or family history of medullary thyroid carcinoma (MTC) or Multiple Endocrine Neoplasia syndrome type 2 (MEN 2). **SIDE EFFECTS** More weight loss and less hypoglycemia than with exenatide; nausea, vomiting, diarrhea, anti-liraglutide antibodies, and pancreatitis **MONITORING** FBG, HbA1C

EXENATIDE COUNSELING

- Take twice daily in the morning and evening, 30-60 minutes before food.

- If you develop nausea, which is common when starting therapy, you must be careful to consume adequate fluids. If you are vomiting or have diarrhea, take fluid replacement drinks and contact your doctor. Nausea generally decreases over time. After a month, if the nausea is manageable, the dose will be increased from 5 mcg twice daily to a more concentrated pen that gives a dose of 10 mcg twice daily.

- Administer (using a fresh needle) by SC injection in thigh, abdomen (preferred) or upper arm. Count to 5 before withdrawing the syringe.

- Never inject after a meal, because of the risk of hypoglycemia.

- The doses are pre-measured in the pen – you do not adjust them.

- After first use, the pen can be kept at a room temperature not to exceed 77°F (25°C).

- Do not freeze *Byetta*. Do not use *Byetta* if it has been frozen. *Byetta* should be protected from light.

- Do not store your *Byetta* Pen with the needle attached. If the needle is left on, *Byetta* may leak from the pen and air bubbles may form in the cartridge.

- When carrying the pen away from home, store the pen at a temperature not to exceed 77°F (25°C) and keep dry. *Byetta* should be protected from light.

- After 30 days of use, throw away the *Byetta* Pen, even if it is not completely empty. Mark the date when you first used your pen and the date 30 days later. *Byetta* should not be used after the expiration date printed on the pen label.

- Keep your pen and needles out of the reach of children.

- Pancreatitis, or inflammation of the pancreas, can rarely happen with the use of this drug. Be seen right away if you develop stomach pain that does not go away, with or without vomiting. The pain can radiate from the abdomen through to the back. Alcohol consumption should be limited.

Pramlintide

Pramlintide is a synthetic analog of the human neuroendocrine hormone, amylin. Amylin is produced by pancreatic beta cells to assist in postprandial glucose control. Amylin helps slow gastric emptying, prevents an increase in serum glucagon following a meal, and increases satiety. This is an amylinomimetic agent.

DRUG	DOSING	SIDE EFFECTS/CONTRAINDICATIONS/MONITORING
Pramlintide *(Symlin)* *SymlinPen 120* (Type 2) *SymlinPen 60* (Type 1) Vial - 0.6 mg/mL (5 mL) - discontinued **Can use in both Types 1 and 2 DM:** ↓ rapid-acting, short-acting, and fixed-mix insulins (70/30) by 50% when starting this drug.	Type 1: Start at 15 mcg immediately prior to meals - can titrate at 15 mcg increments up to 60 mcg if no significant nausea. Type 2: Start at 60 mcg prior to meals - can increase to 120 mcg if no significant nausea. Administered SC in abdomen or thigh <u>prior to each meal</u> (≥ 250 kcal or ≥ 30 grams of carbohydrates).	**Black Box Warning** Co-administration with insulin may induce severe hypoglycemia (usually within 3 hours following administration) **SIDE EFFECTS** <u>Hypoglycemia</u> (when starting therapy, reduce meal-time insulins by 50% to ↓ risk of hypoglycemia), <u>nausea</u> (30%), <u>anorexia</u> (15%), weight loss **CONTRAINDICATIONS** Gastroparesis, hypoglycemia unawareness **MONITORING** FBG, HbA1C Refrigerate pens not in use. Can be stored at room temperature for up to 30 days.

PRAMLINTIDE COUNSELING

- Never mix in the same syringe with insulin.

- Injecting pramlintide is similar to injecting insulin. Inject under the skin (subcutaneously) of your stomach area (abdomen) or upper leg (thigh) and at least 2 inches away from your insulin injection site.

- If you miss or forget a dose, wait until the next meal and take your usual dose at the next meal.

- Do not take if you plan to eat a meal with fewer than 250 calories or fewer than 30 grams of carbohydrates. Do not use if you skip a meal.

- Opened vials can be refrigerated or kept at room temperature for up to 28 days. Pens are good at room temperature for 30 days.

- Low blood sugar (hypoglycemia) is a potentially serious side effect. When starting therapy, your diabetes clinician should instruct you to reduce the dose of insulin you take before or with meals by 50 percent.

- Nausea is the most common side effect. Mild nausea is more likely during the first weeks and usually does not last long. It is very important to start at a low dose and increase only as directed.

Bile Acid Binding Resins

Resins work by binding bile, blocking reabsorption. Bile is produced from cholesterol and cholesterol levels decrease. The mechanism by which colesevelam improves glycemic control in unknown.

DRUG	DOSING	SIDE EFFECTS/CONTRAINDICATIONS/MONITORING
Colesevelam *(WelChol)* 625 mg tabs or 3.75 gram and 1.875 gram packets for oral solution	Take 6 tabs daily or 3 tabs BID WITH a meal AND liquid or take one 3.75 gram packet daily or 1.875 gram packet BID [dissolved in ½ to 1 cup (4-8 oz.) of water] Approved for lipids (↓ LDL ~20%) and DM 2 (↓ A1C 0.5%, ↓ postprandial BG)	**SIDE EFFECTS** Constipation, abdominal pain, dyspepsia, nausea. Can ↑ TGs (~5%) ↓ absorption of other drugs; see below **CONTRAINDICATIONS** Bowel obstruction, TG > 500 mg/dL, history TG-induced pancreatitis **MONITORING** FBG, HbA1C *WelChol* has less GI SEs than the other agents in this class that are used for lipid-lowering.

COLESEVELAM DRUG INTERACTIONS

- The following medications should be taken 4 hours prior to WelChol: phenytoin, levothyroxine, glyburide, cyclosporine and oral contraceptives (E+P).

- With warfarin, monitor INR frequently during initiation.

- Take bile acid resins 4-6 hours before *Niaspan*.

WELCHOL COUNSELING

- Check for other constipating drugs or constipation, and counsel appropriately (laxative, such as senna, or the stool softener docusate, if appropriate). Adequate fluid intake is required.

- May take a multivitamin at other time, due to possible risk of ↓ A, D, E and K (mostly K) absorption.

Bromocriptine

Bromocriptine is indicated as an adjunct to diet and exercise to improve glycemic control in adults with type 2 diabetes. It is a dopamine agonist but it improves glycemic control by working in the CNS to decrease insulin resistance.

DRUG	DOSING	SIDE EFFECTS/CONTRAINDICATIONS/MONITORING
Bromocriptine *(Cycloset)* 0.8 mg tabs	1.6-4.8 mg daily – take with food to ↓ nausea Start at 0.8 mg daily within 2 hours of waking. If miss a dose, do not take later in the day. Titrate in 0.8 mg increments weekly ↓ A1C by 0.5%	**SIDE EFFECTS** Nausea, dizziness due to orthostasis (requires slow dose titration), fatigue, headache, vomiting, rhinitis, risk of psychiatric effects **CONTRAINDICATIONS** Patients allergic to ergot-related drugs, patients with syncopal migraines, and nursing women **MONITORING** FBG, HbA1C

BROMOCRIPTINE DRUG INTERACTIONS

- Bromocriptine is extensively metabolized by CYP 450 3A4 (substrate); inducers or inhibitors of 3A4 can lower or raise the bromocriptine concentration.

- Do not use with other ergot medications. May increase ergot-related side effects or reduce ergot effectiveness for migraines if co-administered within 6 hours of ergot-related drug.

- Monitor for hypoglycemia if patient is using a sulfonylurea – may need dose adjustment.

INSULIN

The 2009 AACE treatment algorithm recommends against the use of regular human insulin ("R"), and the use of NPH insulin ("N") if possible, in view of the fact that these insulin preparations do not have a sufficiently predictable time course that adequately mimics the normal physiologic profile. As a result, the dose required to control hyperglycemia is often associated with an increased risk of hypoglycemia. Basal and rapid-acting insulins should be chosen instead. [Having said that, R and N formulations are less expensive and are commonly written for by many prescribers.]

RAPID-ACTING, OR "MEAL-TIME" INSULIN: LISPRO *(HUMALOG)*, ASPART *(NOVOLOG)*, GLULISINE *(APIDRA)*

These are injected when the person sits down to eat, or up to 15 minutes prior to eating. They are designed to last for a meal, but can last up to 5 hours. The duration of action is shorter than regular insulin.

Rapid-acting insulin is dosed for the amount of carbohydrates in a meal, or is given on a fixed regimen for typical-sized meals. They are clear and can be mixed with other insulins (not glargine or detemir), but they are usually given by themselves with meals. When they are used as mixtures, they are in the pre-mixed formulations (such as *Novolog 70/30, 75/25, 50/50*). They come in pre-filled injection syringes and in 10 mL vials, and are used in insulin pumps and for sliding scales in hospitals (as is regular insulin).

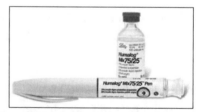

REGULAR OR "SHORT-ACTING" INSULIN: *HUMULIN R, NOVOLIN R*

Regular insulin is usually given as a mixture with the longer-acting NPH (or N) insulin in the mixture NPH/R 70/30. This is 70% NPH, 30% Regular. It is injected 30 minutes before breakfast and dinner. The regular takes ~30 minutes to start to work, which is why the insulin is injected 30 minutes prior to the meal. There is no injection required at lunchtime, because there may be some regular left mid-day, and the NPH will be in effect. Regular insulin lasts 4-6 hours.

In previous days, the regular and NPH were commonly mixed in the same syringe in order to titrate the mixture to control the blood glucose. The regular is drawn up first (the clear insulin) and the NPH (which is cloudy) is drawn up second.

Currently, more people are either using a baseline insulin with oral agents for day-time control, or may be using a "type 1" regimen for tight control: a baseline insulin (such as glargine) with injections of a rapid-acting insulin at meal-times. Regular insulin comes in mixtures (such as *Humulin or Novolin 70/30, 50/50*). The mixtures come in pre-filled injection syringes and in 10 mL vials. Regular insulin (by itself) is usually drawn from a 10 mL vial, or is used in insulin pumps and for sliding scales in hospitals (as are the rapid-acting insulins).

NPH, INTERMEDIATE INSULIN: *HUMULIN N, NOVOLIN N*

This formulation of insulin can last up to 24 hours, but it peaks anywhere from 4-14 hours which can cause hypoglycemic symptoms. If, for example, a patient takes NPH at 7AM, they may get hypoglycemic in the mid-afternoon when they would likely not be taking a meal. This is why the AACE treatment algorithm prefers a basal insulin for long-term control.

BASELINE, 24-HOUR INSULIN: INSULIN GLARGINE *(LANTUS, LANTUS SOLOSTAR)*, INSULIN DETEMIR *(LEVEMIR)*

The baseline insulins are dosed once or twice daily. If dosed once daily, they are usually given at bedtime to ensure no mixing occurs with other insulins (which are usually given at meal times). Insulin glargine has an onset of ~1 hour. Insulin detemir has an onset of ~4 hours. Both last ~24 hours and do not peak. This is important because when insulin peaks, it can cause hypoglycemia. If there is hypoglycemia with a long-acting agent, it can last a long-time and may require re-treatment. Both insulins come in 10 mL vials or can be given by injection pens.

All insulin pens use 3 mL insulin vials and are easier to use and cause less dosing errors, if used correctly. They are easier to use for patients with dexterity problems (arthritis, etc).

INSULIN SIDE EFFECTS

- Hypoglycemia, weight gain, and local skin reactions (to avoid, rotate the injection site). Insulin glargine *(Lantus)* may sting a little when injecting (minor).

INSULIN SLIDING SCALE EXAMPLE

BLOOD SUGAR READING (MG/DL)	INSTRUCTION
BS < 60	Hold insulin; contact MD
150-200	Give 2 units of insulin
201-250	Give 4 units of insulin
251-300	Give 6 units insulin
301-350	Give 8 units of insulin
351-400	Give 10 units of insulin
401-450	Call MD

- Sliding Scales: In the hospital setting, insulin is often dosed as 1-2 baseline injections, plus either regular or rapid-acting insulin, dosed according to a sliding scale. Or, patients can use sliding scales to adjust their own insulin at home.

INSULIN ADMINISTRATION

- Keep unused vials or cartridges in the refrigerator. Vials or pens in current use are good for 30 days at room temperature.

- Do not shake the insulin vial or cartridge; gently roll in the palms to mix the suspension.

- When mixing R or rapid-acting with NPH, inject an equal volume (to the equivalent dose drawn) of air into the vial. Draw the short-acting (clear insulin) 1ˢᵗ, then draw up the NPH.

- The abdomen is the preferred injection site. For alternate sites, see diagram at the end of the chapter. Do not inject within 1 inch of the navel.

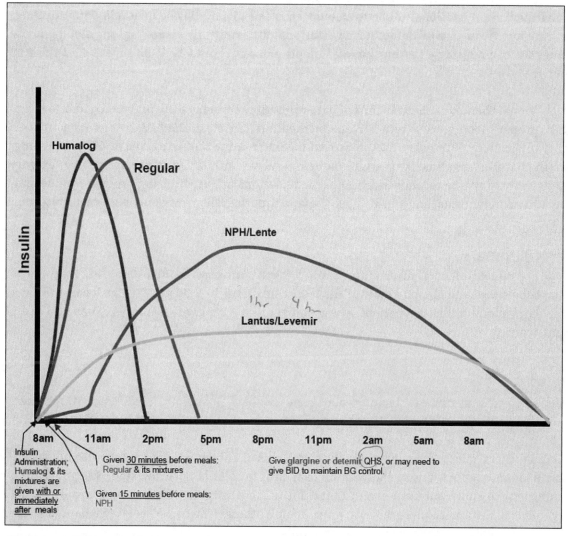

Comparison of Different Insulin Products

- Alternating injection sites around the abdomen should be done regularly to prevent inflammation and atrophy.

- Prior to injecting, clean the injection area (the skin) and the top of the insulin vial (if using) with an alcohol swab. Reduce air bubbles in the syringe.

- To inject subcutaneously, pinch a layer of skin tissue outward and insert the needle at a 90 degree or at a 45 degree (slight) angle. The needle should be inserted between the skin and the muscle tissue.

- Proper needle disposal: Do not break the needle after using because of the risk of poking yourself. There are devices that break off the needle tips for you. Place the needle or entire syringe in an opaque (not clear) heavy-duty plastic (not glass) bottle with a screw cap or a plastic or metal box that closes firmly. These containers can be brought to any proper disposal site (e.g. public health clinic or local needle exchange). Ask the local health department for guidelines or check out the website www.safeneedledisposal.org.

GESTATIONAL DIABETES MELLITUS (GDM)

Treatment for gestational diabetes should keep the blood glucose at levels equal to those of pregnant women who do not have gestational diabetes (this means tighter blood glucose control). In pregnancy, the preprandial blood glucose should be < 95 mg/dL and the A1C should be < 6%.

Nutritional therapy is the standard of care for both the needs of the pregnancy and to maintain proper blood glucose levels. When medication is needed, the ADA recommends insulin therapy. Insulin is the only FDA-approved medication for the treatment of GDM. The long-acting baseline insulins like glargine *(Lantus)* and detemir *(Levemir)* are pregnancy category C and should not be recommended. Other medications are used during pregnancy (like metformin and glyburide) and you will see them in practice. They are not considered first-line.

HYPOGLYCEMIA

Normal fasting blood glucose (in a person without diabetes) is 70-110 mg/dL. Hypoglycemia occurs when the blood glucose falls below this level, or < 70 mg/dL. The lower the level, the more symptomatic the patient. At a blood glucose < 20 mg/dL, seizures, coma and death can occur.

Hypoglycemic Symptoms

Hypoglycemic symptoms include dizziness, headache, anxiety, shakiness, diaphoresis (sweating), hunger, confusion, clumsy or jerky movements, tremors and blurred vision.

Beta blockers can cover up (or mask) the symptoms of shakiness and anxiety (but not sweating or hunger). That is why the beta blocker propranolol is used for stage freight. This is important to know, but keep in mind that this is most notable with the non-cardioselective agents (such as carteolol, carvedilol, propranolol, others). The cardio-selective beta blockers (atenolol, metoprolol) are used more commonly.

Hypoglycemia Treatment

Recommended treatment of hypoglycemia in a conscious individual is <u>15-20 g of rapidly absorbed carbohydrates</u>, which could be: ½ cup (4 oz) of any juice or regular (non-diet) soda, 1 cup (8 oz) milk, 1 tablespoon of sugar or honey, 2 tablespoons of raisins, 4-5 saltine crackers, 3 or 4 glucose tabs, or 1 serving of glucose gel. The blood glucose should be retested 15 minutes after treatment to see if it has reached a safe level. If it has not, the hypoglycemia treatment should be repeated. Once the blood glucose returns to normal, the patient should eat a meal, or a reasonable snack, to prevent recurrence.

Patients often overeat when the blood glucose is low, which causes unnecessary weight gain.

<u>Glucagon is only used if the patient is unconscious.</u> Glucagon 1 mg is given by SC, IM, or IV injection, or glucose can be given intravenously (Dextrose 10%, Dextrose 50%). The patient does not need to be unconscious to receive glucose intravenously.

After treating the low blood glucose, check the BG in 15 minutes. If the BG < 70 mg/dL or if the patient is still symptomatic, repeat the treatment and check the BG again in 15 minutes. All episodes of hypoglycemia are dangerous and should be reported to the physician.

SELF-MONITORING BLOOD GLUCOSE (SMBG)

This is important to prevent hypo- and hyperglycemia, and complications. SMBG should be carried out 3 or more times daily for patients using multiple insulin injections or an insulin pump. For patients using less frequent insulin injections, non-insulin therapies or medical nutrition therapy, SMBG may be useful as a guide to the success of therapy.

Glucometers:

- Some machines require calibration before the 1st use, if a new package of strips is opened, machine is left in extreme conditions, machine is dropped, or if the level does not match how the patient is feeling.

- Check the expiration date of the strip container.

- Close the lid of the strip container after every use, as air and moisture can destroy the strips and affect results.

- Thoroughly wash hands with warm water and mild soap and dry, as wet fingers can affect results and make it harder to form a drop.

- To allow more blood to flow, milk the finger from the base; holding the lanced finger below heart level can also increase blood flow.

- In order to minimize pain, lance the finger at the tips or sides of the fingers where there are fewer nerves, instead of on the finger pads.

- Make sure you have a large enough drop of blood as directed by the meter.

- Clean meter regularly.

- Some meters are approved for testing on other areas, such as lancing the forearm.

- With regards to testing from alternate areas, measurements may be different, such as after meals when BG levels are changing rapidly. A finger may have faster blood flow than other areas. Therefore, alternate testing is best used for fasting BG values.

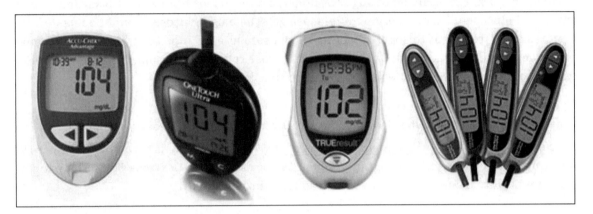

Different Glucometers

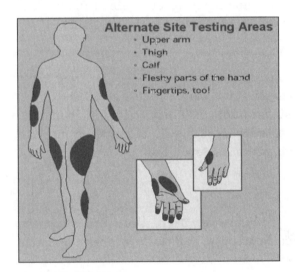

Glucose Testing Sites

Practice Case

Irma is a 44 y/o Hispanic female with dyslipidemia, hypertension and type 2 diabetes. Her father is on dialysis, due to uncontrolled hypertension and diabetes. Her mother and brother have diabetes. Irma is concerned about her family history and wants to "control my sugars better." She has been to a diabetes education class and received instruction in healthy eating and exercise. She has just joined a local exercise club and plans to start soon; until now, she has not had any type of regular physical activity. She has been to the podiatrist and had her feet checked. She has lost some sensation in both feet, but does not have any open cracks or wounds. Her annual vision exam with the ophthalmologist was normal. Her only surgical procedures involved a caesarean section, with sterilization procedure, after the birth of her third child. She does not smoke or drink.

CATEGORY	
Vitals	Blood pressure last visit (1 month ago): 134/74 mmHg, today 136/78 mmHg
	Height 5 feet, 3 inches, weight 152 pounds
Current medications	Metformin extended-release 1,000 mg x 2, with dinner
	Simvastatin 20 mg QHS
	Niacin extended-release 1,000 mg x 2 QHS
	Duloxetine 30 mg BID, for nerve pain in feet
	Amlodipine 10 mg once daily
	Multivitamin daily
Labs	Lipid panel: CH 150, HDL 55, LDL 68, TG 131
	AST 22, ALT 16, BUN/SCr 12/0.8
	Hemoglobin A1C 8.2%
	Urine test for albumin negative

Questions

1. Based on the patient's current hemoglobin A1C, choose the correct statement:

    a. The A1C is elevated; it should be less than 7%, according to the ADA guidelines.

    b. The A1C is elevated; it should be less than 5%, according to the ADA guidelines.

    c. The A1C is well-controlled.

    d. The A1C is a little high, but is acceptable due to her age.

    e. None of the above.

2. The following risk factors for diabetes are present in this patient:

    a. Ethnicity

    b. Overweight

    c. Family history

    d. Low physical activity

    e. All of the above

3. The patient is using niacin therapy. Choose the correct statements:

    a. The use of niacin has likely increased the patient's HDL cholesterol.

    b. Niacin may slightly raise her blood glucose levels.

    c. Niacin extended-release should be taken in the morning, with food.

    d. A and B only.

    e. All of the above.

4. Which microvascular complication of diabetes is present in this patient?

    a. Retinopathy
    b. Nephropathy
    c. Peripheral neuropathy
    d. A and B only
    e. All of the above

5. Irma has brought her fasting blood glucose recordings into the clinic. In the morning before breakfast, she has recorded a range of 111-143 mg/dL. Her postprandial blood glucose (after lunch) recordings have a range of 190-236 mg/dL. Using the American Diabetes Association (ADA) recommendations for blood glucose control, choose the correct statement:

    a. Her morning fasting blood glucose levels are controlled.
    b. Her morning fasting blood glucose levels are not controlled.
    c. Her lunch time postprandial blood glucose levels are not controlled.
    d. A and C
    e. B and C

6. The patient is using amlodipine (*Norvasc*) for hypertension. Choose the correct statement:

    a. She should begin therapy with an ACE Inhibitor (ACE I) or Angiotensin Receptor Blocker (ARB).
    b. Her blood pressure is acceptable; it should be < 140/90 mmHg.
    c. She should try and use the DASH diet (which involves lowering her sodium intake and consuming fresh fruits and vegetables).
    d. A and C only.
    e. B and C only.

7. Irma is not using a daily aspirin therapy. When questioned by the pharmacist, she states she was never told to take aspirin therapy. She has no allergies and no history of GI conditions. Choose the correct advice that should be relayed to Irma:

    a. A daily aspirin would reduce her risk of heart attacks; she should discuss taking aspirin with her doctor.
    b. She does not meet the age criteria for daily aspirin use.
    c. She does not need a daily aspirin because she is female.
    d. B and C only.
    e. None of the above.

8. The physician will begin pioglitazone 30 mg daily. Which of the following statements concerning pioglitazone therapy is correct?

    a. The metformin dose should be increased prior to starting pioglitazone.
    b. The starting dose of pioglitazone should be 4 mg once daily.
    c. Pioglitazone therapy is contraindicated in her due to nerve damage.
    d. Pioglitazone therapy is contraindicated in her due to her weight.
    e. The pioglitazone therapy is appropriate.

9. Irma is using metformin therapy. What is the primary mechanism of action of metformin?

    a. Increases pancreatic insulin secretion
    b. Decreases hepatic glucose output
    c. Increases peripheral insulin sensitivity
    d. Enhances the action of incretins
    e. Alpha glucosidase inhibitor

10. Which of the following medications can cause hypoglycemia?

    a. Insulin
    b. Repaglinide
    c. Glimepiride
    d. A and C only
    e. All of the above

11. A patient has been prescribed *Actoplus Met*. Which would be an acceptable substitution?

    a. Metformin/glipizide

    b. Metformin/glyburide

    c. Metformin/pioglitazone

    d. Glimepiride/pioglitazone

    e. Metformin/repaglinide

ANSWERS

1-a, 2-e, 3-d, 4-c, 5-e, 6-d, 7-b, 8-e, 9-b, 10-e. 11-c

21

THYROID DISORDERS

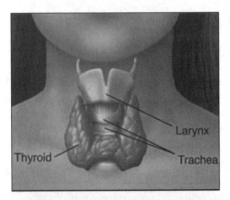

Thyroid

Larynx

Trachea

GUIDELINES

American Association of Clinical Endocrinologists (AACE) Medical Guidelines for Clinical Practice for the Evaluation and Treatment of Hyperthyroidism and Hypothyroidism. Endocrine Practice 2002;8:457-469. (Amended online version 2006)

Background

The thyroid gland is a butterfly-shaped organ composed of two symmetrical lobes which are connected by the isthmus. The thyroid controls how quickly the body burns energy, makes proteins, and controls how sensitive the body should be to other hormones. It is one of the largest organs within the body's endocrine system and is the only organ which contains cells that have the ability to absorb iodine. Hyperthyroidism (overactive thyroid) and hypothyroidism (underactive thyroid) are the most common problems of the thyroid gland. Hypothyroidism is more common (over 10 million in U.S.) and can occur in all age groups.

Pathophysiology

The thyroid produces thyroid hormones, principally thyroxine (T_4) and triiodothyronine (T_3). Iodine and tyrosine are used to form both T_3 and T_4. In a normally functioning system, thyroid-stimulating hormone (TSH) stimulates the secretion of thyroxine (T_4) which is converted to T_3. T_3 is 3-4x more potent than T_4 but has a much shorter half-life. Elevations in T_4 levels will inhibit the secretion of TSH, and a negative feedback loop is created. Since T_3 and T_4 are transported in the blood and bound by proteins, it is important to measure the free T_4 (FT_4) levels as this is the active form. In hypothyroidism, there is a deficiency in T_4, and consequently an elevation in TSH. In hyperthyroidism, there is over-secretion of T_4, and consequently a low level of TSH.

Hypothyroidism

In hypothyroidism, the decrease in thyroid hormone causes the body to slow down and the classic symptoms of low metabolism appear (fatigue, weight gain). The most common cause of hypothyroidism is <u>Hashimoto's disease</u>, an autoimmune condition in which a patient's antibodies attack their own thyroid gland. Drugs can also cause hypothyroidism, most notably <u>lithium and amiodarone</u> – both of which require monitoring of thyroid function tests.

DIAGNOSIS

<u>Low free thyroxine</u> ($\downarrow$ FT_4) (normal range 0.8-1.7 mcg/dL)

<u>High thyroid stimulating hormone</u> ($\uparrow$ TSH) (normal range 0.3 – 3.0 microIU/mL)

MONITORING PARAMETERS

Check free T_4 and TSH levels every 6-8 weeks until levels are normal, then 6 months later, then yearly.

PREGNANCY AND HYPOTHYROIDISM

Levothyroxine is FDA pregnancy category A. Pregnant women with thyroid hormone deficiency or TSH elevation during pregnancy may have children at risk of impairment in their intellectual function and motor skills, unless properly treated. Pregnant women being treated with thyroid hormone replacement will require a 30-50% increase in the levothyroxine dose throughout the course of their pregnancy.

PHARMACOLOGICAL TREATMENT

The goal of therapy is to achieve and maintain a euthyroid (normal) state by both clinical signs and symptoms as well as laboratory values. Counsel the patient regarding clinical symptoms for both hypo and hyperthyroidism – the dose is an estimate and the normal range is wide.

HYPOTHYROIDISM NOTES

Causes of Hypothyroidism
<u>Hashimoto's disease – most common cause</u>

Pituitary failure

Surgical removal of thyroid gland

Thyroid gland ablation with radioactive iodine

External irradiation

Iodine deficiency

<u>Drugs (e.g. lithium, interferon, amiodarone)</u>

Clinical Signs and Symptoms
Cold intolerance

Dry skin

Fatigue

Weight gain

Hoarseness

Coarseness or loss of hair

Heavier than normal menstrual periods

Memory and mental impairment

Goiter (possible)

Myalgias

Hyperlipidemia

Depression

Constipation

Bradycardia

Complications
Cardiovascular disease (cardiomyopathy, HF, hyperlipidemia, CAD)

Goiter

Depression

Infertility

Myxedema – intense cold intolerance, drowsiness, unconsciousness

HYPOTHYROID TREATMENT

DRUG	DOSING	SIDE EFFECTS/CONTRAINDICATIONS/ MONITORING
Levothyroxine (T$_4$) *(Synthroid, Levothroid, Levoxyl, Unithroid, Tirosint, Levo-T)* Check AB-rating of a generic to a brand. Not all generic levothyroxine formulations are AB-rated to various brands. If you change formulations, check signs and symptoms and levels in 6-8 weeks.	25, 50, 75, 88, 100, 112, 125, 137, 150, 175, 200, 300 mcg Start 12.5-25 mcg/day in elderly patients or those with cardiac disease. Younger patients can be started on a higher dose (50 mcg/day or more) Take on an empty stomach, 30 minutes before breakfast, with a full glass of water Usual dosing range: 0.5 mcg/kg/day for elderly 1.7 mcg/kg/day in younger patients (< 50 years of age) **TABLETS** 25 mcg – orange 50 mcg – white 75 mcg – violet 88 mcg – olive 100 mcg – yellow 112 mcg – rose 125 mcg – brown 137 mcg – turquoise 150 mcg – blue 175 mcg – lilac 200 mcg – pink 300 mcg – green	Levothyroxine is preferred over the other agents because of once-daily dosing, is inexpensive, and has more uniform potency **BLACK BOX WARNING** Thyroid supplements are ineffective and potentially toxic when used for weight loss or obesity in euthyroid patients. High doses can produce serious and life-threatening effects **SIDE EFFECTS** If patient is euthyroid, no side effects should exist. If dose is too high, patient will experience hyperthyroid symptoms such as ↑ HR, palpitations, sweating, weight loss, arrhythmias and irritability **CONTRAINDICATIONS** Acute MI, thyrotoxicosis, uncorrected adrenal insufficiency **MONITORING** Check TSH and clinical symptoms every 6-8 weeks, until normalized Pregnancy Category A Highly protein bound (> 99%) **Levothyroxine IV** Must be give upon reconstitution. IV to PO ratio = 1:2
Thyroid USP (T$_3$ and T$_4$) (Armour Thyroid)	60-120 mg daily (usual dose)	**Thyroid USP** Natural porcine-derived thyroid that contains both T$_3$ and T$_4$; less predictable potency and stability. Not preferred, but some feel better using it **Liothyronine** Shorter t ½ leading to fluctuations in T$_3$ levels
Liothyronine (T$_3$) (Cytomel, Triostat)	25-75 mcg daily (usual dose)	
Liotrix (T$_3$ and T$_4$ in 1:4 ratio) (Thyrolar)	60-120 mcg daily (usual dose)	

DRUG INTERACTIONS

The following medications decrease thyroid hormone absorption or levels:

- Cholestyramine, calcium, magnesium, aluminum (antacids), iron supplements, sucralfate, sodium polystyrene (SPS, *Kayexalate)*, orlistat *(Xenical, Alli)*, chromium: all ↓ absorption so separate doses by 2 hours before or 4 hours after

- Estrogen and hepatic inducers (e.g. phenytoin, rifampin, carbamazepine, phenobarbital): ↓ thyroid hormone levels

- Beta-blockers, amiodarone, steroids, and PTU may decrease the effect of levothyroxine by decreasing the conversion of T_4 to T_3

Thyroid hormone can change concentrations/effects of these drugs:

- ↑ effect of anticoagulants (e.g. increased PT/INR with warfarin)

- ↓ digoxin levels

- ↓ theophylline levels

- ↓ effect of antidiabetic agents

PATIENT COUNSELING FOR LEVOTHYROXINE

- Levothyroxine is a replacement for a hormone that is normally produced by your body to regulate your energy and metabolism. Levothyroxine is given when the thyroid does not produce enough of this hormone on its own.

- There are many other medicines that can affect levothyroxine; tell the pharmacist about all medications you are taking. This includes over-the-counter vitamins, supplements and heartburn medicines.

- Different brands of levothyroxine may not work the same. If you get a prescription refill and your new pills look different, ask the pharmacist.

- This medicine is safe to use while you are pregnant. It is also safe to use while you are breast-feeding a baby. It does pass into breast milk, but it is not harmful to a nursing infant.

- Tell your doctor if you become pregnant during treatment; it is likely that your dose will need to be increased during pregnancy or if you plan to breast-feed.

- Take on an empty stomach with a full glass of water 30 minutes before breakfast.

- Some patients will notice a slight reduction in symptoms within 1 to 2 weeks, but the full metabolic response to thyroid hormone therapy is often delayed for a month or two before people start to feel completely normal.

- Even if you feel well, you may still need to take this medicine every day for the rest of your life to replace the thyroid hormone your body cannot produce.

- To be sure this medication is helping your condition, your blood will need to be tested on a regular basis (at least annually).

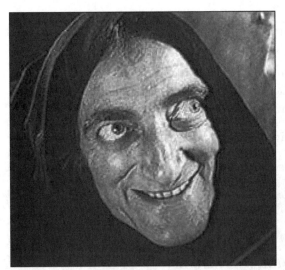

Hyperthyroidism (Thyrotoxicosis)

Hyperthyroidism (overactive thyroid) occurs when there is over-production of thyroid hormone. Instead of low FT_4 and high TSH, you have <u>high FT_4 and low TSH</u> and nearly opposite symptoms. Hyperthyroidism can significantly accelerate the metabolism, causing sudden weight loss, a rapid or irregular heartbeat, sweating, nervousness, irritability, diarrhea and insomnia. Goiter and exopthalmus can occur. Without treatment, hyperthyroidism can lead to tachycardia, arrhythmias, heart failure and osteoporosis. No one should be using thyroid hormone to lose weight – they will be irritable (obnoxious) and can end up with severe cardiac complications. Interestingly, older cats often get hyperthyroidism (more frequently than dogs) and pharmacists occasionally fill scripts for patients with names like Kitty.

HYPERTHYRODISM NOTES

Clinical Signs and Symptoms

Heat intolerance or increased sweating

Weight loss (or gain)

Agitation, nervousness, irritability

Palpitations and tachycardia

Fatigue and muscle weakness

Frequent bowel movements or diarrhea

Insomnia

Light or absent menstrual periods

Goiter (possible)

Tremor

Exopthalmos (exophthalmia), diplopia

CAUSES

The most common cause of hyperthyroidism is <u>Graves' disease</u>, which tends to occur in females in their 30's and 40's. Graves' disease is an autoimmune disorder (like Hashimoto's) but instead of destroying the gland, the antibodies stimulate the thyroid to produce too much T_4. Less commonly, a single nodule is responsible for the excess hormone secretion. Thyroiditis (inflammation of the thyroid) can also cause hyperthyroidism. <u>Drugs that can cause hyperthyroidism include iodide, amiodarone and interferons</u>. Hyperthyroidism can also occur in patients who take excessive doses of any of the available forms of thyroid hormone.

Treatment involves medications or destroying part of the gland via radioactive iodine (RAI-131) or surgery. <u>RAI-131 is the treatment of choice in Graves' Disease</u>. With any option, the patient can be treated with beta blockers first for symptom control (to reduce palpitations, tremor and tachycardia). PTU or methimazole can be used as a temporary measure until surgery is complete.

HYPERTHYROID TREATMENT

DRUG	DOSING	SIDE EFFECTS/CONTRAINDICATIONS/MONITORING

Thionamides - inhibit synthesis of thyroid hormones by blocking the oxidation of iodine in the thyroid gland; PTU also inhibits peripheral conversion of T_4 to T_3

DRUG	DOSING	SIDE EFFECTS/CONTRAINDICATIONS/MONITORING
Propylthiouracil (PTU) (*Propyl-Thyracil*)	50 mg Q8-12H (maintenance dose); initial doses may be higher	**BLACK BOX WARNING** PTU – can cause liver damage and acute liver failure **SIDE EFFECTS** GI upset, rash, itching, fever Hepatitis, agranulocytosis (rare): be se MD at once if develop yellow skin, high fever, or severe sore throat. **MONITORING** CBC, LFTs, and thyroid function tests every 4-6 weeks until euthyroid
Methimazole (*Tapazole*)	5-20 mg daily (maintenance dose); initial doses may be higher	Pregnancy Category D - PTU for women trying to conceive or in 1st trimester – change to methimazole for 2nd and 3rd trimesters PTU is preferred in thyroid storm Take with food to reduce GI upset

Iodides - Inhibit secretion of thyroid hormone; T_4 and T_3 levels will be reduced for several weeks but effect will not be maintained

DRUG	DOSING	SIDE EFFECTS/CONTRAINDICATIONS/MONITORING
Potassium Iodide and Iodine solution (*Lugol's solution*)	4-8 drops Q8H	Do not use in breast-feeding, pregnancy (Pregnancy Category D) **SIDE EFFECTS** Rash, metallic taste, sore throat/gums, GI upset **MONITORING** Thyroid function tests Take with food to reduce GI upset
Saturated solution of potassium iodide (SSKI)	4-5 drops Q8H	

Thyroid Storm

Thyroid storm is rare but serious and can happen in patients with hyperthyroidism due to a particularly stressful event (infection, MI, diabetes, childbirth) and occasionally due to lack of treatment. It can also be due to extreme emotional stress. Thyroid storm can be fatal; patients with hyperthyroidism will need to try and live as stress-free as possible and should be able to recognize the symptoms of thyroid storm. They should understand that this is a medical emergency.

THYROID STORM NOTES
Clinical Signs and Symptoms
Fever (> 103 degrees Fahrenheit)
Tachycardia (> 140 BPM)
Tachypnea
Profuse sweating
Agitation
Psychosis
Coma

TREATMENTS

- PTU 900-1,200 mg PO daily (divided into every 4-6 hrs) PLUS

  - Can crush tablets and administer through NG-tube if needed

  - Given 30 minutes before iodine to block synthesis of thyroid hormone

- SSKI 3-5 drops PO Q8H or Lugol's solution 5-10 drops PO Q8H PLUS

- Propranolol 40-80 mg PO Q6H PLUS

- Dexamethasone 2-4 mg PO Q6H

- Consider other supportive treatments (e.g. antiarrhythmics, insulin, fluids, electrolytes, etc.)

Practice Case

MT is a 45 year old female who comes to the clinic complaining of more fatigue than normal and constipation. On exam, you notice the patient has some dry skin patches and looks a bit depressed. Her past medical history is significant for GERD for which she takes *Dexilant* 30 mg daily and *Maalox*. You order some blood work and it is reported below.

CATEGORY	
Vitals	BP 139/82 mmHg, HR 62 BPM, Temp. 38.0, RR 15 BPM
Labs	TSH: 44 microIU/mL (normal range 0.3 – 3.0 microIU/mL)
	Free T_4: 0.5 mcg/dL (normal range 0.8-1.7 mcg/dL)

QUESTIONS

1. The physician is considering starting thyroid medication for MT. Which of the following options is considered most appropriate for initial therapy?

    a. *Levoxyl*
    b. *Armour Thyroid*
    c. *Thyrolar*
    d. RAI 131
    e. Propranolol

2. What is a reasonable starting dose of Synthroid?

    a. 25 mcg daily
    b. 25 mg daily
    c. 75 mg daily
    d. 150 mcg daily
    e. 2.5 mg daily

3. Which of the following medications can decrease the levels of levothyroxine?

    a. Magnesium-Aluminum hydroxide (Maalox)
    b. Iron
    c. Warfarin
    d. A and B only
    e. A, B, and C

4. Propylthiouracil is associated with which of the following serious adverse effects?

    a. Pregnancy
    b. Liver failure
    c. Renal failure
    d. Rhabdomyolysis
    e. Priapism

5. What is the most common cause of hypothyroidism?

    a. Graves' disease
    b. Hashimoto's disease
    c. Surgery
    d. Amiodarone
    e. Lithium

6. A patient is beginning levothyroxine therapy. Patient counseling points should include the following:

    a. You should feel all better by this afternoon or tomorrow morning.
    b. Your doctor will need to recheck your thyroid hormone levels in 6-8 weeks.
    c. If you get pregnant, stop using this medicine.
    d. A and C only.
    e. All of the above.

7. Which of the following are symptoms of hypothyroidism?

    a. Fatigue
    b. Weight gain or increased difficulty losing weight
    c. Diarrhea
    d. A and B only
    e. All of the above

8. The pharmacist should instruct the patient to take levothyroxine in this manner:

    a. The first thing in the morning, with food
    b. The first thing in the morning, about 30 minutes before food or other medicines
    c. With the largest meal to reduce nausea
    d. With dinner since levothyroxine is sedating
    e. At bedtime

9. A pregnant female is being started on levothyroxine therapy. Levothyroxine has the following pregnancy rating:

    a. Pregnancy Category A
    b. Pregnancy Category B
    c. Pregnancy Category C
    d. Pregnancy Category D
    e. Pregnancy Category X

10. What is the most common cause of hyperthyroidism?

    a. Hashimoto's disease
    b. Pituitary failure
    c. Lithium
    d. Amiodarone
    e. Graves' disease

ANSWERS

1-a, 2-a, 3-d, 4-b, 5-b, 6-b, 7-d, 8-b, 9-a, 10-e

OSTEOPOROSIS & HORMONE THERAPY

Background

Osteoporosis, which means "porous bones," causes bones to become weak and brittle. Falls can cause a bone to fracture. If the bones are extremely porous, coughing or rolling over in bed can cause fractures. The most common location of a fracture is the lower (lumbar) spine. These vertebrae turn over more rapidly (higher rate of cell turnover) than hip bones, and are holding the weight of the upper spine and head.

Hip fractures occur with more severe disease (or bad falls) and can be debilitating. A hip fracture in a woman has a 25% risk of mortality at one year, and is higher in men, since men with osteoporosis are often using long-term steroids or androgen blockers and may be sicker at baseline. Hip fractures, if not fatal, can lead to loss of independence and/or chronic pain. Wrist fracture, which appears often in younger woman, may be an early warning sign of poor bone health.

Diagnosis/Definitions

Osteoporosis is defined by a T-score <-2.5. Osteopenia is lower bone density than normal, but not as low as osteoporosis. Osteopenia is defined by a T-score between -1 and -2.5.

Notice that the scores are negative; a T-score from -1 and higher indicates normal bone density. A higher number correlates with stronger (denser) bones, which are less likely to fracture. The T-score is calculated by comparing the woman's bone mineral density (BMD) to the average peak BMD of a normal, young adult of the same gender.

Osteoblasts are the cells involved in bone formation, and osteoclasts break-down bone. Bone is not "dead tissue"; it is living and constantly remodels, although some types of bone re-models very slowly, and others remodel at a faster rate. The older medications (estrogen, raloxifene, bisphosphonates) slow down bone break-down, or resorption. Newer agents that both prevent bone break-down and help to build-bone are the strongest agents and are re-served for higher-risk patients.

A bone scan is performed by a dual energy x-ray absorptiometry (DEXA, or DXA) scan. The results are reported for several high-risk locations, including hips and the lumbar vertebrae. Ultrasound devices are not optimal, yet they are less expensive and do not emit radiation. An ultrasound reading provides bone density in one location, such as the heel. An ultrasound reading, if low, should encourage the patient to get a DEXA scan.

PHASES OF BONE LOSS

Bone accumulates until approximately age 30. After that, the initial phase of bone loss occurs throughout life. Men lose bone at a rate of 0.2-0.5% per year, unless they use drugs that accelerate bone loss (such as long-term steroids) or prostate cancer agents. Women lose bone slowly after peak bone growth, and then at an increased rate in the 10 years from menopause (1-5% bone loss per year) and then at a slower rate thereafter.

Factors that put a patient at increased fall risk include impaired vision, dementia, poor health/frailty, low physical activity and a history of recent falls.

Calcium Supplementation

All prescription medicines for low bone density require adequate calcium and vitamin D supplementation taken concurrently. Dietary intake of calcium should be assessed first, and supplements used if insufficient. Over half of the US population has low calcium and vitamin D intake. Adequate calcium intake is required throughout life, and is critically important in children (who can build bone stores), in pregnancy (when the fetus can deplete the mother's stores if intake is insufficient) and during the years around menopause, when bone loss is rapid. Vitamin D is required for calcium absorption, and low levels contribute to various health conditions, including autoimmune conditions and cancer. In 2010 there were news reports that calcium supplementation may increase heart attack risk; at present, recommend that patients use the recommended levels and use calcium with vitamin D – the increased risk was seen in patients who did not use vitamin D with calcium.

RISK FACTORS FOR LOW BONE DENSITY

Advanced age

Low bone mineral density (usually evidenced by the T-score)

Previous fracture as an adult (other than skull, facial bone, ankle, finger and toe)

More than 2 alcoholic drinks per day

Oral or IM glucocorticoid use (such as prednisone) for > 3 months at a dose of 7.5 mg prednisone (or equivalent) daily or higher

Body weight < 127 pounds or low BMI < 21 kg/m²

Calcium and vitamin D – low intake over life span

Smoking

DRUGS AND OSTEOPOROSIS RISK

Steroid use, long-term, is the major drug-contributing factor to poor bone health. Other medications that lower bone density include:

Anticonvulsants (carbamazepine, fosphenytoin, phenobarbital, phenytoin, primidone)

Warfarin and heparin

Excess thyroid hormone

Loop diuretics

Aromatase inhibitors used for breast CA

Androgen blockers used for prostate CA

Proton pump inhibitors used chronically (↓ calcium absorption due to ↓ gastric pH)

NIH'S RECOMMENDED ADEQUATE INTAKES (AIs) FOR CALCIUM (2010)

AGE	MALE	FEMALE	PREGNANT	LACTATING
0-6 months	210 mg	210 mg		
7-12 months	270 mg	270 mg		
1-3 years	500 mg	500 mg		
4-8 years	800 mg	800 mg		
9-13 years	1,300 mg	1,300 mg		
14-18 years	1,300 mg	1,300 mg	1,300 mg	1,300 mg
19-50 years	1,000 mg	1,000 mg	1,000 mg	1,000 mg
50+ years	1,200 mg	1,200 mg		

NOTES ON CALCIUM SELECTION & ABSORPTION

- Calcium absorption is saturable; doses should be divided.

- Dietary calcium is generally not sufficient; most women need an additional 600-900 mg/day (2 to 3 dairy portions) to reach recommended levels.

- Calcium requires vitamin D for absorption (see below).

- Calcium citrate *(Citracal*, etc) has better absorption but is a larger pill to swallow and can be taken with or without food; usually tab has 315 mg calcium. It may be preferable with little or no stomach acid – such as with the use of PPIs, which have been shown to increase fracture risk due to impaired calcium carbonate absorption (including the dietary calcium.)

- Calcium carbonate *(Oscal, Tums*, etc) has acid-dependent absorption and should be taken with meals; usually tab is 500-600 mg.

- There is no known benefit of using more expensive formulations – recommend products made by reputable manufacturers, since lead may be present in untested products.

- Both forms come as chewables and in food products.

VITAMIN D SUPPLEMENTATION

- The NIH's recommended intake for vitamin D for people up to age 70 years is 600 IU daily, and 71+ years is 800 IU daily. However, these levels are currently controversial and many endocrinologists are recommending a higher intake of 800-2,000 IU daily. This is based on the recognition that low vitamin D levels is associated with a variety of health conditions – and the fact that many Americans have low vitamin D levels. A few years ago vitamin D levels were not routinely ordered; this has become commonplace.

- The 50,000 unit vitamin D2 supplement (the green capsules) are used in renal disease or short-term in adults with deficiency to replenish stores. Cholecalciferol, or vitamin D3, is the preferred source, although vitamin D2 is often the type in supplements and will provide benefit.

Drug Treatment

Osteoporosis is usually treated with medications, weight-resistant exercise (such as walking) and adequate calcium and vitamin D. Osteopenia should be treated with exercise and calcium and vitamin D, and sometimes, with prescription medications. The decision to use prescription therapy in osteopenia depends on the fracture risk. If a person stays upright, they are at lower risk for fracture than someone who has falls. Any medication or condition that puts the patient at risk for falls (dizziness, mental confusion, gait imbalance) may provide a rationale for prescription therapy. There are calculators that consider the risk factors and estimate the likelihood of major fractures. These can be used to help determine the need for prescription therapy.

Bisphosphonates are used first-line in most patients. They increase bone density more than estrogen and raloxifene, and reduce fracture risk. Teriparatide injection *(Forteo)* is used in patients with osteoporosis who are at high risk for having fractures, or have already had an osteoporotic fracture, or have OP and need to take long-term steroids, or who cannot tolerate bisphosphonates. The newer agent denosumab *(Prolia)* is difficult to administer (it must be given in a doctor's office) and is expensive; it is also reserved for those with high risk.

Estrogen is no longer used first-line for osteoporosis because of health risks. However, if used for menopausal symptoms, estrogen does increase bone density. Raloxifene is used most commonly in women who are at risk or have fear of breast cancer. Calcitonin is used less often than in previous years since the evidence of benefit for bone density improvement is poor.

OSTEOPOROSIS TREATMENT & PREVENTION OPTIONS

DRUG	DOSING	SIDE EFFECTS/MONITORING/ CONTRAINDICATIONS

Bisphosphonates work by inhibiting osteoclast activity

DRUG	DOSING	SIDE EFFECTS/MONITORING/CONTRAINDICATIONS
Alendronate *(Fosamax)* Bisphosphonates are 1st line for most patients	5 mg daily prevention; 10 mg daily treatment 70 mg weekly alone or with vit D3 2,800 or 5,600 IU (cholecalciferol) or 35 mg weekly for prevention 70 mg/75 mL solution – after drink at least 2 oz plain water (tablets need to be taken with 6-8 oz of plain water)	**SIDE EFFECTS** Back pain, arthralgias, dyspepsia, N/V, dysphagia, heartburn, esophagitis (may ↑ esophageal cancer risk long-term) Possible risk of jaw decay/necrosis – get dental work done before starting therapy Risk atypical femur fracture with long-term use; consider stopping after 5 years of therapy (and continue to monitor bone loss), however, if high risk may continue with therapy **CONTRAINDICATIONS** Inability to stand or sit upright for at least 30 minutes (60 minutes with once-monthly *Boniva*)
Risedronate *(Actonel)* *Actonel + Calcium:* 35 mg weekly and Ca²⁺ carb 500 mg x 6 days *Atelvia* is long-acting risedronate that is taken after breakfast. Useful if nausea taking bisphosph on an empty stomach.	5 mg daily, or 35 mg weekly or 75 mg on 2 consecutive days/month 150 mg/once monthly	Hypocalcemia Severe renal impairment Esophageal problems: esophageal ulcer risk Note: with *Atelvia*, no H₂RAs or PPIs. Separate calcium, iron and magnesium supplements (separate time)
Ibandronate *(Boniva)*	150 mg monthly Also available as 2.5 mg daily and 3 mg IV every 3 months.	

Injectable Bisphosphonate

DRUG	DOSING	SIDE EFFECTS/MONITORING/CONTRAINDICATIONS
Zoledronic Acid *(Reclast)* Treatment and prevention OP, Paget's Do not use with *Zometa* (same drug)	5 mg infusion yearly (chemo dose is 4 mg)	**SIDE EFFECTS** No GI problems (bypasses gut), but can cause all others, and TPS (transient post-dose syndrome) in 25-40% of patients on days 2-3 post-injection: flu-like symptoms such as achiness, runny nose, HA. Taking NSAIDs prior and afterwards can ↓ symptoms Do not use in patients with CrCl < 35 mL/min

Osteoporosis Treatment & Prevention Options Continued

DRUG	DOSING	SIDE EFFECTS/MONITORING/ CONTRAINDICATIONS

Raloxifene is a Selective Estrogen Receptor Modulator (SERM) and ↓ bone resorption

Raloxifene *(Evista)* Used often in women at risk (or have fear of) breast CA	60 mg daily Favorable lipid effects (↓ CH and LDL; no effect on HDL and TGs)	**SIDE EFFECTS** Hot flashes, N/V, edema, flushing, HTN, mood changes, amenorrhea, vaginal bleeding/ discharge, skin changes **CONTRAINDICATIONS** Black Box Warning - ↑ risk of thromboembolic events (DVT, PE, MI, stroke) AVOID if risk of blood clots Pregnancy, severe hepatic dysfunction or previous thromboembolism

Calcitonin Nasal Spray and Injection – inhibits osteoclastic bone resorption

Calcitonin *(Miacalcin, Fortical)*	Inhale 1 spray (200 IU) daily (alternate nostril daily)	**SIDE EFFECTS** Rhinitis and other nose irritation effects Dizziness, flu-like symptoms, dyspepsia Possible antibody development to salmon

Teriparatide Injection – stimulates new bone formation and depresses osteoclast activity

Teriparatide *(Forteo)* For patients who are at very high risk for fracture, or who have already had a fracture due to osteoporosis, or for GIO, or if cannot take other medications	20 mcg SC inj daily for max of 2 years If bone pain with bisphosphonates it is less risky (although painful) than with teriparatide; bone pain from this drug could be bone cancer	**SIDE EFFECTS** Dizziness, ↑ HR (especially with 1st few doses), injection site pain, HA, asthenia, arthralgia, rhinitis Mild or transient increase in serum calcium (between 4-16 hours post-dose), ↑ uric acid **CAUTIONS/CONTRAINDICATIONS** Caution in Paget's disease, prior skeletal radiation, bone metastases, and hypercalcemia due to risk of osteosarcoma (Black Box Warning)

Monoclonal Antibody Injectable – binds to nuclear factor-kappa ligand (RANKL) and preventing interaction between RANKL and RANK, preventing osteoclast formation; leads to decreased bone resorption and increased bone mass

Denosumab *(Prolia, Xgeva)* High risk only	60 mg SC inj (in MD's office) every 6 months	Hypocalcemia-check levels prior to using drug Higher risk various infections **SIDE EFFECTS** Anemia, nausea, abdominal pain, risk jaw necrosis

BISPHOSPHONATE COUNSELING

- Take first thing in the morning <u>before you eat or drink anything else except 6-8 ounces</u> (1 cup) of plain water. If you are using formulations that are not once daily (such as weekly), choose the day of the week that is easy to remember (such as Sunday if you going to church, or bridge day, etc.)

- Take the medicine while you are <u>sitting up or standing and stay upright for at least 30 minutes (60 minutes with monthly *Boniva)*</u>. During this time, you cannot eat or drink anything else except more plain water. You cannot take any other medicines or vitamins. Nothing but plain water!

- This medicine must be <u>swallowed whole</u>, and washed down with the water. Do not crush or chew the tablet or keep it in your mouth to melt or dissolve.

- <u>This medicine does not work well if you are not taking enough calcium and vitamin D.</u> Some formulations contain calcium or vitamin D. Discuss with your pharmacist if you need to use calcium or vitamin D supplements.

- If you are using a proton pump inhibitor for heartburn, discuss with your pharmacist. <u>These drugs may increase fracture risk</u>. You may need to use a calcium citrate tablet, with adequate vitamin D.

- Your bone and muscle strength will improve faster if you are doing <u>exercise</u>. Your physician should discuss with you safe and healthy ways to exercise.

- <u>Common side effects include GI upset, joint pain, back pain, dyspepsia or heartburn.</u>

- <u>Stop taking the medicine if</u> you develop difficult or painful swallowing, have chest pain, have very bad heartburn that doesn't get better, or have severe pain in the bones, joints or muscles.

- Some patients have developed serious <u>jaw-bone problems</u> after using this medicine, which may include infection and slower healing after teeth are pulled. Tell your healthcare providers, including your dentist, right away if you have these symptoms. If you have dental work due now, you should have it done before starting the medicine.

Atelvia: This is a long-acting form of risedronate. Take the medicine <u>after breakfast</u>. Sit or stand upright for thirty minutes or longer after taking. <u>Do not use</u> acid suppressing "heartburn" therapy with this medicine. Do not take Calcium, iron, magnesium or multivitamin supplements until later in the day.

MISSED DOSES

- If on weekly schedule and missed one dose, take the following morning (but not 2 doses in 1 day)

- If on daily schedule missed one dose, skip until next dose

- If on monthly *Boniva* and miss a dose, take it as soon as you remember (in the morning before eating) except if it is less than one week to the next dose, skip it (can't take 2 doses in one week.)

For *Reclast* Injection

- Make sure patient is not using *Zometa* (used for hypercalcemia of malignancy) since it is the same drug. Immediately after injection, low serum calcium can occur. This is aggravated if on aminoglycosides, and these should not be used concurrently.

- It is necessary to take 1,500 mg calcium in divided doses (2-3 doses daily) for the 2 weeks after the injection and 1,200 mg the rest of the year, and 800 IU vitamin D throughout the year.

TERIPARATIDE COUNSELING

- Please read the Medication Guide. During the drug testing process, *Forteo* caused some rats to develop a bone cancer called osteosarcoma. Osteosarcoma has been reported rarely in people who took *Forteo*. The warning states that it is not known if people who use *Forteo* have a higher chance of getting osteosarcoma.

- You may feel dizzy or have a fast heartbeat after the first few doses. In case you experience these symptoms, inject this medication where you can sit or lie down right away if necessary.

- Inform your doctor if you develop bone or joint pain.

- The medicine comes in a prefilled SC injection pen that lasts 28 days. Each injection provides a 20-mcg dose. You should change the needle each day.

- The pen should be kept in the refrigerator and re-capped after each use. After 28 days, the pen should be discarded even if some medicine remains. There is a place at the end of the patient's user manual to mark the date when the pen is started and the date (28 days later) when the pen should be thrown away.

- Inject one time each day in your thigh or abdomen (lower stomach area). The injection sites must be rotated.

- Do not transfer the medicine from the delivery device to a syringe. The injection pen is set at the right dose and does not require any dose adjustment.

- You can inject at any time of the day. Take it at about the same time each day.

- If you forget or cannot take the medicine at your usual time, take it as soon as you can on that day. Do not take more than one injection in the same day.

- Do not exceed 2 years of use.

- This medicine does not work well if you are not taking enough calcium and vitamin D. Some formulations contain calcium or vitamin D. Discuss with your pharmacist if you need to use calcium or vitamin D supplements.

- If you are using a proton pump inhibitor for heartburn, discuss with your pharmacist. These drugs may increase fracture risk. You may need to use a calcium citrate tablet, with adequate vitamin D.

CALCITONIN NASAL SPRAY COUNSELING

- This medicine is sprayed in one nostril daily. The other nostril is used the following day.

- A common side effect you may experience are nasal symptoms, including nasal irritation.

- Keep unused bottles in the refrigerator, but not the one being used. When a new bottle is removed it should be allowed to reach room temperature prior to priming. To prime the pump, hold the bottle upright and press the 2 white side arms toward the bottle until a faint spray is seen. Once the pump is primed, it does not have to be re-primed if the bottle is stored in an upright position.

- Before using, allow the product to reach room temperature.

- To use the nasal spray, remove the protective cap, keep head upright and insert the tip into a nostril. Press down firmly on the pump to deliver the medication. Use the other nostril the next day.

- After 30 doses, the pump may not deliver the correct amount of medicine with each spray and should be discarded.

- The bottle should last for 30 doses (even though there may still be product in the bottle after 30 days, subsequent sprays may not deliver full doses). Store the bottle you are using at room temperature and store extra bottles in the refrigerator.

- This medicine does not work well if you are not taking enough calcium and vitamin D. Some formulations contain calcium or vitamin D. Discuss with your pharmacist if you need to use calcium or vitamin D supplements.

- If you are using a proton pump inhibitor for heartburn, discuss with your pharmacist. These drugs may increase fracture risk. You may need to use a calcium citrate tablet, with adequate vitamin D.

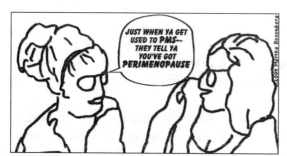

HORMONE THERAPY (HT)

HT is used for women who are in the peri-menopause, or what is commonly referred to as menopause (menopause technically means that menses has ceased for 12 months.) Peri-menopause normally occurs between the ages of 45 and 55. Many women experience vaso-motor symptoms as their ovaries produces less estrogen. A decrease in estrogen causes an increase in luteinizing hormone (LH), which can result in hot flashes and night sweats (hot flashes that occur during sleep). Sleep can be disturbed, and mood changes may be present. Due to a decline in estrogen in the vaginal mucosa, vaginal dryness, burning and painful intercourse may be present.

Some women remain largely asymptomatic during menopause. In others the symptoms can be quite bothersome. Women who have had their ovaries removed, or are receiving anti-estrogen therapy for cancer may experience similar symptoms, but more acutely initially due to a sudden, rather than gradual, estrogen decline.

The most effective therapy for vasomotor symptoms is estrogen, which causes a decrease in LH and more stable temperature control. Estrogen improves bone density and has historically been used to prevent postmenopausal osteoporosis. Estrogen is not a strong enough bone density agent to be used for treatment. Natural products used for vasomotor symptoms include black cohosh, red clover, soy and evening primrose.

In women with a uterus, estrogen should not be given alone. This will put the woman at elevated risk for endometrial cancer – the risk is 5 times higher if using estrogen alone for 3+ years. In practice, progestins can cause mood disturbances in some women, and a woman and her doctor may decide to use estrogen alone, with regular uterine exams. This should not be considered standard therapy.

HORMONE USE HAS HEALTH RISKS – SOME OF WHICH ARE CURRENTLY NOT WELL-DEFINED

Several years ago the data from large trials on hormone therapy became available – these were the Women's Health Initiative (WHI) postmenopausal hormone therapy trials. At first, the news was scary and led to several black box warnings on the use of HT, which including warnings for increased risk of stroke, heart attacks and probable risk of dementia.

As the data was reanalyzed, it became apparent that the majority of risk was highest in older women. At this point there are no clear guidelines as to what age hormones are safest, nor are there useful recommendations available on how to choose specific dosages or formulations.

Many women continue to use the same hormones that were used in the trials. These include *Premarin* (made from conjugated equine estrogens, or CEE), and CEE plus a synthetic progesterone, typically *Prempro* (with medroxyprogesterone acetate, or MPA). Many women are now using estradiol products, such as the generic formulations (often with MPA in women with a uterus) or in brand patches (such as *Vivelle Dot)* and others. Many women and their prescribers feel that the hormone estradiol is safer – since estradiol is produced naturally in (pre-menopausal) women and it was hormone from pregnant mares urine (from female horses) that was used in the WHI trials. Some women find relief with bioidentical hormone replacement therapy (BHRT) that is often compounded specifically for them.

The warnings for HT therapy are based on the analysis of the WHI data and do not distinguish between hormone type. In the future, when more information is available, these warnings should be refined. At present it is safest to assume these warnings apply to all products, although risk appears to be highest among older women:

■ Estrogens increase the risk of endometrial cancer (the warning notes that there is no evidence that "natural" estrogens are safer).

■ The WHI study reported increased risks of myocardial infarction, stroke, invasive breast cancer, pulmonary emboli, and deep vein thrombosis in postmenopausal women (50 to 79 years of age), during 5 years of treatment with oral conjugated estrogens (CE 0.625 mg) combined with medroxyprogesterone acetate (MPA 2.5 mg), relative to placebo. Some data suggest that the risk of heart disease decreases when taken in the early postmenopausal years (in younger women). This is currently being studied in the KEEPS trial.

- The Women's Health Initiative Memory Study (WHIMS), a sub-study of WHI, reported increased risk of developing probable dementia in postmenopausal women 65 years of age or older during 4 years of treatment with oral conjugated estrogens plus medroxyprogesterone acetate, relative to placebo. It is unknown whether this finding applies to younger postmenopausal women or to women taking estrogen alone therapy.

The warning concludes that "other doses of oral conjugated estrogens with medroxyprogesterone acetate, and other combinations and dosage forms of estrogens and progestins were not studied in the WHI clinical trials and, in the absence of comparable data, these risks should be assumed to be similar. Because of these risks, estrogens with or without progestins should be prescribed at the lowest effective doses and for the shortest duration consistent with treatment goals and risks for the individual woman."

In 2010 there were new concerns about cancer risk (particularly lung cancer) in women using estrogen plus a progestin.

Estrogen in any form has the following contraindications:

- Undiagnosed abnormal genital bleeding

- Active or past breast cancer

- Known or suspected estrogen-dependent cancer

- Active or past deep vein thrombosis or pulmonary embolism

- Active or recent arterial thromboembolic disease (e.g., stroke, myocardial infarction)

- Liver dysfunction or disease

- Known or suspected pregnancy

Bioidentical Hormone Replacement Therapy (BHRT)

The term "bioidentical" generally refers to compounds that have the same chemical and molecular structure as hormones that are produced in the human body. Many woman, physicians and compounding pharmacists believe that BHRT is safer, but keep in mind that there are no well-designed studies to confirm risk or benefit. If a woman is using BHRT products and feels better, this is important. She should understand the risks that may be present (it is safest to assume risks known from available trial data (above) for any hormone therapy, until proven otherwise).

Formulation Considerations

Topical formulations, given as a patch, gel or emulsion, bypass first dose metabolism, and lower doses can be used. Topical formulations usually cause less nausea and may expose the woman to lower systemic estrogen. Estrogen use is generally well tolerated, but can cause nausea, dizziness, bloating, weight changes and changes in sexual interest.

Vaginal products are most useful for patients who have vaginal symptoms (dryness, painful intercourse) only, since these do not expose the women to risks from systemic estrogen. These include estrogen vaginal cream or the vaginal ring *(Femring)*. Due to bypassing the liver, topical formulations do not affect cholesterol levels. Estrogen typically ↑ TG and ↑ HDL. In some women the use of estrogen can ↑ TGs about 25% and may put them into a danger zone, but in others the ↑ HDL may be beneficial.

COMMON HRT PRODUCTS (NOT COMPLETE LIST – THERE ARE MANY)

DRUG	COMPONENTS	SIDE EFFECTS/DOSAGE
Activella	estradiol/norethindrone PO	In addition to health risks above, HT can cause dizziness, lightheadedness, headache, stomach upset, bloating, nausea, weight changes, increased/decreased libido, breast tenderness, and if patch, redness/irritation at the application site.
Vivelle, **Vivelle Dot**	estradiol transdermal system Twice-weekly patch	
Alora	estradiol patch	
Climara	estradiol patch	Some formulations come in patches – for all patches instruct patients to remove patches during MRI or the skin can be burned.
Climara Pro	estradiol/levonorgestrel patch	
CombiPatch	estradiol/norethindrone patch	
Estraderm	estradiol patch	
Estrace	17-beta-estradiol micronized tablet	
Estrace vaginal cream	17-beta-estradiol cream	
Estrasorb	estradiol topical emulsion	
Estring	17-beta-estradiol vaginal ring	
Femhrt	ethinyl estradiol/norethindrone acetate PO	
Generic	estradiol	0.5, 1, 2 mg oral tab, 10 mcg vaginal tab
Femring	estradiol acetate vaginal ring	For vaginal symptoms
Provera	medroxyprogesterone	2.5, 5, 10 mg
Premarin	conjugated estrogens tablet	0.3, 0.45, 0.625, 0.9, 1.25 mg
Premarin vaginal cream	conjugated estrogens cream	0.625 mg/gram
Premphase	conjugated estrogens/medroxyprogesterone acetate tablet – P component changes (phasic)	0.625 mg conjugated E continuously + 5 mg medroxyprogesterone (MPA) taken on days 15-28 only
Prempro	conjugated estrogens/medroxyprogesterone acetate tablet (P component stable)	0.3-0.625 conjugated E+1.5-5 MPA
Estratest	esterified estrogens/methyltestosterone tablets (with testosterone – ↑ risk CVD)	

ESTROGEN COUNSELING

- This product does not contain a progestin, which should be dispensed to a woman with a uterus. Estrogens increase the chances of getting cancer of the uterus.

- Report any unusual vaginal bleeding right away while you are taking estrogen. Vaginal bleeding after menopause may be a warning sign of cancer of the uterus (womb). Your healthcare provider should check any unusual vaginal bleeding to find out the cause.

- Do not use estrogens, with or without progestins, to prevent heart disease, heart attacks, or strokes.

- Using estrogens with or without progestins may increase your chances of getting heart attacks, strokes, breast cancer, and blood clots. Using estrogens may increase your risk of dementia. You and your healthcare provider should talk regularly about whether you still need treatment with this product.

- Estrogen use is primarily for menopausal symptoms, and should not be continued indefinitely. When you are ready to stop discuss with your physician the best way to stop the medicine – it will need to be decreased slowly.

- Estrogen can help keep your bones healthy. Ask your pharmacist for help in figuring out if you need to take calcium and vitamin D – these are important for healthy bones.

VIVELLE-DOT PATCH APPLICATION

- Determine Your Schedule for Your Twice-a-Week Application

- Your _Vivelle-Dot_ (estradiol transdermal system) individual carton contains a calendar card printed on its inner flap. Mark the two-day schedule you plan to follow on your carton's inner flap.

- If you forget to change your patch on the correct date, apply a new one as soon as you remember.

- If you forget to change your patch on the correct date, apply a new one as soon as you remember.

VIVELLE dot®
(estradiol transdermal system)
Change your patch only on these two days:
☐ Sun / Wed   ☐ Thu / Sun
☐ Mon / Thu   ☐ Fri / Mon
☐ Tue / Fri   ☐ Sat / Tue
☐ Wed / Sat

- Apply patch to lower abdomen, below the waistline. Avoid the waistline, since clothing may cause the patch to rub off.

- The area must be clean, dry, free of powder, oil or lotion. This applies to all patches. And never apply a patch to cut or irritated skin (unless it is a bandage!)

- DO NOT APPLY PATCH TO BREASTS. (Never apply any estrogen patch to the breasts.)

- If any adhesive residue remains on your skin after removing the patch, allow the area to dry for 15 minutes. Then, gently rub the area with oil or lotion to remove the adhesive from your skin.

Testosterone Therapy

Hypogonadism (low testosterone) is due to diseases, procedures, or to a normal age-related decline in men. If testosterone replacement is due to a medical procedure, that is considered acceptable therapy. Increasingly, older males are requesting testosterone therapy for purported health claims, including increased muscle mass and bone density, improved sexual interest (↑ libido), sharpened memory and concentration, and increased energy. The use of testosterone replacement is controversial: the primary risk is whether the use of testosterone increases prostate cancer risk. Testosterone can also increase cholesterol levels and cause liver damage.

An accepted use for testosterone replacement is in men with low prostate cancer risk who have a low testosterone level and a related condition, such as low muscle mass. It should not be used routinely for normal aging until the health risks are better quantified. [Another reason for the increase in testosterone prescriptions has been due to the restriction on PDE 5 I's in the Medicare formulary – which led men and their physicians to consider other options.]

Reports of virilization of children due to testosterone exposure are serious and proper counseling is required. Men at high risk of prostate cancer should not use testosterone products. BPH symptoms would be expected to worsen with testosterone treatment. If you are giving a 5-α-reductase inhibitor for BPH that blocks the conversion of testosterone to its active form it would not make much sense to give another drug that provides testosterone directly.

TESTOSTERONE PRODUCTS: C III

TESTOSTERONE	COUNSELING	SIDE EFFECTS/MONITORING/ CONTRAINDICATIONS
Testim gel 1% Unit dose tubes with 50 mg testosterone in 5 g of gel **AndroGel 1%, 1.62%** Meter-dose pumps (# of pumps depends on dose) or foil packets of 2.5 g or 5 g gel	See additional counseling below **AndroGel** is to shoulders, arms or both sides of the stomach – each pump to different location. Rinse off bottle and wash hands with soap. Air dry before getting dressed. If woman and child comes into accidental contact wash fast with soap and water. Do not apply to genitals. Do not use if Hx breast or prostate CA. Do not apply **Testim** to abdomen.	**SIDE EFFECTS** Increased creatinine, increased appetite, sensitive nipples, acne, increased risk of hepatotoxicity **BLACK BOX WARNINGS** Patients with benign prostatic hyperplasia (BPH) treated with androgens are at an increased risk for worsening of signs and symptoms of BPH.
Androderm patch Round- 2.5 mg/day Oval- 5 mg/day Remove patches during MRI: can burn skin	Apply to back, abdomen, thighs or upper arms. Apply each evening between 8pm and midnight.	Secondary exposure to testosterone in children and women can occur with use of testosterone. Cases of secondary exposure resulting in virilization of children have been reported. Women and children should avoid contact with any unwashed or unclothed application sites in men using testosterone gel.
Striant buccal tabs 30 mg to the gum region BID	30 mg to the gum region BID	**CONTRAINDICATIONS** Breast or prostate cancer. Never apply to breast or genitals.
Testosterone topical solution (Axiron) Axiron-applied to underarms Fortesta (gel) – applied to thighs Application to thighs, underarms can help reduce accidental exposure	60 mg (2 pumps)	**MONITOR** Testosterone levels, PSA, liver function, some recommend checking hematocrit

ANDROGEL PATIENT COUNSELING

Pump

- Before using the pump for the first time, you will need to prime the pump. To prime *AndroGel*, fully push down on the pump 3 times. Do not use any *AndroGel* that came out while priming. Wash it down the sink or throw it in the trash to avoid accidental exposure to others. Your *AndroGel* pump is ready to use now.

- The doctor or pharmacist will tell you the number of times to press the pump for each dose.

Packets

- Tear open the packet completely at the dotted line.

- Squeeze all of the *AndroGel* out of the packet into the palm of your hand. Squeeze from the bottom of the packet to the top.

For Both

- This medication should not be used by woman or children. Testosterone can cause birth defects in unborn babies. A pregnant woman should avoid coming into contact with testosterone topical gel, or with a man's skin areas where a testosterone topical patch has been worn or the gel has been applied. If contact does occur, wash with soap and water right away.

- Topical testosterone is absorbed through the skin and can cause side effects or symptoms of male features in a child or woman who comes into contact with the medication. Call your doctor if a person who has close contact with you develops enlarged genitals, premature pubic hair, increased libido, aggressive behavior, male-pattern baldness, excessive body hair growth, increased acne, irregular menstrual periods, or any signs of male characteristics.

- The testosterone transdermal patch may burn your skin if you wear the patch during an MRI (magnetic resonance imaging). Remove the patch before undergoing such a test.

How to apply (1+ push from pump/day or 1 packet/day), or topical gels

- Apply the medication as directed to clean, dry skin of the shoulders/upper arms and/or abdomen once daily in the morning. Apply only to areas that would be covered if you were to wear a short sleeve t-shirt. Avoid applying this medication to broken, irritated skin. Do not apply to genitals (penis or scrotum). Do not let others apply this medication to your body.

- After applying, wash your hands thoroughly with soap and water to reduce the risk of accidentally spreading it from your hands to other people. Before dressing, wait a few minutes for the application site to dry completely. Be sure to always wear clothing (such as a t-shirt) to cover the application site until you wash the areas well with soap and water.

- If you expect to have skin-to-skin contact with another person, first wash the application area well with soap and water. For best effect, wait at least 2 to 6 hours before showering.

- This medication is flammable until dry. Let the gel dry before smoking or going near an open flame.

- *Axiron* gel (applied to underarms): Apply deodorant first.

CONTRACEPTION

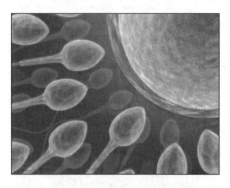

Background

There are 62 million U.S. women in their childbearing years. Seven in 10 women of reproductive age (43 million) are sexually active and do not want to become pregnant, but could become pregnant if they and their partners fail to use a contraceptive method. The typical U.S. woman wants only two children. To achieve this goal, she must use contraceptives for roughly three decades. (source: Guttmacher Institute)

Among the 43 million women who do not want to become pregnant, 89% are practicing contraception. Sixty-three percent of reproductive-age women who practice contraception use nonpermanent methods, including hormonal methods (such as the pill, patch, implant, injectable and vaginal ring), the IUD and condoms. The remaining women rely on female or male sterilization.

Contraceptive choices vary markedly with age. For women younger than 30, the pill is the leading method. Among women aged 30 and older, more rely on sterilization, which is often performed post-partum. Pharmacists have an important role in providing contraceptive health information. We recommend OTC products, including the use of condoms if a risk of STD transmission is present, make emergency contraception services available in the community and provide referral services for pregnancy prevention and STD treatment.

Many women are not aware that birth control pills provide health benefits, including decreased blood loss and a lower incidence of iron-deficiency anemia, reduced cramps, ovarian cysts, ectopic pregnancy, less noncancerous breast cysts/lumps, less acute pelvic inflammatory disease and a decreased risk of ovarian cancer.

Menstrual Cycle Phases/Test Kits

A normal menstrual cycle ranges from 23-35 days (average 28 days). Menstruation starts on day 1 and typically lasts a few days.

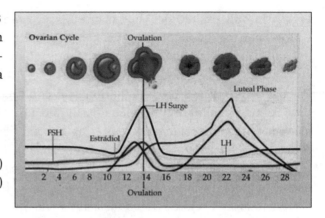

Ovulation

The mid-cycle luteinizing hormone (LH) surge results in release of the oocyte (egg) from the ovary into the fallopian tube.

If the oocyte is not fertilized, it is washed out through menstruation. Ovulation kits test for LH and are positive if LH is present. They predict the best time for a patient to have intercourse in order to try to conceive (get pregnant).

Pregnancy

A female has the highest chance to become pregnant on days 8-16 of her cycle, although pregnancy can occur during any time – no time is considered 100% "safe". Pregnancy test kits are positive if hCG (human chorionic gonadotropin) is in the urine.

If a case indicates hCG+, the patient is pregnant and teratogenic drugs should be discontinued, if possible. Well-known teratogens include alcohol (no drinking during pregnancy), ACE Inhibitors, Angiotensin Receptor Blockers, carbamazepine, isotretinoin, lithium, phenytoin, phenobarbital, topiramate, valproic acid, ribavirin, misoprostol, methotrexate, leflunomide, statins, dutasteride, finasteride, warfarin, lenalidomide and thalidomide. Refer to the pregnancy chapter for a further discussion of teratogenic drugs.

Any woman planning to conceive (and all women of child-bearing age) should be taking a folic acid supplement to help prevent birth defects of the brain and spinal cord (neural tube defects). Folic acid should be taken at least one month before pregnancy, since it takes time to build up adequate body stores. Folic acid is in many healthy foods, including fortified cereals, dried beans, leafy green vegetables and orange juice.

Hormonal Contraceptives

These contain progestin only (pill or injectable) or estrogen/progestin combinations (in pills, a patch, and a ring).

Progestin-only pill (POPs): The use of POPs as a contraceptive method is mostly recommended for lactating (breastfeeding) women, because estrogen reduces the milk production. They are sometimes used for women who cannot tolerate or have a contraindication to estrogen.

Estrogen and progestin combination oral contraceptives (COCs) inhibit the production of both follicle stimulating hormone (FSH) and LH, which prevents ovulation. Contraceptives also may prevent pregnancy by altering the endometrial lining, altering cervical mucus, interfering with fertilization or transport of an egg, or preventing implantation. COCs are used for various indications, including pregnancy prevention, dysmenorrhea, PMS, perimenopausal symptoms (hot flashes, night sweats, as well as pregnancy protection), anemia due to excessive period-related blood loss, and acne (in females). They are sometimes used for reduction in premenstrual migraine (a common migraine in women) although continuous progestin-only contraception is useful for this purpose.

ADVERSE EFFECTS DUE TO ESTROGEN

Estrogen can cause nausea, breast tenderness/fullness, bloating, weight gain or elevated blood pressure. If low-dose estrogen pills are used, or if there is insufficient estrogen (the patient may be a fast metabolizer, or be using an enzyme inducer), then mid-cycle breakthrough bleeding can occur (days 14-21) and may require a higher estrogen dose.

ADVERSE EFFECTS DUE TO PROGESTIN

Progestin can cause breast tenderness, headache, fatigue or changes in mood. If late cycle breakthrough bleeding occurs (after day 21) a higher progestin dose may be required.

Birth control pills do not provide protection from sexually transmitted diseases (STDs). (Condoms provide some protection.)

DRUG INTERACTIONS THAT CAN DECREASE EFFICACY OF ORAL CONTRACEPTIVES

Use back-up while taking the antibiotics listed on the next page (with rifampin, use other form of birth control since the induction will last

WOMEN WITH THE FOLLOWING CONDITIONS SHOULD NOT USE ESTROGEN-CONTAINING BIRTH CONTROL MEDICATIONS

History of blood clot disorders (DVT, PE)

History of stroke or heart attack

Heart valve disease with complications

Severe hypertension

Diabetes that causes blood vessel problems

Poorly controlled diabetes

Severe headaches (for example, migraines – some forms helpful)

Recent major surgery with prolonged bed rest

Breast cancer

Liver cancer or disease

Uterine cancer or other known or suspected estrogen-dependent cancers

Unexplained abnormal bleeding from the uterus

Jaundice during pregnancy or jaundice with prior hormonal contraceptive use

Known or possible pregnancy

If > 35 years old and smoke > 15 cigarettes/day

– if switching back, a back-up method needs to be used for 1½ months after rifampin is stopped).

- Antibiotics (ampicillin, griseofulvin, sulfonamides, tetracycline, rifampin and rifapentine).

- Anticonvulsants (barbiturates, carbamazepine, oxcarbazepine, phenytoin, topiramate and felbamate).

- St John's wort – do not use OC's concurrently – this is a strong enzyme inducer.

- Do not use with the following anti-retrovirals that increase OC metabolism, reducing the efficacy: atazanavir, lopinavir, nelfinavir, nevirapine, ritonavir.

- Bosentan *(Tracleer)* used for pulmonary arterial hypertension.

- Patients should not smoke; may ↓ efficacy and it is dangerous to smoke while using OC's.

- Check the package insert for new drugs you are dispensing to a patient on birth control pills since you don't want to miss counseling on an interaction that could decrease the pill's efficacy.

FORMULATION CONSIDERATIONS

Breastfeeding
Choose progestin only pill.

Clotting disorder or estrogen-contraindication
Choose progestin only pill.

Obesity and age > 35 years consider non-estrogen contraception; higher risk thrombosis.

Estrogenic side effects
Use low estrogen formulation.

Spotting/"breakthrough bleeding"
When starting wait for three cycles before switching. If persists use higher estrogen and progestin if mid-cycle spotting (days 14-21) or more progestin if spotting occurs later in cycle.

Avoiding monthly cycle
Use longer formulation *Seasonale* or *Seasonique* (every 3 months) or *Lybrel* (continuous).

Migraine
Choose among various formulations, if with aura choose POP.

Fluid retention/bloating
Choose *Yasmin* or *Yaz* or newer agent *Natazia*. Progestin component helps reduce water retention.

The progestin component is a mild diuretic. It retains potassium, and is contraindicated with renal or liver disease. Check potassium, renal function and use of other potassium-retaining agents.

Premenstrual dysphoric disorder
Choose *Yaz* or sertraline or fluoxetine *(Sarafem)* – see depression section.

Acne
Can use most formulations; COCs approved for acne include *Ortho Tri-Cyclen*, *Estrostep*, and *Yaz.*

ORAL CONTRACEPTIVES TYPES (REPRESENTATIVE LIST)

Monophasic COCs: all active pills contain the same level of hormones

Desogestrel and Ethinyl Estradiol Tablets *(Apri)*

Ethinyl Estradiol and Ehtynodiol Di-acetate *(Demulen 1/35)*

Ethinyl Estradiol and Ethynodiol Di-acetate *(Demulen 1/50)*

Desogestrel and Ethinyl Estradiol *(Desogen)*

Norethindrone and Ethinyl Estradiol *(Femcon Fe)*

Desogestrel and Ethinyl Estradiol *(Kariva)*

Levonorgestrel and Ethinyl Estradiol *(Levora 21)*

Norethindrone Acetate *(Loestrin 1.5/30)*

Ethinyl Estradiol/Norethindrone *(Loestrin Fe, Loestrin 24 Fe 1/20 – the iron is in the 4 placebo days, Lo Loestrin Fe has 10 mcg estrogen – this very low E dose is not as effective)*

Ethinyl Estradiol and Norgestimate *(Sprintec)*

Norethindrone Acetate and Ethinyl Estradiol *(Loestrin Fe 1.5/30)*

Ethinyl Estradiol and Norgestrel *(Low-Ogestrel)*

Norethindrone/Ethinyl Estradiol *(Necon 0.5/35)*

Norethindrone/Ethinyl Estradiol *(Necon 1/35)*

Mestranol and Norethindrone *(Necon 1/50)*

Ethinyl Estradiol and Norgestimate *(Ortho-Cyclen)*

Ethinyl Estradiol and Norethin-drone *(Ortho-Novum 1/35)*

Norgestrel and Ethinyl Estradiol *(Lo Ovral 28)*

Ethinyl Estradiol and Norethindrone *(Ovcon 35)*

Ethinyl Estradiol/Drospirenone *(Yasmin 28, Ocella – generic)*

Multiphasic COCs: the dose of hormone changes over the course of 21 days

Ethinyl Estradiol and Desogestrel *(Cyclessa)*

Ethinyl Estradiol and Norethindrone *(Estrostep)*

Ethinyl Estradiol and Norethindrone *(Necon 10/11)*

Ethinyl Estradiol and Norethindrone *(Ortho Tri Cyclen)*

Ethinyl Estradiol/Norethindrone *(Tri-Sprintec)*

Ethinyl Estradiol/Norethindrone *(TriNessa)*

Ethinyl Estradiol/Levonorgestrel *(Trivora)*

Ethinyl Estradiol/Norethindrone *(Ortho-Novum 7/7/7)*

Low Estrogen COCs (20 mcg estrogen, compared to ~35 mcg) – Used to ↓ withdrawal symptoms (emotional/physical) and bleeding.

Ethinyl Estradiol/Levonorgestrel *(Alesse-28)*

Ethinyl Estradiol/Desogestrel *(Aviane, Kariva)*

Levonorgestrel/Ethinyl Estradiol *(LoSeasonique)*

Ethinyl Estradiol/Norethindrone *(Loestrin Fe 1/20)*

Ethinyl Estradiol/Desogestrel *(Mircette)*

Ethinyl Estradiol/Norethindrone *(Loestrin 1/20)*

Extended Cycle COCs

Norethindone/Ethinyl Estradiol *(Loestrin Fe 24)* – 24 vs 21 day active pills

Levonorgestrel/Ethinyl Estradiol *(Seasonale)* – 3 months

Levonorgestrel/Ethinyl Estradiol *(Seasonique)* – 3 months, shorter placebo period (and for PMDD)

Estradiol valerate/dienogest *(Natazia)* – 24 vs 21 day active pills, estradiol may be better tolerated

Ethinyl estradiol/drospirenone *(YAZ 24, Gianvi-generic)* – 24 vs 21 day active pills & 20 mcg EE, Yaz formulation with folic acid is called *Beyaz*

Levonorgestrel/Ethinyl Estradiol *(Lybrel)* – 12 months

Levonorgestrel/Ethinyl Estradiol *(LoSeasonique)* – 3 months, with 20 mcg EE

Progestin Only Mini-Pills (POPs)

Norethindrone 35 mcg *(Camila, Errin, Heather, Jolivette, Micronor, Nor-QD, Nora-BE – some names include "nor")*

COUNSELING CONSIDERATIONS

POPs

- All come in 28-d packs and all pills are active.

- Start at any time. Use another method of birth control for the first 48 hours of progestin-pill use – protection begins after two days.

- <u>POPs need to take exactly around the same time of day everyday; if 3 hours have elapsed from the regular scheduled time, back up is needed for 48 hours after taking the late pill. If a dose is missed, patient could be pregnant and EC may be suitable.</u>

COCs

- Start on the <u>Sunday</u> following the onset of menses (will <u>menstruate during the week</u> – most common start is a Sunday start.)

- Start on 1st day of <u>menses – if COCs are started within five days after the start of the period, no back up method of birth control is needed</u>; protection is immediate. If not within 5 days, use back-up for first week of use.

- <u>Missed pills for COCs:</u> First check if it was a placebo pill – no action will be required.

- <u>Missed 1+ pills in week 1:</u> Take as soon as you remember and continue the same pack. Use back-up for 7 days, and consider emergency contraception (EC) if unprotected sex within past 5 days.

- <u>Missed 1-2 pills in week 2 or 3:</u> Take a pill as soon as you remember, and continue the same pack. When you get to the placebo pills, skip them, and go straight to a new pack.

- <u>Missed 3+ pills in week 2 or 3:</u> Take a pill as soon as you remember, and continue the same pack. When you get to the placebo pills, skip them, and go straight to a new pack. Use back-up for 7 days, and consider EC if unprotected sex before 7 consecutive active pills were taken.

Select Different Formulations

Seasonale and *Seasonique* are three month birth control pill formulations.

- They both have a 91-day pill regimen with 84 active pills. The difference is the placebo week: *Seasonale* has 7 days of placebo, and *Seasonique* has 7 days of low dose estrogen. This is not the only formulation where the placebo week has been replaced with low dose estrogen, to ↓ symptoms and bleeding.

- *Seasonale* and *Seasonique* must be started on the Sunday after the period starts, even if the patient is still bleeding. If the period began on Sunday, they should start that same day.

- They must use another method of birth control (such as condom or spermicide) as a back-up method if they have sex anytime from the Sunday they start until the next Sunday (the first 7 days). These formulations require that the pill be taken at the same time each day.

Lybrel is continuous pills with no monthly cycle.

■ *Lybrel* comes in 28 day packets, but there is no placebo week and the packets are taken continuously.

■ With this formulation, it can be difficult to tell if a woman is pregnant.

■ It is important to take *Lybrel* at the same time each day.

■ There is a higher discontinuation rate with *Lybrel* than with other COCs, due to spotting; counsel patients that the spotting should decrease over time.

■ *Lybrel* must be started within 24 hrs of start of period.

Missed pills for extended cycle formulations

If greater than 21 days of consecutive use then up to 7 days can be missed. If greater than 7 days missed use instructions above for missed pills during week 1.

Yasmin, Yaz, Natazia

These are popular COCs, since they decrease bloating, PMS symptoms, weight gain.

This is due to the progestin drospirenone, which is a potassium-sparing diuretic. There is a risk of increased K⁺; and caution must be used with K⁺-sparing agents (potassium-sparing diuretics (spironolactone and others), potassium supplements *(Klor-Con*, etc), salt substitutes (KCl), ACE Is, ARBs, heparin).

Avoid use if kidney, liver, or adrenal gland disease. On a case, check the potassium level. It should be in the safe range of 3.5-5 mEq/L.

This type of progestin may put patients at a slightly higher risk of clotting, and should be avoided in women with clotting risk.

Ortho Evra COC Contraceptive Patch

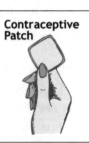

Contraceptive Patch

■ Thin, beige, plastic patch placed on clean, dry skin of buttocks, stomach, upper arm, or upper torso once a week for 21 out of 28 days.

■ Do not apply to the breasts.

■ When starting, a back-up method of contraception is needed for 1 week.

■ If patch becomes loose or falls off ≥ 24 hours or if > 7 days have passed during the 4th week where no patch is required, there is a risk of pregnancy; thus a back-up method should be used for 1 week while a new patch is put in place.

■ Has the same side effects, contraindications and drug interactions as the pills except that the patch causes a higher systemic estrogen exposure (60% more than a 35 mcg pill), which can increase clotting risk; avoid carefully in anyone with clotting risk factors.

■ Less effective in women > 198 pounds. Do not use if smoker and over 35 years old.

NuvaRing Vaginal Contraceptive ring

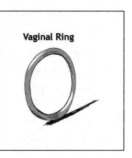

- Small flexible ring inserted into the vagina <u>once a month</u>.

- Similar to OCs in that the ring is inserted <u>in place for 3 weeks</u> and taken out for 1 week before replacement with a new ring.

- For starting: insert the ring between day 1 and day 5 of menses.

- Exact position of ring in vagina does not matter.

- If ring is out > 3 hours during week 1, rinse with cool to luke-warm water and reinsert; use back-up method for 1 week while the ring is in place, consider EC if intercourse within last 5 days.

- If ring is out < 3 hours during week 2 or 3, rinse and re-insert ring.

- If ring is out <u>> 3 hours</u> during week 2 or 3, rinse and re-insert ring and use back-up for 7 days.

- If starting 1st cycle of birth control, use back-up method for the 1st week.

- Has the same side effects, contraindications and drug interactions as the pills.

- Patient can store for up to 4 months at room temperature – refrigerated at pharmacy.

Combination Oral Contraceptives Patient Counseling

- Forgetting to take pills considerably increases the chances of pregnancy.

- <u>The FDA requires that the Patient Package Insert (PPI) be dispensed with oral contraceptives – they are in the product packaging</u>. Tell the patient that the PPI has important safety information and instructions how to use them properly and what to do if pills are missed.

- For the majority of women, oral contraceptives can be taken safely. But there are some women who are at high risk of developing certain serious diseases that can be life-threatening or may cause temporary or permanent disability or death. The risks associated with taking oral contraceptives increase significantly if you:

  - Have or have had clotting disorders, heart attack, stroke, angina pectoris, cancer of the breast or sex organs, jaundice, or malignant or benign liver tumors.

You should not take the pill if you suspect you are pregnant or have unexplained vaginal bleeding.

Cigarette smoking increases the risk of serious adverse effects on the heart and blood vessels from oral contraceptive use. This risk increases with age and with heavy smoking and is quite marked in women over 35 years of age. Women who use oral contraceptives should not smoke.

- Most side effects of the pill are not serious. The most common such effects are nausea, vomiting, bleeding between menstrual periods, weight gain, and breast tenderness. These side effects, especially nausea and vomiting may subside within the first three months of use. Many women have nausea, and some have spotting or light bleeding, during the 1st three months.

- Make sure to discuss with your pharmacist if you start any new medicines, including over-the-counter products, or short-term antibiotics for illness.

- If any of this information is unclear, consult the Patient Information Leaflet or your pharmacist. Your pharmacist will also discuss whether to start your pill on the 1st Sunday following your period (which is done most commonly) or on a different day.

Additional Methods of Birth Control

- <u>Abstinence</u>: Defined as no intercourse. Abstinence is the only 100% way to prevent pregnancy and STDs.

CONDOMS

- Male condoms are a thin latex or plastic sheath to be worn around the penis, thus acting as a barrier to sperm. Female condoms are inserted deep into the vagina; collects semen thus keeping sperm from entering further into the vagina; obtainable OTC, suitable as a back-up method.

- Condoms help protect against many STDs (not plastic condoms).

- Can increase birth control effectiveness of condom with <u>nonoxynol-9 spermicide.</u>

- Do not use spermicide with anal sex and increased risk of STDs.

OTC contraceptive methods (and some condoms) ALL contain the spermicide <u>nonoxynol-9.</u>

- Available as foams, film, creams, suppositories, and jellies.

- Place deep into the vagina right before intercourse where they melt (except for foam, which bubbles).

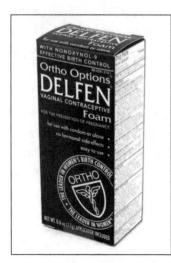
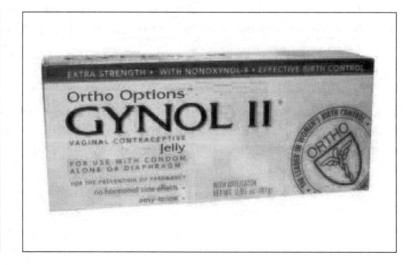

DIAPHRAGM, CAPS & SHIELDS

These 3 options are soft latex or silicone barriers that cover the cervix and prevent sperm passage.

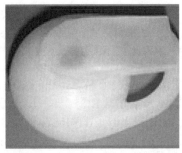

Shield

Diaphragm Directions for Use

- Wash hands thoroughly.

- Place 1 tablespoon of spermicide in the diaphragm and disperse inside and to rim.

- Pinch the ends of the cup and insert the pinched end into the vagina.

- Diaphragms should not be in place greater than 24 hours.

- Leave in for six hours after intercourse.

- Reapply spermicide if intercourse is repeated, by inserting jelly with applicator.

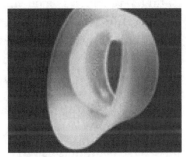

Cap

- Wash with mild soap and warm water after removal, air dry.

- Needs refitting after a greater than 20% weight change and after pregnancy.

Other Forms of Contraception not Dispensed by Pharmacists

- Intrauterine device *(Mirena)*

- Subdermal rod *(Implanon)* – etonogestrel (a progestin)

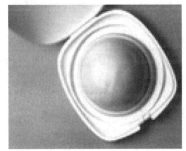

Diaphragm

- Injection *(Depo-Provera)* – medroxyprogesterone acetate, a progesterone IM Q 3 mo inj.

Emergency Contraception (EC)

Emergency contraception (the "morning after pill") is a form of contraception that prevents pregnancy up to 120 hours (5 days) after sexual intercourse. Another option to prevent pregnancy is an IUD insertion.

(Higher-than-normal doses of regular daily oral contraceptives can be used, but are not preferred and are used when the recommended EC products are not available, such 5 tablets of *Aviane* or *Alesse* x 2 doses, taken 12 hours apart.)

The two available formulations are *Plan B One Step* – one 1.5 mg tab levonorgesterol and *Next Choice* – two 0.75 mg tabs. Levonorgesterol EC reduces the risk of pregnancy by 89 percent when started within 72 hours after unprotected intercourse. The sooner it is started, the higher the efficacy. EC has been available for 30 years and there have been no reports of serious complications or birth defects.

EC can be an important resource after unprotected sex, such as from missed pills, a condom breaking during intercourse, a diaphragm or cap that moved out of place during intercourse, or if a woman may have been sexually assaulted.

[Note that EC is not the same as abortion; abortion is used to interrupt an established pregnancy while EC is used to prevent one. This follows the FDA definition of pregnancy as a fertilized egg implanted in the uterine wall. If a person believes that pregnancy occurs at the point of conception (from the time of sexual intercourse) they may not want to use EC. Some pharmacists and patients do not wish to dispense, or use, the EC formulation ulipristal (*Ella*), which is a chemical cousin to misoprostol (*Mifeprex*), one of the components in the "abortion pill" RU-486. They are not the same drugs and are used differently. In RU-486, misoprostol is used to expel the uterine contents (which is why it is pregnancy category X because it causes uterine contractions). In EC, ulipristal is used at a lower dose to delay or inhibit ovulation. It may also prevent implantation and this is a cause of concern for some. All forms of EC, whether ulipristal or levonorgestrel (*Plan B One-Step, etc.*) do not interfere with the fertilized egg after implantation.]

If sexual assault has occurred the woman may require STD treatment, including HIV prevention. Pharmacists should have referrals for other providers available to suggest to patients. Referrals may be needed for regular contraception care.

If a patient vomits within 2 hours of taking the pill/s, they should consider repeating the dose. If easily nauseated, recommend an OTC antiemetic (1 hour prior to use, and caution if driving home).

Occasionally women may be using EC after sex; this may be done when a woman has occasional (not regular) sexual activity. This is not preferred due to a lower efficacy than regular birth control pills and due to changes in the menstrual cycle due to high, intermittent levonorgestrel doses. Depending on insurance coverage, it may also be more expensive.

Levonorgestrel EC

EC products are OTC if over 17 years old and prescription (Rx) if under 17 years old. It is legal to sell OTC to men 17+ as well. Both sexes require proof of age. The FDA approved EC under the "CARE" Program: Convenient Access, Responsible Education program.

EC has dual-labeled (OTC & Rx) behind-the-counter labeling. This is the first time the FDA has approved the same product package for both OTC and prescription use. The approved packaging includes room for a prescription label (to be used when the product is dispensed by prescription), as well as the required Drug Facts box for OTC sales.

Pharmacies must have a pharmacist on duty and available for consumer consultation in order to sell EC. Although the pharmacist must be available, it is not required that the pharmacist be the person who sells the product, or for the consumer to consult with the pharmacist. Any member of the pharmacy staff working behind the pharmacy counter may sell the products to eligible consumers as long as a pharmacist is on duty and available for consultation if requested by the purchaser.

Retail outlets with pharmacies where the retail store has longer hours of business than the pharmacy are not able to sell EC when the pharmacy is closed. Medical clinics may also sell EC if there is a licensed health care provider on the premises for consumer consultation at the time of sale. There is no requirement for purchasers of EC to sign a registry in the pharmacy or to provide photo identification for purchases – although the staff may request proof of age. They can receive multiple packets and ACOG recommends an additional packet for future use, if needed, since EC is more effective the sooner it is used.

- Mechanism of action: similar to other hormonal contraceptives. All of them act by one or more of the following mechanisms: altering the endometrial lining, altering cervical mucus, interfering with fertilization or transport of an egg, or preventing implantation. There is evidence that levonorgestrel primarily works by preventing or delaying ovulation, but other mechanisms may be involved.

- This type of EC is indicated for up to 3 days after unprotected intercourse (and is used longer off-label).

- Take 1.5 mg as a single dose *(Plan B One Step)*, or in two divided doses (0.75 mg) separated by 12 hours.

- Primary side effect is nausea.

- If the period is more than a week late, a pregnancy test should be taken.

Ulipristal *(Ella)*

- Requires a prescription.

- Works primarily by delaying ovulation. May also prevent implantation in the uterus – this mechanism is more controversial than levonorgestrel – make sure procedure in place at pharmacy.

- Indicated for up to 5 days after unprotected intercourse.

- Primary side effects are headache, nausea and abdominal pain. Some women have changes in their menstrual cycle, but all should get their period within a week. If the period is more than a week late, they should get a pregnancy test. If they have severe abdominal pain, they may have an ectopic pregnancy (outside of the uterus) and need immediate medical attention.

- Use contraception the rest of the cycle as ovulation may occur later than normal.

Resuming Contraception after EC

Regular hormonal contraceptives (OCs, the shot, the ring, or the patch), should be started on the following day after completing the last EC dose. The patch and the ring can also be started on the first day of menses.

PAIN

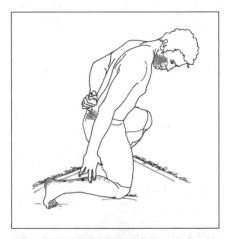

Background

Pain is an unpleasant sensory and emotional experience. It is due to tissue damage, either actual or potential, or both. Pain can be acute (usually due to an injury that just occurred, such as a cut), or chronic (which lasts beyond the expected time of tissue healing).

Chronic pain can be due to an injury such as chronic back or joint pain or due to a disease, such as cancer or diabetes. Many patients, and especially elderly patients, live with daily, chronic pain, and many die in pain. This is a tragic problem in medicine. As pharmacists, we are concerned about inadequate pain treatment <u>and</u> the abuse potential of some of these medicines <u>and</u> side effect management.

<u>Joint Commission standards require that pain be treated as a "vital sign,"</u> making is compulsory for health care professionals in accredited facilities to enquire about, measure and treat pain as they would blood pressure, pulse and respiratory rate. Pain is now commonly referred to as the "fifth vital sign."

PHARMACISTS ROLE IN PAIN MANAGEMENT

Our profession provides pain management care to patients in various settings, including community pharmacies and dedicated pain management clinics. In the community setting the use of OTC products requires careful consideration – these drugs are toxic and overdose or use in the wrong patient population must be avoided. On the other hand, proper use of OTC agents can be beneficial for pain management and is generally more affordable than the use of prescription agents. Counseling for opioids and other prescription drugs is essential. In clinical settings pharmacists are involved in choosing appropriate medications, or selecting combinations of medicines, and assisting patients with monitoring and side effect management. They assist with reducing risk potential and tolerance management via opioid dose conversions. Pharmacists also help with cost management via conversion to more affordable agents, or with assistance in applying for patient assistance programs.

TREATMENT PRINCIPLES & TERMINOLOGY

Pain is subjective and the primary measurement for assessing pain is the patient's own report. Patients should be monitoring their pain. This

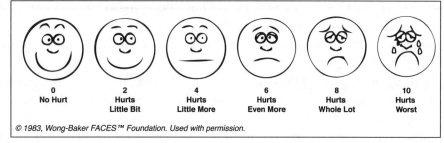

© 1983, Wong-Baker FACES™ Foundation. Used with permission.

will enable the clinician to adjust the medications. Pain scales such as shown here can be used as guides to assess the pain severity. The patient should record the pain level, pain type (using words such as burning or stabbing for a neuropathic presentation) and the time of day. Timing is important – for example, when the pain control may be adequate, but the pain medication may not last long enough. The frequency of use of breakthrough pain medications is important – this can indicate the need for a higher baseline (long-acting) pain medication dose.

It is preferable to treat severe pain at initial onset since delays require a higher analgesic dose. The lowest dose that treats the pain in the right dose. Using mechanisms with multiple mechanisms of action can be useful, and providing access to non-medication techniques, such as physical therapy, is essential. Opioid agents, in particular, can be hard to take even for the patient that needs them and an appropriate goal may be to try and lessen or avoid the use of opioids, if reasonable.

OPIOID TERMINOLOGY

Patients taking opioids chronically (including tramadol and tapentadol, which have dual mechanisms of action) will develop physiological adaptation and live "dose to dose." Although this can be necessary, they will suffer withdrawal symptoms (anxiety, tachycardia, shakiness, shortness of breath) if a dose is missed or late.

It is important to distinguish between physiological adaptation and addiction. All patients, including addicts, become "physiologically" adapted to opioids. Addiction is quite different and involves a strong desire or sense of compulsion to take the drug and difficulties in controlling drug-seeking behavior.

Occasionally, we see a patient in the pharmacy who suffers from "pseudo-addiction." This is when the patient is quite anxious for the drug and may have used up the medication too quickly – which will appear as addiction, but is actually due to poorly treated pain. The response to this type of patient is not to scold – but to counsel them that if they used up the medicine too fast and continue to remain in pain they need to return to the doctor (or find a new one!) to get help with proper pain management. If the drug being taken too quickly is a hydrocodone/acetaminophen combo such as *Vicodin*, over-use will put the patient at risk of hepatotoxicity.

Tolerance usually develops over time to opioids and necessitates a higher dose for the same analgesic response. Sometimes, the condition causing the pain has worsened and it may be hard to tell why the medication is no longer as effective. Is it tolerance, a worsening of disease, or both? Full opioid agonists have no upper dose (no ceiling effect) and we see in practice patients on very high opioid doses due to tolerance. In some cases it is prudent to switch them to a different opioid to reduce tolerance and improve pain control.

Break-through pain (BTP) is acute pain that "breaks through" the control provided by a long-acting opioid. It is treated with a fast relief agent – such as an injection or fentanyl sub-lingual (such as Fentora). In practice BTP is often treated with generic hydrocodone/acetaminophen – this will take time for oral absorption but is less expensive than a faster-acting SL formulation. If many doses of BTP medication are needed, then the baseline opioid dose should be increased. Baseline opioids should be dispensed with a BTP medication, and constipation prophylaxis.

PAIN SEVERITY AND THE USE OF ADJUVANTS

Pain agents can be chosen based on severity and type. Severity is categorized as mild, moderate or severe. Mild pain can be self-treated at the pharmacy and usually responds to acetaminophen, or an NSAID. Moderate pain is often treated with combination agents, such as hydrocodone and acetaminophen. Severe pain may require opioids. Multiple therapies may be needed in moderate and severe pain. In any level of pain the use of adjuvant agents, which are primarily antidepressants and anticonvulsants, can be used. Adjuvants can reduce the amount of regular pain medicine required.

Specifying the pain type is important in choosing the right therapy. For neuropathic pain, you might choose an antidepressant such as amitriptyline or duloxetine and/or an anticonvulsant, such as pregabalin, with or without other classes of agents. For severe pain due to an injury, cancer, or other indications, the patient might need to start on an opioid.

MILD PAIN AGENTS IF USED AS SINGLE AGENTS, AVAILABLE RX AND OTC: ACETAMINOPHEN AND NSAIDS

Acetaminophen MOA: Inhibits the synthesis of prostaglandins in the CNS and peripherally blocks pain impulse generation. Note that IV APAP and Ibuprofen can treat more severe pain – and enable lower opioid doses. Ketorolac is also used for more severe pain and can be given by injection.

DRUG	DOSING	SIDE EFFECTS/MONITORING/ CONTRAINDICATIONS
Acetaminophen *(Tylenol, APAP)* The following come in generics and brands: **+ hydrocodone *(Vicodin, Norco, Lortab)*** + oxycodone *(Percocet, **Endocet**)* Norco is safer hydrocodone/ APAP combo – has 325 mg APAP **+ codeine:** *(Tylenol #2, 3, 4)* **+ tramadol** *(Ultracet)* … and many OTC combos + diphenhydramine *(Tylenol PM)* And in multiple cough and cold products IV Acetaminophen *(Ofirmev)* – used inpatient to enable lower opioid doses	325 mg, max 6/day (3,250 mg) 500 mg, max 5/day (3,000 mg) 650 ER, max 6/day (3,900 mg) Children 's Dosing 10-15 mg/kg Q4-6H, max 5 doses/d Children's Feverall rectal supp 120 mg Infant drops have been 80 mg/0.8 mL but are being replaced with the same concentration as the children's suspension (160 mg/5 mL) to ↓ toxicity risk Use dosing syringe or cup that comes with the medicine Do NOT use APAP on labels so that patients know what they are getting to help avoid toxicity	**SIDE EFFECTS** Rare (and can rarely cause renal damage but safer than other agents in renal disease – primary issue is liver toxicity.) **Liver** With overdose-liver damage can be fatal. Heavy drinkers should not exceed 3 g/day All do not exceed 3,000-3,900 mg/d FDA (Jan 2011) requested manufacturers do not exceed 325 mg APAP in combo drugs to ↓ toxicity risk – they have 3 years to comply. DOC for pain in pregnancy **Antidote for Overdose** N- Acetylcysteine (NAC) MOA: Restores intracellular glutathione (acts as a glutathione substitute) NAC should be administered immediately, even before the results of APAP level are obtained. The loading dose is 140 mg/kg PO. 70 mg/kg Q4H x 17 doses, unless the APAP level is non-toxic. It smells like rotten eggs and causes nausea. IV form *(Acetadote)* can be used as an alternative.

APAP DRUG INTERACTIONS

- Considered DOC for use with warfarin; however, if used chronically, can change INR – monitor.

- None or moderate alcohol due to risk of hepatotoxicity – see counseling section.

APAP COUNSELING

- Contact your doctor right away for any condition that is being self-treated if the condition worsens, if it lasts for more than two days, if there is a high fever (> 102.5), rash, nausea, vomiting or blood in the stool. These are true also for children. Infants should be seen by the pediatrician.

- Many products contain the same drug, including prescription pain medicines and over-the-counter pain and cough-and-cold products. The name may be written as acetaminophen, Tylenol, APAP, non-aspirin pain reliever etc. The total daily dose of all products should not exceed the limits above.

- Too much acetaminophen can cause kidney damage, and can permanently harm the liver. This can be exacerbated by the use of too much alcohol. Women should not exceed more than 1 drink per day, and men should not exceed more than 2 drinks per day.

Aspirin/NSAIDs

Aspirin binds irreversibly, and other NSAIDs reversibly, to cyclooxygenase-1 and 2 (COX-1 and 2) enzymes, thus inhibiting prostaglandin (PG) synthesis, which are involved in pain impulse generation, and preventing formation of thromboxane A_2, which ↓ platelet aggregation.

NSAID Black Box Warnings

CV: NSAIDS may cause ↑ risk of serious CV thrombotic events, MI, and stroke, which can be fatal. Risk may be ↑ with duration of use. Patients with CV disease or risk factors for CV disease may be at greater risk.

GI: NSAIDS cause an increased risk of serious GI adverse events including bleeding, ulceration, and perforation of the stomach or intestines, which can be fatal. These events can occur at any time during use and without warning. Elderly patients are at greater risk for serious GI events.

CABG: CI for peri-op pain in the setting of CABG surgery

NSAID MOA

Inhibit the cyclooxygenase-1 (COX-1) and cycloxygenase-2 (COX-2) enzymes. These enzymes catalyze prostaglandins (PG) and thromboxane from arachadonic acid. PGs have various functions, including increasing inflammation. By suppressing PG formation NSAIDs decrease inflammation. Both acetaminophen and NSAIDs treat pain and fever. NSAIDs also treat inflammation. COX-1 inhibition increases bleeding risk. The COX-2 selective agents have lower bleeding risk.

DRUG	DOSING	SIDE EFFECTS/MONITORING/ CONTRAINDICATIONS
Aspirin – primarily used for cardioprotection ***Bayer, Bayer "Advanced" Aspirin (dissolves slightly faster), Ascriptin, Bufferin*** (↓ stomach upset), ***Ecotrin, Excedrin*** (ASA + APAP + caffeine) EC (enteric-coated) and buffered products ↓ nausea	81-325 mg ALL NSAIDs: know risk factors for GI bleeding: Elderly, previous bleed, chronic or high dose use, hypoxic gut – check for dark, tarry stool, stomach upset, weakness, coffee-ground emesis (indicates a more serious, fast GI bleed) Highest risk of GI damage with higher doses and the long-acting agents. Ketorolac and piroxicam are the most GI-toxic Celecoxib has the lowest risk Ibuprofen is relatively low-risk and has less risk than the other OTC agent naproxen Patients may be using PPIs to protect the gut from chronic NSAID use. If done, consider the risk from chronic PPIs (decreased bone density, increased infection risk)	**SIDE EFFECTS** Dyspepsia, heartburn (more with aspirin, but also with others – EC products, or buffered ASA, can help) – take NSAIDs with food to ↓ nausea! Blood pressure may increase (monitor) GI irritation/bleeding, renal (caution in patients with renal impairment, such as high SCr), CNS effects (fatigue, confusion, dizziness), photosensitivity Due to antiplatelet effects, stop all NSAIDs at least a week prior to elective surgery. Aspirin (salicylate) overdose can be seen as tinnitus. All NSAIDs, even OTC that came in on a script, require a med guide **CONTRAINDICATIONS** Pregnancy C/D (avoid, esp 3rd trimester) Avoid with any NSAID hypersensitivity (past reaction with trouble breathing), nasal polyps, asthma Avoid aspirin (not other NSAIDs) in children (< 16 y/o) with any viral infection due to potential risk Reye's syndrome (symptoms include sleepiness, nausea, lethargy, confusion)
Ibuprofen *(Motrin, Advil)* IV *Caldolor*, also for mild-mod pain, can ↓ opioid dose	OTC 200-400 mg Q6-8H Rx 600-800 mg TID OTC: mild-mod pain Rx: moderate pain or inflammation	
Naproxen Na+ *Treximet* (Sumatriptin-Naproxen 85-500 mg) *Vimovo* (Naproxen-Esomeprazole) – the PPI is used to protect the gut from damage caused by the NSAID.	ALL BID OTC Naproxen Na+ *(Aleve)* 220 mg BID Rx *Naprosyn* 250-375-500 mg *Naprosyn EC* 375-500 mg *Naprelan* 375-500 mg *Anaprox* 275 mg *Anaprox DS* 550 mg	Although slightly higher GI risk and higher cardiac risk, prescribers and patients sometimes prefer naproxen since it is BID versus Q6-8H for ibuprofen. Naproxen: DO NOT USE DOSES > 440 mg/day in patients with CVD risk.

NSAID MOA Continued

DRUG	DOSING	SIDE EFFECTS/MONITORING/CONTRAINDICATIONS
Other Non-Selective NSAIDs		
Diclofenac *(Cataflam, Voltaren XR)* *Arthrotec* (50 mg-200 mcg misoprostol) *Voltaren* gel *Flector* patch (topical formulations)	50-75 mg BID Misoprostol is used to replace the gut-protective prostaglandin, in order to reduce the risk of GI damage from the NSAID. This used to be a more popular agent before the advent of PPIs.	Preg Cat X due to misoprostol component in *Arthrotec* – which causes diarrhea, cramping. Topical forms of diclofenac for mild pain, possibly ↑ GI/renal issues
Indomethacin *(Indocin IR, CR)*	IR 25-50 mg CR 75 mg Approved for gout; others can be used	High risk for CNS SEs (avoid in psych conditions) and GI toxicity
Piroxicam *(Feldene)*	10-20 mg daily	High risk for GI toxicity and severe skin reactions, including SJS/TEN. Use if failed other NSAIDs, and may need agent to protect gut (PPI, misoprostol)
Ketorolac *(Toradol)*	10-20 mg (oral) Always start IV or IM and continue with oral, if necessary. Not to be used in any situation with increased bleeding risk. Start with injection and switch to oral for <u>5-days total max treatment.</u>	Can cause severe adverse effects including GI bleeding and perforation, post-op bleeding, acute renal failure, liver failure and anaphylactic shock. For short-term moderate-severe acute pain (<u>max 5 days in adults</u>), usually in post-op setting and NEVER pre-op.
Other less-commonly used NSAIDs include: meclofenamate *(Meclomen)*, tolmectin *(Tolectin)*, sulindac *(Clinoril* – this one may be a little better with reduced renal function), oxaprozin *(Daypro* – caution similar to piroxicam – higher risk side effects).		

COX-2 SELECTIVE - Lower risk for GI complications (but still present), ↑ risk MI/stroke (avoid with CVD risk – which is dose related, do not use higher doses in CVD-risk patients), same risk for renal complications

Celecoxib *(Celebrex)*	OA: 200 mg daily-BID RA: 100-200 mg BID Other indications: acute pain, ankylosing spondylitis, Familial Adenomatous Polyposis (FAP)	Highest COX-2 selectivity Contraindicated with sulfa allergy Same Black Box Warnings as NSAIDS above Pregnancy Category C prior to 30 weeks gestation; Category D starting at 30 weeks gestation
Meloxicam *(Mobic)*	7.5-15 mg/d	Agents that have some COX-2 selectivity (but not as high as celecoxib)
Etodolac *(Lodine)*	300-500 mg Q6-8H	
Nabumetone *(Relafen)*	1,000-2,000 mg daily	

NSAID DRUG INTERACTIONS

- Caution for additive bleeding risk with the use of concurrent agents that are antiplatelets, such as aspirin, clopidogrel *(Plavix)*, prasugrel *(Effient)*, ticagrelor *(Brilinta)*, dipyridamole *(Persantine)* and with warfarin, dabigatran, rivaroxaban, ginkgo biloba, and others.

- There is no reason to use two different NSAIDs concurrently (exception: low dose aspirin for cardioprotection).

- NSAIDs can increase the level of lithium (avoid concurrent use) and methotrexate.

- Caution with use of aspirin and other ototoxic agents (vancomycin, etc.)

NSAID COUNSELING

- Take with food if this medicine upsets your stomach.

- This medicine may increase the chance of a heart attack or stroke that can lead to death. The risk increases in people who have heart disease. If you have heart disease, please discuss using this medicine with your doctor.

- Do not use this medicine before any elective surgery.

- Do not use after coronary heart surgery, unless you have been instructed to do so by your doctor.

- This medicine can cause ulcers and bleeding in the stomach and intestines at any time during treatment. The risk is highest if you use the drugs at higher doses, and longer-term. To help reduce the risk, limit alcohol use while taking this medicine, and use the lowest possible dose for the shortest possible time. This medicine should not be used with medicines called "steroids" (such as prednisone) and "anticoagulants" (such as warfarin, *Pradaxa* or *Xarelto)*. [There are some exceptions in very high risk (clotting) patients who use both aspirin and warfarin. In general, using them together is not recommended.]

- Do not use this medicine if you have experienced breathing problems or allergic-type reactions after taking aspirin or other NSAIDs.

- This medicine can raise your blood pressure. If you have high blood pressure, you will need to check your blood pressure regularly.

- This medicine can cause fluid and water to accumulate particularly in your ankles. If you have heart disease, discuss the use of this medicine with your doctor and monitor your weight.

- Photosensitivity: Limit sun exposure, including tanning booths, wear protective clothing, use sunscreen that blocks both UVA and UVB (this really applies to just some of the NSAIDs, but the system usually prints the sticker for all of them).

- Do not use this medicine if you are pregnant.

OPIOIDS

<u>OPIOIDS IN COMBINATION (such as with APAP) are used for moderate pain, and single opioid agents are used for severe pain. Codeine, fentanyl, hydrocodone, hydromorphone, methadone, morphine, oxycodone, and oxymorphone are classified as full opioid receptor agonists. The primary receptor for pain relief is the <u>mu receptor</u>. Full agonists are used for acute and chronic pain and have no ceiling effect – the dose can go up. However, opioids at <u>high doses should be rotated with other opioids to reduce tolerance.</u></u>

<u>MANY MORE LONG-ACTING OPIOIDS ARE getting REMS requirements</u> (see medication safety section).

DRUG	DOSING	SIDE EFFECTS/MONITORING/ CONTRAINDICATIONS
Morphine (long-acting brands: *MS Contin, Avinza, Kadian, Oramorph SR, Roxanol*) C II Morphine/Naltrexone *(Embeda)* **OPIOID AUX LABELS** Controlled substance. Cannot be refilled without a written prescription. May cause drowsiness. Do not operate machinery. Do not share: can be fatal to others. Keep away from children and animals. If long-acting: Do not crush or chew – swallow whole. Do not drink alcoholic beverages. Take with food or milk.	Common dosing – opioids have no ceiling dose and some need high doses due to tolerance IR 10-30 mg Q4H prn ER 15, 30, 60, 100, 200 mg Q8-12H *Avinza* daily *Kadian* daily or BID <u>DO NOT CRUSH OR CHEW LONG-ACTING OPIOIDS</u> *Avinza*: <u>NO alcohol, can shorten ER duration. Can sprinkle on applesauce</u> *Kadian*: <u>can be opened and the beads put down a NGT for control over 24 hrs, or can sprinkle on applesauce</u> Do not write MSO4 or MS for morphine or magnesium – due to risk of errors If renally impaired, start at a lower dose. *Embeda*: if drug altered (for abuse) then naltrexone, an opioid blocker, is released. The capsule contents can be sprinkled on applesauce. Injection of crushed capsule contents can be fatal. 2 week washout required between *Embeda* (and *Exalgo*, below) and MAO-Is. Requires MedGuide. **Allergy Information** Cross-reactivity with these agents (if allergy to 1 of the following, do not use another: morphine, codeine, hydrocodone, hydromorphone, oxycodone) <u>If morphine-group allergy, choose (if appropriate)</u>: fentanyl, meperidine, methadone, tramadol, tapentadol (meperidine & fentanyl cross react) <u>Opioid Allergy Symptoms (NOT just nausea!)</u>: Difficulty breathing, severe drop in BP, serious rash, swelling of face, lips, tongue, larynx – use an agent in a different chemical class	**SIDE EFFECTS** **GI effects** Constipation, nausea, vomiting (May need anti-emetics, such as prochlorperazine, ondansetron, etc.) **CNS effects** Sedation (somnolence), dizziness, changes in mood, confusion **Skin reactions** Flushing, pruritis, diaphoresis – may need antihistamine **Constipation notes** Tolerance usually develops to opioid side effects <u>except</u> constipation. When opioids are ATC, constipation will likely require stimulant laxatives (e.g. senna, bisacodyl) or osmotic laxatives (e.g. MOM). Sometimes, docusate (DSS) alone may be enough, or in DSS + stimulant laxative. Methylnaltrexone (*Relistor*) is a laxative for constipation due to opioids (it blocks gut opioid-receptors) The patient must have failed DSS + laxative (senna, bisacodyl). Administered by SC every other day. **Respiratory depression** Caused by opioid overdose and can be fatal (see opioid antagonist section that follows)

Opioids Continued

DRUG	DOSING	SIDE EFFECTS/MONITORING/ CONTRAINDICATIONS
Fentanyl *(Duragesic)* C II *Sublimaze* injection *Actiq SL lozenge* on a stick "lollipop": always start with 200 mcg, can titrate to 4 BTP episodes/d. Only for cancer BTP **Abstral, Fentora SL** pills *Onsolis* SL film *Lazanda* nasal spray -keep in child-resistant box. -empty unused drug into carbon lined pouch.	<u>Patch: 12, 25, 50, 75, 100 mcg/h transdermal patch – change patch Q 3 d (occas. Δ Q48H – do not ↑ dose if pain is controlled but doesn't last long enough – in this case you shorten the interval</u>, as you would do with any long-acting opioid. Otherwise, you risk overdose or high degree of side effects.) <u>Fentanyl, in any form, is for chronic pain management only</u>: can transfer patient who has been using morphine 60 mg daily or equivalent – not used prn and not used as initial opioid agent PATCH Analgesic effect of patch can be seen 8-16 hrs after application – do not stop other analgesic at first (decrease dose 50% for the first 12 hrs). <u>Do not apply > 1 patch each time and do not heat up patch or skin area before applying. Do not cover with heating pad or any bandage. Caution with fever (tell patient to call doctor if they have a fever). Do not cover with heating pads.</u> Apply to hairless skin (cut short if necessary) on flat surface (chest, back, flank, upper arm) and change every 72 hrs. Press in place for 30 seconds.	Cut off stick and flush unused/ unneeded *Actiq* sticks. Do not switch generic fentanyl patches – try to use the same one. Do not use soap, alcohol, or other solvents to remove transdermal gel if it accidentally touches skin. Use large amount of water. <u>Dispose patch in toilet or cut it up and put it in coffee grounds.</u> <u>Keep away from children and animals, including used patches.</u> Contraindications Cannot use in opioid-naïve patients – especially the potent SL forms; these are for cancer BTP. <u>The SL forms are REMS drugs</u> (Onsolis Focus program, etc.) Caution with 3A4 Inhibitors, use lower doses initially
Hydromorphone **Dilaudid** *Exalgo* (hydromorphone extended release) REMS drug C II	2, 4, 8 mg *Exalgo* contraindicated in opioid-naïve patients. 2 week washout required between *Exalgo* and MAO-Is.	Opioid-naïve patients should start with no more than 2 to 4 mg orally or 1 to 2 mg by injection every four to six hours Potent; start low, convert carefully Caution with 3A4 Inhibitors, use lower doses initially
Oxycodone **IR: oxycodone,** *Oxenta* **CR:** *OxyContin, Oxycontin OP)* **Endocet, Percocet, Roxicet (oxycodone/ APAP)**, also comes in ibuprofen comb called *Combunox*. C II – full opioids and oxycodone combos CR formulations are REMS drugs. *Oxenta IR* – see right column	IR - 5, 10, 15, 20, 30 mg CR - 10,15, 20, 30 mg (60, 160 mg only for opioid-tolerant patients) Avoid high fat meals with higher doses	BOXED WARNINGS: <u>Report abuse</u>, misuse and diversion. <u>Avoid use with 3A4 inhibitors</u> – will increase oxycodone levels. Due to abuse potential, prescribers receive training. New formulation called "*Oxycontin OP*" contains polyethylene oxide to deter abuse – substance forms a gel when mixed with water. *Oxenta* is IR form that cannot be crushed into powder & contains nasal irritant (also to deter abuse)

Opioids Continued

DRUG	DOSING	SIDE EFFECTS/MONITORING/ CONTRAINDICATIONS
Oxymorphone *(Opana, Opana ER, Opana Injectable)* C II	*Opana ER* (BID) 5-30 mg BID *Opana IR* 5-10 mg prn Take on empty stomach (most other analgesics are with food to help avoid stomach upset) No alcohol	MUST use low doses in elderly, renal or mild liver impairment – there will be higher drug concentrations in these patients. Contraindicated with moderate-to-severe liver impairment.
Methadone *(Dolophine)* *(Methadose*- liquid) C II	Start at 2.5-10 mg Q8-12H Methadone 40 mg is indicated for detox and maintenance treatment of opioid-addicted patients. It's not FDA-approved for pain	Due to variable half life (it varies widely and can range from 15-55 hours) methadone is hard to dose safely AND has a risk of QT prolongation (pro-arrhythmic) – which will be aggravated if dosed incorrectly. Should be prescribed by professionals who know requirements for safe use. Can ↓ testosterone, contribute to sexual dysfxn
Meperidine *(Demerol)* C II	50-150 mg Q2-4H Short duration of action (pain control for max 3 hrs) Avoid as agent for chronic pain management and do not use at all chronically, even short-term in elderly. OK drug for short-term acute use (e.g. sutures in ER) In combo with other drugs, it is serotonergic and can raise risk of serotonin syndrome	Renal impairment/elderly at risk for CNS toxicity Normeperidine (metabolite) is renally cleared and can accumulate and cause CNS toxicity, including seizures. ISMP (2007) discourages use as analgesic – especially in elderly and renally impaired.

Opioids used primarily in combination

Hydrocodone **+ acetaminophen** *Lorcet, Lortab, Vicodin, Norco* (325 mg APAP – safer combo) + ibuprofen *(Vicoprofen)* Hydrocodone is C II, combos (w/APAP, ibuprofen) are C III	2.5, 5, 7.5, 10 mg in combo with APAP Watch for APAP max dosing – higher doses of APAP can result in liver toxicity; APAP doses higher than 325 mg being phased out – should be gone mid-2012	
Codeine **+ acetaminophen** *(Tylenol #2, 3, 4)* Codeine is C II, combos (w/ APAP) are C III Used as antitussive (anti-cough) agent – codeine cough syrups are C V	Usually 30 mg Q4-6H prn, range 15-120 mg Use with caution if CYP 2D6 variants; may have increased conversion codeine to morphine; do not dispense to lactating women as baby may receive excessive morphine and could be fatal	Drowsiness, high degree GI side effects: constipation, nausea

COMBINATION OPIOID AGONISTS/NOREPINEPHRINE REUPTAKE INHIBITORS – AND TRAMADOL ALSO INHIBITS 5HT REUPTAKE

DRUG	DOSING	SIDE EFFECTS/MONITORING/CONTRAINDICATIONS
Tramadol (Ultram, Ultram ER, Ryzolt – ER tabs) Not controlled by DEA, but C IV in a few states (AR, KY, TN – TN also has carisoprodol as V IV) **+ acetaminophen (Ultracet)**	50 mg, or with APAP 37.5-325 mg 1-2 Q4H prn, max 400 mg/d	↑ seizure threshold – avoid in patients with seizure history Serotonin syndrome risk if used in combination with others, such as SSRIs, etc. and is dose-dependent Dizziness, nausea, constipation, loss of appetite, flushing insomnia (some patients find tramadol sedating but for most it is not sedating; this can be an advantage over hydrocodone), possible headache, ataxia Respiratory depression (rare), like opioids, can cause physiological dependence
Tapentadol (Nucynta, Nucynta ER) C II	50-100 mg Q4-6H prn ER up to 250 mg	Dizziness, drowsiness, nausea but less GI side effects than opioids Like opioids, can cause physiological dependence

OPIOID DRUG INTERACTIONS

- Caution with use of concurrent agents that are CNS depressants: Additive sleepiness (somnolence), dizziness, confusion. These include alcohol, hypnotics, benzodiazepines, muscle relaxants, etc.

- With methadone, caution with agents that worsen cardiac function or increase arrhythmia risk. ↑ QT

- With meperidine, caution with agents that worsen renal function, elderly and those with seizure history. Caution with other serotonergic agents.

- With tramadol, caution with other agents that lower seizure threshold. Caution with other serotonergic agents.

- With *Opana* and *Avinza*: no alcohol. *Opana*: take on empty stomach.

OPIOID COUNSELING

- Do not crush, chew, break, or open controlled-release forms. Breaking them would cause too much drug to be released into your blood at one time.

- *Avinza* and *Kadian* must be swallowed whole (not chewed, crushed, or dissolved) or may be opened and the entire bead contents sprinkled on a small amount of applesauce immediately prior to ingestion. The beads must NOT be chewed, crushed, or dissolved due to the risk of exposure to a potentially toxic dose of morphine. *Kadian* can be put down a G-tube.

- *Opana*: take on empty stomach.

- *Avinza and Opana*: No alcohol.

- To ensure that you get a correct dose, measure liquid forms with a special dose-measuring spoon or cup, not with a regular tablespoon. If you do not have a dose-measuring device, ask your pharmacist.

- This medicine will cause drowsiness and fatigue. Avoid alcohol, sleeping pills, antihistamines, sedatives, and tranquilizers that may also make you drowsy, except under the supervision of your doctor.

- Take with a full glass of water. Take with food or milk if it upsets your stomach.

- Do not stop taking suddenly if you have been taking it continuously for more than 5 to 7 days. If you want to stop, your doctor will help you gradually reduce the dose.

- This medicine is constipating. Increase the amount of fiber and water (at least six to eight full glasses daily) in your diet to prevent constipation (if not fluid restricted due to heart failure). Your pharmacist or doctor will recommend a stronger agent for constipation if this is not adequate. (If asked, recommend stool softener if hard stool, stimulants for most scheduled opioid patients.)

- Do not share this medication with anyone else.

- Never take more pain medicine than prescribed. If your pain is not being adequately treated, talk to your doctor.

OPIOID DOSE CONVERSIONS

For opioid conversions (not methadone) you can use ratio conversion to solve. Make sure the units <u>and</u> route in the numerator match, and the units <u>and</u> route in the denominator match. You can technically convert with fentanyl (note no oral dose conversion as fentanyl is not absorbed orally) but it is sometimes done differently using a dosing table.

When converting one opioid to another, estimate down (don't round up) and use breakthrough doses for compensation. A patient may respond better to one agent than another (likely due to less tolerance) and estimating lower will reduce the risk of overdose.

DRUG	IV/IM (mg)	ORAL (mg)
Morphine	10	30
Hydromorphone	1.5	7.5
Oxycodone	–	20
Hydrocodone	–	30
Codeine	130	200
Fentanyl	0.1	–
Meperidine	75	300

<u>If the medicine works, but runs out too fast, do not increase the dose.</u> You will risk respiratory depression. Rather, shorten the dosing interval.

To convert

- Calculate total 24 hr dose of the current drug.

- Use ratio-conversion to calculate the dose of the new drug: make SURE the numerators and denominators match in both drug and route of administration.

- Calculate 24 hr dose of new drug and <u>reduce dose at least</u> 25%. (If the problem on the exam does not tell you to reduce it but just to find the equivalent dose then don't reduce it.)

- Divide to attain appropriate interval and dose for new drug.

- Always have breakthrough pain (BTP) medication available while making changes. Guideline recommendation for BTP dosing ranges from 5-17%.

Example:

A hospice patient has been receiving 12 mg/d of IV hydromorphone. You are instructed to convert the hydromorphone to morphine extended-release, to be given Q12. The hospice policy for opioid conversion is to reduce the new dose by 50%, and to use 5-15% of the total daily dose for breakthrough pain.

The conversion factors (the left fraction) are taken from the above table. The right fraction has your total daily IV dose of hydromorphone in the denominator, and you are calculating the total daily dose of morphine in the numerator.

$$\frac{30 \text{ mg oral morphine}}{1.5 \text{ mg IV hydromorphone}} = \frac{X \text{ mg oral morphine}}{12 \text{ mg IV hydromorphone}}$$

Multiply the top left numerator (30) by the bottom right denominator, and then divide by the left denominator. This will give a total daily dose of morphine (PO) of 240 mg. Reduce by 50%, as instructed. The correct dose of morphine extended-release would be 60 mg BID.

Morphine IR can be given for BTP as 10 mg Q 4 h prn. Other agents commonly used for BPT include the combo agents, such as acetaminophen/hydrocodone. In an inpatient setting, injections can be given – injections will have a faster onset and since BTP is typically severe, it may be preferable. However, if the patient does not have a port, the injection itself will cause discomfort.

Methadone Conversion: Not straight-forward; should be done by pain specialists

Methadone conversion from morphine ranges from 1-20 for conversion; this is highly variable due to patient tolerance and duration of therapy. The half-life of methadone varies widely. There are separate conversion charts for pain specialists to estimate methadone dosing. This is done by specialists. Note the variable half-life, pro-arrhythmic effect and other side effects of methadone. Methadone is used for both treatment of addictions (heroin and other opioid addiction) and for general use in chronic pain by those familiar with this agent.

Opioid Antagonist (Blockers) For Use in Overdose

Opioid Antagonists are rescue agents for respiratory depression. They block the opioid from binding to the opioid receptor.

DRUG	DOSING	SIDE EFFECTS/MONITORING/ CONTRAINDICATIONS
Naloxone *(Narcan)* Nalmefene *(Revex)* Morphine + naltrexone *(Embeda)* – designed to ↓↓ high from crushing morphine – option in opioid-abuser	Naloxone-Initially, 0.4 mg-2 mg Q2-3 min or IV infusion at 100 mL/hr (0.4 mg/hr) Repeat dosing may be required (opioid may last longer than blocking agent) Will cause an acute withdrawal syndrome (pain, anxiety, trouble breathing, etc) in patients physically dependent on opioids *Embeda*-avoid alcohol-can cause death Naltrexone is an opioid blocker normally used to help treat alcoholism; the IV form *(Vivitrol)* is used for alcohol and opioid dependence	**ACUTE OVERDOSE SIGNS AND SYMPTOMS** Somnolence, respiratory depression with shallow breathing, cold and clammy skin and constricted (pinpoint, miosis) pupils. Can lead to coma and death. Highest risk of respiratory depression in opioid-naïve patients (new users), if dose is ↑ too rapidly, and in illicit substance abuse (e.g., heroin).

Buprenorphine is an opioid agonist and naloxone is an opioid antagonist. Higher doses used to treat addiction, lower doses used to treat pain

DRUG	DOSING	SIDE EFFECTS/MONITORING/ CONTRAINDICATIONS
Buprenorphine **+ naloxone (to block opioid if used)** *(Suboxone* Tabs and Sublingual Film – slightly higher drug conc, not bioequiv to tabs) Buprenorphine transdermal *(Butrans)* – only for mod-severe pain in patients who need ATC opioid Buprenorphine *(Buprenex Inj)* C III Buprenorphine formulations are REMS drugs	*Suboxone*: Used as alternative for methadone (so patients can get from a regular doctor and filled at any pharmacy and can get over opioids since withdrawal Sx are reduced). Used daily for addiction. To prescribe *Suboxone* Prescribers need Drug Addiction Treatment Act (DATA 2000) waiver. If they have it, the DEA number will start with X.	**SIDE EFFECTS** CNS depression: sleepiness, confusion, mental and physical impairment Respiratory depression in overdose Buprenorphine reduces patients' opioid cravings and withdrawal symptoms. In addition, buprenorphine may discourage use of nonprescribed opioids by binding to the mu receptor, thereby blocking other opioids' effects. ***Butrans* black box warning (patch)** Do not exceed a dose of one 20 mcg/ hour *Butrans* system due to the risk of QT prolongation. Do not expose to heat. Side effects from patch: nausea, headache, application site pruritus, dizziness, constipation, somnolence, vomiting, application site erythema, dry mouth, and application site rash.

BUPRENORPHINE DRUG INTERACTIONS

- Caution with use of concurrent agents that are CNS depressants: Additive sedation (somnolence), dizziness, confusion. These include alcohol, hypnotics, benzodiazepines, skeletal muscle relaxants, etc.

- Prolongs the QT interval – do not use with other QT-prolonging agents or in patients at risk of arrhythmia.

BUPRENORPHINE COUNSELING *(BUTRANS* PATCH)

- Butrans is not for pain that you only have once in awhile ("as needed"). It is only for people who have regular, daily pain and need a long-lasting pain medicine.

- Do not place direct heat on the patch. This can lead to overdose and death. Do not put a heating pad over it or sunbathe or go to tanning booths.

- Do not cut the patch. Wear 1 patch for 7 days continuously.

- Do not drink alcohol while using this or any other opioid-like medication.

- Your doctor should prescribe a short-acting opioid pain medicine for you to use while your dose is being adjusted to treat your moderate to severe continuous around-the-clock pain

- This medicine can make you sleepy. Using drugs like sleeping pills and alcohol should be avoided, but if you do use them, do NOT drive.

- Your friends and family should be advised that an ambulance should be called right away in the event that you become extremely sleepy, the pupils of your eyes become like pin-points, you feel faint or dizzy, or your breathing becomes much slower than normal.

Muscle Relaxant/Spasticity Agents

Muscle Relaxant MOA: Various; some work as sedatives, others via effects on spinal reflexes.

DRUG	DOSING	SIDE EFFECTS/MONITORING/CONTRAINDICATIONS
Carisoprodol *(Soma)* C IV (due to dependence, withdrawal symptoms, and diversion and abuse)	250-350 mg QID, prn	Excessive sedation, dizziness, confusion Aux Labels: May cause drowsiness. Do not operate machinery.... Notes Do not overdose in elderly (e.g., start low, titrate carefully), watch for additive side effects
Baclofen *(Lioresal)*	5-20 mg TID-QID, prn	
Cyclobenzaprine *(Flexeril,* Amrix ER)	5-10 mg TID, prn	
Metaxalone *(Skelaxin)*	800 mg TID-QID, prn	
Methocarbamol *(Robaxin)*	1,500-2,000 mg QID, prn	
Tizanidine *(Zanaflex)*	2-4 mg Q6-8H, prn (max 3/d)	
Valium *(Diazepam)* C IV	2-10 mg TID-QID, prn	Same CNS Effects Abuse potential, tolerance MOA: Potentiates GABA

Less-rarely used muscle relaxants include Dantrolene *(Dantrium*-also used for malignant hyperthermia), Chlorzoxazone *(Parafon Forte)*, Orphenadrine *(Norflex)*

MUSCLE RELAXANT DRUG INTERACTIONS

- Caution with use of concurrent agents that are CNS depressants: Additive sedation (somnolence), dizziness, confusion. These include alcohol, hypnotics, benzodiazepines, opioids, etc.

MUSCLE RELAXANT COUNSELING

- This medicine will cause <u>drowsiness and fatigue</u> and can impair your ability to perform mental and physical activities.

- <u>Avoid alcohol</u>, sleeping pills, antihistamines, sedatives, pain pills and tranquilizers that may also make you drowsy, except under the supervision of your doctor.

COMMON NEUROPATHIC PAIN AGENTS

DRUG	DOSING	SIDE EFFECTS/MONITORING/CONTRAINDICATIONS
Pregabalin *(Lyrica)* C-V category – produces slight euphoria, which can help patients with anxiety	Usually 75 to 150 mg two times a day, or 50 to 100 mg three times a day (150 to 300 mg/day) ↑ with CrCl < 60 mL/min Diabetic neuropathic pain Postherpetic neuralgia Fibromyalgia Adjunctive therapy for adult patients with partial onset seizures	**SIDE EFFECTS** Dizziness, somnolence, mild euphoria, blurred vision, peripheral edema, weight gain MedGuide required
Duloxetine *(Cymbalta)*	30-60 mg/day Peripheral neuropathic pain Fibromyalgia Chronic musculoskeletal pain Depression Generalized Anxiety Disorder	**SIDE EFFECTS** **Common to all SNRIs** ↑ BP, HR, sexual side effects: (20-50%) include ↓ libido, ejaculation difficulties, anorgasmia, increased sweating (hyperhydrosis), restless leg (see if began when therapy was started) Possibility of mood changes – requires MedGuide and monitoring **Duloxetine-Specific Side Effects** Nausea, Dry mouth; somnolence, fatigue, ↓ appetite
Gabapentin *(Neurontin)*	600-3,600 mg/day ↓ dose 50% if CrCl < 60 mL/min Not indicated and not very useful, used off-label for neuropathic pain.	**SIDE EFFECTS** Fatigue, somnolence, dizziness, confusion, ataxia, blurred vision (poor pain efficacy)
Gabepentin extended-release *(Gralise)* For postherptic neuralgia pain	Start 300 mg, titrate to 1,800 mg, taken at night with dinner	Similar to gabapentin (above), decrease in renal disease. (A different formulation of long-acting gabapentin was released in 2011 for restless leg *(Horizant)*, this one is taken 2 hours prior to sleep. *Gralise* is taken with dinner. Generic gabapentin IR is divided BID-TID.)

Common Neuropathic Pain Agents Continued

DRUG	DOSING	SIDE EFFECTS/MONITORING/CONTRAINDICATIONS
Amitriptyline *(Elavil)*	10-50 mg QHS, sometimes higher Not indicated, but has clinical evidence for neuropathic pain and commonly used	**SIDE EFFECTS** Are uncommon with low doses used for pain, but could include: **Cardiotoxicity** (QT-prolongation) with overdose – can be used for suicide- counsel carefully Orthostatic hypotension, tachycardia, anticholinergic – dry mouth, blurred vision, urinary retention, constipation

FIBROMYALGIA: SEROTONIN AND NOREPINEPHRINE REUPTAKE INHIBITOR (SNRI)

DRUG	DOSING/ INDICATIONS	SIDE EFFECTS/MONITORING/CONTRAINDICATIONS
Milnacipran *(Savella)*	Day 1: 12.5 mg daily Days 2-3: 12.5 mg BID Days 4-7: 25 mg BID Then 50 mg BID (CrCl < 30 mL/min, max dose is 25 mg BID)	**SIDE EFFECTS** Nausea, headache, constipation, dizziness, insomnia, hot flashes, dry mouth, ↑ HR, ↑ BP **DRUG INTERACTIONS** ↑ risk mydriasis; contraindicated in narrow angle glaucoma Possibly ↑ LFTs; monitor, hyponatremia, seizures. Monitor for worsening of mood (as with all antidepressants) If discontinuing must taper off. CI with MAO Is, wash out period required. Caution with other serotonergic agents.
Pregabalin *(Lyrica)*	See above neuropathic pain section.	
Duloxetine *(Cymbalta)*	See above neuropathic pain section.	

TOPICAL PAIN AGENTS, FOR LOCALIZED PAIN

DRUG	DOSING/ NOTES	SIDE EFFECTS/MONITORING/ CONTRAINDICATIONS
Lidocaine 5% patches *(Lidoderm)*	Apply to affected area 1-3 times/d for 12 hrs Approved for shingles (postherpetic neuralgia)	SEs: minor topical burning, itching, rash Can cut into smaller pieces (before removing backing). Do not apply more than 3 patches at one time. Caution with used patches; can harm children and pets; fold patch in half and discard safely. Do not cover with heating pads/electric blankets.
Capsaicin 0.025% and 0.075% *(Zostrix, Zostrix HP)* *Qutenza 8%* – Rx capsaicin patch	Apply to affected area TID-QID MOA: ↓ TRPV1- expressing nociceptive nerve endings (↓ substance P)	Topical burning, which dissipates with continued use. *Qutenza* is given in the doctor's office only – it causes topical burning and requires pre-treatment with lidocaine – it's applied for 1 hour and lasts for months – works in ~40% of patients to reduce pain, indicated for shingles pain.

Topical Pain Agents, For Localized Pain Continued

DRUG	DOSING/ NOTES	SIDE EFFECTS/MONITORING/ CONTRAINDICATIONS
Diclofenac topical *Voltaren* gel *Flector* patch	Apply to affected area TID-QID NSAIDs, for OA	
Salonpas, and others Methyl salicylate plus other ingreds. -comes alone or in combo w/capsaicin	OTC NSAID patch	

LIDODERM DRUG INTERACTIONS

- Use with caution in patients receiving Class I antiarrhythmic drugs (such as tocainide and mexiletine) since the toxic effects are additive and potentially synergistic. Excessive absorption can be pro-arrhythmic.

LIDODERM PATIENT COUNSELING

- Patches may be cut into smaller sizes with scissors before removal of the release (plastic) liner.

- Safely discard unused portions of cut patches where children and pets cannot get to them.

- Apply up to three (3) patches at one time to cover the most painful area. Apply patches only once for up to 12 hours in a 24-hour period (12 hours on and 12 hours off).

- Remove patch if skin irritation occurs.

- Fold used patches so that the adhesive side sticks to itself and safely discard used patches or pieces of cut patches where children and pets cannot get to them. Even a used patch contains enough medicine to harm a child or pet.

CAPSAICIN PATIENT COUNSELING

- Apply a thin film of cream to the affected area and gently rub in until fully absorbed.

- Apply 3 to 4 times daily

- Best results typically occur after 2 to 4 weeks of continuous use. Do not use as-needed, since frequent, long-term use is required for benefit.

- Unless treating hands, wash hands thoroughly with soap and water immediately after use.

- If treating hands, leave on for 30 minutes, then wash hands as above.

- Do not touch genitals, nasal area, mouth or eyes with the medicine; it will burn the sensitive skin.

- The burning pain should dissipate with continual use; starting at the lower strength will help.

- Never cover with bandages or a heating pad; serious burning could result.

PRACTICE CASE

PATIENT PROFILE

Patient Name	Gene Schneider
Address	11188 Countryclub Drive

Age	50	**Sex**	Male	**Race**	White	**Height**	5'6"	**Weight**	239lbs

Allergies	NKDA

DIAGNOSES

Hypertension

Osteoarthritis

MEDICATIONS

Date	No.	Prescriber	Drug & Strength	Quantity	Sig	Refills
12/09	57643	Suhlbach	Atenolol 100 mg *BB*	30	1 PO daily	11
12/09	57647	Suhlbach	Amlodipine 5 mg *CCB*	30	1 PO daily	11
12/09	57648	Suhlbach	HCTZ 25 mg	30	1 PO daily	11
OTC			Acetaminophen 500 mg		1-2 PO prn, 4-5x daily	
OTC			Capsaicin cream 0.025%		Apply QID	

LAB/DIAGNOSTIC TESTS

Test	Normal Value	Results Date 1/11/2010	Date	Date
↑ GLU	65-99 mg/dL	118		
↓ Na	135-146 mEq/L	130		
K	3.5-5.3 mEq/L	3.7		
Cal	98-110 mEq/L	104		
C02	21-33 mmHg	28		
↑ BUN	7-25 mg/dL	26		
Creatinine	0.6-1.2 mg/dL	1.5		

ADDITIONAL INFORMATION

Date	Notes
1/12/2010	BP today 152/92, Pt reports pain at 5-7 throughout day, describes knee as "grating." Capsaicin and APAP used regularly; asking for stronger pain medicine.

QUESTIONS

1. Gene's wife asks if OTC ibuprofen would be useful when the pain is not relieved with acetaminophen. You counsel Gene and his wife that this may be unsafe due to the following reason/s:

   a. It could cause acute kidney problems
   b. It could cause his blood pressure to increase
   c. It could cause an interaction with the acetaminophen
   d. A and B only
   e. None of the above is correct

2. Gene's physician prescribes *Ultracet*. This drug contains the following ingredients:

   a. Tramadol-acetaminophen
   b. Tramadol-ibuprofen
   c. Hydrocodone-acetaminophen *lorcet*
   d. Hydrocodone-ibuprofen
   e. Codeine-acetaminophen

3. Gene's wife uses *Darvocet*, and she suggests that this might help Gene. Which of the following statements is correct?

   a. This drug contains an NSAID
   b. It is no more effective for pain than aspirin and can be dangerous
   c. There are no significant side effects
   d. It may increase weight
   e. It may raise blood pressure

4. Gene fills a prescription for *Ultracet*, and finds that the pain relief is satisfactory for about one year. After this time, the physician tries *MS Contin*, and eventually switches Gene over to the *Duragesic* patch. You call the physician and suggest the following:

   a. *Duragesic* is the brand name for hydromorphone
   b. This is a poor choice due to his degree of renal insufficiency
   c. This medication can only be used in patients who have dysphagia
   d. The correct dosing frequency is one patch daily
   e. The correct dosing frequency is one patch every 3 days

Questions 5-11 are NOT based on the above case.

5. Tramadol is not a safe choice in a patient with this condition in their profile:

   a. Renal insufficiency
   b. Aspirin allergy
   c. Seizures
   d. Peptic ulcer disease
   e. Gout

6. A physician has called the pharmacist. He has a patient on morphine sulfate extended-release who is having difficulty with regular bowel movements. The patient is using docusate sodium 100 mg BID. The patient reports that his stools are difficult to expel, although they are not particularly hard or condensed. Which of the following recommendation is most appropriate to prevent the constipation?

   a. Senna
   b. Bismuth subsalicylate
   c. *Relistor*
   d. Mineral oil
   e. Phosphate soda

7. A patient with cancer is using the fentanyl patch along with the *Actiq* transmucosal formulation for breakthrough pain. Which statement is correct?

   a. The starting dose of *Actiq* is 400 mcg
   b. No more than 4 BTP episodes per day should be treated with *Actiq*; if more are required, the patient should consult with their physician.
   c. A patient who is not taking an extended-release version of an opioid may still use *Actiq* for occasional, breakthrough cancer pain
   d. This drug should not be given with *MS Contin* at doses greater than 100 mg daily
   e. This drug is contraindicated in patients older than 65 years of age.

8. Which of the following brand-generic combinations is correct?

   a. Celecoxib *(Mobic)*
   b. Naproxen *(Motrin)*

c. Morphine *(Opana)*

d. Hydromorphone *(Dilaudid)*

e. Methadone *(Demerol)*

9. Choose the correct statement regarding the pain medication *Celebrex*:

   a. This may be a safer option for patients with GI bleeding risk

   b. This may be a safer option for patients with reduced renal function

   c. This is a non-selective NSAID, and has a better safety profile

   d. This drug is safe to use in patients with any type of sulfonamide allergy

   e. The maximum dose for inflammatory conditions, such as RA, is 200 mg daily

10. A pain patient with poor control has been taking hydrocodone-acetaminophen 10mg-500mg 8 tablets daily. The physician will convert the patient to *Avinza* to provide adequate pain relief and to reduce the risk of acetaminophen toxicity. Using the hydrocodone component only, calculate the total daily dose of *Avinza* that is equivalent to the hydrocodone dose, and then reduce the dose by 25% (to lessen the possibility of excessive side effects from the initial conversion). The final daily dose of *Avinza* is:

    a. 10 mg *Avinza*

    b. 40 mg *Avinza*

    c. 60 mg *Avinza*

    d. 80 mg *Avinza*

    e. 110 mg *Avinza*

11. Which is the correct antidote for acetaminophen toxicity?

    a. Flumazenil

    b. N- Acetylcysteine

    c. Pyridoxine

    d. Physostigmine

    e. Atropine

ANSWERS

1-d, 2-a, 3-b, 4-e, 5-c, 6-a, 7-b, 8-d, 9-a, 10-c, 11-b

MIGRAINE

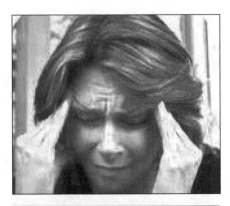

GUIDELINES

Treatment: Evidence-Based Guidelines for Migraine Headache in the Primary Care Setting: Pharmacological Management for Prevention of Migraine, American Academy of Neurology. Available at www.aan.com

ICSI Health Care Guideline: Diagnosis and Treatment of Headache, 2011. Available at: http://www.icsi.org/headache/headache__diagnosis_and_treatment_of_2609.html

Background

Headache treatment is a common concern in the community pharmacy, one of the most common patient complaints in neurologists' offices and the most common pain complaint seen in family practice. Most headaches are migraine and tension-type headaches.

Migraines are chronic headaches that can cause significant pain for hours or days. In addition to severe pain, most migraines cause nausea, vomiting, and sensitivity to light and sound. Some migraines are preceded or accompanied by sensory warning symptoms or signs (auras), such as flashes of light, blind spots or tingling in the arms or legs. Most migraines do not have an aura.

Rarely, a migraine could be occurring with a serious cardiovascular, cerebrovascular or infectious event. Patients should be seen at once if the headache is accompanied with fever, stiff neck, rash, mental confusion, seizures, double vision, weakness, numbness, chest pain, trouble breathing or trouble speaking.

Migraine Causes

Migraines may be caused by changes in the trigeminal nerve and imbalances in neurotransmitters, including serotonin, which decreases during a migraine causing a chemical release of neuropeptides that trigger vasodilation in cranial blood vessels. Triptan drugs are serotonin-receptor agonists and cause vasoconstriction of cranial blood vessels.

The cause of migraines is not well-understood but "trigger" identification can be useful to help the patient avoid triggers and reduce migraine incidence.

Treatment

A common type of migraine is a menstrual-associated migraine in women. These may be treated with hormone therapy to decrease migraine frequency. Common treatments include the estradiol patch or birth control pills. Acute treatment may occasionally be needed.

Children get migraines and may ask the pharmacist for advice. OTC agents, usually ibuprofen, are used first. Triptans are used in children.

Non-pharmacologic interventions involve avoiding triggers, mental relaxation, stress management, or applying cold compresses to the head.

Pharmacologic interventions include OTC medicines (such as *Advil Migraine*, which is plain ibuprofen), *Excedrin migraine* (aspirin, acetaminophen and caffeine) or other agents, including generics of these options. Some patients get more relief from OTC products, some from triptans or other prescription agents (including hydrocodone or other opioid combos or tramadol) and others need to use combinations of both OTC and prescription agents.

If a patient has migraines > 1x/month, or has severe symptoms, or requests prophylaxis, an agent can be used to decrease migraine frequency. These agents can be antidepressants, anticonvulsants, vitamins or natural products, and should be tried at a reasonable dose for 2-6 months. All prophylactic agents can ↓ frequency by 50%, but a patient may need to try several options before finding an agent (or combination of agents) that works for them.

The pharmacist should understand which drugs are useful for both treating an acute attack and which drugs are used for preventing further attacks (prophylaxis).

NATURAL PRODUCTS

Feverfew, willow bark (a salicylate), butterbur, guarana (a caffeine product), fish oils, magnesium, coenzyme Q10 and riboflavin may be helpful, alone or in combination.

COMMON MIGRAINE TRIGGERS

Hormonal changes in women
Fluctuations in estrogen trigger headaches in many women. Some women will use monophasic birth control pill formulations to keep estrogen levels more constant and help reduce pre-menstrual migraines, the most common type of female migraine. ACOG recommends progestin-only bcp's for women with migraine.

Foods
Common offending agents include alcohol, especially beer and red wine, aged cheeses, chocolate, aspartame, overuse of caffeine, monosodium glutamate (MSG), salty foods and processed foods.

Stress
Stress is a major instigator of migraines.

Sensory stimuli
Bright lights, sun glare, loud sounds and scents (which may be pleasant or unpleasant odors).

Changes in wake-sleep pattern
Either missing sleep or getting too much sleep (including jet lag).

Changes in the environment
A change of weather or barometric pressure.

ACUTE TREATMENT

Triptans are used commonly for migraines but some patients find better relief with NSAIDs or *Excedrin Migraine* or generics (acetaminophen+aspirin+caffeine). OTC agents, in some patients, are the best option. Other patients find that using an NSAID and triptan together provides stronger relief.

TRIPTANs: are $5HT_1$ receptor agonists. Blood vessels in the brain become dilated during a migraine attack and the triptans, by binding to $5HT_1$-receptors, causes cranial vessel constriction, inhibiting neuropeptide release and ↓ pain transmission.

DRUG	DOSING	SIDE EFFECTS/FORMULATIONS/CONTRAINDICATIONS
Naratriptan *(Amerge)*	1 and 2.5 mg, can repeat x 1 after 4 hr	**SIDE EFFECTS** Somnolence, nausea, paresthesias (tingling/numbness), throat/neck pressure, dizziness, hot/cold sensations, chest pain/tightness
Almotriptan *(Axert)*	6.25 and 12.5 mg, can repeat x 1 after 2 hr	Triptan sensations include pressure in the chest or heaviness or pressure in the neck region and usually dissipate after administration.
Frovatriptan *(Frova)*	2.5 mg, can repeat x 1 after 2 hr	**CONTRAINDICATIONS** Serious but rare cerebrovascular and cardiovascular events can occur; because of this, triptans are contraindicated in patients with cerebrovascular disease or uncontrolled hypertension.
Sumatriptan *(Imitrex)* Needleless sumatriptan injection *(Sumavel DosePro*- 6 mg – injection by air pressure – may hurt)* **Imitrex STATdose SC injection** **Imitrex** nasal spray Sumatriptan + naproxen 85-500 mg *(Treximet)*	PO: 25, 50 and 100 mg, can repeat x 1 after 2 hr Nasal Spray: 5, 20 mg, can repeat x 1 after 2 hr SC inj: 4, 6 mg, can repeat x 1 after 1 hr *Treximet* max 2 tabs/24 hr	A few are contraindicated with MAOIs (see below). All must be used with caution with concurrent use of other serotonergic drugs. **Formulations** ■ All of the triptans are available in tablet formulation. ■ Rizatriptan and zolmitriptan also have disintegrating tablets that dissolve on the tongue: *good if N/V, dysphagia.*
Rizatriptan *(Maxalt,* **Maxalt-MLT** *disint tabs)*	5 mg and 10 mg, can repeat x 1 after 2 hr *Maxalt MLT* 5 mg, no water needed	Sumatriptan has a nasal spray and a SC injection – fast onset for migraines that come on quickly, and avoids oral route. Zolmitriptan has an intranasal spray (and the disintegrating tablet).
Eletriptan *(Relpax)*	20 mg and 40 mg, can repeat after 2 hr	**Duration of Action** The longest-acting triptans (longer acting, but slower onset) are frovatriptan (the longest – has 26 hr t½ – and naratriptan. Choose if HA recurs after dosing, lasts a long time. Can use agents with shorter durations of action if fast onset required. The ones with a shorter half-life have a faster onset: almotriptan, eletriptan, rizatriptan, sumatriptan and zolmitriptan.
Zolmitriptan *(Zomig,* *Zomig-ZMT* disint tabs*)* *Zomig* nasal spray (NS)	PO: 2.5 and 5 mg, can repeat after 2 hr NS: 5 mg, can repeat after 2 hr *Zomig-ZMT* dissolving tabs 2.5, 5 mg, no water needed	Study: eletriptan (*Relpax*) 40 mg was more effective than sumatriptan (*Imitrex*) 100 mg in relieving pain.

TRIPTAN DRUG INTERACTIONS

- FDA warning about combining triptans with serotonergic drugs such as SSRIs and SNRIs. Counsel patients on both medications to report restlessness, sweating, poor coordination, confusion, hallucinations. However, many patients take both types together. It may present a problem when another serotonergic agent is added to the combination.

- *Imitrex, Maxalt* and *Zomig* are contraindicated with MAO-Is, the others are not.

- Eletriptan *(Relpax)* is contraindicated with strong CYP 3A4 inhibitors.

PATIENT COUNSELING FOR TRIPTANS

- Side effects that you may experience include sleepiness, nausea, numbness, throat or neck pressure, dizziness, hot or cold sensations, and a heaviness or pressure in the chest or neck region. These usually occur after the drug is taken and go away shortly.

- If nausea prevents you from swallowing or holding down your medicine, your doctor can prescribe a tablet that dissolves in your mouth or an injection or nasal spray.

- If you have migraines that come on very quickly, a nasal spray or SC injection will provide faster relief.

- Serious, but rare, side effects such as heart attacks and strokes have occurred in people who have used this type of medicine; because of this, triptans cannot be used in patients who have had a stroke, have heart disease or have blood pressure that is not well-controlled. If any of this applies to you, please let your pharmacist know so the doctor can be contacted.

- Take the medicine with or without food, at the first sign of a migraine. The migraine treatment will not work as well if you wait to use it.

- If you use the orally disintegrating tablets *(Maxalt-MLT and Zomig-ZMT)*, peel open the blister pack and place the orally disintegrating tablet on your tongue, where it will dissolve and be swallowed with saliva. You do not need to use water with the medicine. These formulations should not be used in patients with phenylketonuria, due to the sweetener.

- If your symptoms are only partly relieved, or if your headache comes back, you may take a second dose in the time period explained to you by the pharmacist.

- If you have migraines more than once a month or if they are severe, you should be using a daily medicine to help reduce the number of migraines. Please discuss using a "prophylaxis" medicine with your doctor if you are not using one.

IMITREX INJECTION COUNSELING USING THE STATDOSE SYSTEM

Imitrex injections can be administered by prefilled SC syringe, or commonly using the STAT-dose injection device.

- Inject the medication just below the skin (always SC, never IM or IV) as soon as the symptoms of your migraine appear.

- Use the STATdose system to administer your injection. This system includes a carrying case and two syringes which will assist you in taking your subcutaneous shot. The shot is relatively mild as it is not a large needle.

- Clean the area of skin, usually in the upper outside arm, with rubbing alcohol prior to administering the injection.

- Open the *Imitrex* injection carrying case and pull off the tamper-proof packaging from one of the cartridge packs. Open the lid of the cartridge. Pull the unused STATdose cartridge from the carrying case.

- Load the STATdose pen by inserting it into the cartridge and turning it clockwise. The cartridge is loaded when you are no longer able to turn the pen clockwise.

- Gently pull the loaded pen out of the carrying case. The blue button on the side triggers the injection. There is a safety feature that does not allow the injection to be triggered unless it is against your skin

- Hold the loaded pen to the area that you have cleaned to receive the shot. Push the blue button on the side of the pen. To make sure you receive all of the medicine, you must hold the pen still for 5 seconds.

- Follow safety procedures and return the used injection needle to the cartridge. Insert the pen once again into the cartridge. This time turn it counterclockwise to loosen the needle. Remove the empty STATdose pen from the cartridge and store it in the carrying case.

- Replace the cartridge pack after both doses of have been used. Discard the pack and insert a new refill.

ZOMIG NASAL SPRAY COUNSELING

- Blow your nose gently before use.

- Remove the protective cap.

- Hold the nasal sprayer device gently with your fingers and thumb as shown in the picture to the right.

- There is only one dose in the nasal sprayer. Do not try to prime the nasal sprayer or you will lose the dose.

- Do not press the plunger until you have put the tip into your nostril or you will lose the dose.

OTC Migraine Agents

If recommending an OTC product, any OTC NSAID such as *Advil Migraine* (ibuprofen only, or generics), or *Excedrin Migraine* (acetaminophen+aspirin+caffeine) are reasonable options. Aspirin would not be a good choice due to nausea. Always ask the patient what they have tried in the past, and if it was useful.

LESS COMMONLY USED ACUTE MIGRAINE MEDICATIONS

Acetaminophen/ butalbital/ caffeine (*Fioricet*) C III, also comes *Fioricet* with codeine.

- *Fioricet* generic is popular drug. It contains a barbiturate and if using regular, and long-term, must taper off or patient will get worsening of headache, tremors, and be put at risk of delirium and seizures.

- Aspirin/butalbital/caffeine *(Fiorinal)* C III, also comes *Fiorinal* with codeine.

- If using codeine formulation, counsel on possible nausea, constipation.

- Do not mix with alcohol.

- Do not exceed safe doses of acetaminophen.

Can also use hydrocodone/APAP combinations *(Vicodin* etc), or other opioid combo products.

Butorphanol *(Stadol NS)*, C IV, intranasal intranasal spray may provide fast and effective relief of migraine. Onset in 15 mins.

Ergotamine Products

- <u>Pregnancy Category X BLACK BOX WARNING</u>: DO NOT USE with strong/moderate CYP 3A4 Inhibitors due to risk of cerebral ischemia with higher levels of the ergotamine drug.

- Ergoloid mesylates *(Ergomar, Ergostat)*, ergotamine/caffeine *(Cafergot*, generics), Dihydroergotamine *(DHE-45, Migranal Nasal Spray)*.

- Ergotamine side effects include nausea/vomiting, muscle pain, tingling in periphery, angina-like pain, weakness in legs, tachycardia, bradycardia.

MIGRAINE PROPHYLAXIS

Consider using a prophylactic agent if the patient has > 1 migraine per month, or if the patient wants to use prophylaxis, or if they have severe migraines. This is an agent taken daily. Typically, the reduction in migraines is ~50%, but a patient may have to try more than one agent to find one that works well for them. A full trial, at a reasonable dose, should be 2-6 months. Topiramate is being used commonly since it has a better side effect profile than most of the other agents, and causes weight loss.

First-line therapies for migraine prophylaxis in adults include:

- Propranolol *(Inderal)*, timolol *(Blocadren)*, amitriptyline *(Elavil)*, divalproex *(Depakote)*, sodium valproate, and topiramate *(Topamax)*.

Second-line therapy for migraine prophylaxis (there are many) include:

- Other beta blockers, ACE Inhibitors, antidepressants, natural products (see introduction section), birth control pills (for premenstrual migraine) and botulinum toxin type A *(Botox)* injections.

FIRST-LINE AGENTS FOR MIGRAINE PROPHYLAXIS

DRUG	TYPICAL DOSING RANGE	COMMENTS/SIDE EFFECTS
Beta-blockers		
Propranolol (*Inderal*)	40-120 mg, divided BID	Typical DOC for migraine prophylaxis if side effects are tolerated: fatigue, ↓ HR, possible depression with propranolol (most lipophilic)
Timolol (*Blocadren*)	10-15 mg twice daily	Both propranolol and timolol are non-selective beta blockers; do not use in COPD, emphysema, asthma
TCAs		
Amitriptyline (*Elavil*)	10-150 mg per day, usually given QHS	Dry mouth, sedation, constipation, urinary retention, dry/blurry vision, weight gain, caution with other QT-prolonging agents or in pre-existing CVD
Anticonvulsants		
Divalproex (*Depakote*) Avoid in women of childbearing age	250-500 mg twice daily	Liver toxicity, pancreatitis, sedation, weight gain, tremor, teratogenicity, thrombocytopenia, alopecia
Topiramate (*Topamax*)	50-200 mg once daily	Nephrolithiasis, open angle glaucoma, hypohydrosis (children), depression, metabolic acidosis, 6-8% weight loss

<u>Medication-overuse ("rebound") headaches</u> result from overuse of most headache medicines: NSAIDs, narcotics, analgesic combination products, triptans, and ergotamines (except DHE). Slow taper of offending agents is required. Pharmacists are in a position to see many patients who are chronically using headache medicines, and have daily headaches. It may be best to discuss this with a doctor if the patient seems at risk or is unlikely to try and cut down analgesic use independently. To prevent medication-overuse headaches, educate patients to limit acute treatment medications to 2 or 3 times per week, at most.

RHEUMATOID ARTHRITIS (RA) & SYSTEMIC LUPUS ERYTHEMATOSUS (SLE)

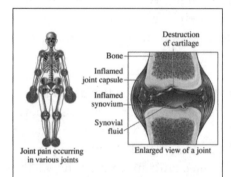

Destruction of cartilage

Bone

Inflamed joint capsule

Inflamed synovium

Synovial fluid

Joint pain occurring in various joints

Enlarged view of a joint

GUIDELINE

American College of Rheumatology 2008 Recommendations for the Use of Nonbiologic and Biologic Disease-Modifying Antirheumatic Drugs in Rheumatoid Arthritis. Arthritis and Rheumatism 2008.59;6:762-784. Available at www.rheumatology.org.

Background

Rheumatoid arthritis (RA) is an autoimmune disease. Autoimmune diseases are illnesses that occur when the body's tissues are attacked by the person's own immune system. The immune system is a complex organization of cells and antibodies designed normally to "seek and destroy" invaders of the body, particularly infections. Patients with autoimmune diseases have antibodies in their blood that target their own body tissues.

RA causes chronic inflammation of the joints and other organs in the body, including the kidneys, eyes, heart and lungs. This is a chronic, symmetrical, systemic and progressive disease – although the disease course is variable and some have much more aggressive disease than others. RA typically presents first in the hands and feet. Macrophages, cytotoxins, and free oxygen radicals promote cellular damage and inflammation. The inflammation leads to cartilage and bone destruction, resulting in the classic symptoms of RA: joint swelling, stiffness, pain and, eventually, bone deformity.

Clinical Presentation

The disease process is highly variable, progressing rapidly in some and slow in others. Many symptoms are constitutional, such as morning fatigue, fever, weakness, loss of appetite, and joint and muscle pain. Patients experience articular manifestations and they are almost always polyarticular and symmetrical. Any synovial joint can be involved, but the finger joints of the hand are most often affected. The wrists, knees and toe joints are also frequently involved. Morning stiffness, swelling, redness, edema, pain, decreased range of motion, muscle atrophy, weakness, and deformity are typical articular symptoms.

DIAGNOSIS

Criteria 1-4 must be present for ≥ 6 weeks and 4 or more criteria must be present.

Diagnostic Criteria

1. Morning stiffness around joints lasting > 1 hour

2. Soft tissue swelling (arthritis) in 3 or more joints

3. Swelling (arthritis) of hand, foot, or wrist joints

4. Symmetric involvement

5. Subcutaneous nodules

6. Positive serum rheumatoid factor (~70% of pts)

7. Radiographic erosions or periarticular osteopenia in hand or wrist joints

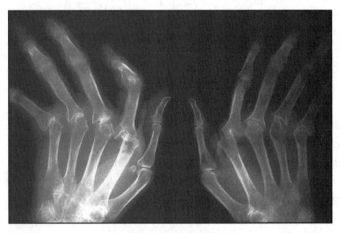

Patients may also experience extra-articular manifestations which include subcutaneous nodules of the skin (20-30%), vasculitis, pulmonary complications (fibrosis, effusions, nodules), lymphadenopathy, splenomegaly, eye inflammation, pericarditis/myocarditis, and atherosclerosis.

Treatment

Non pharmacological treatments include rest, physical therapy, occupational therapy, exercise, diet and weight control, and the possibility of surgical intervention (e.g., a joint replacement).

The goal is to have the patient on a Disease-Modifying Antirheumatic Drug (DMARD) within 3 months of diagnosis. DMARDs work by various mechanisms to slow down the disease and help prevent further joint damage.

In addition, patients may require bridging therapy (short-term) or, in some cases, long-term use of the anti-inflammatory medications such as NSAIDs or steroids. NSAIDs and steroids have significant health risks with long-term use.

Patients with milder symptoms may be able to live acceptably on the old standard DMARD methotrexate, or on other older agents, such as hydroxychloroquine or sulfasalazine. Often times these older agents are used in combination.

For patients with more severe disease, the advent of the newer biologic agents including etanercept, adalimumab and infliximab, each of which can be used with methotrexate, have been life-saving. The biologics have adverse effects, are costly, and do not work well for everyone but for many patients they significantly increase mobility and the quality of life.

AGENTS USED FOR PAIN AND INFLAMMATION

DRUG	DOSING	SIDE EFFECTS/CONTRAINDICATIONS/MONITORING

Non-Selective NSAIDs (for more complete information, see pain chapter)

DRUG	DOSING	SIDE EFFECTS/CONTRAINDICATIONS/MONITORING
Ibuprofen *(Motrin, Advil)* and others	**OTC** 200-400 mg Q6-8H Mild-moderate pain **Rx** 600-800 mg TID Moderate pain or inflammation, such as with RA. Need Rx doses for pain relief	**NSAID BLACK BOX WARNINGS (2)** **1) Cardiovascular (CV)** NSAIDs are associated with an ↑ risk of adverse CV thrombotic events including fatal MI and stroke. Risk may be ↑ with duration of use. Patients with CV disease or risk factors for CV disease may be at greater risk Contraindicated for Coronary Artery Bypass Graft (CABG) peri-operative pain. **2) Gastrointestinal (GI)** NSAIDs may ↑ the risk of GI adverse events including irritation, inflammation, bleeding, ulceration, and perforation which can be fatal. These events can occur at any time during use and without warning. Elderly patients are at greater risk for serious GI events. **SIDE EFFECTS** Dyspepsia, heartburn (take with food to ↓ GI upset), ↑ BP, GI bleeding, renal impairment **CONTRAINDICATIONS** ASA or NSAID- induced asthma or urticaria, pregnancy 3rd trimester (> 30 weeks = Pregnancy Category D), CABG surgery peri-operative use **Cautions** Avoid use in advanced renal disease **Pregnancy** Category C = < 30 weeks gestation Category D = > 30 weeks gestation (3rd trimester)

COX-2 Selective Inhibitor - Lower risk for GI complications (but still present), ↑ risk MI/stroke (avoid with CVD risk – which is dose related, do not use higher doses in CVD-risk patients), same risk for renal complications

DRUG	DOSING	SIDE EFFECTS/CONTRAINDICATIONS/MONITORING
Celecoxib *(Celebrex)*	OA: 200 mg daily-BID RA: 100-200 BID Other indications: acute pain, ankylosing spondylitis, Familial Adenomatous Polyposis (FAP)	Highest COX-2 selectivity Contraindicated with sulfa allergy Same Black Box Warnings as NSAIDs above Pregnancy Category C/D ≥ 30 weeks gestation

DRUG	DOSING	SIDE EFFECTS/CONTRAINDICATIONS/MONITORING

Steroids, using prednisone as an example

| Prednisone *(Deltasone)* Initial dose 5-60 mg daily, some use Alternate Day Therapy (ADT) dosing regimen in which twice the usual daily dose is given every other day to ↓ adrenal suppression. | Indicated for acute inflammation/ pain – steroids are not supposed to be used long-term – however, many patients use chronically due to severity of disease. If used long-term, assess bone density and consider use of bisphosphonates and optimize calcium and vitamin D intake. If used longer than 2 weeks, need to taper dose off to avoid withdrawal symptoms. | **SIDE EFFECTS** **Short-term** Fluid retention, stomach upset, emotional instability (euphoria, mood swings, irritability), ↑ appetite, weight gain. If high dose , then acute rise in blood glucose, possible rise in blood pressure. **Long-term** Adrenal suppression/Cushing's syndrome, impaired wound healing, hypertension, hyperglycemia, cataracts, osteoporosis, hypokalemia, growth suppression in children, muscle wasting, dermal thinning, bruising, cane, menstrual irregularities (and others). More complete list in asthma section. |

NON-BIOLOGIC DISEASE-MODIFYING ANTI-RHEUMATIC DRUGS (DMARDs)

DRUG	DOSING	SIDE EFFECTS/CONTRAINDICATIONS/MONITORING
Methotrexate *(Rheumatrex)* Folate antimetabolite that inhibits DNA synthesis	7.5-22.5 mg/week Low WEEKLY doses are used for RA, (the weekly dose can be split into smaller doses taken over 12-36 hours); never dosed daily for RA	**MANY BLACK BOX WARNINGS** (many apply when using higher doses for cancer) Fetal death and/or congenital abnormalities; do not use in pregnancy Hepatotoxicity Life-threatening pneumonitis Bone marrow suppression Malignant lymphomas have occurred on therapy Severe and fatal dermatologic reactions Renal damage (with high doses) **SIDE EFFECTS** (most common) - nausea, vomiting, diarrhea, GI upset, anorexia, reddening of skin, stomatitis **CONTRAINDICATIONS** Pregnancy, alcoholism, chronic liver disease, blood dyscrasias **MONITORING** CBC, LFTs, and SCr (baseline and every 2-4 weeks for first 3 months, then less frequently), hepatitis B and C prior to starting therapy Pregnancy Category X
Hydroxychloroquine *(Plaquenil)* Used in mild RA	400-600 mg/day initially, then 200-400 mg/d for maintenance dose Take with food or milk	**SIDE EFFECTS** Decreased visual acuity, photophobia, blurred vision, corneal deposits, nausea, vomiting, irritability, pruritus, rashes (including SJS), ataxia, alopecia, pigmentation of skin and hair (bleaching of hair), neuromyopathy with long-term use **MONITORING** Obtain eye exam within first year of treatment, CBC, LFTs, and SCr Mainly eliminated by the kidney

Non-biologic Disease-Modifying Anti-Rheumatic Drugs continued

DRUG	DOSING	SIDE EFFECTS/CONTRAINDICATIONS/MONITORING
Sulfasalazine (*Azulfidine, Azulfidine EN-tabs, Sulfazine, Sulfazine EC*)	500 – 1,000 mg BID (max 3 grams/day) Take with food and 8 oz of water to prevent cystalluria Impairs folate absorption, may give 1 mg/day folate supplement	**SIDE EFFECTS** Headache, GI upset, nausea, vomiting, anorexia, dyspepsia, oligospermia (reversible), rash (all > 10%) **CONTRAINDICATIONS** Patients with a sulfa or salicylate allergy, GI or GU obstruction **MONITORING** CBC, LFTs, and SCr Can cause yellow-orange coloration of skin/urine; metabolized to sulfapyridine and 5-ASA
Minocycline (*Minocin*) Used in mild RA	100 mg BID	**SIDE EFFECTS** GI upset, nausea, vomiting, ↑ LFTs, rash (exfoliative dermatitis, SJS), photosensitivity, others **MONITORING** CBC, LFTs, and SCr Do not use in pregnancy or in children ≤ 8 years of age
Leflunomide (*Arava*)	20 mg daily Must have negative pregnancy test before starting this medication and use 2 forms of birth control. If want to get pregnant, wait 2 years after discontinuation or give cholestyramine	**BLACK BOX WARNINGS** Women of childbearing potential should not receive leflunomide until pregnancy has been excluded and hepatotoxicity **SIDE EFFECTS** Hepatotoxicity, diarrhea, upper respiratory tract infections (URTIs), alopecia, rash **CONTRAINDICATION** Pregnancy **MONITOR** LFTs and CBC at baseline and monthly for first 6 months, SCr, hepatitis B and C prior to starting therapy Pregnancy Category X Can use +/- MTX

ACE J G

BIOLOGIC DMARDS

DRUG	DOSING	SIDE EFFECTS/CONTRAINDICATIONS/MONITORING

Tumor Necrosis Factor (TNFα) Inhibitors

DRUG	DOSING	SIDE EFFECTS/CONTRAINDICATIONS/MONITORING
Etanercept *(Enbrel, Enbrel Sureclick autoinjector)*	50 mg SC once/week	**BLACK BOX WARNINGS** Serious infections and malignancies (lymphoma) **SIDE EFFECTS** Infections and injection site reactions (redness, rash, swelling, itching, or bruising) **CONTRAINDICATIONS** Sepsis (severe infection)
Adalimumab *(Humira, Humira Pen)*	40 mg SC every other week (If not taking MTX, can ↑ dose to 40 mg SC weekly)	**MONITORING** Signs of infection, WBCs, signs of heart failure, LFTs *Enbrel* and *Humira* are self-injectable (SC) and are usually considered first within the biologics. Do not shake. Requires refrigeration (biologics will denature if hot). Do not freeze. Allow to reach room temperature before injecting (15-30 min). Usually, MTX is used 1st-line and these agents are add-on therapy. However, if the initial presentation is severe, these can be started as initial therapy. Do not use biologics in combination. Do not use live vaccines if using these drugs.
Infliximab *(Remicade)* -given with MTX	3 mg/kg IV at weeks 0, 2, and 6, and then every 8 weeks (can ↑ dose to 10 mg/kg based on need but ↑ infection risk) Infusion reactions: hypotension, fever, chills, pruritus (may benefit w/ pre-treatment w/APAP, antihistamine, steroids) Delayed hypersensitivity reaction 3-10 days after administration (fever, rash, myalgia, HA, sore throat)	**Dispense MedGuide** All TNF inhibitors carry a black box warning for risk of serious infections, including tuberculosis, and invasive fungal and other opportunistic infections. All patients should be evaluated for TB before starting these drugs. Patients with latent TB should start prophylactic treatment. Retest TB annually. Precautions: TNF inhibitors can cause neurological reactions, demyelinating disease, malignancies, hepatitis B reactivation, HF, auto-immunity (lupus), and immunosuppression. They should not be used in combo with other biologics or live vaccines.
Certolizumab pegol *(Cimzia)*	400 mg SC at weeks 0, 2, and 4. Then, 400 mg every 4 weeks (or 200 mg every other week)	Infection: All TNF-blockers require TB test prior to admin (and annually), Can cause heart failure, new onset or worsening may occur; may ↑ LFTs. Antibody induction: ↓ usefulness of drug
Golimumab *(Simponi)* -given with MTX	50 mg SC once/month	

Biologic DMARDs continued

DRUG	DOSING	SIDE EFFECTS/CONTRAINDICATIONS/MONITORING

Other Biologics

DRUG	DOSING	SIDE EFFECTS/CONTRAINDICATIONS/MONITORING
Rituximab (Rituxan) -given with MTX Depletes CD20+ B cells	1 gram IV on day 1 and 15 in combination with MTX need to pre-medicate with a steroid start infusion at 50 mg/hr; can to 400 mg/hr if no reaction	**BLACK BOX WARNINGS (4)** Severe and fatal infusion related reactions, usually with the first infusion Progressive multifocal leukoencephalopathy (PML) due to JC virus infection Tumor lysis syndrome leading to acute renal failure and dialysis may occur following the first dose Severe and fatal mucocutaneous reaction (SJS, TEN, etc.) can occur **SIDE EFFECTS** Fever, chills, headache, pain, rash, pruritus, angioedema, abdominal pain, bone marrow suppression, infusion related reactions **MONITORING** Cardiac monitoring during and after infusion, vital signs, infusion reactions, CBC, CD20+ cells, renal function
Anakinra *(Kineret)* IL-1 receptor antagonist	100 mg SC daily	**SIDE EFFECTS** Headache, injection site reactions, infections, bone marrow suppression **CONTRAINDICATIONS** Active infection **MONITORING** CBC, SCr, signs of infection
Abatacept *(Orencia)* T lymphocyte inhibitor	500 mg – 1,000 mg IV based on body wt; given IV over 30 min. Give at 0, 2, and 4 weeks, then every 4 weeks thereafter	**SIDE EFFECTS** Headache, injection site reactions, infections Caution in those with COPD- may worsen symptoms
Tocilizumab *(Actemra)* IL-6 inhibitor	4 mg/kg IV every 4 weeks given over 60 min (may ↑ to 8 mg/kg based on clinical response)	**BLACK BOX WARNING** Risk of serious infections **SIDE EFFECTS** ↑ LFTs, infections, bone marrow suppression, GI perforation, ↑ LDL **MONITORING** CBC and LFTs (every 4-8 weeks), LDL

Pointers for All Immune Modulators

If hypersensitivity to a drug develops, further use is contraindicated (this is true for other drugs as well but these drugs cause more hypersensitivity). Consider varicella vaccination prior to the start of treatment. The patients should monitor for infections and for liver damage (see the counseling section). Note the injection information at the top of the dosing column. If you dispense a self-injectable, counseling must include how to store the medication, reconstitute (if a powder), and where to inject. If the vial or syringe is kept refrigerated, the patient should wait until the drug is at room temperature (cold injections are painful) but should not use external heat sources; holding the medication or slowly rolling it in the hand is acceptable.

If the drug is a powder that is reconstituted, the drug powder may be required to be refrigerated or be kept at room temperature (they vary). If a drug is reconstituted, it has to be used right away (at most within a few hours, a few reconstituted injections permit short storage in the refrigerator; others do not). Some of the powders that are reconstituted contain albumin and some patients will not wish to or cannot use albumin-containing products. Dispense MedGuides and instruct patients to read them. If pregnancy occurs during treatment, the patient should be referred to pregnancy registry as the fetal effects of these newer drugs is not well known.

Systemic Lupus Erythematosus (SLE)

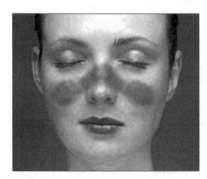

BACKGROUND
Systemic lupus erythematosus (SLE), or lupus, is a systemic autoimmune disease that can affect any part of the body. Like RA, the immune system attacks the body's cells and tissues, resulting in inflammation and tissue damage. Similarly, the course of the disease is unpredictable, with periods of illness, called flares, followed by periods of remission. SLE often affects the heart, joints, lungs, skin, blood vessels, liver, kidneys, and nervous system. The disease predominantly occurs in women, particularly those between 15 - 45 years of age.

The hallmark of SLE is the development of auto-antibodies by B cells to cellular components that leads to a chronic inflammatory autoimmune disease. This abnormal auto-antibody formation can attack multiple types of cells in various organ systems leading to a highly variable disease process with multiple organ involvement. Many antibodies can be produced including antinuclear antibodies and antiphospholipid antibodies and these antibodies are often present many years before the diagnosis of SLE.

<u>Drug-induced lupus has been most commonly associated with procainamide, hydralazine, isoniazid, quinidine, chlorpromazine, methyldopa, and minocycline</u>. Other drugs have been implicated in causing lupus but the incidence is low.

CLINICAL PRESENTATION
Patients with SLE can develop different combinations of symptoms and organ involvement. The most common symptoms include fatigue, fever, anorexia, weight loss, muscle aches, arthritis, rash (butterfly rash), photosensitivity, and joint pain and stiffness. Over half of the

people with SLE develop a characteristic red, flat facial rash over the bridge of their nose. Because of its shape, it is frequently referred to as the "butterfly rash" of SLE. The rash is painless and does not itch. The facial rash, along with inflammation in other organs, can be precipitated or worsened by exposure to sunlight. Arthritis and cutaneous manifestations are most common, but renal, hematologic and neurologic manifestations contribute largely to morbidity and mortality. Lupus nephritis develops in over 50% of patients with SLE.

TREATMENT

Non-pharmacologic therapy consists of rest and proper exercise to manage the fatigue these patients experience. Also, smoking cessation is encouraged since tobacco smoke can be a trigger for disease. Many patients experience photosensitivity, therefore, using sunscreens and avoiding sunlight may help better manage their disease. Drug therapy for SLE consists of immunosuppressants, cytotoxic agents, and/or anti-inflammatory agents. Treatment approaches emphasize using a combination of drugs to minimize chronic exposure to corticosteroids. The goal of therapy is to suppress the immune system to avoid disease flares and keep the patient in remission.

Patients with mild disease may do well on an NSAID (dosed at anti-inflammatory doses) but caution as these patients are more sensitive to the GI and renal side effects. Concurrent use with a PPI is generally recommended. Other agents are discussed below.

AGENTS USED IN LUPUS

DRUG	DOSING	SIDE EFFECTS/CONTRAINDICATIONS/MONITORING

Antimalarial agents

DRUG	DOSING	SIDE EFFECTS/CONTRAINDICATIONS/MONITORING
Hydroxychloroquine	200 - 400 mg daily	Hydroxychloroquine is safer (preferred); takes 6 months to see maximal effect Effective for cutaneous symptoms and arthralgias, fatigue and fever - more for mild disease; chronic (not acute) therapy See more information in RA lecture above
Chloroquine	250 - 500 mg daily	

Corticosteroids

DRUG	DOSING	SIDE EFFECTS/CONTRAINDICATIONS/MONITORING
Prednisone (or methylprednisolone IV if life-threatening disease)	1 - 2 mg/kg/day PO; then taper	Used acutely to control flares at higher doses; taper to lower doses for chronic, suppressive therapy See more information in RA lecture above

Agents Used In Lupus Continued

DRUG	DOSING	SIDE EFFECTS/CONTRAINDICATIONS/MONITORING

Cytotoxic agents - used in severe disease

DRUG	DOSING	SIDE EFFECTS/CONTRAINDICATIONS/MONITORING
Cyclophosphamide	500 - 1,000 mg/m² IV monthly for 6 months, then every 3 months for 2 years; or 1-3 mg/kg if using PO daily	**SIDE EFFECTS** Bone marrow suppression, infections, hemorrhagic cystitis (give mesna therapy and keep patient well hydrated), malignancy, sterility, and teratogenesis **MONITORING** CBC and urinalysis monthly Can use IV or oral therapy; used for flares as induction therapy; very toxic for chronic therapy
Azathioprine	1 - 3 mg/kg PO daily	**SIDE EFFECTS** Bone marrow suppression, infections (including herpes zoster), malignancy, hepatotoxicity **MONITORING** CBC and LFTs Not used acutely; may be used after cyclophosphamide induction; less toxic than cyclophosphamide
Mycophenolate mofetil *(Cellcept)*	1 - 3 grams PO daily	**SIDE EFFECTS** Bone marrow suppression, hepatotoxicity, malignancy, nausea, vomiting, GI upset **MONITORING** CBC, LFTs See more information in the transplant lecture

Biologic

DRUG	DOSING	SIDE EFFECTS/CONTRAINDICATIONS/MONITORING
Belimumab *(Benlysta)* inhibits B cells	10 mg/kg at 2 week intervals for the first 3 doses, then 4 week intervals thereafter, infuse over 1 hour	**SIDE EFFECTS** Higher risk of infection, depression, anaphylaxis and infusion reactions, malignancy, ↑ mortality in clinical trials compared to placebo Consider giving premedication for infusion reactions and hypersensitivity reactions Live vaccines should not be given 30 days prior or concurrently with therapy Only modestly effective; use after standard therapy has failed

PATIENT COUNSELING

Methotrexate   *liver / lung / kidney*

- Patients should be encouraged to read the Patient Instruction sheet within the Dose Pack. Prescriptions should not be written or refilled on a PRN basis.

- If you are receiving this medicine for rheumatoid arthritis or psoriasis, the dosage is usually given <u>once weekly</u>. Some patients are told to divide the once weekly dose in half and take it over two days per week. <u>Do NOT use this medicine daily</u> or double-up on doses. Serious side effects could occur if it is used more frequently than directed. Choose a day of the week to take your medicine that you can remember.

- Methotrexate has caused birth defects and death in unborn babies (Preg Categ X). If you are pregnant or have a chance of becoming pregnant, you should not use this medicine. Use an effective form of birth control, whether you are a man or a woman. Tell your doctor if you or your sexual partner become pregnant during treatment.

- Do not use methotrexate if you are breast-feeding.

- If you have kidney problems or excess body water (ascites, pleural effusion), you must be closely monitored and your dose may be adjusted or stopped by your doctor.

- Your liver will need to be tested (a blood test) on a regular basis to make sure it stays healthy.

- Methotrexate (usually at high dosages) has rarely caused severe (sometimes fatal) bone marrow suppression (decreasing your body's ability to fight infections) and stomach/intestinal disease (e.g., bleeding) when used at the same time as non-steroidal anti-inflammatory drugs (NSAIDs). Therefore, NSAIDs should not be used with high-dose methotrexate. Caution is advised if you also take aspirin. NSAIDs/aspirin may be used with low-dose methotrexate such as for the treatment of rheumatoid arthritis if directed by your doctor. If you are using low-dose aspirin (81-325 milligrams per day) for heart attack or stroke prevention, continue to take it unless directed otherwise. Consult your doctor regarding safe use of these drugs (e.g., close monitoring by your doctor, maintaining stable doses of NSAIDs). Do not use additional OTC NSAIDs (such as ibuprofen or naproxen).

- In rare instances, this drug may also cause liver problems when it is used for long periods of time. If you are using methotrexate long-term, a liver biopsy may be recommended.

- Do not drink alcohol when using this medicine, since alcohol can also damage the liver.

- Methotrexate use has rarely resulted in serious (sometimes fatal) side effects, such as <u>lung problems</u>, lung infections *(Pneumocystis carinii* pneumonia), skin reactions, diarrhea, and mouth sores (ulcerative stomatitis).

- Tell your doctor right away if you develop any new or worsening symptoms, including black, tarry stools; dry, nonproductive cough; mouth sores; red, swollen, or blistered skin; severe or persistent diarrhea or vomiting; shortness of breath or trouble breathing; signs of infection (e.g., fever, chills, sore throat); stomach pain; unusual bruising or bleeding; unusual tiredness or weakness; or yellowing of the skin or eyes.

Etanercept

- Read the medication guide that comes with this medicine. You will be given a medication guide the first time you get the medicine, and with each refill.

- This medication is used alone or in combination with an immunosuppressant (such as methotrexate) to treat certain types of arthritis (e.g., rheumatoid, psoriatic, and ankylosing spondylitis), as well as a skin condition called psoriasis. These conditions are caused by an overactive immune system (autoimmune disease).

- People taking etanercept should not get live vaccines. Make sure your vaccines are up-to-date before taking this medicine. You can continue to take the annual influenza shot (but not the nasal mist vaccine, since this is a live vaccine).

- Because etanercept works by blocking the immune system, it may lower your ability to fight infections. This may make you more likely to get a serious (rarely fatal) infection or can make any infection you have worse. You should be tested for tuberculosis (TB skin test or chest X-ray) before and during treatment with etanercept. If you have been exposed to TB (but do not have active disease) you will need to start taking a daily TB medicine to prevent TB before starting *Enbrel*. Tell your doctor immediately if you have any signs of infection such as a cough, night sweats or fever.

- This medicine has a possibility of causing liver damage. Call your doctor right away if you have any of these symptoms: feel very tired, skin or eyes look yellow, poor appetite or vomiting, pain on the right side of your stomach (abdomen).

- This medicine may worsen congestive heart failure (CHF). Notify your doctor if you experience a sudden weight gain or shortness of breath.

- Common side effects include injection site reactions such as redness, swelling, itching, or pain. These symptoms usually go away within 3 to 5 days. If you have pain, redness or swelling around the injection site that doesn't go away or gets worse, call your doctor.

- Other side effects can include upper respiratory infections (sinus infections), headache, dizziness or coughing.

- Etanercept is injected subcutaneously (SC) under the skin of the thigh, abdomen, or upper arm, once or weekly exactly as prescribed by your doctor.

- Store the medication (single-use syringes or multiple-use vials) in the refrigerator. Allow the medicine to warm to room temperature before injecting (takes 15-30 minutes). Do not shake the medicine. Before using, check for particles or discoloration. If either is present, do not use the medicine.

- Before injecting each dose, clean the injection site with rubbing alcohol. It is important to change the location of the injection site each time you use this drug to prevent problems under the skin. New injections should be given at least 1 inch (2.5 centimeters) from the last injection site. Do not inject into areas of the skin that are sore, bruised, red, or hard.

PRACTICE CASE

PATIENT PROFILE

Patient Name	Gina Calderon						
Address	1954 Milton Drive, San Gabriel						
Age	44	**Sex** Female	**Race** Hispanic	**Height** 5'3"	**Weight** 140 lbs		
Allergies	None known						

DIAGNOSES

Rheumatoid Arthritis	Poor exercise tolerance
Hypertension	
Depression	
Chronic fatigue	

MEDICATIONS

Date	No.	Prescriber	Drug & Strength	Quantity	Sig	Refills
4/20/10	55287	Casey	Lisinopril 20 mg	30	1 PO daily	11
4/20/10	55288	Casey	Methotrexate 7.5 mg	8	2 tabs Q weekly	3
4/20/10	55289	Casey	Prednisone 10 mg	45	1 PO daily	3
4/20/10	55292	Casey	Alendronate 70 mg	4	1 PO Q weekly	3
		(OTC)	Calcium 500+ D 400 IU		1 tab Q AM	

LAB/DIAGNOSTIC TESTS

Test	Normal Value	Results		
		Date 5/12/09	Date	Date
Rheum Fact	< 40 IU/mL	88 IU/mL		
ESR	≤ 30 mm/hr	81.1 mm/hr		
Alk Phos	33-115 u/L			
AST	10-35 IU/L	48 IU/L		
ALT	6-40 IU/L	76 IU/L		
GLU	65-99 mg/dL			
Na	135-146 mEq/L			
K	3.5-5.3 mEq/L			
Cl	98-110 mEq/L			
C02	21-33 mmHg			
BUN	7-25 mg/dL			
Creatinine	0.6-1.2 mg/dL			
Calcium	8.6-10.2 mg/dL			
WBC	4-11 cells/mm^3	5.8 cells/mm^3		
TB test, PPD		Negative		

ADDITIONAL INFORMATION

Date	Notes
7/31/10	BP 122/78 mmHg. Patient reports morning stiffness for past 2 months which improves as the day progresses. Reports that wrists, arms and leg joints are swollen and tender. States she is physically exhausted. No chest pain, breathing problems.

QUESTIONS

1. The physician is deciding whether to change the dose of methotrexate to daily therapy or begin etanercept. Choose the correct response:

   a. The methotrexate can be increased safely to 50 mg daily for rheumatoid arthritis.

   b. The methotrexate can be increased safely to 100 mg daily for rheumatoid arthritis.

   c. The methotrexate can be increased safely to 150 mg daily for rheumatoid arthritis.

   d. The methotrexate can be increased safely to 200 mg daily for rheumatoid arthritis.

   e. Methotrexate is not given daily for this condition.

2. The pharmacist will counsel the patient on her methotrexate therapy. She should include the following counseling points:

   a. Common side effects include GI upset, nausea and diarrhea.

   b. She should not get pregnant while using this medication.

   c. Her liver will need to be checked periodically with a blood test.

   d. Choose a day of the week that you will remember to take the medicine.

   e. All of the above.

3. The patient is using prednisone 10 mg daily and weekly bisphosphonate therapy. Choose the correct statement:

   a. She does not need supplemental calcium and vitamin D with the alendronate.

   b. The prednisone may improve her blood pressure control.

   c. If she is able, her doctor should try and help her decrease the prednisone dose.

   d. Prednisone is not bad for bones; in fact, it builds strong bones.

   e. A, B and C.

4. The physician decides to begin etanercept therapy. Choose the correct administration route for this medication:

   a. Oral tablets

   b. Suppository

   c. Subcutaneous injection

   d. Intramuscular injection

   e. Intravenous injection

5. The pharmacist will counsel the patient on the etanercept therapy. She should include the following counseling points:

   a. Store the medication at room temperature.

   b. Inject subcutaneously in the deltoid muscle.

   c. This medication can activate latent tuberculosis; you will need to have a TB test prior to starting therapy.

   d. This medication does not cause increased risk of infections, except for tuberculosis.

   e. You can receive live vaccines, but not the annual influenza vaccine.

6. A physician has written a prescription for *Humira*. Choose the appropriate therapeutic interchange:

   a. Adalimumab

   b. Etanercept

   c. Rituximab

   d. Anakinra

   e. Infliximab

7. A physician has written a prescription for *Remicade*. Choose the appropriate therapeutic interchange:

   a. Adalimumab

   b. Etanercept

   c. Rituximab

   d. Anakinra

   e. Infliximab

ANSWERS

1-e, 2-e, 3-c, 4-c, 5-c, 6-a, 7-e

GOUT

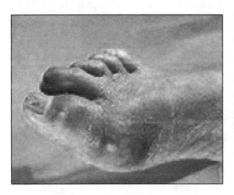

Background

Gout is a disease that usually presents with recurrent attacks of acute inflammatory arthritis. Gout attacks are sudden with severe pain, burning, and swelling. Gout typically occurs in one joint, which is most often the metatarsophalangeal joint (MTP, the big toe). If left untreated, the attacks can occur over and over, and will eventually damage the joints, tendons and other tissues.

Causes

Uric acid is produced as an end-product of purine metabolism (see chart to the right). Under normal conditions, uric acid is excreted ⅔ renally and ⅓ by the GI tract. When uric acid builds up in the blood, the patient may remain asymptomatic (many people with high uric acid, or hyperuricemia, never get gout) or the uric acid can crystallize in the joints, resulting in a severe, painful gout attack. Gout typically strikes after many years of persistent hyperuricemia.

RISK FACTORS

Risk factors for gout include male sex, overweight (2-3 x ↑ risk), excessive alcohol consumption (particularly beer), hypertension, renal insufficiency, advanced age and using medications that increase uric acid. Studies confirm that total protein intake (purine rich foods) is not associated with ↑ uric acid levels.

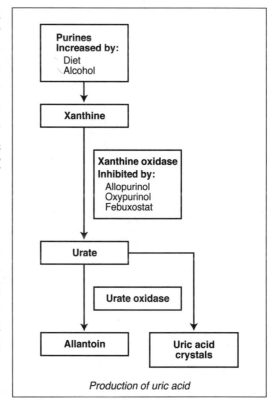

Production of uric acid

LABORATORY PARAMETERS

A normal serum uric acid level is ~2.0 – 7.2 mg/dL. If you are given a case with elevated uric acid, do not choose treatment unless a gout attack has occurred. Asymptomatic hyperuricemia is not treated.

Treatment Goals

The goal of treatment is to treat acute attacks, prevent future flare-ups, and reduce UA levels. Note that the drugs used to treat an acute attack (colchicine, NSAIDs, steroids) are different than

MEDICATIONS THAT INCREASE URIC ACID
diuretics (thiazides, loops)
niacin
aspirin
cyclosporine
ethambutol
levodopa (possibility higher with levodopa alone than with levodopa/carbidopa)
pyrazinamide

the drugs used to prevent attacks. Colchicine, however, is sometimes used during the initiation of prophylactic therapy to reduce the risk of acute attacks which can occur when uric acid is lowered rapidly.

Acute Gout Attack Treatment

DRUG	DOSING	SIDE EFFECTS

Colchicine

DRUG	DOSING	SIDE EFFECTS
Colchicine (*Colcrys*) + probenecid (*Colbenemid*)	1.2 mg orally (this is two 0.6 mg tablets) followed by 0.6 mg in 1 hour (do not exceed a total of 1.8 mg – or 3 doses) IV colchicine is highly toxic, has a narrow therapeutic index, and is considered a HIGH risk drug by ISMP. It is rarely used. It cannot be used in renal or hepatic disease.	Nausea, vomiting, abdominal pain, diarrhea (~80% of patients) Rare side effects: myelosuppression and neuromyopathy and death possible if overdosed – check dosing and enzyme inhibitors.

NSAIDs

DRUG	DOSING	SIDE EFFECTS
Indomethacin (*Indocin*)	50 mg TID until pain is tolerable – then taper down to avoid risk of rebound attack	(See pain section; avoid use in severe renal disease (uric acid is renally cleared and gout patients may have renal insufficiency); consider risk of bleeding, however risk of GI bleeding is less due to short duration of therapy), CVD risk (most with celecoxib)
Naproxen (*Naprosyn, others*)	750 mg x 1, then reduce to 250 mg Q8H until attack resolved	Indomethacin was 1st NSAID approved and is the traditional DOC, however, it is more toxic than ibuprofen (↑ risk for GI toxicity) and has psychiatric side effects including confusion, depression, psychosis.
Sulindac (*Clinoril*)	300-400 mg daily	
Celecoxib (*Celebrex*)	Used, not FDA-approved	All NSAIDs cause nausea, take with food

Acute Gout Attack Treatment Continued

DRUG	DOSING	SIDE EFFECTS

Steroids: Can be given PO, IM, IV, intra-articular or via ACTH (adrenocorticotropic hormone) which triggers endogenous glucocorticoid secretion.

| Prednisone (orally) | 0.5 mg/kg/day x 1, then ↓ by 5 mg each day or 2-60 mg daily x 5-7 days (taper is not required if treatment is short-term, such as 5-7 days therapy) | Acute steroid use side effects (not an issue if injected into joint): increased blood glucose, elevated blood pressure, nervousness, insomnia, increased appetite, edema. |
| Methylprednisolone *(Solu-Medrol)*
 Triamcinolone | Intra-articular injection (into joint); systemic side effects unlikely | |

COLCHICINE DRUG INTERACTIONS

- Colchicine is a substrate of CYP 3A4 and the efflux transporter P-glycoprotein (P-gp). Fatal toxicity can occur if colchicine is combined with strong 3A4 inhibitors, such as clarithromycin or a strong inhibitor of P-gp, such as cyclosporine. Check for inhibitors prior to dispensing drug. If using a moderate 3A4 inhibitor, the maximum dose is 2 tablets (x 1) – and wait at least 3 days prior to an additional dose.

- Myopathy and rhabdomyolysis have been reported in patients taking colchicine with a statin or fibrate; try not to use with gemfibrozil and have patients monitor muscle pain/soreness.

COLCHICINE COUNSELING

- At the first sign of an attack, take 2 tablets. You can take 1 more tablet in one hour. Do not use more than this amount. Taking too much colchicine can lead to serious side effects.

- You should not take the 2nd dose if you have upset stomach, nausea or diarrhea.

- Report any serious stomach upset, or other issues, to your doctor.

- Wait at least 3 days before initiating another course of therapy.

PROPHYLACTIC TREATMENT

MOA: Allopurinol and febuxostat are <u>xanthine oxidase</u> inhibitors (block UA production).

Chronic UA- Lowering Therapy

DRUG	DOSING	SIDE EFFECTS/MONITORING/CONTRAINDICATIONS
Use colchicine at daily dose of 0.6 mg once or twice daily or NSAIDs for at least 6 months to reduce the risk of acute flares when beginning UA-lowering acid therapy.		

Xanthine Oxidase Inhibitors

Allopurinol *(Zyloprim)*	50-200 mg daily, (Prophylaxis for hyperuricemia due to cancer drugs that cause tumor lysis syndrome requires very high doses of allopurinol used short-term, or the IV agent rasburicase)	**SIDE EFFECTS, ALLOPURINOL** Precipitation of acute attacks, nausea and skin rash. The rash can be serious – it may appear benign but can rarely develop into more serious reactions including toxic epidermal necrolysis or Steven-Johnson Syndrome Allopurinol dose adjustment if CrCl < 20 mL/min.
Febuxostat *(Uloric)* For resistant cases, and possibly in renal disease, or if reaction to allopurinol	40-80 mg daily	Febuxostat: much more expensive than allopurinol ($20K more/year), may be safer in severe renal impairment (no dose adjustment in moderate renal disease) and has ↓ risk for hypersensitivity reactions (↓ risk of serious skin rash). Check LFTs at 2 and 4 months and periodically thereafter.

rash (handwritten note)

Uricosuric

Probenecid	500-1,000 mg BID	Uricosurics <u>require adequate renal function</u>. They are not commonly used, but may be used in younger patients with good renal function (> 60 mL/min) or if taking agents that increase uric acid, such as diuretics.
Sulfinpyrazone		

Uricase – breaks down uric acid

Pegloticase *(Krystexxa)* – IV medication, costly, <u>resistant cases only</u>	8 mg IV Q 2 weeks > $20K/year	Risk severe infusion reactions (6.5%) – give in medical setting only. Can precipitate acute attack, may worsen heart failure

PROBENECID DRUG INTERACTIONS

- Probenecid may decrease the renal clearance of other medications taken concurrently, including aspirin, methotrexate, theophylline, penicillins, etc.

- Probenecid used to be given with penicillins to ↑ the penicillin plasma concentrations; this will ↑ adverse reactions associated with the beta lactam.

ALLOPURINOL COUNSELING (PROBENECID IS USED LESS COMMONLY)

- Take once daily with a meal to reduce stomach upset (higher doses used for tumor lysis prophylaxis can be divided).

- It may take up to several weeks for this medicine to have an effect and you may have more gout attacks for several months after starting this medicine while the body removes extra uric acid. If this happens, you can use different medicine for the acute attack.

- If you get a rash, notify your doctor. The rash could become serious. If the rash looks serious, you should be seen quickly.

Practice Case

Brian is a 62 year-old male with hypertension. His blood pressure has a daily range of 155-178/88-98. He is using amlodipine 10 mg once daily, lisinopril 10 mg once daily and HCTZ 25 mg once daily. He takes several OTC products, including aspirin EC 81 mg once daily, fish oils and coenzyme Q10. He reports "weekend" alcohol use (3-4 beers on Saturday/Sunday). No past or present history of tobacco use. Brian is presenting at the clinic with pain described as 10/10. He is trying to avoid putting weight on his right foot. Physical exam reveals a swollen, tender, enlarged big toe.

CATEGORY	
Vitals	Height 5'11", weight 255"
	AST 12 U/L, ALT 14 U/L, BUN/SCr 22/1.4, Uric Acid 18.3 mg/dL

QUESTIONS

1. What is Brian's creatinine clearance (in ml/min), using the Cockcroft-Gault equation and his ideal body weight?

   a. 89
   b. 71
   c. 58
   d. 34
   e. 11

2. The physician is considering allopurinol therapy to treat the acute attack. Choose the correct statement:

   a. This is not appropriate therapy for an acute attack.
   b. He should receive a starting dose of 50 mg once daily.
   c. He should receive a starting dose of 75 mg once daily.
   d. He should receive a starting dose of 100 mg once daily.
   e. He should receive a starting dose of 150 mg once daily.

3. Brian will receive a short-course of prednisone therapy, with taper, that will last less than 2 weeks. Which of the following adverse effects are possible and should be explained to Brian?

   a. Growth suppression
   b. Insomnia/spaciness
   c. Osteoporosis
   d. Cataracts
   e. All of the above

4. Choose the correct dosing regimen for colchicine for an acute gout attack:

   a. 1.2 mg followed by 0.6 mg every 2 hours, not to exceed 6 tablets/24 hours
   b. 1.2 mg followed by 0.6 mg every 2 hours, not to exceed 8 tablets/24 hours
   c. 1.2 mg followed by 0.6 mg in 2-4 hours (total 1.8 mg)
   d. 1.2 mg followed by 0.6 mg in 1 hour, then as-needed for 3 additional doses (total 3.6 mg)
   e. 1.2 mg followed by 0.6 mg in 1 hour (total 1.8 mg)

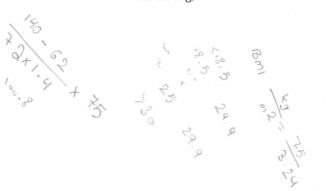

5. A pharmacist receives a prescription for *Zyloprim*. Which medication is an acceptable alternative?

   a. Probenecid
   b. Colchicine
   c. Allopurinol
   d. Naproxen
   e. Febuxostat

6. A physician wants to prescribe prednisone to a patient with an acute gout attack. He calls the pharmacy to ask if a taper is required, and if so, the reason why. The pharmacist should provide the following information to the prescriber:

   a. No taper is required if the steroid therapy is less than 2 weeks duration.
   b. A taper is required with prednisone therapy to prevent an additional attack.
   c. NSAID therapy may also require the initial dose to be decreased when used for acute gout.
   d. Colchicine will also require a taper if used for acute gout.
   e. B and C only.

7. Which of the following side effects are likely to occur with colchicine therapy?

   a. Nausea
   b. Stomach upset
   c. Mental confusion
   d. A and B only
   e. All of the above

8. A pharmacist has just attended an education program on the use of Febuxostat *(Uloric)*. He wants to present the main points about this new drug to his pharmacy colleagues. He should include the following points:

   a. Febuxostat (like allopurinol) is a xanthine oxidase inhibitor.
   b. Febuxostat appears to have lower risk of hypersensitivity reactions than allopurinol, including less of a risk of serious rash.
   c. Febuxostat costs much more than generic allopurinol and provides little extra benefit in the majority of patients.
   d. A and B only.
   e. All of the above.

9. A pharmacist is going to counsel a patient beginning allopurinol therapy. Which counseling statement should be included?

   a. This medication should be taken on an empty stomach.
   b. Allopurinol can cause blood pressure changes; hold onto the bed or rail when changing from a sitting to a standing position.
   c. If you notice a rash, contact your doctor at once. If the rash looks serious, you should not use the medicine and should be seen right away.
   d. A and C.
   e. All of the above.

10. The patient in this case has several known risk factors for gout. Which of the following risk factors increase his risk of gout?

    a. Consuming alcohol, especially beer
    b. His weight
    c. His hypertension history, and the use of HCTZ
    d. A and B only
    e. All of the above

ANSWERS

1-c, 2-a, 3-b, 4-e, 5-c, 6-e, 7-d, 8-e, 9-c, 10-e

HYPERTENSION

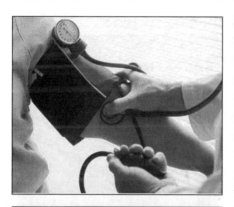

GUIDELINES

Seventh Report of the Joint National Committee (JNC 7) on Prevention, Detection, Evaluation, and Treatment of High Blood Pressure. U.S. Department of Health and Human Services. Dec. 2003. JNC 8 expected release spring, 2012.

Treatment of Hypertension in the Prevention and Management of Ischemic Heart Disease. *Circulation* 2007;115:2761-2788.

Background

Nearly 1 in 3 adults have hypertension. If left untreated, the patient is at increased risk of heart disease, stroke and kidney disease. Hypertension is largely asymptomatic, and often is untreated. Only when the blood pressure is very high (such as with hypertensive crisis) are symptoms (throbbing headache, fatigue and shortness of breath) likely to appear. Pharmacists should help patients identify hypertension and advise them to stick with medication therapy. One in four patients discontinue antihypertensive therapy within 6 months. Beta blockers can cause fatigue (and sometimes sexual problems), diuretics can increase urination and ACE inhibitors can cause cough. Some patients get edema from calcium channel blockers, especially if high doses are used. These side effects can each lead to discontinuation, but the major cause of patients stopping their medicines is a <u>lack of understanding</u> of the necessity for treatment <u>and</u> cost. If a brand is prescribed, see if a generic can be used.

Counseling should include recommendations to follow healthy lifestyle measures that can decrease blood pressure, such as sodium restriction, a healthy diet, physical activity, maintaining a healthy weight, smoking cessation, etc. Recommending a home blood pressure monitoring device can help the patient get involved and improve motivation and success of therapy.

Pathophysiology

Most cases of hypertension are essential hypertension, which means they are not known to be caused by an identifiable factor, although poor lifestyle and genetics are contributory. Secondary hypertension is linked to a specific cause, such as renal disease, adrenal disease and/or drug-induced hypertension.

Drug-induced hypertension can be caused by corticosteroids, excessive alcohol (> 1-2 drinks daily), NSAIDs (selective and non-selective), ACTH, amphetamines, appetite suppressants, caffeine, cyclosporine, erythropoietin, estrogen (such as contraceptives with higher estrogen doses), oral decongestants (e.g. pseudoephedrine), thyroid hormone (if given too much), duloxetine and venlafaxine (at higher doses), and chemo drugs [e.g. bevacizumab *(Avastin)*, sorafenib *(Nexavar)*, others].

CLASSIFICATION OF BLOOD PRESSURE IN ADULTS ACCORDING TO JNC 7

CLASSIFICATION	SYSTOLIC BP/DIASTOLIC BP (mmHg)
Normal	Less than 120/80
Pre-hypertension	120-139/80-89
Stage 1	140-159/90-99
Stage 2	≥ 160 / ≥ 100

COMPELLING INDICATION AND TREATMENT CHOICE PER JNC-7

INDICATION	TREATMENT CHOICE
Heart Failure	ACEI, ARB, BB, diuretic, aldosterone antagonist
S/P MI	ACEI, BB, aldosterone antagonist
High risk of CAD	ACEI, BB, diuretic, CCB
Diabetes	ACEI, ARB, BB, CCB, diuretic
CKD	ACEI, ARB
Recurrent stroke prevention	ACEI, diuretic

NOTES

If Stage 1 HTN, consider thiazide-type diuretics for most. May consider ACEI, ARB, BB, CCB, or combo.

If Stage 2 HTN, start with two drugs (usually thiazide-type diuretic and ACEI, or ARB, or BB, or CCB).

Beta blockers are not 1st line for general coronary artery disease (CAD) prevention.

High risk is defined as having diabetes mellitus, chronic kidney disease (CKD), known CAD or CAD equivalent (carotid artery disease, peripheral arterial disease, abdominal aortic aneurysm), or a 10-year Framingham risk score > 10%.

Lifestyle modification is recommended at ALL levels.

BP goal per JNC-7 is < 140/90 mmHg, unless patient has DM or CKD, then BP goal is < 130/80 mmHg.

TREATMENT BASED ON AHA GUIDELINES

CONDITION	GOAL (mmHg)	DRUG CHOICE
General CAD prevention	< 140/90	Any drug or combo
High CAD risk	< 130/80	ACEI or ARB or CCB or thiazide diuretic or combo
Stable angina	< 130/80	Beta-Blocker and ACEI or ARB
Unstable Angina/NSTEMI	< 130/80	Beta-Blocker (if patient is hemodynamically stable) and ACEI or ARB
STEMI	< 130/80	Beta-Blocker (if patient is hemodynamically stable) and ACEI or ARB
LVD	< 120/80	ACEI or ARB and beta blocker and aldosterone antagonist and thiazide or loop diuretic and hydralazine/isosorbide dinitrate (black patients)

LIFESTYLE MODIFICATIONS

Always encourage if needed!

Weight
Maintain normal BMI and waist circumference

Eating
Recommend the Dietary Approaches to Stop HTN (DASH) eating plan, which is high in fruits and vegetables, and recommends low-fat dairy products with reduced saturated and total fat

Reduce Na+
Healthy adults should be ≤ 2.4 grams sodium/day. But if hypertensive, the goal is < 1.5 grams/day

Increase Physical Activity
Engage in regular aerobic physical activity such as brisk walking (at least 30 min per day, most days of the week)

Moderate Alcohol Consumption
Alcohol should be limited to 1 drink/day (most women) and 2 drinks/day (most men)

Smoking Cessation
Pharmacists should be able to recommend how to quit and assist with therapy (nicotine replacement, gum, etc.)

Control Blood Glucose And Lipids To Reduce Cardiovascular Disease Risk!

Diuretics

- Thiazides (HCTZ, others) are cheap, effective, have mild side effects and are often used first.

- Loop diuretics (furosemide, others) are used mostly in heart failure. Loops cause more sodium excretion, and are thus more potent fluid depletors (greater water loss), which provides benefit in HF. They also waste much more potassium than thiazides and run a risk of ototoxicity (auditory damage/hearing loss). Loops usually require K^+ supplements (potassium ext-release, or *Klor-Con*). Used long-term, they can lower bone density.

- Thiazides work on the distal convoluted tubule of the nephron, however the long-term blood pressure lowering effect is thought to be due to vasodilation ($\downarrow$ resistance). Loops work on the ascending loop by blocking sodium reabsorption – this causes water to follow sodium into the urine, resulting in volume depletion.

- Potassium-sparing diuretics (triamterene, others) are not as effective and are not used as monotherapy for BP, but they are commonly used in combo with HCTZ *(Maxzide/Dyazide)* to counter the thiazide's mild potassium loss and help (a little) with BP. If any potassium-retaining agent is used, there will be a risk of hyperkalemia, especially with reduced renal function. Spironolactone and eplerenone are used for HF (and HTN), and $\uparrow K^+$ is a considerable risk with these agents.

DRUG	DOSING	SIDE EFFECTS/CONTRAINDICATIONS/ MONITORING

Thiazides - inhibit Na⁺ reabsorption in the distal tubules causing increased excretion of Na⁺ and water as well as K⁺ and H⁺ ions

DRUG	DOSING	SIDE EFFECTS/CONTRAINDICATIONS/MONITORING
Chlorothiazide *(Diuril)*	125-500 mg/d	**SIDE EFFECTS** Hypokalemia (can usually be avoided with regular intake of potassium rich foods) Can contribute to hyperuricemia ($\uparrow$ UA), elevated lipids ($\uparrow$ CH, $\uparrow$ TG), hyperglycemia ($\uparrow$ BG), hypercalcemia ($\uparrow$ Ca²⁺), hyponatremia, hypomagnesemia, photosensitivity, rash.
Chlorthalidone *(Thalitone)*	12.5-25 mg, max 50 mg/d	
Hydrochlorothiazide *(Microzide* – capsule, *Oretic, Esidrix)*	12.5-25 mg, max 50 mg/d	**CONTRAINDICATIONS** Hypersensitivity to sulfonamide-derived drugs, anuria, and renal decompensation Sulfa Allergy – may not cross-react, but first dose should be given under supervision if allergic.
Indapamide *(Lozol)*	1.25-5 mg/d	Thiazides may not be as effective if CrCl < 30 mL/min) – exception; metolazone may work in patients with reduced renal function.
Metolazone *(Zaroxolyn)*	2.5-5 mg, max 20 mg/d	
Methylclothiazide	2.5-5 mg/d	

Diruetics Continued

DRUG	DOSING	SIDE EFFECTS/CONTRAINDICATIONS/ MONITORING

Loop diuretics - inhibit reabsorption of Na⁺ and Cl⁻ in the <u>ascending loop of Henle</u> and distal renal tubule, interfering with the chloride binding co-transport system thus causing increased excretion of water, Na^+, Cl^-, Mg^{2+}, and Ca^{2+}

Loop diuretics are used more for edema (for fluid depletion) in HF; occasionally for BP if ↓ renal function

DRUG	DOSING	SIDE EFFECTS/CONTRAINDICATIONS/ MONITORING
Furosemide *(Lasix)* – most patients take divided doses: take 2nd dose early	20-80 mg daily, or divided, can go higher. <u>Oral loop dose equivalency =</u> <u>40 mg</u>	**BLACK BOX WARNING** Can lead to profound diuresis resulting in fluid and electrolyte depletion **SIDE EFFECTS** <u>Hypokalemia, orthostatic hypotension, ↓ Na⁺, ↓ Mg²⁺, ↓ Cl⁻, ↓ Ca²⁺ (different than thiazides which ↑ Ca²⁺), metabolic alkalosis, hyperuricemia (↑ UA), hyperglycemia (↑ BG), photosensitivity, ototoxicity (MORE with ethacrynic acid)</u>
Bumetanide *(Bumex)*	0.5-2 mg daily <u>Oral loop dose equivalency =</u> <u>1 mg</u>	**CONTRAINDICATIONS** Anuria Caution in patients with a sulfa allergy (except ethacrynic acid) **MONITORING** <u>Renal function (SCr, BUN), fluid status (in's and out's, weight), BP, electrolytes, hearing with high doses or rapid IV administration</u> IV formulations are light-sensitive (in amber bottles)
Torsemide *(Demadex)*	5-20 mg daily <u>Oral loop dose equivalency =</u> <u>20 mg</u>	
Ethacrynic Acid *(Edecrin)*	25, 50 mg tabs; 50 mg inj.	

Diruetics Continued

DRUG	DOSING	SIDE EFFECTS/CONTRAINDICATIONS/MONITORING

Potassium-Sparing Diuretics - compete with aldosterone for receptor sites in the distal renal tubules, increasing Na⁺, Cl⁻, and water excretion while conserving K⁺ and H⁺ ions

DRUG	DOSING	SIDE EFFECTS/CONTRAINDICATIONS/MONITORING
Amiloride *(Midamor)*	5-20 mg	**BLACK BOX WARNINGS** Tumor risk with spironolactone; tumorigenic in chronic rat toxicity studies. Only used in approved indications and avoid unnecessary use. Hyperkalemia potentially fatal with amiloride or triamterene. 10% incidence when not coadministered with K⁺ depleting diuretic. ↑ incidence in elderly, diabetes or renal impaired patients. Check K⁺ at the start of treatment dose increases and with illnesses that affect renal function. **SIDE EFFECTS** Hyperkalemia, ↑ serum creatinine. For spironolactone, gynecomastia, breast tenderness, impotence, menstrual changes, hirsutism, hyperchloremic metabolic acidosis. **CONTRAINDICATIONS** Anuria, K⁺ > 5.5 mEq/L at initiation, CrCl < 30 mL/min; concomitant use of 3A4 inhibitors (eplerenone) **MONITORING** Check K⁺ before starting and periodically thereafter. Stop if K⁺ > 5.5 mEq/L. BP, SCr/BUN Pregnancy Category C
Triamterene *(Dyrenium)* **+ HCTZ** *(Maxzide, Dyazide)*	50-100 mg BID, max 300 mg/d	
Spironolactone *(Aldactone)*	NYHA 3 and 4 HF 25-50 mg/d HTN 50-100 mg/d	
Eplerenone *(Inspra)*	CHF, post MI: 25-50 mg/d HTN 50-100 mg/d	

DRUG INTERACTIONS

- All antihypertensives can add to or potentiate the therapeutic effect of other blood pressure-lowering drugs; always carefully monitor when adding-on therapy, particularly with diuretics.

- Loop diuretics can increase the ototoxic potential of aminoglycoside antibiotics, especially in the presence of impaired renal function. Except in life-threatening situations, avoid this combination.

- Do not use ethacrynic acid with other loop diuretics due to the risk of additive ototoxicity.

- Lithium generally should not be given with diuretics because diuretics reduce lithium's renal clearance and add a high risk of lithium toxicity.

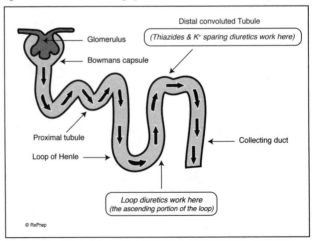

Renin-Angiotensin Aldosterone System (RAAS) Inhibitors

- All RAAS inhibitors ↓ vasoconstriction, ↓ aldosterone release, and have benefit in renal protection and heart failure. Some patients are receiving ACEI-ARBs together: as both ↑ K⁺, this requires careful monitoring. Potassium should remain within the safe level of 3.5-5 mEq/L.

- ARBs are given if patient is intolerant to ACE-I (e.g. cough that is dry, intermittent), and are also first-line.

- Angioedema is more common in black patients. Although angioedema is more likely with ACEIs than ARBs, if a person had angioedema with either class of agents, all others are contraindicated since angioedema can quickly be FATAL. Counsel to report any swelling of lips, mouth, tongue, face, or neck immediately.

- Patients on these medicines should not use salt substitutes (which contain KCl, rather than NaCl).

- Captopril has more side effects than other agents (taste disturbances, rash). It is not an optimal agent due to frequent dosing (BID or TID). The others are daily or BID.

- When used in pregnancy, fetal/neonatal morbidity/mortality can occur with any drug class that directly act on renin-angiotensin system (ACE-I, ARB, direct renin inhibitor); discontinue drug as soon as possible when pregnancy is detected.

DRUG	DOSING	SIDE EFFECTS/CONTRAINDICATIONS/MONITORING

ARBs - block angiotensin II (AT II) from binding to the angiotensin II type-1 (AT₁) receptor on vascular smooth muscle.

DRUG	DOSING	SIDE EFFECTS/CONTRAINDICATIONS/MONITORING
Valsartan *(Diovan)*	80-320 mg/d	**BLACK BOX WARNING** Can cause injury and death to developing fetus; discontinue as soon as pregnancy is detected
Losartan *(Cozaar)*	25-100 mg/d and generic	**SIDE EFFECTS** Hyperkalemia, angioedema (if occurs, drug is CI), hypotension, headache, dizziness
Irbesartan *(Avapro)*	150-300 mg/d	**CONTRAINDICATIONS** Angioedema. Do not use in bilateral renal artery stenosis; renal function will worsen.
Candesartan *(Atacand)*	8-32 mg/d	
Olmesartan *(Benicar)*	20-40 mg/d	**MONITORING** BP, K⁺, renal function Pregnancy Category C (1st trimester) /D (2nd & 3rd trimester)
Telmisartan *(Micardis)*	40-80 mg/d	Pregnancy category D: Valsartan
Eprosartan *(Teveten)*	400-800 mg/d	
Azilsartan *(Edarbi)*	40-80 mg/d	

Renin-Angiotensin Aldosterone System (RAAS) Inhibitors Continued

DRUG	DOSING	SIDE EFFECTS/CONTRAINDICATIONS/MONITORING

ACE Inhibitors - inhibit the angiotensin converting enzyme, preventing the conversion of angiotensin I (Ang I) to angiotensin II (Ang II), a potent vasoconstrictor, thereby reducing BP

DRUG	DOSING	SIDE EFFECTS/CONTRAINDICATIONS/MONITORING
Benazepril *(Lotensin)*	10-40 mg/d	**Black Box Warning** Can cause injury and death to developing fetus; discontinue as soon as pregnancy is detected
Captopril *(Capoten)*	25-50 mg BID-TID Take 1 hour before meals	**SIDE EFFECTS** Cough, hyperkalemia, angioedema (if occurs, drug is CI), hypotension. Captopril has more SEs (taste perversion, rash).
Enalapril, Enalaprilat IV injection *(Vasotec)*	5-40 mg/d	
Fosinopril *(Monopril)*	20-80 mg/d	**CONTRAINDICATIONS** Angioedema. Do not use in bilateral renal artery stenosis; renal function will worsen.
Lisinopril *(Prinivil, Zestril)*	10-40 mg/d	**MONITORING** BP, K+, renal function
Moexipril *(Univasc)*	7.5-30 mg/d	Pregnancy Category C (1st trimester) /D (2nd & 3rd trimester)
Perindopril *(Aceon)*	4-16 mg/d	
Quinapril *(Accupril)*	40-80 mg/d	
Ramipril *(Altace)*	5-20 mg/d	
Trandolapril *(Mavik)*	2-8 mg/d	

Renin Inhibitor - directly inhibits renin which is responsible for the conversion of angiotensinogen to angiotensin I (Ang I)

DRUG	DOSING	SIDE EFFECTS/CONTRAINDICATIONS/MONITORING
Aliskiren *(Tekturna)*	150-300 mg/d Avoid high fat foods. Take with or without food and take the same way each day.	**Black Box Warning** Can cause injury and death to developing fetus; discontinue as soon as pregnancy is detected **SIDE EFFECTS** Hyperkalemia, angioedema (if occurs, drug is CI), hypotension. **CONTRAINDICATIONS** Angioedema. Do not use in bilateral renal artery stenosis; renal function will worsen. **MONITORING** BP, K+, renal function Pregnancy Category C (1st trimester) /D (2nd & 3rd trimester)

DRUG INTERACTIONS

- Most critical drug interactions are additive effects on potassium: monitor with concurrent drugs that increase levels, and with reduced renal function since potassium is renally cleared.

- Aliskiren is metabolized by CYP 450 3A4; concentration is affected by 3A4 inducers and inhibitors. Do not use with cyclosporine due to increased aliskiren levels. Atorvastatin increases aliskiren level.

- Aliskiren decreases the level of furosemide; monitor effectiveness.

β–Blockers, α+β–Blockers (Carvedilol/Labetolol), β–Blocker/ Nitric Oxide (Nebivolol)

- β–blockers are used for HTN, post-MI, angina, HF and migraine prophylaxis. 1st-line use for HTN now being discouraged; risk may be higher with atenolol (currently unknown).

- The primary α+β–blocking agent (carvedilol) is used for HF and HTN; note different dosing/titration schedules for the indications and formulation. Metoprolol XL is also commonly used for HF and HTN.

- Nebivolol, the β–blocker/ Nitric Oxide agent, is indicated for HTN, and used off-label for HF.

- β–blockers with intrinsic sympathomimetic activity (ISA): CAPP (carteolol, acebutolol, penbutolol, pindolol). ISA β–blockers can show antagonism (blocker) and low level agonist (stimulate) activity at the beta receptor. These agents are useful in patients with excessive bradycardia who need β–blocker therapy.

- Beta-1 selectivity: AMEBBA (atenolol, metoprolol, esmolol, bisoprolol, betaxolol, acebutolol).

- Lipid solubility (more CNS side effects): Propranolol has high lipid solubility. More sedation, cognitive effects, and depression seen with lipid-soluble agents.

- Take carvedilol with food (even the CR version).

- Carvedilol CR is less bioavailable than carvedilol IR, therefore, dose conversions are not mg per mg.

- Labetolol is often used 1st-line for HTN in pregnancy. Nifedipine is also used. Methyldopa can be used and was used historically, but has many side effects.

- Beta blockers can cover up the symptoms of shakiness and anxiety with hypoglycemia; this occurs mostly with the non-selective agents. This is why the beta blocker propranolol is used for stage freight. They do not, however, cover up sweating (diaphoresis) and hunger.

- Use caution in patients with breathing problems (asthma, COPD). Choose beta-1 selective agents, and keep at selective dosing.

DRUG	DOSING	SIDE EFFECTS/CONTRAINDICATIONS/ MONITORING

β1-selective blockers

DRUG	DOSING	SIDE EFFECTS/CONTRAINDICATIONS/MONITORING
Acebutolol *(Sectral)*	200-800 mg/d	**SIDE EFFECTS** ↓ HR, hypotension, fatigue, dizziness. Less common: depression, ↓ libido
Atenolol *(Tenormin)*	25-100 mg/d	**CONTRAINDICATIONS** Severe bradycardia, 2nd or 3rd degree heart block, cardiogenic shock, sick sinus syndrome, Do not initiate in patients with active asthma bronchospasm
Betaxolol *(Kerlone)*	5-40 mg/d	
Bisoprolol *(Zebeta)*	2.5-20 mg/d	**MONITORING** HR, BP, titrate Q 2 wks (as tolerated); ↓ dose if HR < 55 Caution use in patients with asthma
Metoprolol tartrate *(Lopressor)*, Metoprolol succin ext rel *(Lopressor XL, Toprol XL)*	HTN: 25-400 mg/d IR BID; XL daily HF: Start 12.5-25 mg/d (max 200 mg/d)	Avoid abrupt discontinuation – must taper Caution in those with diabetes who have recurrent hypoglycemia, asthma, severe COPD, and resting limb ischemia

β1-selective blocker and Nitric Oxide

DRUG	DOSING	SIDE EFFECTS/CONTRAINDICATIONS/MONITORING
Nebivolol *(Bystolic)*	5-40 mg/d. CrCl < 30 mL/min or liver impairment, start 2.5 mg/d	**SIDE EFFECTS** Headache, fatigue, dizziness, diarrhea, and nausea Nitric oxide causes peripheral (arterial) vasodilation; clinical benefit unclear

β1 & β 2 (non-selective) blockers

DRUG	DOSING	SIDE EFFECTS/CONTRAINDICATIONS/MONITORING
Carteolol *(Cartrol)*	2.5-10 mg/d	ISA Agents – acebutolol, carteolol, penbutolol, pindolol (CAPP): Do not ↓ HR as much as others.
Nadolol *(Corgard)*	20-320 mg/d	
Penbutolol *(Levatol)*	10-80 mg/d	
Pindolol *(Visken)*	10-60 mg/d	
Propranolol *(Inderal LA, InnoPran XL)*	40-480 mg/d	
Timolol *(Blocadren)*	10-60 mg/d	

Non-selective α & β blockers

DRUG	DOSING	SIDE EFFECTS/CONTRAINDICATIONS/MONITORING
Carvedilol **(Coreg, Coreg CR)**	HTN: 20-80 mg CR, or 6.25 mg BID HF: Start IR 3.125 mg BID (max 50 mg BID) or CR 10 mg/d (max 80 mg)	Same as above Take carvedilol – all forms – with food Pregnancy Category C
Labetalol *(Trandate, Normodyne)*	200-2,400 mg/d	

DRUG INTERACTIONS

- Beta blockers can enhance the effects of insulin and oral hypoglycemic (sulfonylureas, etc), monitor BG carefully.

- Use caution when administering other drugs that slow HR, such as digoxin.

- Some (carvedilol, etc) are substrates of various CYP enzymes; check for drug interactions. For example, rifampin lowers the serum level of carvedilol by ~70%.

Calcium Channel Blockers

- There are 2 types of CCBs: the dihydropyridines: DHPs, which end in "pine" and include amlodipine, nifedipine, etc. and the NON-DHPs, which are diltiazem and verapamil.

- They are used quite differently: the DHPs are used primarily for HTN and angina.

- Diltiazem and verapamil are used primarily for arrhythmias to control/slow HR, and sometimes for HTN and angina. Diltiazem and verapamil are negative inotropes (↓ contraction force) and negative chronotropes (↓ HR). The DHPs do not have these properties.

- Diltiazem and verapamil are CYP 3A4 inhibitors and can have significant DIs (can increase other drugs), and they are also 3A4 substrates. The DHPs do not have significant drug interactions.

- Side effects differ among the types: in addition to slowing HR, the non-DHPs can cause troublesome constipation (especially verapamil) and may cause gingival hyperplasia.

- The DHPs cause peripheral vasodilation, which can lead to reflex tachycardia, headache, flushing, and peripheral edema. Some agents are worse than others: amlodipine is used commonly since it does not commonly cause these problems.

- *Covera HS, Adalat CC,* and *Sular* have capsular shells that can be seen in feces (ghost shells).

- Clevidipine is contraindicated in soy or egg allergy.

- With CCBs, you need to be careful to check the orange book since there is such a variety of long-acting formulations; choose a generic that is AB-rated to the brand.

DRUG	DOSING	SIDE EFFECTS/CONTRAINDICATIONS/ MONITORING

DHP CCBs - inhibit Ca²⁺ ions from entering the "slow" channels or voltage-sensitive areas of vascular smooth muscle resulting in peripheral arterial vasodilation and decreasing peripheral vascular resistance

DRUG	DOSING	SIDE EFFECTS/CONTRAINDICATIONS/ MONITORING
Amlodipine *(Norvasc)*	2.5-10 mg/d	**SIDE EFFECTS** Peripheral edema, reflex tachycardia, headache, flushing
Felodipine ER *(Plendil)*	2.5-10 mg/d	**MONITORING** BP, HR, peripheral edema
Isradipine ER *(DynaCirc CR)* Isradapine IR is BID	5-10 mg/d	Do not use sublingual nifedipine – may ↑ risk of MI
Nifedipine ER *(**Adalat CC, Procardia XL, Afeditab CR**)*, **Nifedipine IR** *(**Procardia**)*	30-90 mg/d	
Nisoldipine ER *(Sular)*	8.5-34 mg/d	
Nisoldipine ER	20-60 mg/d	
Nicardipine ER *(Cardene SR)* Nicardipine IR *(Cardene)* is TID	30-60 mg (BID)	

Non-DHP CCBs - inhibit Ca²⁺ ions from entering the "slow" channels or voltage-sensitive areas of vascular smooth muscle and myocardium, resulting in coronary vasodilation.

DRUG	DOSING	SIDE EFFECTS/CONTRAINDICATIONS/ MONITORING
Diltiazem *(Cardizem, Cardizem CD, Cardizem LA, Dilacor XR, Dilt-CD, Dilt-XR, Cartia XT, Tiazac, Taztia XT)*	QDs are 120-420 mg/d BIDs are 60-240 mg TID is 30-120 mg	**SIDE EFFECTS** Edema, AV block, bradycardia, hypotension, arrhythmias, HF, headache, constipation (more with verapamil), gingival hyperplasia **CONTRAINDICATIONS** Severe hypotension, 2ⁿᵈ or 3ʳᵈ degree heart block, cardiogenic shock, sick sinus syndrome, acute MI and pulmonary congestion
Verapamil *(Calan, Calan SR, Isoptin SR, Verelan, Verelan PM, Covera HS)*	QDs are 100-300 mg/d BIDs are 120-180 mg TID is 40-120 mg	**MONITORING** BP, HR, ECG

Inpatient Acute Care DPH CCB

DRUG	DOSING	SIDE EFFECTS/CONTRAINDICATIONS/ MONITORING
Clevidipine *(Cleviprex)* IV only Other CCBs are used acutely: diltiazem, verapamil, nicardipine	1-16 mg/hr In 20% Intralipid	**SIDE EFFECTS** Headache, nausea/vomiting **CONTRAINDICATIONS** Do not use in soy or egg allergy, acute pancreatitis, severe aortic stenosis **MONITORING** BP, HR

DRUG INTERACTIONS

- Diltiazem and verapamil are both CYP 450 3A4 substrates <u>and</u> moderate inhibitors. They will raise the concentration of many other drugs, and 3A4 inducers and inhibitors will affect their concentration; check for interactions prior to dispensing. Avoid grapefruit juice.

Centrally Acting Alpha-2 Adrenergic Agonists

- Clonidine is used commonly for resistant hypertension and in patients who can not swallow (due to dysphagia, dementia) since it comes as a patch formulation. Since the patch is changed weekly, it can help with adherence.

- Clonidine has many side effects, including sedation, dizziness, lethargy, dry mouth, and can aggravate depression and contribute to sexual dysfunction. If it is used first-line without a valid reason, it may be inappropriate prescribing.

- Clonidine is sometimes used off-label for opioid withdrawal to block nervousness, anxiety and help with sleep.

- If stopped abruptly, especially at higher doses, a withdrawal syndrome with very high blood pressure, headache, anxiety, and tremors will result. Must taper over 2-5 days.

DRUG	DOSING	SIDE EFFECTS/CONTRAINDICATIONS/ MONITORING

Centrally-Acting Alpha$_2$ Agonists - stimulate alpha$_2$-adrenergic receptors in the brain which results in reduced sympathetic outflow from the CNS

DRUG	DOSING	SIDE EFFECTS/CONTRAINDICATIONS/ MONITORING
Clonidine (Catapres, Catapres-TTS patch, *Duraclon inj, Clonidine ER oral susp)*	0.1-0.3 mg BID Catapres-TTS-1 = 0.1 mg/24 hr Catapres-TTS-2 = 0.2 mg/24 hr Catapres-TTS-3 = 0.3 mg/24 hr	**SIDE EFFECTS** Bradycardia, dry mouth, drowsiness, fatigue, lethargy, depression, psychotic reactions, nasal stuffiness, impotence, and exacerbation of Parkinson's Rebound hypertension (with sweating/anxiety/tremors), if stopped abruptly
Guanabenz *(Wytensin)*	4 and 8 mg tabs	Skin irritation (with patches) Methyldopa has same as above plus hypersensitivity reactions, hepatitis, myocarditis, hemolytic anemia, positive Coombs test, drug-induced fever and lupus-like syndrome
Guanfacine *(Tenex)*	1 and 2 mg tabs	**MONITORING** BP, HR, mental status Clonidine patch is applied weekly. Do not stop abruptly, must taper.
Methyldopa *(Aldomet)*	125, 250, and 500 mg tabs 50 mg/mL PO susp 50 mg/mL inj	

Centrally Acting Alpha-2 Adrenergic Agonists Continued

DRUG	DOSING	SIDE EFFECTS/CONTRAINDICATIONS/ MONITORING

Direct Vasodilators - direct vasodilation of arterioles with little effect on veins

Drug	Dosing	Side Effects/Monitoring
Hydralazine *(Apresoline)*	10-75 mg TID 20 mg/mL inj.	**SIDE EFFECTS** <u>Lupus-like syndrome (dose and duration related -report fever, joint/muscle aches, fatigue)</u>, reflex tachycardia **MONITORING** HR, BP
Minoxidil	2.5-40 mg/d	**SIDE EFFECTS** Fluid retention, tachycardia, aggravation of angina, pericardial effusion, hirsutism (used for hair growth)

Alpha Blockers- bind to alpha$_1$-adrenergic receptors which results in vasodilation of arterioles and veins; used mostly for BPH. Not 1st line therapy for HTN.

Drug	Dosing	Side Effects
Prazosin *(Minipress)*	1-5 mg BID-TID	**SIDE EFFECTS** Orthostatic hypotension, syncope with 1st dose, dizziness, fatigue Caution with concurrent use with the PDE-5 inhibitors (sildenafil, tadalafil and vardenafil) due to additive effects on BP, dizziness
Terazosin *(Hytrin)*	1-20 mg QHS	
Doxazosin *(Cardura)*	1-16 mg QHS	

SELECT COMBO AGENTS	BRAND NAME	GENERIC DRUGS
ACE-I and CCB	*Lotrel*	Amlodipine and benazepril
	Lexxel	Enalapril and felodipine
	Tarka	Trandolapril and verapamil
ARB and CCB	*Twynsta*	Amlodipine and telmisartan
	Exforge	Amlodipine and valsartan
	Azor	Amlodipine and olmesartan
DRI and CCB	*Tekamlo*	Aliskiren and amlodipine
DRI and diuretic	*Tekturna HCT*	Aliskiren and HCTZ
DRI, CCB, and diuretic	*Amturnide*	Aliskiren, amlodipine and HCTZ

Centrally Acting Alpha-2 Adrenergic Agonists Continued

SELECT COMBO AGENTS	BRAND NAME	GENERIC DRUGS
DRI and ARB	*Valturna*	Aliskiren and valsartan
ACE-I and diuretic	***Lotensin HCT***	Benazepril and HCTZ
	Capozide	Captopril and HCTZ
	Vaseretic	Enalapril and HCTZ
	Prinzide, Zestorectic	Lisinopril and HCTZ
	Uniretic	Moexipril and HCTZ
	Accuretic	Quinapril and HCTZ
	Monopril HCT	Fosinopril and HCTZ
ARB's and diuretic	*Atacand HCT*	Candesartan and HCTZ
	Edarbyclor	Azilsartan and chlorthalidone
	Teveten HCT	Eprosartan and HCTZ
	Avalide	Irbesartan and HCTZ
	Hyzaar	Losartan and HCTZ
	Micardis HCT	Telmisartan and HCTZ
	Diovan HCT	Valsartan and HCTZ
	Benicar HCT	Olmesartan and HCTZ
Beta-blocker and diuretic	***Tenoretic***	Atenolol and chlorthalidone
	Ziac	Bisoprolol and HCTZ
	Inderide	Propranolol and HCTZ
	Lopressor HCT	Metoprolol and HCTZ
	Corzide	Nadolol and bendroflumethiazide
	Timolide	Timolol and HCTZ
Centrally acting drug and diuretic	*Aldoril*	Methydopa and HCTZ
	Diupres	Reserpine and chlorothiazide
	Hydropres	Reserpine and HCTZ
Diureitc and diuretic	*Moduretic/Midamor*	Amiloride and HCTZ
	Aldactazide	Spironolactone and HCTZ
	Dyazide, Maxzide	Triamterene and HCTZ
Vasodilator and diuretic	*Alpresazide*	Hydralazine and HCTZ
CCB and ARB and diuretic	*Exforge HCT*	Amlodipine, valsartan and HCTZ
	Tribenzor	Amlodipine, olmesartan and HCTZ

HYPERTENSIVE URGENCIES AND EMERGENCIES

	URGENCY: NOT LIFE-THREATENING	EMERGENCY: POTENTIALLY LIFE-THREATENING
Definition	BP (generally ≥ 185/110) without acute target organ damage	BP (generally ≥ 185/110) with acute target organ damage (such as encephalopathy, MI, unstable angina, pulmonary edema, eclampsia, stroke, aortic dissection, etc).
Treatment	Oral medication with an onset of action of 15-30 minutes; reduce BP gradually over 24-48 hrs.	Reduce SBP or MAP by 10-15% within the first 30-60 minutes, continue to lower BP gradually over the next day. Use IV medication.

Drugs Used in Hypertensive Urgencies

DRUG	DOSE	SIDE EFFECTS
Captopril (Capoten)	25 mg, repeat in 1-2 hrs PRN	Hypotension, ↑ K$^+$, angioedema
Clonidine (Catapres)	0.1-0.2 mg, repeat in 1-2 hrs PRN	Hypotension, drowsiness, sedation, dry mouth, etc.
Labetalol (Normodyne, Trandate)	100-400 mg, repeat in 2-3 hrs PRN	Hypotension, heart block, bronchoconstriction

Of note, do not use nifedipine SL for HTN urgency!

Drugs Used in Hypertensive Emergencies

DRUG	MOA
Clevidipine (Cleviprex) *	DHP-CCB
Sodium Nitroprusside (Nipride)	Arteriole and Venous Vasodilator – nitrate
Nicardipine (Cardene)	DHP-CCB
Fenoldopam (Corlopam)	Dopamine-1 receptor agonist
Nitroglycerin **	Venous vasodilator - nitrate
Enalaprilat (Vasotec IV)	ACEI
Hydralazine	Arteriole vasodilator
Labetalol	Alpha and beta-blocker
Esmolol	Beta-blocker

* Cleviprex comes in a lipid emulsion (milky white in color), therefore, maintain strict aseptic technique. Hung vials need to be discarded after 4 hours.

**Nitroglycerin (by injection) will absorb into plastic. Keep in glass bottles and do not use PVC tubing. It can decrease BP dramatically; careful monitoring is required.

PATIENT COUNSELING

All Hypertension Medications

- Hypertension often has no symptoms, so you may not even feel that you have high blood pressure. Continue using this medicine as directed, even if you feel well. You may need to use blood pressure medication for the rest of your life. If cost prevents you from obtaining the medicine, please ask the pharmacist for help finding a lower priced alternative. They exist!

- To be sure this medication is helping your condition, your blood pressure will need to be checked on a regular basis. It is important that you do not miss any scheduled visits to your doctor.

- This medicine is only part of a complete program of treatment for hypertension that may also include diet, exercise, and weight control. Follow your diet, medication, and exercise routines very closely if you are being treated for hypertension.

Diuretics

- This medication will cause you to urinate more throughout the day. This is expected from your medication.

- This medicine may make you feel dizzy and lightheaded when getting up from a sitting or lying position. Get up slowly. Let your feet hang over the bed for a few minutes before getting up. Hang on to the bed or near dresser when standing from a sitting position.

- Be sure that all objects are off the floor as you make your way to the bathroom. It is best to prevent any risks of falls.

- Potassium supplements may be needed while you are on this medication to ensure you have enough potassium for your heart. (not for potassium-sparing diuretics)

- If you have diabetes, your blood sugar may have to be monitored more frequently in the beginning as this medication can affect your blood sugar.

ACE Inhibitors, ARBs, and Aliskiren

- Do not use this medicine without telling your doctor if you are pregnant or planning a pregnancy. This medicine could cause birth defects in the baby if you take the medication during pregnancy. Use an effective form of birth control. Stop using this medication and tell your doctor right away if you become pregnant during treatment.

- Take the missed dose as soon as you remember. If it is almost time for your next dose, skip the missed dose and take the medicine at the next regularly scheduled time. Do not take extra medicine to make up the missed dose.

- Do not use salt substitutes or potassium supplements while taking this medication, unless your doctor has told you to do so. Be careful of your potassium intake.

- Get emergency medical help if you have any of these signs of an allergic reaction: hives; difficulty breathing; swelling of your face, lips, tongue, or throat.

- Tell your doctor if you develop a bothersome, dry occasional cough while taking this medicine (with ACE-I's only).

Beta Blockers

- Remember to take at the same time every day.

- Do not skip doses. If you miss a dose, take the missed dose as soon as you remember. If your next dose is less than 8 hours away, skip the missed dose and take the medicine at the next regularly scheduled time.

- Do not discontinue your medication without consulting your physician. Stopping this medicine suddenly may make your condition worse.

- Avoid operating automobiles and machinery or engaging in other tasks requiring alertness until you are use to the medicine's effects.

- Contact your physician if you experience any difficulty in breathing (for non-selective beta blockers).

- If taking *Coreg*: Take *Coreg* with food.

Clonidine

- Do not stop clonidine suddenly; this can cause your blood pressure to become dangerously high. Make sure you do not run out of medicine.

- Clonidine can cause a variety of side effects, including sedation, dizziness, fatigue, dry mouth, and can aggravate depression and contribute to sexual dysfunction. If the side effects bother you, please let your doctor know.

- The clonidine patch *(Catapres-TTS)* is changed weekly: Apply the patch to a hairless area of the skin on the upper outer arm or chest every 7 days. Do not use on broken or irritated skin. After 7 days, remove the used patch and apply a new patch to a different area than the previous one to avoid skin irritation.

Practice Case

FP is a 58 year old black male who comes into your clinic for a routine follow up visit. He states that he feels fine and does not understand why he has to take any medications.

CATEGORY	
PMH	Chronic lower back pain, Hypertension
Vitals	BP 162/95 mmHg, HR 88 BPM, RR 18 BPM, Temp 38.0 Pain 3/10
Current medications	*Lortab* 1-2 tabs NTE 8 tabs/day *Prinzide* 20/25 mg 1 tab daily
Labs	Na⁺ 141 mEq/L, K⁺ 3.8 mEq/L, BUN 35 mg/dL, SCr 1.2 mg/dL Glucose (non-fasting) 180 mg/dL

AcE I, Hctz

QUESTIONS

1. Which of the following medication combinations is *Prinzide*?

   a. Benazepril and hydrochlorothiazide
   b. Enalapril and hydrochlorothiazide
   c. Irbesartan and hydrochlorothiazide
   d. Lisinopril and hydrochlorothiazide
   e. Triamterene and hydrochlorothiazide

2. FP has a risk factor for developing angio-edema. Which of the following increases his risk?

   a. Age
   b. Gender
   c. Ethnicity
   d. Concurrent medications
   e. Electrolyte profile

3. FP needs better BP control. Which of the following medications would be the best recommendation to add to his profile?

   a. Lasix
   b. Zaroxolyn
   c. Bumex
   d. Avalide
   e. Norvasc

4. FP is started on his new therapy. He should also be counseled to keep his daily sodium intake BELOW this level:

   a. 10 g daily
   b. 5 g daily
   c. 1 g daily
   d. 5 mg daily
   e. 1.5 g daily

Questions 5-10 do not apply to the above case.

5. What is the mechanism of action for *Bystolic*?

   a. Beta 2- selective blocker
   b. Beta-1 selective blocker
   c. Increases nitric oxide production
   d. A and C
   e. B and C

6. Choose the correct statement concerning *Coreg CR*:

   a. The generic name is labetalol.
   b. The starting dose for heart failure is 20 mg BID.
   c. The drug is a non-selective beta and alpha blocker.
   d. The drug increases heart rate.

e. The drug should be taken without food.

7. A 77 year old patient comes into the pharmacy and takes their BP reading. It is 155/105. She mentions her BP has been around that reading for a while. What is the best recommendation to give this patient?

    a. You should have your BP checked by your doctor and it is likely you will need to be started on 2 medications to control your BP.

    b. You should have your BP checked by your doctor and it is likely you may need to be started on 1 medication to control your BP.

    c. You should go to the urgent care center since you are in hypertensive urgency and need immediate treatment.

    d. Your BP is fine given your age.

    e. As long as you are not symptomatic, you do not need to treat your BP with medicines.

8. A patient comes in with a new prescription for *Valturna*. Which of the following medications are the correct match for this prescription?

    a. Aliskiren and hydrochlorothiazide

    b. Aliskiren and valsartan

    c. Amlodipine and benazepril

    d. Valsartan, amlodipine, and hydrochlorothiazide

    e. Valsartan and hydrochlorothiazide

9. A patient develops angioedema while taking *Altace*. Which of the following medications should this patient be switched to?

    a. *Tenormin*

    b. *Atacand*

    c. *Exforge*

    d. *Mavik*

    e. *Tekturna*

10. Which one of the following beta blockers has intrinsic sympathomimetic activity (ISA)?

    a. Atenolol

    b. Amlodipine

    c. Carvedilol

    d. Pindolol

    e. Metoprolol

11. A patient is prescribed diltiazem. Choose the correct statement:

    a. Heart rate would be expected to slow.

    b. The correct reference to check for an AB-rated generic is the *Red Book*.

    c. Diltiazem is an enzyme inducer.

    d. Diltiazem is a beta blocker.

    e. Diltiazem is a dihydropyridine calcium channel blocker.

ANSWERS

1-d, 2-c, 3-e, 4-e, 5-e, 6-c, 7-a, 8-b, 9-a, 10-d, 11-a

DYSLIPIDEMIA

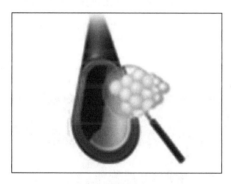

GUIDELINES

Third report of the National Cholesterol Education Program (NCEP) Expert Panel on Detection, Evaluation, and Treatment of High Blood Cholesterol in Adults, Adult Treatment Panel III, 2001.

Grundy SM, Cleeman JI, Merz CN, Brewer HB Jr, Clark LT, Hunninghake DB, Pasternak RC, Smith SC Jr, Stone NJ. Implications of recent clinical trials for the National Cholesterol Education Program Adult Treatment Panel III guidelines. Circulation 2004 Jul 13;110(2):227-39.

Miller M, Stone NJ, Ballantyne C, et al. Triglycerides and cardiovascular disease: a scientific statement from the American Heart Association. Circulation 2011;DOI:10.1161/CIR.0b013e3182160726.

Background

Cholesterol is produced in the liver or intestines and comes from our diet, including dairy products (whole milk), eggs, meat and many types of prepared foods. We need cholesterol for cell membrane formation, hormone synthesis, and fat soluble vitamin production. However, excess intake of cholesterol is thought to lead to a build-up of plaque (atherosclerosis) in the arteries. This may result in conditions such as Coronary Heart Disease (CHD). Lipids, being water immiscible, are not present in the free form in the plasma, but rather circulate as lipoproteins. Dyslipidemia is defined as an elevation of total cholesterol, elevation in LDL cholesterol, elevation in triglycerides or low HDL cholesterol concentration, or some combination of these abnormalities.

Complications

The risk for CHD is increased when the LDL is elevated. If the triglycerides are elevated, this can lead to pancreatitis (acutely), along with an increased risk for heart disease. Having a low HDL can further increase the risk of CHD. CHD can cause anginal pain due to reduced blood flow to the heart (from narrowing of the arteries due to plaque formation). If the plaque ruptures in the coronary arteries, it can cause a heart attack (myocardial infarction, or MI). CHD is a systemic condition and plaque may be identified elsewhere, including in the carotid arteries [the arteries in the neck that bring blood to the brain; plaque rupture can cause a stroke, (cerebrovascular accident, or CVA)] and in the leg arteries (this can lead to leg pain from peripheral arterial disease, or PAD).

Causes of a Poor Lipid Profile

PRIMARY

- Familial

SECONDARY

- High dietary intake of cholesterol and saturated fat (saturated fat should be < 7% of total calories)

- Low physical activity (exercise will ↑ HDL and ↓ LDL)

- Diseases: diabetes, hypothyroidism, liver disease, transplantation, renal disease (e.g. nephrotic syndrome), obesity, anorexia, and others

- Drugs: Protease inhibitors, atypical antipsychotics, anabolic and corticosteroids (prednisone, etc), isotretinoin, beta-blockers, thiazide diuretics, azole antifungals, mirtazapine, cyclosporine, tacrolimus and some types of birth control pills

CHOLESTEROL (LIPOPROTEIN) TYPES AND RECOMMENDED HEALTHY LEVELS

TYPE	DESCRIPTION	LEVEL (MG/DL)	COMMENTS
LDL	Low density or "bad" cholesterol	< 100	Optimal
		100-129	Near or above optimal
HDL	High density, or "good" cholesterol	< 40	Low
		≥ 60	High
TG	Triglycerides	< 150	Normal
		150-199	Borderline high
		200-499	High
		> 500	Very high
CH	Total cholesterol	< 200	Desirable
		200-239	Borderline high
		≥ 240	High

Treating Dyslipidemias

STEP 1

- Obtain lipoprotein levels after a 9-12 hour fast (if patient did not fast, the levels may be falsely elevated). See chart above for normal ranges. You may need to calculate LDL if it is not given using the Friedewald equation:

- LDL = CH − HDL − (TG/5) (Cannot use this formula if the TGs are > 400 mg/dL)

STEP 2

- Identify presence of clinical athero-sclerotic disease that confers high risk for CHD events and look for CHD risk equivalents

- Clinical CHD – history of MI, angina, coronary procedures (e.g., angioplasty)

- Symptomatic carotid artery disease (TIA, stroke)

- Peripheral arterial disease (PAD)

- Abdominal aortic aneurysm (AAA)

- Diabetes

- Multiple (≥ 2) risk factors that confer ≥ 20% risk of CHD at 10 years (determined by the Framingham Risk Score)

STEP 3

- Determine presence of major risk factors (other than LDL).

MAJOR RISK FACTORS FOR CHD

Age
men ≥ 45 y/o; women ≥ 55 y/o

Cigarette smoking

Hypertension
BP ≥ 140/90 mmHg or on antihypertensive medication

HDL-C < 40 mg/dL

Family history of premature CHD
< 55 years old in first-degree male relative (father, brother)

< 65 years old in first-degree female relative (mother, sister)

Negative Risk Factor (get to subtract 1 risk factor if have high HDL)
HDL ≥ 60 mg/dL

STEP 4

- Using the cumulated risk factors, determine risk category and corresponding LDL goal.

CATEGORIES OF RISK AND LDL GOALS

RISK CATEGORY	LDL GOAL (MG/DL)	INITIATE TLCs (MG/DL)	CONSIDER DRUG TX (MG/DL)
High Risk: CHD or CHD risk equivalents (10-yr risk > 20%)	< 100 **(optional goal : < 70)**	≥ 100	≥ 100 < 100 (consider drug therapy)
Moderately High Risk: ≥ 2 risk factors (10-yr risk 10%-20%)	< 130 **(optional goal: < 100)**	≥ 130	≥ 130 100-129 (consider drug therapy)
Moderate Risk: ≥ 2 risk factors (10-yr risk < 10%)	< 130	≥ 130	≥ 160
Low Risk: 0-1 risk factor	< 160	≥ 160	≥ 190 160-189 (consider drug therapy)

STEP 5

Initiate therapeutic lifestyle changes (TLC) if LDL is above goal.

In all patients with dyslipidemia, therapeutic lifestyle changes are recommended (see below). However, lifestyle changes are difficult to maintain and may not provide enough benefit. Most of the time, TLC are started concurrently with drug therapy. TLC should be emphasized, monitored and reinforced.

- Total fat 25-35% of total calories

- Saturated fat < 7% of calories

- Cholesterol < 200 mg/day

- Increase fiber intake (20-30 g/day) and plant stanols/sterols (2 g/day) to enhance LDL lowering – helps bind fats in the gut

- Weight management – maintain a normal BMI (< 25)

- Increase physical exercise – should be doing 30 minutes/day on most days of the week

- Stop smoking

CHD RISK EQUIVALENTS
Diabetes
Atherosclerotic Disease peripheral artery disease carotid artery disease
Abdominal Aortic Aneurysm
Clinical CHD (defined as a Framingham calculated CHD 10-year risk > 20%)

STEP 6

- Select Appropriate Drug Therapy

- LDL lowering is the primary goal, except when TG are > 500 mg/dL. If TG > 500 mg/dL, then TG reduction becomes the primary goal.

TARGETING DIFFERENT LIPIDS

LIPID TARGET	DRUG CHOICE
LDL	Statins (most effective)
HDL	Niacin (in Rx strength); Fenofibrates
TG	Fenofibrates or *Lovaza* (omega-3 fish oils)
2010 AHA recommendation to use TLC first-line to ↓ TGs. Use drugs when TG > 500.	

NATURAL PRODUCTS

Red Yeast Rice is the product of yeast grown on rice that contains naturally occurring HMG-CoA reductase inhibitors and is commercially available in capsules. The amount of statin in each product can vary. Both myalgias and myopathy have been reported with the use of the product. Garlic may have a very small beneficial effect on cholesterol. Over-the-counter fish oils (to ↓ TGs) and plant sterols/stanols may provide additional benefit.

DRUG THERAPY

Statins are the primary drugs used to ↓ LDL (they also ↓ TG, ↑ HDL), with additional benefits besides lipid-lowering (such as ↓ risk of developing CHD, slowing disease progression, ↓ risk MIs). The other agents are used if the TGs are high (fibrates, fish oils), or for additional

LDL-lowering (if a statin alone isn't enough), or if a statin cannot be tolerated (e.g., myalgias, liver enzyme elevations). There are some exceptions, such as using niacin to ↑ HDL or using a resin to ↓ cholesterol and postprandial blood glucose. Note: Many of the drug classes used for cholesterol management are potentially hepatotoxic (statins, niacin, potentially fibrates and ezetimibe). Liver enzymes should be monitored and the drug stopped if AST (10-35 units/L) or ALT (6-40 units/L) become > 3 times the upper limit of normal.

Statins

Statins inhibit the enzyme 3-hydroxy-3-methylglutaryl coenzyme A (HMG-CoA) reductase preventing the conversion of HMG-CoA to mevalonate (the rate-limiting step in cholesterol synthesis). Statins are the most potent LDL lowering agents.

DRUG	DOSING	SIDE EFFECTS/MONITORING/CONTRAINDICATIONS
Atorvastatin _(Lipitor)_ + amlodipine _(Caduet)_	10-80 mg Equiv dose = 10 mg	**Statins** ↓ LDL ~20-55% ↑ HDL ~5-15% ↓ TG ~10-30% Doubling the dose of a statin will ↓ LDL level by 3-6%
Simvastatin _(Zocor)_ **+ ezetimibe _(Vytorin)_** + sitagliptin _(Juvisync)_	10-80 mg Note: see paragraph below on label limits for 80 mg dose. 2011 FDA Medwatch Safety Alert, 6/8/2011 Equiv dose = 20 mg Take at bedtime	**SIDE EFFECTS** Myalgias, arthralgias, myopathy, rhabdomyolysis (↑ risk with higher doses), ↑ LFTs
Rosuvastatin _(Crestor)_	5-40 mg Equiv dose = 5 mg	**Muscle Damage** If present, should be seen right away, may get CPK checked; may have statin stopped or changed. Factors that ↑ risk of myopathy include higher doses, age > 65, renal impairment, untreated hypothyroidism, and use of fibrates. Use of potent 3A4 inhibitors should be avoided
Pravastatin _(Pravachol)_	10-80 mg Equiv dose = 40 mg	
Lovastatin _(Mevacor, Altoprev)_	20-80 mg Take _Mevacor_ (immediate release) with Meal (dinner) Take _Altoprev_ (extended release formulation) at bedtime Equiv dose = 40 mg	**Monitoring Liver** Check LFTs at the start (baseline) and at 3 months, and periodically afterwards (such as at annual physical) **Renal** Use lower doses if CrCl < 30 mL/min, except with _Lescol_ and _Lipitor_. With _Livalo_, use lower doses when CrCl < 60 mL/min
Fluvastatin _(Lescol, Lescol XL)_	20-80 mg Take at bedtime, or take XL (80 mg) at any time Equiv dose = 80 mg	**CONTRAINDICATIONS** Active Liver Disease (including any unexplained elevations in hepatic transaminases) Pregnancy Category X
Pitavastatin _(Livalo)_	1-4 mg Most potent statin Contraindicated with concomitant cyclosporine Equiv dose = 2 mg CrCl < 60 mL/min: 2 mg/d max	Nursing mothers Can take _Crestor, Lipitor, Livalo_ and _Pravachol_ at any time of day.

DRUG INTERACTIONS

Lovastatin, simvastatin & atorvastatin

- Simvastatin and lovastatin undergo extensive first-pass metabolism by CYP 3A4. Atorvastatin undergoes less first-pass metabolism by 3A4; therefore, most 3A4 inhibitors cause a smaller ↑ in plasma concentration.

- Increased risk of muscle damage with amiodarone and other 3A4 inhibitors such as azole antifungals, grapefruit products, cyclosporine, diltiazem, verapamil, macrolide antibiotics, protease inhibitors, etc – see our DI chapter.

- Use of simvastatin is contraindicated in patients taking azole antifungals, macrolides, protease inhibitors, gemfibrozil, cyclosporine, and danazol. Do not exceed 10 mg/d of simvastatin in patients taking amiodarone, verapamil, or diltiazem (or 40 mg/d of lovastatin immediate release or 20 mg lovastatin extended release). Do not exceed 20 mg/d of simvastatin in patients taking ranolazine and amlodipine.

Do not use simvastatin 80mg/day → profound ↑ in risk of myopathy (~ 6 fold increase). Package insert states: *Due to the increased risk of myopathy, including rhabdomyolysis, associated with the 80-mg dose of simvastatin, patients unable to achieve their LDL-C goal utilizing the 40-mg dose of ZOCOR should not be titrated to the 80-mg dose, but should be placed on alternative LDL-C-lowering treatment(s) that provides greater LDL-C lowering. Also, due to the increased risk of myopathy, including rhabdomyolysis, use of the 80-mg dose of ZOCOR should be restricted to patients who have been taking simvastatin 80 mg chronically (e.g., for 12 months or more) without evidence of muscle toxicity.*

Rosuvastatin

- Warfarin: may ↑ INR, monitor.

- Cyclosporine may ↑ rosuvastatin; do not exceed 5 mg/d of rosuvastatin.

- Lopinavir/ritonavir and atazanavir/ritonavir: do not exceed 10 mg/d of rosuvastatin.

- Gemfibrozil: combo should be avoided; do not exceed 10 mg/day of rosuvastatin.

- Concomitant lipid-lowering therapies: use with fibrates and niacin products may ↑ risk of myopathies.

Fluvastatin

- Metabolized mainly by 2C9 – monitor patients taking warfarin.

Pitavastatin

- Minimal CYP450 metabolism. Contraindicated with cyclosporine. Limit dose to 1 mg daily with erythromycin or 2 mg daily with rifampin. Consider dosage reduction with niacin. Monitor PT/INR in patients taking warfarin.

COUNSELING

For <u>all</u> cholesterol medicines: Your doctor should start you on a low-fat diet.

- Contact your doctor right away if you have muscle problems such as weakness, tenderness, or pain that happens without a good reason, especially if you also have a fever or feel more tired than usual.

- Contact your doctor right away if you are passing brown or dark-colored urine, have pale stools, feel more tired than usual or if your skin and/or whites of your eyes become yellow. These may be signs of liver damage.

- Grapefruit and grapefruit juice may interact with this medicine. This could lead to incorrect amounts of drugs in your body. Do not change the amount of grapefruit products you consume without discussing with your doctor. (for lovastatin, simvastatin, atorvastatin)

- <u>Do not use</u> if pregnant or think you may be pregnant, or are planning to become pregnant. This drug may harm your unborn baby. If you get pregnant, stop taking and call doctor right away.

Ezetimibe

Intestinal cholesterol absorption inhibitor.

DRUG	DOSING	SIDE EFFECTS/MONITORING/CONTRAINDICATIONS
Ezetimibe *(Zetia)* **+ simvastatin** *(Vytorin)* Used alone (usually when a statin cannot be tolerated) or in combo with a statin or fenofibrate for additional ↓ LDL.	10 mg daily ↓ LDL 18-23% ↑ HDL 1-3% ↓ TG 8-10%	**SIDE EFFECTS** Well-tolerated; may cause upper RTI's, diarrhea, arthralgias, myalgias, pain in extremities **MONITORING** When used with a statin, obtain liver function tests at baseline and then according to the recommendations of the statin **CONTRAINDICATIONS** None, however use caution with any liver issue, especially if using statins concurrently. Liver enzymes increase more with the combo than with a statin alone. Clinical trial results showed a ↓ in LDL, but no reduction in clinical outcomes seen.

EZETIMIBE DRUG INTERACTIONS

- When ezetimibe and cyclosporine are given together, the concentration of both can ↑; monitor levels of cyclosporine.

- Concomitant bile acid resins ↓ ezetimibe. Separate doses by 4-6 hours.

- When used with statins, monitor liver enzymes and have patient monitor clinical symptoms.

- If using warfarin, monitor INR/bleeding.

EZETIMIBE COUNSELING

- <u>Especially if with statin</u>: Contact your doctor right away if you are passing brown or dark-colored urine, have pale stools, feel more tired than usual or if your skin and/or whites of your eyes become yellow. These may be signs of liver damage.

■ Take this medicine once daily, with or without food.

Bile Acid Sequestrants/Bile Acid Binding Resins

Binds bile acids in the intestine forming a complex that is excreted in the feces. This non-systemic action results in a partial removal of the bile acids from the enterohepatic circulation, preventing their reabsorption.

DRUG	DOSING	SIDE EFFECTS/MONITORING/CONTRAINDICATIONS
Cholestyramine (*Questran* 4 g/dose, *Questran Light* 4 g/dose) Also approved for relief of pruritis associated with partial biliary obstruction	2 to 4 packets or scoopfuls daily, divided BID – <u>mix</u> the powder with water or other non-carbonated liquid (2-6 oz.)	↓ LDL ~10-30% ↑ HDL ~3-5% No change or ↑ TG (~5%) **SIDE EFFECTS** <u>Constipation</u> (may need dose reduction or laxative, most is transient – but watch for pre-existing constipation because these drugs will worsen it), <u>abdominal pain, cramping, gas, bloating</u>, heartburn (<u>less GI side effects with *WelChol*</u>) ↓ absorption of other drugs (less, but still present, with *WelChol*) – see below
Colesevelam (*WelChol*) Also approved for DM Type 2 (↓ A1C~ 0.5%)	625 mg, take 6 tabs daily or 3 tabs BID <u>with</u> a meal <u>and</u> liquid (8 oz.). Also comes in oral susp.	**CONTRAINDICATIONS (WELCHOL)** Bowel obstruction
Colestipol *(Colestid)*	Start with 2 g tablet daily or BID, can increase to 16 g, swallow tablet whole, one at a time, with adequate liquid. Comes in granules as well (5-30 grams/day)	TG > 500 mg/dL History of hypertrigylceridemia-induced pancreatitis *WelChol* is preg category B, others are preg category C.

DRUG INTERACTIONS

WelChol has less drug interactions than the other 2 bile acid resins and is more commonly used. For *Questran* or *Colestipol*, separate all other drugs by 1 hour before and 4-6 hours after (statins, fibrates, etc).

■ The following medications should be taken 4 hours prior to *WelChol*: phenytoin, levothyroxine, glyburide, and oral contraceptives (E+P).

■ With warfarin, monitor INR frequently during initiation.

■ Take bile acid resins 4-6 hours before *Niaspan*.

COUNSELING

See dosing for instructions regarding food/fluid intake for specific agents.

■ For cholestyramine: sipping or holding the suspension in your mouth can lead to tooth decay.

■ Check for other constipating drugs or constipation itself and counsel appropriately (laxative, such as senna, or the stool softener docusate, if appropriate). Maintain adequate fluid and fiber intake.

- Take multivitamin at another time, due to possible risk of ↓ A,D,E and K (mostly K) absorption.

- These medications ↓ folate levels; supplement in women and children.

Fibrates

Fibrates are peroxisome proliferator receptor alpha (PPARα) activators. By activating PPARα, there is enhanced elimination and ↓ synthesis of VLDL (causing ↓ TGs) and an ↑ in HDL – this causes an increase in apolipoprotein lipase, which may ↓ LDL – <u>however, when TGs are high, reducing TGs can ↑ LDL</u> – be careful to monitor LDL when reducing TGs.

DRUG	DOSING	SIDE EFFECTS/MONITORING/ CONTRAINDICATIONS
Fenofibrate, Fenofibric Acid (several, see dosing, all in mg)	Come in different strengths – and the delivery technology may be different. If you want to dispense a generic, you may need to call prescriber for a close mg strength – and try to match one with a similar delivery technology, using the orange book. **FORMULATIONS** Micronized formulations and other modes are used to improve bioavailability – to get more TG reduction (which is dose dependent). *TriCor* 48, 145 *Lofibra* (with meals) 54, 67, 134, 160, 200 *Lipofen* (with meals) 50, 100, 150 *Antara* 43, 130 *Fenoglide* (with meals) 40, 120 *Trilipix* 45, 135 *Triglide* 50, 67, 134, 160, 200	↓ TGs ~20-50% ↑ HDL ~15% ↓ LDL ~5-20% (but can ↑ LDL when TG are high) **SIDE EFFECTS** ↑ LFTs (dose related), ↑ CPK, myopathy, abdominal pain, dyspepsia, constipation, rhinitis; rarely can cause cholelithiasis (calculi, or gallstones in the gallbladder) Risk of myopathy and rhabdomyolysis ↑ when co-administered with a statin (esp with gemfibrozil), particularly in elderly patients, and in those with diabetes, renal failure, or hypothyroidism. **MONITORING** Regular, periodic monitoring of LFTs **CONTRAINDICATIONS** Severe liver disease Severe renal disease Gallbladder disease Nursing mothers Pregnancy Category C
Gemfibrozil *(Lopid)*	600 mg BID, 30 minutes before breakfast and dinner	

DRUG INTERACTIONS

- When used in combination with statins, fenofibrates can ↑ the risk of myopathies (and rhabdomyolysis), especially gemfibrozil. <u>Only *Trilipix*</u> has the indication for use with a statin although others (except gemfibrozil) may have a similar safety profile. Monitor liver enzymes with all fibrates, statins, and when the 2 drug classes are used in combination.

- Fibrates may increase the effects of sulfonylureas and warfarin.

- Fibrates may ↑ cholesterol excretion into the bile, leading to cholelithiasis.

COUNSELING

- *Antara, TriCor, Triglide* and *Trilipix*: Take once daily, with or without food.

- *Fenoglide, Lofibra and Lipofen*: Take once daily, with food.

- *Lopid*: Take twice daily, 30 minutes before breakfast and dinner.

- Do not crush or chew. Contact your doctor if you experience muscle aches.

- Contact your doctor right away if you experience abdominal pain, nausea or vomiting. These may be signs of inflammation of the gallbladder or pancreas.

- Contact your doctor right away if you are passing brown or dark-colored urine, feel more tired than usual or if your skin and/or whites of your eyes become yellow. These may be signs of liver damage.

- *TriLipix* (fenofibric acid) has not been shown to lower you risk of having heart problems or a stroke.

Niacin

Decreases the rate of hepatic synthesis of VLDL (↓ TGs) and LDL; may also ↑ rate of chylomicron TG removal from plasma.

DRUG	DOSING	SIDE EFFECTS/MONITORING/CONTRAINDICATIONS
Immediate release (crystalline) niacin (*Niacor*) – OTC Formulations of niacin are not interchangeable	500 mg (start ½ tablet with dinner), can ↑ weekly; max 6 g/d, divided	↓ LDL 5-25% ↑ HDL 15-35% ↓ TG 20-50% The difficulty with niacin is poor tolerability due to flushing/itching. Extended-release forms (CR and SR) have less (but still significant) flushing/itching.
Extended-Release **Niacin** (**Niaspan**) **500, 750, 1,000 mg** + lovastatin (*Advicor*) **+ simvastatin** (*Simcor*)	500 mg QHS x 4 wks 1,000 mg QHS x 4 wks Can ↑ to 1,500-2,000 mg QHS MAX 2 g daily	*Slo-Niacin* (OTC) has more hepatotoxicity. Therefore, the best clinical choice is *Niaspan* (↓ side effects, without increased risk liver damage) – but it is the most expensive. **SIDE EFFECTS** Flushing, pruritis (itching), diarrhea, GI distress, hyperglycemia, hyperuricemia (or gout), hepatotoxicity, orthostatic hypotension **Monitoring Liver** Check LFTs at the start (baseline), every 6 to 12 weeks for the first year, and periodically thereafter (e.g., at approximately 6-month intervals).
Controlled (or sustained) release Niacin (*Slo-Niacin, OTC*) Do not use OTC flush-free niacin – ineffective (inositol hexaniacinate or hexanicotinate)	250, 500, 750 mg	**CONTRAINDICATIONS** Active liver disease Active PUD Arterial bleeding Use with caution with gout Pregnancy Category C *Niaspan* is approved for use with simvastatin and lovastatin if statin alone is not enough – however, risk must outweigh benefit due to ↑ risk of myopathy, rhabdomyolysis – if used in combo, use lower doses of statins; also approved for use with any of the resins.

DRUG INTERACTIONS

- Watch for other drugs that are potentially hepatotoxic being used concurrently. This includes combo use with statins – stick to lower statin doses. The combo drug lovastatin/niaspan *(Advicor)* has a max dose of 2,000/40 mg and simvastatin/niaspan *(Simcor)* has a max dose of 2,000/40 mg.

- Separate dosing from bile acid resins by 4-6 hours.

COUNSELING

- *Niaspan*: Take at bedtime after a low-fat snack. Other niacins: Take with food.

- With long-acting formulations: Do not crush or chew.

- Contact your doctor right away if you are passing brown or dark-colored urine, feel more tired than usual or if your skin and/or whites of your eyes become yellow. These may be signs of liver damage.

- Flushing (warmth, redness, itching and/or tingling of the skin) is a common side effect that may subside after several weeks of consistent use. You can pre-treat with up to 325 mg uncoated aspirin (or 200 mg of ibuprofen) 30 min before dose (for a few weeks) to ↓ flushing. With *Niaspan*, flushing will occur mostly at night; use caution if awakened due to possible dizziness.

- Avoid using alcohol or hot beverages or eating spicy foods around the time of taking this medicine to help reduce flushing.

- If you have diabetes, check your blood sugar when starting this medicine because there may be a mild increase. Niacin is good for people with diabetes because it raises the good cholesterol (and lowers the bad types).

Lovaza

Various mechanisms to ↓ TGs, including reducing TG synthesis and transport.

DRUG	DOSING	SIDE EFFECTS/MONITORING/ CONTRAINDICATIONS
Omega-3 Acid Ethyl Esters (*Lovaza*) For TG: use when TGs are ≥ 500 mg/dL in addition to a low-fat diet	Start at 2 capsules daily, can ↑ to 4 daily 1 g capsule contains 465 mg EPA (eicosapentaenoic acid) and 375 mg DHA (docosahexaenoic acid)	↓ TGs up to 45% ↑ HDL ~9% Can ↑ LDL up to 44% **SIDE EFFECTS** Eructation (burping), dyspepsia, nausea Use with caution in patients with known hypersensitivity to fish and/or shellfish

DRUG INTERACTIONS

- Omega-3-acids may prolong bleeding time. Monitor INR if patients are taking warfarin. Caution with other medications that can ↑ bleeding risk.

COUNSELING

- Use a low-fat diet in addition to this medicine.

- Can take once daily, or split BID.

- Take with or without food, but you may find it more comfortable to take with food.

- This medicine does not usually cause side effects, but may cause indigestion (stomach upset), burping, or a distorted sense of taste.

PRACTICE CASE

PATIENT PROFILE

Patient Name	David Armistead					
Address	1882 Peekaborn					
Age	57	**Sex** Male	**Race** White	**Height** 5'11"	**Weight** 246 lbs	
Allergies	NKDA					

DIAGNOSES

Coronary Heart Disease, stent placement 7/09	
Dyslipidemia	
Hypertension	
Diabetes Type 2	

MEDICATIONS

Date	No.	Prescriber	Drug & Strength	Quantity	Sig	Refills
5/15/09	77328	Gallagher	Actos 45 mg	#30	1 PO daily	2
7/28/09	77001	Sulyman	Lipitor 80 mg	#30	1 PO daily	4
5/15/09	73768	Gallagher	Metformin 1000 mg	#60	1 PO BID	2
5/15/09	73554	Gallagher	Lisinopril-HCT 20-25 mg	#30	1 PO daily	2
			Fish oils 1000 mg cap		1 PO BID	
			Aspirin 81 mg EC		1 PO daily	
			Multivitamin		1 PO daily	

LAB/DIAGNOSTIC TESTS

Test	Normal Value	Results Date 5/12/09	Date	Date
Protein, T	6.2-8.3 g/dL			
Albumin	3.6-5.1 g/dL			
Alk Phos	33-115 units/L			
AST	10-35 units/L	32		
ALT	6-40 units/L	20		
CH, T	125-200 g/dL	224 ↑ TC		
TG	<150 g/dL	248 ↑ TG		
HDL	g/dL	36 ↓ HDL		
LDL	g/dL			
GLU	65-99 mg/dL	114 ↑ Glucose		
Na	135-146 mEq/L	131 ↓ Na		
K	3.5-5.3 mEq/L	3.8		
Cl	98-110 mEq/L	105		
C02	21-33 mmHg	28		
BUN	7-25 mg/dL	18		
Creatinine	0.6-1.2 mg/dL			
Calcium	8.6-10.2 mg/dL			
WBC	4-11 cells/mm³	4.6		
RBC	3.8-5.1 mL/mm³			
Hemoglobin	Male: 13.8- 17.2 g/dL Female: 12.1-15.1 g/dL	14.2		
Hematocrit	Male: 40.7-50.3% Female: 36.1- 44.3%	38		
MCHC	32-36 g/dL			
MCV	80-100 µm			
Platelet count	140-400 x 10³/mm³	210		
TSH	0.4-4.0 mIU/L			
FT4	4.5- 11.2 mcg/dL			
Hgb A1c	4-6%	7.2% ↑ A1C		

ADDITIONAL INFORMATION

Date	Notes
11/11/09	Patient reports walking more since heart surgery. He lost 13 lbs in last 5 months. Decreasing "donuts and sugar." No EtOH, no tobacco use (past Hx smoking). Patient states he prefers not to take more pills, and is scared about his heart.

QUESTIONS

1. What is David's calculated LDL?

   a. 188

   b. 176

   c. 138

   d. 105

   e. 99

2. Is his LDL at goal?

   a. Yes, he is at goal.

   b. No, he needs to be below 130.

   c. No, he needs to be below 100.

   d. No, he needs to be below 70.

   e. It's close to goal, but since he is losing weight, he can be left on the current therapy.

3. What modification would you make to David's lipid therapy?

   a. Move the *Lipitor* dosing to bedtime

   b. Change *Lipitor* to simvastatin, taken at bedtime

   c. Add on gemfibrozil

   d. Add on fenofibrate

   e. No change is required

4. David states he has not received counseling on the *Lipitor*, and is wondering if this type of drug is safe to take. You should include the following in your discussion with the patient:

   a. The statins are considered safe, but can rarely cause problems that he should note.

   b. This medication may cause muscle aches and any unusual muscle aches should be reported promptly to his doctor.

   c. When using this type of medicine, the doctor should occasionally check his liver to make sure that the drug is being handled safely by his body. If it is not, the doctor can discuss changing the medicine.

   d. This medicine may interact with other medication. Tell your doctor and pharmacist all the medications you are currently taking.

   e. All of the above.

5. The doctor decides to begin therapy with *Lopid*. Which of the following statements is <u>correct?</u>

   a. This is a better choice than *Trilipix*, which has a higher risk of toxicity with concurrent statin therapy.

   b. The dosing for *Lopid* is 145 mg once daily, taken with or without food.

   c. *Lopid* should be taken 30 minutes before breakfast and dinner.

   d. The generic name is fenofibrate, micronized.

   e. *Lopid* should be crushed and given with a carbonated beverage.

Questions 6-11 do not relate to the case.

6. Which of the following cholesterol medicines should be taken with dinner?

   a. *Niaspan*

   b. *Zetia*

   c. *Mevacor*

   d. *Zocor*

   e. *Altoprev*

7. A patient is going to be started on *Niaspan* therapy. Which of the following statements is <u>correct?</u>

   a. *Niaspan* is immediate release niacin.

   b. *Niaspan* has a higher degree of hepatotoxicity than all the other niacin formulations.

   c. *Niaspan* causes less flushing than immediate release niacin.

   d. *Niaspan* is taken with breakfast.

   e. *Niaspan* must be taken on an empty stomach.

8. A physician has called the pharmacist. He has a patient on phenytoin who cannot tolerate statins. He wishes to begin *WelChol*. Which of the following statements is correct?

   a. The phenytoin should be given 4 hours before *WelChol*.
   b. He cannot use this class of drugs with phenytoin.
   c. *Questran* would be a better option due to a lower risk of drug interactions.
   d. The dose of *WelChol* is 5 g twice daily, with food and water.
   e. There is no drug interaction between phenytoin and *WelChol*.

9. Which of the following drug classes is used primarily for triglyceride reduction:

   a. Fibrates
   b. Fish oils
   c. *Zetia*
   d. Statins
   e. A and B

10. Which of the following generic/brand combinations is correct?

   a. Amlodipine/Atorvastatin (*Vytorin*)
   b. Fenofibric Acid (*Trilipix*)
   c. Amlodipine/Rosuvastatin (*Caduet*)
   d. Fluvastatin (*Mevacor*)
   e. Fenofibric Acid (*Lopid*)

11. A prescription is written for *Altoprev*. Which of the following medications should be used to fill the prescription?

   a. Niacin
   b. Colesevelam
   c. Ezetimibe
   d. Lovastatin extended release
   e. Simvastatin extended release

ANSWERS

1-c, 2-d, 3-d, 4-e, 5-c, 6-c, 7-c, 8-a, 9-e, 10-b, 11-d

HEART FAILURE

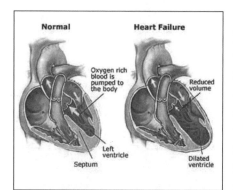

GUIDELINES

2009 Focused Update Incorporated Into the ACC/AHA 2005 Guidelines for the Diagnosis and Management of Heart Failure in Adults can be found at: http://circ.ahajournals.org/cgi/reprint/CIRCULATIONAHA.109.192065

Executive Summary: HFSA 2010 Comprehensive Heart Failure Practice Guideline. Journal of Cardiac Failure. June 2010;16(6):475-539.

Background

Heart failure is a syndrome where the heart is not able to supply sufficient blood flow (or cardiac output) to meet the metabolic needs of the body. The heart fails as a "pump" and the ventricle's ability to fill with or eject blood is compromised. This syndrome is characterized by high mortality, frequent hospitalizations, reduced quality of life, and a complex therapeutic regimen. Heart failure is a leading cause of hospitalizations in the elderly. Many of the hospital admissions are not new onset heart failure cases but are attributable to medication discontinuation and/or lifestyle non-adherence. This is a major cause of increased health care dollars, and consequently it is necessary to make sure that patients know how to use their medicines appropriately and are assisted with cost concerns. Heart failure is one of the most important conditions to include lifestyle counseling, such as the necessity to restrict sodium intake, to monitor weight on a daily basis (a sudden water-weight gain can indicate that the condition has become acutely "decompensated", or worsened), the need to discontinue tobacco use, limit alcohol, and improve nutrition and physical activity.

Causes of Heart Failure

Heart failure is a progressive syndrome caused by cardiac dysfunction, generally resulting from myocardial muscle dysfunction or muscle loss, and characterized by either left ventricular dilation or hypertrophy or both. Hypertension may cause heart failure since the heart has to pump against a high pressure – this results in an enlarged ventricle and eventually a reduced cardiac output. Other medical conditions can cause the heart to over-work, including hypothyroidism and diabetes. Coronary artery disease is a major cause of heart failure when the disease results in a reduced blood flow to heart muscle. Myocardial infarction can result in heart failure when a section of the heart muscle is damaged from the ischemia. Congenital heart defects are another important cause of heart failure, although not as common. There are other less-common causes, including the use of cardiotoxic drugs.

Pathophysiology

The heart has four chambers: a right atrium and ventricle and a left atrium and ventricle. The right atrium collects oxygen-poor blood, which passes into the right ventricle – then the right ventricle contracts and pushes the blood through the pulmonary artery and into the lungs to be replenished with oxygen. After gas-exchange occurs in the lungs, the oxygen-rich blood travels back through the pulmonary veins to the left side of the heart into the left atrium, and then into the left ventricle. The left ventricle is the starting point for oxygen-rich blood to be sent to the rest of the body. When the left ventricle contracts, it pushes blood through the aorta and into the systemic circulation.

The heart has four valves which open and close to keep the blood flowing in one direction – but sometimes the valves "leak" and blood is allowed to flow back (regurgitate) the wrong way. If this occurs, the valve may need to be replaced, which will put the patient at risk for clots and require long-term anticoagulation. Normal heart sounds make a "lub-dub, lub-dub" sound. The normal S1 heart sound (the "lub") is the sound of the tricuspid and mitral valves closing in the right atrium and left atrium, and the S2 sound (the "dub") is the sound of the pulmonary valves and aortic valves closing in the right ventricle and left ventricle. Other heart sounds generally indicate an abnormality.

Each time the left ventricle contracts a volume of blood is ejected. This is called the cardiac output (CO). The CO is determined by the stroke volume (SV) x the number of beats per minute (the heart rate, or HR). The CO is expressed as:

- CO = SV x HR [written in mL or L (of blood volume) per minute]

Cardiac output can be individualized to a patient's body surface area (BSA) and this value is known as the cardiac index (CI).

- CI = CO/BSA

Heart failure occurs when the left ventricle (and sometimes the right, or both ventricles) does not fill with or eject blood properly. Consequently, the heart fails to pump sufficient blood to meet the body's metabolic (oxygen and nutrient) needs.

In early stages of failure, the heart responds to diminished output by stretching (to hold more blood) and by growing thicker muscular walls in order to pump harder. This will improve the situation short-term, but eventually the chamber inside the left ventricle becomes smaller due to expanding muscle, and the muscle walls weaken. This results in a ↓ CO.

In an attempt to compensate, the body tries to maintain normal arterial pressure through constricting arterial vessels by activation of the sympathetic (adrenergic) nervous system

(SNS). SNS activation causes the kidneys to release renin, which activates the renin-angiotensin-aldosterone system (RAAS), resulting in increased systemic vascular resistance via ↑ angiotensin II and ↑ vasopressin (antidiuretic hormone, or ADH). This, in turn, causes an increase in aldosterone, which results in ↑ renal reabsorption of sodium and water. Therefore, blood volume increases and helps maintain CO, but it is harmful because it raises venous pressure and causes pulmonary and systemic edema. The excess fluid causes the body to become "congested" and classic symptoms of "congestive" heart failure appear, including dyspnea (shortness of breath, or SOB), fatigue, pulmonary congestion (fluid back-up into the lungs – which contributes to the SOB) and peripheral edema. In severe cases, a lack of organ perfusion can lead to organ failure, including renal failure.

NON-PHARMACOLOGIC THERAPY

- Monitor body weight daily, preferably in the morning before eating and after voiding. Weight should be documented.

- Patients should have instructions on what to do if HF symptoms worsen and what to do when body weight increases.

- Limit sodium intake to < 2 grams/d in moderate to severe HF. If the patient also has hypertension, limit sodium intake to ≤ 1,500 mg/day.

- Consider daily multi-vitamin due to dietary restrictions and diuretic therapy.

- Use of n-3 polyunsaturated fatty acids (PUFA), or fish oils (1 gram/day), may ↓ mortality in Class II-IV HF.

- Avoid using products containing ephedra (ma huang) or ephedrine due to ↑ morbidity and mortality.

- Avoid NSAIDS, including COX-2 inhibitors, due to the risk of renal insufficiency and fluid retention.

- Stop smoking. Limit alcohol intake. Avoid illicit drug use.

- Pneumococcal vaccine and annual influenza vaccination is recommended.

- Encourage weight reduction to BMI < 30. Exercise 30 minutes/day, 3-5 days a week

DRUGS THAT CAUSE OR WORSEN HEART FAILURE

Chemotherapeutic agents, particularly anthracyclines and derivatives (doxorubicin, daunorubicin, etc.). Also trastuzumab. (*Herceptin*) Imatinib *(Gleevec)* and docetaxol *(Taxotere)* – cause fluid retention.

Amphetamines and other sympathomimetics. Also, itraconazole can cause HF.

Negative inotropic drugs (such as verapamil and diltiazem) can exacerbate heart failure. Avoid in heart failure.

Anti-arrhythmic drugs (lower risk with amiodarone and dofetilide). Do NOT use class I antiarrhythmic agents (mexiletine, tocainide, procainamide, quinidine, disopyramide, flecainide and propafenone)

Heart valve disease can be caused by these drugs: fenfluramine *(Pondimin)*, dexfenfluramine *(Redux)*, ergot derivatives including ergotamine *(Ergostat)*, dihydroergotamine *(Migranal)*, methysergide *(Sansert)*, and others.

Immunomodulators, including interferons, etanercept (TNF-blockers can worsen heart failure), rituximab and others.

NSAIDs, including the selective COX-2 inhibitor celecoxib *(Celebrex)* – avoid use of NSAIDs especially if advanced renal disease – use can cause renal dysfunction, fluid retention and worsen heart failure. Glucocorticoids can worsen heart failure.

Triptan migraine drugs (*contraindicated* with history of cardiovascular disease or uncontrolled hypertension).

Thiazolidinediones – particularly rosiglitazone *(Avandia)*; and pioglitazone *(Actos)*

Excessive alcohol use: modest use may have mild cardiovascular benefit, but excessive use does not.

Pharmacotherapy

Two classes of agents have become the recommended cornerstone of therapy to delay or halt the progression of cardiac dysfunction and improve mortality: ACE inhibitors and beta blockers. These medications should be utilized in everyone with heart failure who does not have a contraindication or intolerance to their use. Other agents have shown a positive impact on mortality (e.g., ARBs, aldosterone antagonists, and the combination of hydralazine and a nitrate) and these are added on top of standard therapy of ACEIs and beta blockers when patients are still symptomatic.

CHF → loop diuretics

Patients with "congestive" heart failure receive diuretics (primarily loop diuretics) to reduce fluid retention. Diuretic therapy is recommended to restore and maintain normal volume status in patients with clinical evidence of fluid overload, generally manifested by signs of elevated filling pressures (jugular venous distention, peripheral edema, rales, etc.) and by congestive symptoms (orthopnea, edema, and shortness of breath). Digoxin is another agent that can be used to treat symptomatic HF in patients already controlled on standard therapy.

SIGNS AND SYMPTOMS OF HEART FAILURE

Dyspnea at rest or on exertion

Weakness/fatigue

Shortness of Breath (SOB)

Orthopnea *difficulty breathing lying down*

Paroxysmal nocturnal dyspnea (PND) or nocturnal cough

Jugular venous distention (JVD)

Hepatojugular reflux (HJR)

Bibasilar rales

Edema

Ascites

Reduction in exercise capacity

S3 gallop

LVH

EF < 40% -if systolic dysfunction (> 40% in diastolic dysfunction)

↑ BNP (B-type Natriuretic Peptide (normal < 100 pg/mL)

Hepatomegaly

HEART FAILURE CLASSIFICATION

ACC/AHA STAGING SYSTEM	NYHA FUNCTIONAL CLASS
A. At high risk for development of HF, but have no structural heart disease or symptoms of heart failure (i.e., patients with HTN, CHD, DM, obesity, metabolic syndrome)	No corresponding category
B. Structural heart disease present, but no signs or symptoms of HF (i.e., LVH, low EF, valvular disease, previous MI)	1. No limitations of physical activity. Ordinary physical activity does not cause undue fatigue, palpitation, or dyspnea.

Heart Failure Classification Continued

ACC/AHA STAGING SYSTEM	NYHA FUNCTIONAL CLASS
Clinical Diagnosis of HF	
C. Structural heart disease with prior or current symptoms of HF (i.e., patients with known structural heart disease, SOB and fatigue, reduced exercise tolerance)	2. Slight limitation of physical activity. Comfortable at rest, but ordinary physical activity results in fatigue, palpitations, or dyspnea
	3. Marked limitation of physical activity. Comfortable at rest but minimal exertion (bathing, dressing) causes symptoms (fatigue, palpitation, or dyspnea)
D. Advanced structural heart disease with symptoms of HF at rest despite maximal medical therapy	4. Unable to carry on any physical activity without discomfort. Symptoms of HF present at rest.

RENIN-ANGIOTENSIN ALDOSTERONE SYSTEM (RAAS) INHIBITORS

- Titrate the drug to target doses, if possible. Titrate dose to reduce symptoms, not BP.

- Some patients may receive ACEI-ARBs together. Both can $\uparrow$ K$^+$, careful monitoring is required. Potassium should remain within the safe level of 3.5-5 mEq/L.

- ARBs are given if a patient is intolerant to ACEI (due to cough, etc.), or can be used 1st-line.

- There is an increased incidence of angioedema in black patients. Angioedema is more likely with ACEIs than ARBs, but if a person had angioedema with either class of agents, both are contraindicated since angioedema can be fatal. Counsel to report any swelling of lips, mouth, tongue, face or neck immediately.

- Patients on these medicines should not use salt substitutes (which contain KCl, rather than NaCl) or potassium supplements.

- Captopril has more side effects than other agents (taste disturbances, rash). It is not an optimal agent due to frequent dosing (TID). The other agents are once daily or BID.

ACEIs AND ARBs

These agents are used to decrease RAAS system activation, thereby $\downarrow$ cardiac remodeling and $\downarrow$ morbidity and mortality. These agents $\downarrow$ preload and afterload.

ACE inhibitors block the conversion of angiotensin I (AT I) to angiontensin II (AT II) by inhibiting the ACE-converting enzyme. ARBs block the AT II receptors on the smooth muscle wall of the vessel.

DRUG	DOSING	SIDE EFFECTS/CONTRAINDICATIONS/MONITORING

ACE Inhibitors - only those mentioned in the guidelines (See complete list in Hypertension lecture)

Captopril *(Capoten)*	25-50 mg BID-TID Target dose: 50 mg TID Take 1 hour before meals	**BLACK BOX WARNING** Can cause injury and death to developing fetus; discontinue as soon as pregnancy is detected
Enalapril, Enalaprilat injection *(Vasotec)*	5-40 mg/d Target dose: 10 mg BID	**SIDE EFFECTS** Cough, hyperkalemia, angioedema (if occurs, drug is CI), hypotension. Captopril has more SEs (taste perversion, rash).
Fosinopril *(Monopril)*	20-80 mg/d Target dose: 80 mg daily	
Lisinopril *(Prinivil, Zestril)*	10-40 mg/d Target dose: 20 mg daily	**CONTRAINDICATIONS** Angioedema. Do not use in bilateral renal artery stenosis; renal function will worsen.
Quinapril *(Accupril)*	40-80 mg/d Target dose: 80 mg daily	**MONITORING**
Ramipril *(Altace)*	2.5-20 mg/d Target dose: 10 mg daily	BP, K+, renal function; signs and symptoms of HF Pregnancy Category C (1st trimester) /D (2nd & 3rd trimester)
Trandolapril *(Mavik)*	2-8 mg/d Target dose: 4 mg daily	

ARBs - only those mentioned in the guidelines (See complete list in Hypertension lecture)

Candesartan *(Atacand)*	8-32 mg/d Target dose: 32 mg daily	**BLACK BOX WARNING** Can cause injury and death to developing fetus; discontinue as soon as pregnancy is detected **SIDE EFFECTS** Hyperkalemia, angioedema (if occurs, drug is CI), hypotension, headache, dizziness
Losartan *(Cozaar)*	25-100 mg/d and generic Target dose: 150 mg daily	**CONTRAINDICATIONS** Angioedema. Do not use in bilateral renal artery stenosis; renal function will worsen. **MONITORING** BP, K+, renal function; signs and symptoms of HF
Valsartan *(Diovan)*	80-320 mg/d Target dose: 160 mg BID	Pregnancy Category C (1st trimester) /D (2nd & 3rd trimester) Pregnancy category D: Valsartan

ALDOSTERONE RECEPTOR ANTAGONISTS

These agents inhibit the effects of aldosterone (part of the RAAS system) and ↓ cardiac re-modeling, ↓ Na+/water retention, and ↓ morbidity and mortality. These agents are used in Class III and Class IV HF, in addition to standard therapy.

Spironolactone is a non-selective aldosterone receptor blocker (also blocks androgen and progesterone receptors). Eplerenone is a selective aldosterone blocker; therefore, it has less side effects.

DRUG	DOSING	SIDE EFFECTS/CONTRAINDICATIONS/MONITORING

Potassium-Sparing Diuretics - only those mentioned in the guidelines (See complete list in Hypertension lecture)

| Spironolactone *(Aldactone)* | 12.5-25 mg/d

Target dose: 25 mg daily | **SIDE EFFECTS**
Hyperkalemia, ↑ serum creatinine (eplerenone). For spironolactone, gynecomastia, breast tenderness, impotence, menstrual changes, hirsutism.

CONTRAINDICATIONS
K⁺ > 5.0 mEq/L (per CHF guidelines), SCr > 2.5 mg/dL, CrCl < 30 mL/min; concomitant use of 3A4 inhibitors (eplerenone)

MONITORING
Check K⁺ before starting and periodically thereafter. Stop if K⁺ > 5.5 mEq/L. BP, SCr/BUN; signs and symptoms of HF

To minimize risk of hyperkalemia in patients treated with aldosterone blockers:

Higher risk if ↓ renal function (CI if CrCl < 30mL/min)

Do not start if K⁺ > 5 mEq/L. Stop if K⁺ > 5.5 mEq/L |
| Eplerenone *(Inspra)* | 25-50 mg/d

Target dose: 50 mg daily | Use low doses – and must start low. Higher risk when concurrent ACEIs or ARBs used at higher doses.

Do not use NSAIDs concurrently (which should be avoided in HF anyway).

Monitor frequently.

Counsel patient about ↑ risk if dehydration occurs (due to vomiting, diarrhea or ↓ fluid intake).

Pregnancy Category C |

Drug Interactions

- All RAAS inhibitors can ↑ the risk of hyperkalemia (most significant side effect). Monitor K⁺ and renal function frequently.

- The triple therapy of an ACEI, ARB, and aldosterone antagonist is not recommended due to high risk of hyperkalemia.

- All RAAS inhibitors can have additive antihypertensive effects - monitor BP.

- Lithium should not be given with diuretics (aldosterone antagonists) because diuretics ↓ lithium's renal clearance and ↑ the risk of lithium toxicity.

BETA-BLOCKERS

These agents inhibit the sympathetic nervous system (SNS) and ↓ cardiac remodeling and ↓ morbidity and mortality. Used in Class II-IV HF. Avoid beta-blockers with intrinsic sympathomimetic activity (ISA) as these agents may worsen survival.

DRUG	DOSING	SIDE EFFECTS/CONTRAINDICATIONS/MONITORING

β blockers - only those mentioned in the guidelines (See complete list in Hypertension lecture)

DRUG	DOSING	SIDE EFFECTS/CONTRAINDICATIONS/MONITORING
Bisoprolol *(Zebeta)* – benefit in clinical trials but no FDA indication	Start 1.25-2.5 mg/d Target dose: 10 mg daily	**SIDE EFFECTS** ↓ HR, hypotension, fatigue, dizziness. Less common: depression, ↓ libido **CONTRAINDICATIONS** Severe bradycardia, 2nd or 3rd degree heart block, cardiogenic shock, sick sinus syndrome, Do not initiate in patients with active asthma bronchospasm
Metoprolol, Metoprolol succin ext rel *(Lopressor XL, Toprol XL)*	Start 12.5-25 mg/d (long acting usual choice in HF) Target dose: 200 mg daily	**MONITORING** HR, BP, titrate Q 2 wks (as tolerated); ↓ dose if HR < 55; signs and symptoms of HF Caution use in patients with asthma Avoid abrupt discontinuation – must taper Caution in those with diabetes with recurrent hypoglycemia, asthma, severe COPD, and resting limb ischemia

Non-selective α & β blocker

DRUG	DOSING	SIDE EFFECTS/CONTRAINDICATIONS/MONITORING
Carvedilol *(Coreg, Coreg CR)*	Start IR 3.125 mg BID or CR 10 mg/d Target dose: 25 mg BID/80 mg daily (CR)	Same as above Take carvedilol – all forms – with food Pregnancy Category C

Drug Interactions

- Caution with diabetes: beta blockers can cover up the symptoms of shakiness and anxiety with hypoglycemia – this occurs mostly with the non-selective agents. They do not, however, cover up sweating (diaphoresis) and hunger.

- Beta blockers can enhance the effects of insulin and oral hypoglycemic (sulfonylureas, etc) – monitor BG carefully.

- Use caution when administering other drugs that slow HR, such as digoxin.

- Carvedilol is a substrate of CYP 450 2D6; check for drug interactions.

- Carvedilol can ↑ digoxin and cyclosporine levels; may require dose reduction.

HYDRALAZINE/NITRATES

Hydralazine is a direct arterial vasodilator which reduces afterload. Nitrates are venous vasodilators and reduce preload. The combination product, *BiDil*, is indicated in black patients with Class III and Class IV HF who are symptomatic despite optimal therapy with ACEIs and beta blockers. Hydralazine and nitrates are also used in patients who cannot tolerate ACEIs or ARBs due to poor renal function, angioedema, or hyperkalemia. Do not use nitrates alone; hydralazine is used with nitrates to improve efficacy and reduce nitrate tolerance.

DRUG	DOSING	SIDE EFFECTS/CONTRAINDICATIONS/MONITORING
Hydralazine and Nitrates		
Isosorbide dinitrate/ hydralazine *(BiDil)*	20-37.5 mg – start 1 TID, ↑ to 2 TID (target dose), as tolerated. No nitrate tolerance Target dose: 75 mg hydralazine/ 40 mg ISDN TID	**SIDE EFFECTS** Lupus-like syndrome (report fever, joint/muscle aches, fatigue), headache, dizziness, reflex tachycardia **CONTRAINDICATIONS** CI with PDE-5 Is **MONITORING** HR, BP; signs and symptoms of HF
Hydralazine *(Apresoline)*	37.5 mg QID Target dose: 75 mg QID	**SIDE EFFECTS** Lupus-like syndrome (report fever, joint/muscle aches, fatigue), reflex tachycardia **MONITORING** HR, BP; signs and symptoms of HF
Isosorbide mononitrate (*Imdur, Ismo, Monoket*) Isosorbide dinitrate (*Isordil*)	Given daily or BID (mononitrate); TID-QID (dinitrate) Target dose: 40 mg QID	**SIDE EFFECTS** Headache, dizziness, tachyphylaxis (need 10-12 hour nitrate free interval) **CONTRAINDICATIONS** CI with PDE-5 Is **MONITORING** HR, BP; signs and symptoms of HF

DIURETICS

Loops are used to reduce congestive symptoms and restore euvolemia (or "dry" weight). These agents ↓ fluid retention, volume status, and venous pressure. Relief of congestive signs and symptoms (orthopnea, edema, shortness of breath) must be achieved without causing side effects (i.e. symptomatic hypotension or worsening renal function). If needed more diuresis, may ↑ dose, switch to IV, or add metolazone.

DRUG	DOSING	SIDE EFFECTS/CONTRAINDICIATIONS/MONITORING
Loops		
Furosemide *(Lasix)* Most patients take divided doses: take 2nd dose early	20-80 mg daily, or divided, can go higher with all loops <u>Oral loop dose equivalency = 40 mg</u>	**SIDE EFFECTS** Hypokalemia, orthostatic hypotension, ↓ Na+, ↓ Mg2+, ↓ Cl-, ↓ Ca2+ (different than thiazides which ↑ Ca2+), metabolic alkalosis, hyperuricemia (↑ UA), hyperglycemia (↑ BG), photosensitivity, ototoxicity (MORE with ethacrynic acid) **CONTRAINDICATIONS** Anuria and caution in patients with a sulfa allergy (except ethacrynic acid) **MONITORING** Renal function (SCr, BUN), fluid status (in's and out''s, weight), BP, electrolytes, hearing with high doses or rapid IV administration IV formulations are light-sensitive (in amber bottles)
Bumetanide *(Bumex)*	0.5-2 mg daily <u>Oral loop dose equivalency = 1 mg</u>	
Torsemide *(Demadex)*	5-20 mg daily <u>Oral loop dose equivalency = 20 mg</u>	
Ethacrynic Acid *(Edecrin)*	25, 50 mg tabs; 50 mg inj.	

Drug Interactions

- All antihypertensives can have additive blood pressure-lowering effects. Always carefully monitor BP when adding-on therapy, <u>particularly with diuretics.</u>

- Loop diuretics can increase the ototoxic potential of aminoglycoside antibiotics, especially in the presence of impaired renal function. Except in life-threatening situations, avoid this combination.

- Lithium generally is not used concurrently because diuretics ↓ lithium's renal clearance and ↑ risk of lithium toxicity.

- <u>Do not use NSAIDS</u> in patients with HF. Also NSAIDS can cause sodium and water retention and reduce the effect of the loop diuretics.

HF CI: NSAIDS
Na + H₂O retention (opposite action of loop)

DIGOXIN

Digoxin can be used in patients with symptomatic HF who are receiving standard therapy, including ACEIs and beta-blockers. In HF, digoxin leads to symptom improvement, ↑ exercise tolerance, and ↑ QOL. Dosing should be based on renal function, concomitant medications and should be dosed at 0.125 mg daily in most patients.

Digoxin inhibits Na^+/K^+ ATP-ase pump; acts as a positive inotrope (↑ contractility and cardiac output), and as a negative chronotrope (↓ HR).

DRUG	DOSING	SIDE EFFECTS/CONTRAINDICIATIONS/MONITORING
Digoxin **(Lanoxin, Digitek)** – *tabs, solution, inj*	0.125-0.25 mg daily Loading doses not needed in HF Therapeutic range for CHF = 0.5-0.9 ng/mL (higher range for Afib) Watch for renal impairment ↓ in renal dysfunction; can be given 0.125 mg every other day, or even less frequently ↓ 20-25% when going from oral tabs to IV Antidote: *Digibind* or *DigiFab*	**SIDE EFFECTS** Dizziness, headache, diarrhea, nausea, vomiting, rash, mental changes **CONTRAINDICATIONS** 2nd or 3rd degree heart block without a pacemaker, Wolff-Parkinson-White syndrome (WPW) with A Fib, **MONITORING** HR, BP, electrolytes (K^+, Ca^{2+}, Mg^{2+}), renal function. ECG and drug level (if suspect toxicity) **TOXICITY** First signs of toxicity are nausea/vomiting and loss of appetite and bradycardia. Other signs of toxicity include blurred or "yellow" vision, abdominal pain, confusion, delirium, prolonged PR interval, accelerated junctional rhythm, bidirectional ventricular tachycardia Pregnancy Category C

Drug Interactions

- Beta-blockers and non-DHP calcium channel blockers may have additive effects on ↓ HR.

- Digoxin is mostly renally cleared and partially cleared hepatically. Decreased renal function requires a ↓ digoxin dose, or, if acute renal failure, the digoxin should be held.

- Digoxin levels may ↑ with amiodarone, quinidine, verapamil, erythromycin, clarithromycin, azole antifungals, cyclosporine, propafenone, PIs and a few others: a dose reduction likely required.

- Digoxin levels may ↓ with bile acid resins, St. John's wort and others.

- Hypokalemia (K^+ < 3.5 mEq/L) may ↑ risk of digoxin toxicity. Hypercalcemia may also ↑ risk of digoxin toxicity.

ACUTE DECOMPENSATED *(INPATIENT)* HEART FAILURE TREATMENT

- B-type natriuretic peptide (BNP) or N-terminal pro-B-type natriuretic peptide (NT-proB-NP) should be measured in patients being evaluated for dyspnea in which the contribution of HF is unknown. A final diagnosis requires interpreting these results in the context of all available clinical data and should not be used as a stand-alone test.

- Patients with fluid overload should be treated with IV loop diuretics.

- In the (absence of symptomatic hypotension,) IV nitroglycerin, nitroprusside or nesiritide may be considered in addition to diuretic therapy for rapid improvement of congestive symptoms. Frequent BP monitoring is required (↓ dose if hypotensive or worsening renal function develops)

- IV inotropic drugs such as dobutamine or milrinone might be reasonable if patient has low BP and low cardiac output (CO) to maintain systemic perfusion. (See ICU drug lecture for more information on dobutamine and milrinone).

Vasodilators

Nesiritide *(Natrecor)* is a B-type natriuretic peptide that binds to vascular smooth muscle and ↑ cGMP resulting in smooth muscle cell relaxation. Also produces dose-dependent reductions in systemic arterial pressure and pulmonary capillary wedge pressure (PCWP). No tachyphylaxis.

Nitroglycerin is more of a venous vasodilator, particularly at low doses. Nitroglycerin dilates coronary arteries and improves collateral blood flow to ischemic regions. Nitroprusside is an arterial and venous vasodilator and has more pronounced effects on blood pressure. Careful and continuous BP monitoring is essential.

DRUG	DOSING	SIDE EFFECTS/MONITORING/CONTRAINDICATIONS
Nesiritide *(Natrecor)*	Draw bolus only from prepared (reconstituted) infusion bag and monitor BP during treatment: give 2 mcg/kg IV bolus followed by a continuous infusion at 0.01 mcg/kg/min	**SIDE EFFECTS** Hypotension, ↑ SCr, others **CONTRAINDICATIONS** SBP < 90 mmHg Caution with other drugs that lower BP **MONITORING** BP, SCr, BUN, urine output
Nitroglycerin *(NTG)*	Prepare in glass bottles, PAB™, EXCEL™ (polyolefin) containers. Soft plastic-like PVC can cause adsorption of drug. Use administration sets intended for NTG.	**SIDE EFFECTS** Hypotension, headache, lightheadedness, tachycardia, tachyphylaxis **CONTRAINDICATIONS** SBP < 90 mmHg, CI with PDE-5 Is, ↑ intracranial pressure **MONITORING** BP, HR, SCr, BUN, urine output
Nitroprusside *(Nipride)*	Need to protect infusion bag from light (cover with opaque material or aluminum foil). A blue-color solution indicates degradation to cyanide – do not use	**SIDE EFFECTS** Hypotension, headache, tachycardia, cyanide/thiocyanate toxicity (especially in renal impairment) **CONTRAINDICATIONS** SBP < 90 mmHg, CI with PDE-5 Is, ↑ intracranial pressure **MONITORING** BP, HR, SCr, BUN, urine output, cyanide/thiocyanate toxicity, acid-base status

PATIENT COUNSELING

All Heart Failure Patients

- Monitor body weight daily, preferably in the morning before eating and after using the restroom. Weight should be documented.

- Patients should have instructions on what to do if HF symptoms worsen and what to do when body weight increases.

- Follow a sodium restricted diet.

- Avoid cigarette smoking, alcohol, and illicit drug use.

- Do not use NSAIDS or COX-2 inhibitors (or negative inotropic drugs such as verapamil, diltiazem, etc.) unless you check with your doctor first. Also, do not use nutritional supplements for HF without discussion of safety s with your health-care provider.

- Stay compliant with all medications – discuss with the pharmacist if cost-barrier exists.

Beta Blockers in HF

Using *Coreg CR* as an example – as this one has specific info about opening the CR capsules

- Take exactly as prescribed. *(Coreg* specifically is taken with food, to help reduce dizziness by delaying absorption).

- Swallow *Coreg CR* capsules whole. Do not chew or crush the capsules. If you have trouble swallowing *Coreg CR* whole:

  - The capsule may be carefully opened and the beads sprinkled over a spoonful of applesauce which should be taken right away. The applesauce should not be warm. Do not use other foods…only applesauce.

- Do not stop taking the medication unless your doctor tells you to do so.

- If you miss a dose, take your dose as soon as you remember, unless it is time to take your next dose. Do not double the dose.

- This medication can cause you to feel dizzy, tired, or faint. Do not drive a car, use machinery, or do anything that requires you to be alert until you adjust to the medication and the symptoms subside.

- This medication may make your feel more tired and dizzy at first. These effects will go away in a few days. However, call your doctor if the symptoms feel severe or you have weight gain or increased shortness of breath.

- This medication can cover up some of the signs and symptoms of low blood sugar (hypoglycemia); make sure to test your blood sugar often, and take a fast-acting sugar source if needed.

- This medication may cause worsening symptoms of peripheral vascular disease like pain, numbness and cold legs/feet.

- Medications used to treat severe allergic reaction may not work as well while taking this medication.

For *Toprol XL*

- If your doctor has instructed you to cut the *Toprol XL* or its generic equivalent tablet in half, you must use a pill cutter and cut only at the score line. Otherwise, the medicine will enter your body too quickly. Swallow the ½ tablet whole. The tablets cannot be crushed or chewed.

Digoxin

- This medicine helps make the heart beat stronger and with a more regular rhythm. Keep taking as directed, even if you feel well.

- Do not stop taking this medicine without talking to your doctor. Stopping suddenly may make your condition worse.

- Avoid becoming overheated or dehydrated as an overdose can more easily occur if you are dehydrated.

- Symptoms of overdose may include nausea, vomiting, diarrhea, loss of appetite, blurred vision, seeing halos around lights or objects, uneven heartbeats, and feeling like you might pass out. If any of these occur, see a doctor right away.

- There are many medications that can interact with digoxin. Check with your physician or pharmacist before starting any new medicines, including over the counter, vitamin, and/or herbal products.

- If your doctor has asked you to monitor heart rate, please do so as directed. A lower heart rate can indicate that the drug level in your body has become too high.

- To be sure that this medication is not causing harmful effects, your blood may need to be tested on a regular basis. Your kidney function will also need to be tested.

Practice Case

Janice is a 74 year old white female (60 kg) who came into the ICU with acute decompensated heart failure. Per her husband's report, Janice had been doing well over the past few months with her heart failure regimen. Her symptoms started on Easter night after she ate her daughter's ham, canned vegetables, and other dishes. She mentioned her weight was up a bit more and she seemed more short of breath, but thought these symptoms would go away by themselves.

CATEGORY	
PMH	CHF – NYHA Class III
	Hypertension, Depression
Vitals	BP:83/52 HR:134 RR:23 Temp:38.4°C
Test Results	

Item	Normal Range	Patient Value
Glucose	70-110 mg/dL	218
Na⁺	135-145 mEq/L	151
K⁺	3.5-5.0 mEq/L	4.7
Cl⁻	96-106 mEq/L	99
HCO₃	23-28 mEq/L	22
BUN	10-24 mg/dL	39
Creatinine	0.6-1.2 mg/dL	1.8

Digoxin level: 1.8 ng/mL

ECG: Normal sinus rhythm (NSR) with slight artifact

Medications prior to hospitalization	Lisinopril 40 mg daily
	Lasix 40 mg daily
	Digoxin 0.25 mg daily
	Toprol XL 100 mg daily
	Citalopram 20 mg daily

QUESTIONS

5. The medical team will start a dobutamine drip on this patient at 10 mcg/kg/min. The standard concentration of dobutamine in the pharmacy is a 250 mg/250 mL bag. Calculate how many hours the bag will last at the prescribed infusion rate.

    a. 3 hours
    b. 5 hours
    c. 7 hours
    d. 10 hours
    e. 15 hours

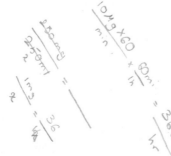

6. The patient is using digoxin. She has experienced an acute decline in renal function. Choose the correct statement concerning the patient's digoxin therapy:

    a. The patient's current potassium level will put her at risk for digoxin toxicity.
    b. The patient's renal function will put her at risk for digoxin toxicity.
    c. The patient should receive *Digibind* as soon as possible.
    d. A and B only.
    e. All of the above.

7. While in the hospital, Janice is started on a furosemide drip to try and pull off some fluid that has accumulated around her lungs. Choose the correct statement concerning the patient's furosemide therapy:

   a. If the patient experiences ototoxicity, she should be switched to ethacrynic acid.
   b. Furosemide is not effective as a diuretic if the creatinine clearance is < 30 mL/min.
   c. The furosemide will increase her risk of hyperkalemia.
   d. A and B only.
   e. None of the above.

8. Janice is ready to be discharged to home. Choose the correct counseling statement for her digoxin therapy:

   a. Monitor your pulse daily (preferably apical); a low rate can mean that the digoxin level is too high.
   b. If you lose your appetite or become nauseated, contact your doctor – this may indicate that the digoxin level is too high.
   c. Stop all use of potassium supplements while taking digoxin as potassium supplements will cause digoxin toxicity.
   d. A and B only.
   e. All of the above.

9. Janice has been home for 1 month and goes in for her first doctor's appointment since her hospitalization. She states she is taking all her medications which include lisinopril 40 mg daily, *Lasix* 40 mg daily, *Toprol XL* 100 mg daily, and digoxin. She is following a sodium restricted diet and monitoring her weight but she still feels symptomatic. The doctor decides to increase her *Toprol XL* dose to 200 mg daily. Which of the following patient counseling points should be discussed with Janice regarding this change in therapy?

   a. The increase in medication may make you feel more tired and dizzy at first. These effects will likely improve in a few days – if they do not, contact the doctor.
   b. This increase in medication can cause a loss of appetite, blurred vision, and seeing halos around lights or objects.
   c. This medication may be cut in half (if directed to do so), but do not crush or chew the tablets.
   d. A and C.
   e. All of the above.

Questions 6-10 do not pertain to the above case.

10. A patient is beginning carvedilol therapy for heart failure. The starting dose is 3.125 mg BID. Choose the correct statement:

    a. The medication should be taken on an empty stomach.
    b. If the CR formulation is used instead, the equivalent dose would be 7.5 mg daily.
    c. Carvedilol is a selective beta1-blocker and an alpha-blocker.
    d. Carvedilol capsules should never be opened. The contents cannot be exposed to light.
    e. Carvedilol should be titrated to 25 mg BID, as tolerated.

11. A patient with heart failure develops atrial fibrillation. Which agent represents the least dangerous option for treatment of the arrhythmia?

    a. Quinidine
    b. Propafenone
    c. Amiodarone
    d. Flecainide
    e. Mexiletine

12. A patient comes to the emergency department with acute decompensated heart failure. His vital signs include a respiratory rate (RR) of 24, HR of 130, and a BP of 80/57. Which of the following medications would be a good choice for this patient?

    a. Milrinone
    b. Nitroprusside
    c. Nesiritide
    d. Furosemide infusion
    e. Nesiritide

13. Which of the following medications should generally be avoided in patients with heart failure?

    a. Celecoxib
    b. Verapamil
    c. Amiodarone
    d. A and B
    e. All of the above

14. What is the trade name for eplerenone?

    a. Invega
    b. Invanz
    c. Invirase
    d. Isuprel
    e. Inspra

ANSWERS

1-c, 2-b, 3-e, 4-d, 5-d, 6-e, 7-c, 8-a, 9-d, 10-e

ANTICOAGULATION

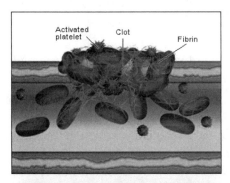

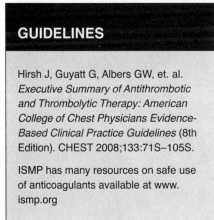

GUIDELINES

Hirsh J, Guyatt G, Albers GW, et. al. *Executive Summary of Antithrombotic and Thrombolytic Therapy: American College of Chest Physicians Evidence-Based Clinical Practice Guidelines* (8th Edition). CHEST 2008;133:71S–105S.

ISMP has many resources on safe use of anticoagulants available at www.ismp.org

Background

Anticoagulants are used to prevent blood clots from forming and to keep existing clots from becoming larger or expanding. They do not break down existing clots (that is done by drugs such as tissue plasminogen activator, or tPA). Anticoagulant therapy must be intensively monitored as the risks of not using anticoagulants correctly can lead to patient harm. A deep vein thrombosis (DVT) is a blood clot (thrombus) in a vein. DVTs can oc-

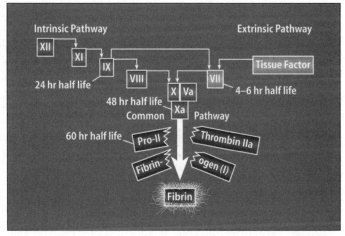

cur anywhere in the body but are most frequently found in the deep veins of the legs, thighs, and pelvis. When a DVT forms in a deep vein, a piece from the clot can break off and travel back to the heart and be pumped into the arteries of the lung. This can cause a pulmonary embolism (PE). The blood clot is called an embolus (plural emboli). Anticoagulants are also used for the prevention of stroke, and in the treatment of acute coronary syndrome (ACS).

HOW CLOTS ARE FORMED

Coagulation is the process by which blood forms clots – and anticoagulants inhibit this process at some point in the pathway. Damaged blood vessel walls activate platelets and the clotting cascade, leading to fibrin formation and a stable clot to prevent continued bleeding. Coagulation begins as soon as an injury is sustained to a blood vessel and the lining of the vessel wall is damaged. The coagulation cascade has two pathways which lead to fibrin formation. These are called the contact activation pathway (or the intrinsic pathway) and the tissue factor pathway (or the extrinsic pathway).

Pharmacological Treatment

Anticoagulants work by various mechanisms. Unfractionated heparin, low molecular weight heparins (LMWHs), and fondaparinux work by binding to antithrombin III (AT) causing a conformational change which increases ATs activity a 1000-fold. AT inactivates thrombin and other proteases involved in blood clotting, including factor Xa. LWMHs inhibit factor Xa more specifically than unfractionated heparin. Fondaparinux *(Arixtra)* selectively inhibits Factor Xa, but it's not a LMWH. It is a synthetic pentasaccharide that still requires AT binding for its pharmacologic action.

Direct thrombin inhibitors (which block thrombin, as the name suggests) decrease the amount of fibrin available for clot formation. The intravenous direct thrombin inhibitors have been very important clinically since they do not cross-react with heparin-induced thrombocytopenia (HIT) antibodies. Once HIT develops from the use of heparin (or less commonly from the LMWHs), the injectable direct thrombin inhibitors are the drugs of choice. The oral direct thrombin inhibitor, dabigatran *(Pradaxa)*, does not require blood tests to monitor for effectiveness and is not subject to food interactions and very little drug interactions. This is an advantage over warfarin.

Rivaroxaban *(Xarelto)*, a Factor Xa inhibitor, was recently approved. This oral agent is taken once daily and requires no laboratory monitoring for efficacy. However, it is associated with some drug interactions.

Warfarin is a vitamin K antagonist. Vitamin K is required for the carboxylation of clotting factors II, VII, IX, and X. Without adequate vitamin K, the liver produces the factors – but they have reduced coagulant activity. Warfarin requires careful patient monitoring – with frequent blood tests to measure the INR (international normalized ratio), the test used to measure warfarin's effectiveness. Warfarin has a narrow range of effectiveness and the INR is highly variable and affected greatly by the addition of many medicines or changes in dietary vitamin K intake. It has a high risk of bleeding and is contraindicated in pregnancy (pregnancy category X).

FOODS HIGH IN VITAMIN K	
Broccoli	Mustard greens
Brussels sprouts	Parsley
Cabbage	Soybean Oil
Canola oil	Spinach
Cauliflower	Swiss chard
Chickpea	Tea (green or black)
Cole Slaw	
Collard Greens	Turnip greens
Coriander	Watercress
Endive	
Green kale	
Lettuce (red leaf or butterhead)	

TREATMENT SAFETY CONCERNS & PHARMACIST'S ROLE

All of the anticoagulants can cause significant bleeding and are classified as "High Alert" medications by the Institute for

Safe Medication Practices (ISMP). Bleeding events associated with anticoagulants put the patient at risk for increased mortality, including higher risk for stroke and myocardial infarction. Ten percent of all adverse drug events treated in the emergency room are due to anticoagulants. The Joint Commission's National Patient Safety Goals require the implementation of policies and protocols to properly initiate and manage anticoagulant therapy. Patients receiving anticoagulants should receive individualized care through a defined process that includes standardized ordering, dispensing, administration, monitoring and education (for treatment doses). When pharmacists are involved in managing anticoagulants, patient care and outcomes are improved and costs are decreased. Pharmacists are also involved with ensuring that patients who need anticoagulants–such as orthopedic and cardiac surgical patients – receive them for DVT prophylaxis.

Unfractionated Heparin (UFH)

Binds to antithrombin III (AT III) and inactivates thrombin (Factor IIa) and Factor Xa (as well as factors IXa, XIa, XIIa, and plasmin) and prevents the conversion of fibrinogen to fibrin

DRUG	DOSING	SIDE EFFECTS/CONTRAINDICATIONS/MONITORING
Heparin (AKA unfractionated heparin)	**PREVENTION OF VTE:** 5,000 units SC Q8-12H **TREATMENT OF VTE** 80 units/kg IV bolus (or 5,000 units); 18 units/kg/hr (or 1,300 units/kg/hr) infusion ACS/STEMI 60 units/kg IV bolus (max 4,000 units); 12 units/kg/hr (max 1,000 units/hr) infusion Use actual body weight for dosing Onset: IV-immediate; SC- 30 min-2 hrs t ½ = ~1.5 hrs Unpredictable anticoagulant response - has variable and extensive binding to plasma proteins and cells Heparin induced thrombocytopenia (HIT) type II (IgG mediated) – heparin antibody complexes form and bind to platelets, causing aggregation and clots. Look for a drop in platelet count of > 50% from baseline HIT has cross-sensitivity with LMWHs Antidote: Protamine – 1 mg protamine will reverse ~100 units of heparin; max dose 50 mg	**CONTRAINDICATIONS** Uncontrolled active bleed, severe thrombocytopenia, ICH, history of HIT Do not give IM due to hematoma risk **SIDE EFFECTS** Bleeding (epistaxis, ecchymosis, gingival, GI, etc.), thrombocytopenia, heparin induced thrombocytopenia (HIT), hyperkalemia and osteoporosis (with long-term use) **MONITORING** Heparin is monitored via the aPTT (or anti-Xa level: 0.3-0.7 units/mL) Taken 6 hours after initiation and every 6 hrs until therapeutic range of 1.5-2.5 x control (patient's baseline) is reached; also check aPTT at every rate change; then daily Platelet count, Hgb, Hct at baseline and daily to monitor for thrombocytopenia and bleeding **SAFETY NOTE** Heparin "lock-flushes" (*Hep-Lock, HepFlush*) are used to keep IV lines open (patent). They are not used for anticoagulation. There have been fatal errors made by choosing the incorrect heparin strength. (Heparin injection 10,000 units/mL and Hep-Lock 10 units/mL have been confused with each other). Using a higher dose to flush a line could cause significant bleeding, including fatal hemorrhage. Many of the dosing errors have occurred in neonates. Heparin comes in different strengths. To help avoid errors, heparin should not be stocked in unfamiliar concentrations. The concentration must be verified by the pharmacist prior to dispensing the dose. Never rely on color as a sole indicator to differentiate product identity. Commercially prepared premixed heparin infusions are preferred. Having the pharmacy prepare the flush syringes (rather than busy nurses) can help reduce errors.

HEPARIN DRUG INTERACTIONS

Most drug interactions are due to additive effects with other agents that can ↑ bleeding risk, such as antiplatelet drugs, NSAIDS, anticoagulants, thrombolytics, dextran, dipyridamole, SSRIs, SNRIs, natural products, and others. See drug interactions chapter for more information on drugs that can increase bleeding.

Low Molecular Weight Heparins

Similar mechanism to heparin except that the inhibition is much greater for Factor Xa than Factor IIa

DRUG	DOSING	SIDE EFFECTS/CONTRAINDICATIONS/ MONITORING
Enoxaparin *(Lovenox)* Comes in multidose vials or these prefilled syringes: 30 mg/0.3 mL, 40 mg/0.4 mL, 60 mg/0.6 mL, 80 mg/0.8 mL, 100 mg/mL, 120 mg/0.8 mL, 150 mg/mL	**PROPHYLAXIS** 30 mg SC Q12H or 40 mg SC daily CrCl < 30 mL/min: use 30 mg SC daily **TREATMENT** 1mg/kg SC Q12H or 1.5 mg/kg SC daily CrCl < 30 mL/min: use 1mg/kg SC daily **TREATMENT FOR STEMI** In patients < 75 years: 30 mg IV bolus plus a 1 mg/kg SC dose followed by 1 mg/kg SC Q12H (max 100 mg for the 1st two doses only) In patients ≥ 75 years: 0.75 mg/kg SC Q12H (no bolus - max 75 mg for the 1st two doses only) CrCl < 30 mL/min: use 1mg/kg SC daily In patients managed with percutaneous coronary intervention (PCI): if the last SC dose was given more than 8 hours before balloon inflation, give 0.3 mg/kg IV bolus	**BLACK BOX WARNING** Patients receiving neuraxial anesthesia (epidural, spinal) or undergoing spinal puncture are at risk of hematomas and subsequent paralysis **CONTRAINDICATIONS** History of HIT Active major bleed Hypersensitivity to pork Sulfite allergy (tinzaparin) **SIDE EFFECTS** Bleeding, thrombocytopenia, anemia, injection site reactions, priapism with tinzaparin **MONITORING** Anti-Xa levels can be used to monitor but monitoring is not routine. Monitoring is recommended in pregnancy, and may be done in renal insufficiency or in morbidly obese patients. aPTT is not used. Check platelet count, Hgb, Hct @ baseline and every 2-3 days (if inpatient); stool occult blood tests More predictable anticoagulant response (therefore do not need to monitor LMWHs in most cases.) Less monitoring and more cost effective, even though actual drug costs more than unfractionated heparin. Pregnancy Category B
Dalteparin (*Fragmin*)		
Tinzaparin (*Innohep*)		

LMWH DRUG INTERACTIONS

- Most drug interactions are due to additive effects with other agents that can ↑ bleeding risk, such as antiplatelet drugs, NSAIDS, anticoagulants, thrombolytics, dextran, dipyridamole, etc.

ENOXAPARIN PATIENT COUNSELING

- Proper instructions on self injection should be discussed with the patient (see below).

- This medication can cause bleeding. Ask your health care provider before starting any new medications including aspirin and other pain relief medication, herbal products, etc.

- This medication can cause you to bruise and/or bleed more easily. Report any unusual bleeding, bruising, or rashes to your physician

- Tell physicians and dentists that you are using this medication before any surgery is performed.

Proper Subcutaneous Administration of Enoxaparin

- First, wash and dry hands.

- Choose an area on the right or left side of your abdomen, at least 2 inches from the belly button.

- Clean the injection site with an alcohol swab. Let dry.

- Remove the needle cap by pulling it straight off the syringe and discard it in a sharps container. (Do not twist the cap off as this can bend the needle)

- <u>Do not expel the air bubble in the syringe prior to injection (unless your doctor has advised you to do so).</u>

- With your other hand, pinch an inch of the cleansed area to make a fold in the skin. Insert the full length of the needle straight down – at a 90 degree angle- into fold of skin.

- Press the plunger with your thumb until the syringe is empty.

- Pull the needle straight out at the same angle that it was inserted.

- Point the needle down and away from yourself and others, and push down on the plunger to activate the safety shield.

- Do not rub the site of injection as this can lead to bruising. Place the used syringe in the sharps collector.

Fondaparinux *(Arixtra)*

Synthetic pentasaccharide that selectively inhibits Factor Xa via antithrombin III (AT III)

DRUG	DOSING	SIDE EFFECTS/CONTRAINDICATIONS/MONITORING
Fondaparinux *(Arixtra)*	**Prophylaxis of DVT/PE:** 2.5 mg SC daily **Treatment of DVT/PE:** 5 mg SC daily (body wt < 50 kg) 7.5 mg SC daily (50-100 kg) 10 mg SC daily (> 100 kg) Do not expel air bubble from syringe prior to injection No antidote	**BLACK BOX WARNING** Patients receiving neuraxial anesthesia (epidural, spinal) or undergoing spinal puncture are at risk of hematomas and subsequent paralysis **CONTRAINDICATIONS** CrCl < 30 mL/min (poor renal function), active major bleed, bacterial endocarditis, thrombocytopenia with positive test for anti-platelet antibodies in presence of fondaparinux, or body wt < 50 kg (for prophylaxis only) **SIDE EFFECTS** Bleeding (epistaxis, ecchymosis, gingival, GI, etc.), local injection site reactions (rash, pruritus, bleeding), thrombocytopenia, SCr, stool occult blood tests **MONITORING** Platelet count, Hgb, Hct at baseline and daily to monitor for thrombocytopenia and bleeding; SCr Pregnancy Category B

Direct Thrombin Inhibitors

These agents directly inhibit thrombin (Factor IIa)

DRUG	DOSING	SIDE EFFECTS/CONTRAINDICATIONS/MONITORING

Direct Thrombin Inhibitors (IV)

Lepirudin *(Refludan)* Recombinant hirudin for HIT with thrombosis	Intravenous drugs Used in patients with a history of HIT/TS	No cross-reaction with HIT **CONTRAINDICATIONS** Active major bleeds **SIDE EFFECTS** Bleeding, anemia, hematoma **MONITORING** aPTT, and/or ACT (for bivalirudin); platelets, Hgb, Hct No antidote
Argatroban *(Novastan)* HIT with thrombosis and patients undergoing PCI who are at risk for HIT		
Bivalirudin *(Angiomax)* For patients with ACS undergoing PTCA and are at risk for HIT		

Direct Thrombin Inhibitors Continued

DRUG	DOSING	SIDE EFFECTS/CONTRAINDICATIONS/MONITORING

Direct Thrombin Inhibitor (oral)

DRUG	DOSING	SIDE EFFECTS/CONTRAINDICATIONS/MONITORING
Dabigatran *(Pradaxa)* Reduce the risk of stroke and systemic embolism in patients with non-valvular atrial fibrillation	150 mg BID; 75 mg BID if CrCl 15-30 mL/min Comes in 75, 150 mg caps Swallow capsules whole. Do not break, chew, or crush. Take missed dose ASAP unless it is within 6 hours of next scheduled dose; do not double up Once bottles are opened, the product must be used within 4 months. Keep bottle tightly closed. Store in original package to protect from moisture. Blister packs are good until the date on the pack (usually 6-12 months)	**CONTRAINDICATIONS** Active pathological bleed **SIDE EFFECTS** Gastritis-like symptoms, bleeding (including more GI bleeding) No monitoring of efficacy required. Pregnancy Category C Dabigatran prevents 5 more strokes per 1,000 patients/year than warfarin If switching from warfarin to dabigatran, discontinue warfarin and start dabigatran when INR < 2.0. Start dabigatran 0-2 hrs before the next dose of parenteral drug, like *Lovenox*, or just after discontinuation of heparin infusion. Discontinue if going for invasive surgery (1-2 days before if normal renal function, 3-5 days before if CrCl < 50 mL/min) No antidote **MONITORING** Renal function at baseline and yearly in patients > 75 years of age or in patients with a CrCl < 50 mL/min

DRUG INTERACTIONS

Dabigatran – avoid concurrent use with rifampin and other P-glycoprotein inducers. In patients with moderate renal impairment (CrCl 30-50 mL/min), concomitant use of P-gp inhibitor dronedarone or systemic ketoconazole can be expected to increase dabigatran levels.

See drug interactions chapter for more information on drugs that can increase bleeding risk.

FACTOR Xa INHIBITOR

DRUG	DOSING	SIDE EFFECTS/CONTRAINDICATIONS/MONITORING
Rivaroxaban *(Xarelto)* Prophylaxis of deep vein thrombosis (DVT) which may lead to pulmonary embolism (PE) in patients undergoing knee or hip replacement surgery Also indicated for stroke prevention in patients with non-valvular atrial fibrillation	**Non-Valvular A Fib** CrCl > 50 mL/min: 20 mg PO daily with the evening meal CrCl 15-50 mL/min: 15 mg PO daily with the evening meal CrCl < 15 mL/min: avoid use **Prophylaxis for DVT (after knee/hip replacement)** 10 mg PO daily - without regards to meals Do not use in CrCl < 30 mL/min First dose given 6-10 hours after surgery Take for 35 days after hip replacement surgery; Take for 12 days after knee replacement surgery	**BLACK BOX WARNING** Patients receiving neuraxial anesthesia (epidural, spinal) or undergoing spinal puncture are at risk of hematomas and subsequent paralysis Discontinuation of rivaroxaban in patients with non-valvular A. Fib can put patients at increased risk of thrombotic events, like stroke **CONTRAINDICATIONS** Active major bleeding, avoid use in patients with moderate to severe hepatic impairment or with any degree associated with coagulopathy **SIDE EFFECTS** Bleeding No monitoring required Pregnancy Category C No antidote

DRUG INTERACTIONS

Avoid concomitant use with drugs that are combined P-glycoprotein and strong 3A4 inducers (e.g. carbamazepine, phenytoin, rifampin, St. John's wort). A dose increase of rivaroxaban to 20 mg should be considered if these drugs must be co-administered. The 20 mg dose should be taken with food.

Avoid concomitant use with drugs that are combined P-glycoprotein and strong 3A4 inhibitors (e.g. ketoconazole, itraconazole, lopinavir/ritonavir, ritonavir, indinavir/ritonavir, and conivaptan). Use caution with concomitant 3A4 inhibitors in patients with mild to moderate renal impairment.

Avoid concurrent use with other anticoagulants as this may increase bleeding risk. Avoid concurrent use with clopidogrel unless benefit outweighs the risk of bleeding.

Warfarin *(Coumadin, Jantoven)*

Inhibits the C1 subunit of the vitamin K epoxide reductase (VKORC1) enzyme complex, thereby reducing the regeneration of vitamin K epoxide causing depletion of clotting factors II, VII, IX and X and proteins C and S.

Per the ACCP guidelines (*Chest, 2008*): Initial starting doses between 5-10 mg for the first 1-2 days, then adjust per INR values. A starting dose of ≤ 5 mg is recommended for the following patient populations: elderly, debilitated, malnourished, those patients taking meds that increase sensitivity to warfarin (e.g. amiodarone), liver disease, recent major surgery, CHF. Presence of CYP2C9*2 or *3 allele and/or polymorphism to the VKORC gene ↑ risk of bleeding. Lower doses may be required in these patients and genetic testing may be useful in determining the appropriate dose.

DRUG	DOSING	SIDE EFFECTS/CONTRAINDICATIONS/ MONITORING
Warfarin (*Coumadin, Jantoven*) Racemic mixture of R- and S- enantiomers with the S- enantiomer being more potent (3-5x more) Please see foods high in vitamin K on page 448 – be consistent with intake	**Initial starting doses** between 5-10 mg for the first 1-2 days, then adjust per INR values. Doses of 5 mg or less made be an appropriate starting dose; see information above the chart 1 mg (pink) 2 mg (lavender) 2.5 mg (green) 3 mg (tan) 4 mg (blue) 5 mg (peach) 6 mg (teal) 7.5 mg (yellow) 10 mg (white) Highly protein bound (99%) Antidote: vitamin K	**BLACK BOX WARNING** May cause major or fatal bleeding **CONTRAINDICATIONS** Hemorrhagic tendencies, blood dyscrasias, cerebrovascular hemorrhage, pregnancy, predisposition to bleeding, uncontrolled hypertension, bacterial endocarditis, pericarditis, pericardial effusions, an unreliable, non-compliant patient, alcoholism, history of falls, and many others. **SIDE EFFECTS** Bleeding, skin necrosis, purple toe syndrome Pregnancy Category X **MONITORING** PT/INR should be 2.0-3.0 for most indications (DVT, A. fibrillation) and should be 2.5-3.5 for some high-risk indications, including patients with a mechanical heart valve. INR monitoring to begin after the initial 2 or 3 doses, or if on chronic warfarin therapy, monitor at an interval no longer than monthly.

WARFARIN – PHARMACOKINETIC DRUG INTERACTIONS

- Warfarin is a substrate of CYP 2C9 (major), 1A2 (minor) and 3A4 (minor) and an inhibitor of 2C9 (moderate). Avoid use with tamoxifen.

- 2C9 inducers – including phenobarbital, phenytoin, primidone, rifampin (large ↓ INR), and St. John's Wort - may ↓ INR.

- 2C9 inhibitors - including amiodarone, *Bactrim*, azole antifungals, macrolide antibiotics, and metronidazole - may ↑ INR. See drug interactions chapter.

- Check for 1A2 and 3A4 interactions; these occur, but usually have less of an effect on INR.

WARFARIN – PHARMACODYNAMIC DRUG INTERACTIONS

- The most common pharmacodynamic interaction is with NSAIDs, including aspirin and ibuprofen (but not selective agents such as celecoxib), and with antiplatelet agents. These interactions ↑ bleeding risk, but the INR will be in the usual range.

- Ginkgo biloba increases bleeding risk with no effect on the INR. Other natural products that can also pose a risk include bromelains, danshen, dong quai (this product may ↑ INR), vitamin E, evening primrose oil, high doses of fish oils, garlic, ginseng, glucosamine, grapefruit, policosanol, and willow bark.

- SSRIs and SNRIs, with the use of an anticoagulant, can increase bleeding risk without increasing the INR. Use extreme caution with the drugs in combination.

- Nutritional products, including drinks and supplements, can include vitamin K (e.g. green tea). Coenzyme Q10 may reduce the effectiveness of warfarin. Any additions of vitamin K will lower the INR. Check the product for vitamin K content.

WARFARIN PATIENT COUNSELING

- Take warfarin at the same time every day as prescribed by your doctor. You can take warfarin either with food or on an empty stomach.

- Warfarin lowers the chance of blood clots forming in your body.

- If you miss a dose, take the dose as soon as possible on the same day. Do not take a double dose the next day to make up for a missed dose.

- Call your healthcare provider if you are sick with diarrhea, an infection, or have a fever.

- Tell your healthcare provider about any planned surgeries, medical or dental procedures. Your warfarin may have to be stopped for a short time or you may need the dose adjusted.

- Call your healthcare provider right away if you fall or injure yourself, especially if you hit your head.

- You will need to have your blood tested frequently to monitor your response to this medication. This test is called an INR. Your dose may be adjusted to keep you INR in a target range.

- Check with your doctor or pharmacist before taking any other medication, including over the counter medications, vitamins, and herbal products.

- Do not start, stop, or change any medicine without talking with your healthcare provider.

- This medication is very important for your health, but it can cause serious and life-threatening bleeding problems.

- Call your healthcare provider right away if you get any of these symptoms:

  - Pain, swelling, or discomfort

  - Headaches, dizziness, or weakness

  - Unusual bruising (bruises that develop without known cause or grow in size)

  - Nosebleeds

  - Bleeding gums

  - Bleeding from cuts takes a long time to stop

  - Menstrual bleeding or vaginal bleeding that is much heavier than normal

  - Pink or brown urine

  - Red or black stools

  - Coughing up blood

  - Vomiting blood or material that looks like coffee grounds

- Do not make changes in your diet, such as eating large amounts of green, leafy vegetables. Be consistent with the amount of leafy green vegetables and other foods rich in vitamin K.

- Do not change your weight by dieting, without first checking with your healthcare provider.

- Avoid drinking alcohol.

- Other side effects besides bleeding include purple toe syndrome that can cause your toes to become painful and purple in color. Also, death of skin tissue can occur. Report either of these immediately to your health care professional.

Use of Vitamin K for High (Supratherapeutic) INRs

Variable INRs are a norm of clinical practice. Elevated INRs can scare the clinician due to the risk of bleeding. It is important to know the difference between recommended treatments for mildly elevated INRs versus very high INRs. Bleeding, at any INR, will warrant more serious intervention.

It is dangerous when vitamin K injections are over-used when oral formulations could be safely used instead, or when the wrong route of administration is chosen. Subcutaneous injection (SC) can produce a variable response and may end up leaving the patient with a subtherapeutic INR (and now at risk for clotting, rather than bleeding) for an extended time period. SC injections of vitamin K should not be used. Intravenous or intramuscular injections should be avoided – except when IV is recommended (see chart below) in life-threatening bleeding. Both types can cause severe anaphylaxis. If given IV, the vitamin K should be diluted and rapid infusion should be avoided.

Note that the algorithm does not recommend vitamin K at an INR < 5 if bleeding is not present. Even at an INR of 5-9, if no bleeding is present, it may be viable to hold doses and monitor more frequently. When vitamin K is used, if a stat reversal is not required, <u>oral is the preferred formulation.</u>

Use of Vitamin K for Overanticoagulation

SYMPTOMS/INR VALUE	WHAT TO DO
For patients with a supratherapeutic INR but INR < 5.0 with no significant bleeding:	Lower the dose or omit a dose, monitor more frequently, and resume therapy at a lower dose when the INR is therapeutic.
For patients with INR ≥ 5.0 but < 9.0 and no significant bleeding:	Omit the next 1-2 doses, monitor more frequently, and resume therapy at an appropriately adjusted dose when the INR is therapeutic OR Omit 1 dose and give oral vitamin K <u>1-2.5 mg</u>, particularly if patient is at ↑ risk of bleeding (correction takes place within 24 hours).

Use of Vitamin K for Overanticoagulation Continued

SYMPTOMS/INR VALUE	WHAT TO DO
For patients with INR ≥ 9.0 and no significant bleeding:	Hold warfarin therapy and give oral vitamin K 2.5-5 mg with the expectation that the INR will be reduced in 24-48 hrs. Monitor more frequently, give more vitamin K if necessary, and resume therapy at an appropriately adjusted dose when the INR reaches therapeutic range.
In patients with serious bleeding and an elevated INR:	Hold warfarin therapy and give vitamin K 10 mg by slow IV infusion supplemented with fresh frozen plasma, prothrombin complex concentrate, or recombinant factor VIIa, depending on the urgency of the situation. Repeat vitamin K administration Q12H for persistent INR elevations.
In patients with life-threatening bleeding (e.g. ICH) and elevated INR:	Hold warfarin therapy and give fresh frozen plasma, prothrombin complex concentrate, or recombinant factor VIIa supplemented with vitamin K 10 mg by slow IV infusion, repeated, if necessary, depending on the INR

Do not give vitamin K via IM route (due to risk of hematoma formation) or SC (variable absorption)

PERIOPERATIVE MANAGEMENT OF PATIENTS ON WARFARIN

- Stop warfarin therapy approximately 5 days before major surgery. If patient is moderate to high risk for thromboembolism, then bridge with therapeutic LMWH given SC (or UFH IV). Discontinue the LMWH 24 hours before surgery (4 hours before if using UFH IV).

- If INR is still elevated 1-2 days before surgery, give low-dose vitamin K (1-2 mg).

- If reversal of warfarin is needed in a patient requiring an urgent surgical procedure, give low-dose (2.5-5 mg) IV or oral vitamin K.

- Resume warfarin therapy 12-24 hours after the surgery, when there is adequate hemostasis.

- Resume therapeutic dose of LMWH therapy 24 hours after surgery, when there is adequate hemostasis.

- Continue warfarin or ASA in patients undergoing minor dental, dermatologic, or cataract surgery.

- Antiplatelet therapies (such as clopidogrel or prasugrel) may need to be stopped 5-10 days prior to major surgery. The risks/benefit of stopping therapy must be evaluated on a case-by-case basis.

Anticoagulation for Patients with Atrial Fibrillation (Chest Guidelines 2008)

- Anticoagulation for patients with A Fib. who are going to undergo cardioversion:

- Those patients with A Fib of 48 hrs in duration or longer, or when the duration is unknown, anticoagulation (INR 2.0-3.0) is recommended for at least 3 weeks prior to and 4 weeks after cardioversion (regardless of method – electrical or pharmacological) when normal sinus rhythm is restored.

- Those patients staying in atrial fibrillation, chronic anticoagulation therapy is needed for stroke prevention. Therapy depends on the number of risk factors the patient has. See tables below.

ANTITHROMBOTIC THERAPY FOR PATIENTS WITH ATRIAL FIBRILLATION

RISK CATEGORY	RECOMMENDED THERAPY
No risk factors	ASA 75-325 mg daily
One moderate risk factor	ASA 75-325 mg daily or warfarin (INR 2.0-3.0; target 2.5) or dabigatran (or rivaroxaban)
Any high-risk factor or ≥ 2 moderate risk factors	Warfarin (INR 2.0-3.0; target 2.5)* or dabigatran (or rivaroxaban)

If mechanical valve, target INR greater than 2.5

HIGH RISK FACTORS	MODERATE RISK FACTORS
Prior stroke, TIA, or systemic embolism	Age > 75 years old
	Hypertension
	Heart Failure (EF ≤ 35%)
	Diabetes

RISK FACTORS FOR VENOUS THROMBOEMBOLISM

- Surgery

- Major trauma or lower extremity injury

- Immobility

- Cancer or chemotherapy

- Venous compression (tumor, hematoma, arterial abnormality)

- Previous venous thromboembolism

- Increasing age

- Pregnancy and postpartum period

- Estrogen-containing medications or selective estrogen receptor modulators

- Erythropoietin-stimulating agents

- Acute medical illness

- Inflammatory bowel disease

- Nephrotic syndrome

- Myeloproliferative disorders

- Paroxysmal nocturnal hemoglobinuria

- Obesity

- Central venous catheterization

- Inherited or acquired thrombophilia

CHADS$_2$ SCORING SYSTEM
Each risk factor = 1, except for stroke/TIA which = 2. Add up the total number of risk factors for a patient.
C – CHF
H – HTN
A – Age (> 75)
D – Diabetes
S$_2$ – prior Stroke/TIA

Options for patients who cannot receive anticoagulation (due to a contraindication)

Graduated compression stockings (GCS) and intermittent pneumatic compression (IPC) devices are 2 non-pharmacologic measures used to prevent venous thromboembolism.

Practice Case

Alice is a 47 year old female (5′ 6″, 176 lbs.) who has been admitted to the hospital with shortness of breath, problems breathing, chest pain, coughing, and sweating. She may have a pulmonary embolism so the medical team started her on heparin therapy.

CATEGORY	
Past Medical History	Atrial Fibrillation HTN – Stage 1
Vitals	BP 155/89 HR 155 RR 25 Temp 38°
Labs	SCr 1.8 mg/dL; K 4.2 mEq/L; Glucose 241 mg/dL
Current Medications	Amiodarone 200 mg daily ASA 325 mg daily
Allergies	Sulfites

QUESTIONS

Heparin protocol for St. Mary's Hospital

INDICATION	REGIMEN
Treatment of DVT/PE	80 units/kg (max 10,000 units bolus); 20 units/kg/hr (max 2,300 units/hr)

APTT (SEC.)	DOSE ADJUSTMENT
< 35	80 units/kg bolus then ↑ infusion by 4 units/kg/hr
35-50	40 units/kg bolus then ↑ infusion by 2 units/kg/hr
51-71	No change
72-93	Decrease infusion by 2 units/kg/hr
> 93	Hold infusion for 1 hour then ↓ by 3 units/kg/hr

1. The medical team asks you to dose the heparin for Alice per hospital protocol. The protocol is to the left. What should the correct bolus and infusion rate of heparin be for Alice?

   a. 10,000 units bolus, followed by 2,300 units/hr infusion
   b. 14,000 units bolus, followed by 3,500 units/hr infusion
   c. 7,000 units bolus, followed by 1,400 units/hr infusion
   d. 6,400 units bolus, followed by 1,600 units/hr infusion
   e. None of the above

2. The bolus and infusion are given. After 6 hours, the aPTT comes back at 48 sec. What is the correct dose adjustment to make to the heparin according to the protocol?

   a. Give a 6,400 unit bolus now and increase the infusion rate to 1,900 units/hr
   b. Give a 3,200 unit bolus now and increase the infusion rate to 1,760 units/hr
   c. Make no change to the dose
   d. Do not give a bolus and reduce the infusion rate to 1,500 units/hr
   e. None of the above

3. The pulmonary embolism was confirmed. It is Alice's third day in the hospital, and the medical team would like her discharged. She is going to be transitioned to warfarin. She receives 5 mg of warfarin at her bedside. Which of the statements is true regarding warfarin?

   a. Warfarin is a direct thrombin inhibitor that helps to prevent clot formation.
   b. Warfarin has a high risk of bleeding. Careful monitoring is advised.
   c. Warfarin should be taken with a low fat meal and never double up on the dose.
   d. Warfarin is a racemic mixture and the R-isomer is more potent than the S-isomer.
   e. None of the above statements are true.

4. Alice needs another medication as a "bridge" therapy until her warfarin becomes therapeutic. Select the appropriate agent, route of administration, and dose for Alice's treatment of PE.

   a. Lovenox 30mg SC daily
   b. Lovenox 30mg SC Q12H
   c. Lovenox 80mg SC Q12H
   d. Lovenox 80mg SC daily
   e. Innohep 14,000 anti-Xa units SC daily

5. Alice will need proper counseling on subcutaneous administration of enoxaparin. All of the following points regarding enoxaparin administration are correct except:

   a. Place the used syringe in a sharps container.
   b. Insert half the length of the needle at a 45 degree angle.
   c. Place injection in the abdomen area at least 2" from the navel.
   d. Wash hands thoroughly.
   e. The patient should clean the injection site with alcohol.

6. Alice should be careful not to take other products that can increase the bleeding risk while taking warfarin. Which of the following would not increase her risk of bleeding?

   a. Calcium with Vitamin D
   b. Large amounts of garlic
   c. Dong quai
   d. Fish oils
   e. Ginkgo biloba

Questions 7-10 do not relate to the case.

7. Which of the following medications can significantly interact with warfarin?

   a. Amiodarone
   b. Morphine
   c. Rifampin
   d. A and C
   e. All of the above

8. A patient comes to the hospital with a DVT. He has developed HIT with thrombosis in the past. Which of the following agents is considered first line for treatment in this patient?

   a. Arixtra
   b. Argatroban
   c. Innohep
   d. Dalteparin
   e. None of the above.

9. Which of the following is not a side effect of heparin therapy?

   a. Xerostomia
   b. Thrombocytopenia
   c. Osteoporosis
   d. Hyperkalemia
   e. Bleeding

10. Which of the following parameters need to be monitored during heparin therapy?

    a. Hematocrit, hemoglobin, platelets, AST, and ALT
    b. Hematocrit, hemoglobin, platelets, and aPTT
    c. Hematocrit, hemogloblin, platelets, and PT
    d. CBC and Chem 7 panel
    e. Chem 7 panel and aPTT

ANSWERS

1-d, 2-b, 3-b, 4-c, 5-b, 6-a, 7-d, 8-b, 9-a, 10-b

CHRONIC ANGINA

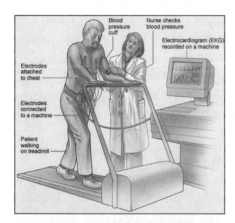

Blood pressure cuff
Nurse checks blood pressure
Electrocardiogram (EKG) recorded on a machine
Electrodes attached to chest
Electrodes connected to a machine
Patient walking on treadmill

GUIDELINES

2007 Chronic Angina Focused Update of the ACC/AHA 2002 Guidelines for the Management of Patients with Chronic Stable Angina. J Am Coll Cardiol 2007;50:2264-74.

ACC/AHA/ACP-ASIM Guidelines for the Management of Patients with Chronic Stable Angina; Executive Summary and Recommendations. Circulation 1999;99:2829-2848.

Background

Angina is chest pain or discomfort that typically occurs with routine physical activity, exertion, or stress. Pain usually begins during or after the activity, comes on slowly and gets worse over the next few minutes before subsiding. The pain generally lasts 5-15 minutes and goes away with nitroglycerin or rest, but may recur with additional activity or stress. This angina is caused by the heart muscle needing more oxygen to meet the demands of the body. The most common cause of angina is coronary heart disease (CHD). Symptoms of angina occur when the coronary arteries are narrowed by plaque lining the arteries (atherosclerosis) or by a blood clot. This type of angina is known as stable angina and is associated with predictable chest pain. Although it is less serious than acute coronary syndrome, it can be very painful and uncomfortable.

Angina can also be present in patients with normal coronary arteries, where symptoms are the result of vasospasm in the arteries. This type of angina is known as Prinzmetal's (variant or atypical) angina.

Angina attacks can also be triggered by exercise, extreme cold or heat, large meals, cigarette smoking, air pollution, or heavy meals – all of which can place extra demands on the heart.

Some patients (women in particular) do not develop the classic symptoms of angina and may not recognize they have cardiac risk and need medical attention.

Different Types of Angina

STABLE ANGINA
- Decreased myocardial O_2 supply due to reduced blood flow, mainly due to atherosclerotic plaque

- Symptoms have been occurring for weeks but without worsening

PRINZMETAL'S ANGINA
- Decreased myocardial O_2 supply due to vasospasm

SILENT ISCHEMIA
- Transient ischemic attacks without symptoms of angina

- Silent ischemia often detected during activity (such as with exercise testing)

- ST elevation or depression during activity

UNSTABLE ANGINA
- Severe, crushing chest pain due to ischemia; acute medical care is needed

Non-Pharmacologic Treatment for Chronic Stable Angina

Patients should be encouraged to follow a heart healthy lifestyle. Encourage patients to stop smoking, maintain a BMI < 25 kg/m², and maintain a waist circumference < 35 inches in females and < 40 inches in males. It is important for patients to engage in physical activity of 30-60 minutes, 7 days/week (minimum 5 days). Medically supervised programs, like cardiac rehabilitation, are recommended for at-risk patients (recent ACS or HF patients).

Pharmacologic Treatment for Chronic Stable Angina

The treatment goals for chronic angina are to reduce the risk of an acute coronary syndrome (unstable angina/myocardial infarction) and provide symptomatic relief from the angina pain. Therefore, an antiplatelet agent and an antianginal regimen are used together. The antiplatelet agent recommended in the guidelines is aspirin. Clopidogrel *(Plavix)* is considered in patients with a contraindication to aspirin. The antianginal agents are beta blockers, calcium channel blockers, nitrates, and sometimes ranolazine *(Ranexa)*. In addition to these agents, patients should be considered for other therapies when they may derive benefit, such as ACEIs in patients at risk for HF, annual influenza vaccine given their chronic disease. Patients should also be aggressively managed if they have concurrent hypertension, hyperlipidemia, and diabetes. Here is an acronym to remember the non-pharmacologic and pharmacologic therapies in chronic angina:

DIAGNOSTIC PROCEDURES
History and physical
Labs
CBC, CK-MB, troponin (T or I), aPTT, PT/INR, lipid panel, glucose
ECG (at rest and during chest pain)
Exercise tolerance test
Stress imaging
Cardiac catheterization/angiography

A - Aspirin, antianginal drugs, and ACE-I

B - Blood pressure and beta-blockers

C - Cholesterol and cigarettes

D - Diet and diabetes

E - Exercise and education

Antiplatelet Agents

Aspirin (ASA) binds irreversibly to cyclooxygenase-1 and 2 (COX-1 and 2) enzymes which results in decreased prostaglandin (PG) precursors; irreversibly inhibits thromboxane A_2 (TxA$_2$), a platelet-aggregating substance. ASA has anti-platelet, antipyretic, analgesic and anti-inflammatory properties. Clopidogrel inhibits P2Y$_{12}$ ADP-mediated platelet activation and aggregation.

DRUG	DOSING	SIDE EFFECTS/CONTRAINDICATIONS/MONITORING
Aspirin *(Bayer, Ascriptin, Bufferin)* Caution: EC products must be chewed if patient is having ACS	75-162 mg daily	**SIDE EFFECTS** Dyspepsia, heartburn, GI upset, GI bleed/ulceration, bleeding, renal impairment, hypersensitivity – see pain chapter for further information. **CONTRAINDICATIONS** Allergy or hypersensitivity; active bleeding **MONITORING** Signs and symptoms of bleeding Shown to decrease incidence of MI, CV events, and death; to be used in all acute and chronic CAD patients
Clopidogrel *(Plavix)*	75 mg daily	**Black Box Warning** Diminished Effectiveness in poor metabolizers Effectiveness depends on the activation to an active metabolite mainly by 2C19. Poor metabolizers exhibit higher cardiovascular events than patients with normal 2C19 function. Tests to check CYP 2C19 genotype can be used as an aid in determining a therapeutic strategy. Consider alternative treatment strategies in patients identified as 2C19 poor metabolizers. The CYP2C19*1 allele corresponds to fully functional metabolism while the CYP2C19*2 and *3 alleles are nonfunctional. **CONTRAINDICATIONS** Active pathological bleed (e.g. PUD, ICH) **SIDE EFFECTS** Bleeding, bruising, rash, TTP (rare) Thrombotic thrombocytopenic purpura (TTP) – rare but serious - have patients report fever, weakness, extreme skin paleness, purple skin patches, yellowing of the skin or eyes, or neurological changes. **MONITORING** Signs of bleeding. Hgb/Hct as necessary Do not start in patients likely to undergo CABG surgery and discontinue 5 days prior to any major surgery. Used in patients with a contraindication to aspirin

ASPIRIN DRUG INTERACTIONS

- Caution with the use of concurrent medications that ↑ bleeding risk (antiplatelets, anticoagulants, dipyridamole *(Persantine)*, herbals (ginkgo biloba), other NSAIDS, etc. See drug interactions chapter for drugs that can increase bleeding risk.

- NSAIDs (like ASA) can increase the level of lithium (avoid concurrent use) and methotrexate.

- Caution with use of aspirin and other ototoxic agents (vancomycin, loop diuretics).

CLOPIDOGREL DRUG INTERACTIONS

- Avoid use, if possible, with other agents that ↑ bleeding risk, including other antiplatelets (although clopidogrel is used with low-dose aspirin), NSAIDs, anticoagulants, SSRIs, ginkgo and others. See drug interactions chapter for drugs that can increase bleeding risk.

- Clopidogrel is a prodrug metabolized mainly by CYP2C19. Avoid concomitant use with strong or moderate 2C19 inhibitors (cimetidine, fluconazole, ketoconazole, voriconazole, fluoxetine, fluvoxamine and others). Omeprazole, a moderate 2C19 Inhibitor, has been shown to reduce the pharmacological activity of clopidogrel if given concomitantly or if given 12 hours apart. Consider using another PPI with less 2C19 inhibitory activity.

Anti-Anginal Therapy

DRUG	MECHANISM	CLINICAL NOTES
Beta-Blockers Used 1st line See hypertension chapter for a complete review of these agents	Inhibit catecholamine effects, ↓ HR (negative chronotropic effect); negative inotropic effect which ↓ contractility; ↓ BP	Start low, go slow; titrate to resting HR of 50-60 BPM; avoid abrupt withdrawal. Do not use a beta-blocker with intrinsic sympathomimetic activity (ISA) More effective than nitrates and CCBs in silent ischemia; avoid use in Prinzmetal's angina; effective as monotherapy or in combo with nitrates and/or CCBs
Calcium Channel Blockers Preferred agent for Prinzmetal's (variant) angina See hypertension chapter for a complete review of these agents	Produces vasodilation, ↓ SVR and BP; non-dihydropyridines (NDHPs) ↓ contractility and HR	Used when beta-blockers are contraindicated or as add on therapy Slow-release or long-acting DHP and NDHP CCBs are effective; avoid short-acting agents. NDHP's may be more effective

Anti-Anginal Therapy Continued

DRUG	MECHANISM	CLINICAL NOTES
Nitrates	Reduces cardiac oxygen demand by ↓ left ventricular pressure and preload; causes vasodilation of veins and arteries (minor effect)	**SL tablets or spray** Call 911 if chest pain doesn't go away after the first dose of SL or spray **For long-acting nitrates** Requires a nitrate-free interval with the dosing. See dosing below. Nitrates used for immediate relief of angina (SL or spray). These agents are not used alone for chronic therapy but can be used in combo with beta-blockers and CCBs as add on therapy
Ranolazine (Ranexa)	Selectively inhibits the late Na^+ current; ↓ intracellular Na^+ and Ca^{2+}; may ↓ myocardial O_2 demand 500 mg BID (max 1,000 mg BID)	**SIDE EFFECTS** Dizziness, constipation, QT prolongation, headache, nausea **CONTRAINDICATIONS** Liver cirrhosis, concurrent use of strong 3A4 inhibitors and inducers **MONITORING** ECG, BP, K^+ Has little to no clinical effects on HR or BP More effective in males than females

NITRATE DRUG INTERACTIONS

Avoid concurrent use with PDE-5 I's; use caution with other antihypertensive medications and alcohol as these can potentiate the hypotensive effect and cause a significant drop in blood pressure.

RANOLAZINE DRUG INTERACTIONS

Ranolazine is a major 3A4 substrate and minor 3A4 inhibitor. Do not use with strong 3A4 inhibitors (e.g. itraconazole, ketoconazole, clarithromycin, nefazodone, nelfinavir, ritonavir, indinavir, saquinavir). Limit the dose to 500 mg BID in patients taking moderate CYP3A4 inhibitors (diltiazem, verapamil, aprepitant, erythromycin, fluconazole, and grapefruit juice). Do not use with CYP3A4 inducers.

NITROGLYCERIN FORMULATIONS	SIDE EFFECTS/CONTRAINDICATIONS/MONITORING
Nitroglycerin SL tabs *(Nitrostat)* 0.3, 0.4, 0.6 mg	**SIDE EFFECTS** Headache, flushing, hypotension, tachycardia, dizziness **CONTRAINDICATIONS** Hypersensitivity to organic nitrates, concurrent use with PDE-5 inhibitors; increased intracranial pressure; severe anemia **MONITORING** BP (continuously if receiving IV), HR, chest pain
Nitroglycerin sublingual spray 0.4 mg/spray *(Nitromist, Nitrolingual Pump Spray)*	Counsel patients to dose so they have a 10-12 hour nitrate free period to ↓ tolerance (some products require longer than 12 hours of a nitrate free interval).
Nitroglycerin ointment 2% (*Nitro-Bid*)	**Nitroglycerin patch** On for 12-14 hours, off for 10-12 hours **Nitroglycerin ointment 2%** Dosed BID, 6 hours apart with 10-12 dose-free interval
Nitroglycerin transdermal patches *(Nitro-Dur, Minitran)*	**Isosorbide mononitrate** Dosed daily or BID. Immediate release (IR) is BID at least 7 hours apart (for example 9AM and 4PM). Extended release is the same (if divided) or daily in the morning.
Nitroglycerin extended release caps (*Nitro-Time*, generics)	**Isosorbide dinitrate** IR is dosed BID-TID. If TID, give at 7AM, 12PM and 5PM for a 14 hour dose-free interval (or similar). SR/ER is daily in the morning or divided BID for an 18 hour dose-free interval.
Nitroglycerin IV	
Isosorbide mononitrate tabs/caps *(Ismo, Monoket)*	
Isosorbide mononitrate ER tabs/caps (*Imdur*, generics)	
Isosorbide dinitrate *(Isordil IR and SL)* – preferred for HF	
Isosorbide dinitrate SR tabs/caps *(Dilatrate-SR)* – preferred for HF	

PATIENT COUNSELING

Sublingual or Spray Nitroglycerin

- <u>Contact EMS immediately if pain persists after one dose of sublingual NTG.</u> You can continue to take additional doses (up to three) at five minute intervals while waiting for the ambulance to arrive. Explain to patients that many of the patient inserts provided with sublingual NTG products may not reflect these updated recommendations.

- <u>Nitroglycerin tablets should be kept in the original amber glass bottle, which is kept tightly capped.</u>

- Patients should be reminded that the reformulated NTG tablets have extended potency and stability. Previous recommendations to replace sublingual tablets every six months are no longer valid. <u>If NTG products are stored at room temperature and properly handled; the tablets should be stable until the manufacturer provided expiration date.</u>

- If the tablets start to get powdery, instruct patients to get a new bottle.

- You may feel a slight burning or stinging in your mouth when you use this medication. However, this sensation is not a sign of how well the medication is working. Do not use more medication just because you do not feel a burning or stinging sensation. Newer formulations of these products are less likely to have this side effect.

- Patients should take the medicine while sitting down to avoid dizziness, lightheadedness or fainting which may be associated with use. Patients should not eat, drink, or smoke for at least five to ten minutes after use of the product or while experiencing chest pain.

- <u>For the Nitrolingual Pumpspray:</u> Instruct patients to spray 5 times into the air to prime the pump the first time they use it and prime once if they have not used the medicine for 6 weeks or more. Do not shake. Press the button firmly with the forefinger to release the spray on or under the tongue. Close your mouth after each spray. Do not inhale the spray and try not to swallow too quickly afterwards. Do not shake the spray before or during use. You can use 1 spray every 5 minutes but no more than 3 sprays in 15 minutes.

- <u>Nitostat</u> tablets come in 0.3, 0.4, and 0.6 mg. Instruct patients to place 1 tablet under the tongue and allow it to dissolve completely. Do not chew or swallow the tablet.

- If a patient has recently used a phosphodiesterase-5 inhibitor like sildenafil *(Viagra, Revatio)*, tadalafil *(Cialis, Adcirca)*, or vardenafil *(Levitra, Staxyn)*, he/she should avoid use of nitroglycerin and inform medical professionals of this use immediately.

Nitroglycerin Patches

- Remove the patch from its pouch and peel off the protective clear liner as directed. Usually, you will wear the patch on the upper arm or chest. Keep the patch above the elbows when wearing on the arm. If placing on the legs, keep patch above the knees.

- Apply the patch to a clean, dry, and hairless area. Hair in the area may be clipped, but not shaved. Avoid areas with cuts or irritation. Do not apply the patch immediately after bathing or showering. Wait until your skin is completely dry. However, you may bathe, shower, and swim while wearing the patch.

- Press the patch firmly in place with the palm of your hand. Wash your hands after applying the patch.

- You will usually use 1 patch a day and wear it for 12 to 14 hours or as directed. The dosage is based on your medical condition and response to treatment.

- For the medicine to work well, there must be a 10-12 hour "patch free" interval between patches (where the patch is left off).

- To reduce skin irritation, apply each new patch to a different area of skin. After removing the old patch, fold it in half with the sticky sides together, and discard out of reach of children and pets.

Isosorbide Mononitrate

Take this medication by mouth, usually twice daily or as directed by your doctor. Take the first dose of the day when you wake up, then take the second dose 7 hours later. It is important to take the drug at the same times each day. Do not change the dosing times unless directed by your doctor.

- Side effects may include headache (can be severe), dizziness, lightheadedness, redness, mild warmth, or nausea. The redness and mild warmth is called flushing and this will go away when your body adjusts to the medicine. Headache is often a sign that this medication is working. Your doctor may recommend treating headaches with an over-the-counter pain reliever (such as acetaminophen). The headache also should become less bothersome as your body gets used to the medicine. If the headaches continue or become severe, tell your doctor promptly.

- This drug may make you dizzy. Do not drive, use machinery, or do any activity that requires alertness until you are sure you can perform such activities safely. Limit alcoholic beverages.

- To reduce the risk of dizziness and lightheadedness, get up slowly when rising from a sitting or lying position. Hold onto the side of the bed or chair to avoid falling.

- This drug should not be used with the following medications: sildenafil *(Viagra, Revatio)*, tadalafil *(Cialis, Adcirca)*, or vardenafil *(Levitra, Staxyn)*. A dangerous drop in blood pressure could occur.

Ranolazine

- Ranolazine is used with other medications to treat a certain type of chest pain (chronic stable angina). It decreases the number of times you may get chest pain. Relieving symptoms of angina can increase your ability to exercise and perform more strenuous work.

- Ranolazine works differently than other drugs for angina, so it can be used with your other angina medications (e.g., nitrates, calcium channel blockers such as amlodipine, beta blockers such as metoprolol). It is thought to work by improving how well the heart uses oxygen so that it can do more work with less oxygen.

- Take this medication by mouth, usually twice daily with or without food or as directed by your doctor. Swallow the tablet whole. Do not crush or chew the tablets. Doing so will destroy the slow release mechanism of the drug, which may decrease its effectiveness and increase your risk of side effects.

- Use this medication regularly in order to get the most benefit from it. To help you remember, take it at the same times each day. This medication must be taken regularly to be effective. It should not be used to treat angina when it occurs. Use other medications (e.g., sublingual nitroglycerin) to relieve an angina attack as directed by your doctor.

- Inform your doctor if your condition does not improve or if it worsens (e.g., your chest pain happens more often).

- Dizziness, headache, lightheadedness, nausea, tiredness, and constipation may occur. If any of these effects persist or worsen, notify your doctor or pharmacist promptly.

- Avoid eating grapefruit or drinking grapefruit juice while being treated with this medication. Grapefruit can increase the amount of certain medications in your blood.

- Ranolazine may cause a condition that affects the heart rhythm (QT prolongation). This heart rhythm can infrequently result in serious (rarely fatal) fast/irregular heartbeat and other symptoms (such as severe dizziness, fainting) that require immediate medical attention. The risk may be increased if you are taking other drugs that may affect the heart rhythm. Check with your doctor or pharmacist before using any herbal, over the counter or other medication.

- Low levels of potassium or magnesium in the blood may also increase your risk of QT prolongation. This risk may increase if you use certain drugs (such as diuretics/"water pills") or if you have conditions such as severe sweating, diarrhea, or vomiting.

ACUTE CORONARY SYNDROMES

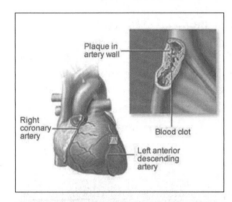

Plaque in artery wall

Right coronary artery

Blood clot

Left anterior descending artery

GUIDELINES

2011 ACCF/AHA Focused Update of the Guidelines for the Management of Patients with Unstable Angina/Non ST-Elevation Myocardial Infarction (Updating the 2007 Guideline). J Am Coll Cardiol 2011;57(19):1920-1959.

2009 Focused Updates: ACC/AHA Guidelines for the Management of Patients with ST-Elevation Myocardial Infarction (Updating the 2004 Guideline and 2007 Focused Update). J Am Coll Cardiol 2009;54:2205-41.

Background

Acute Coronary Syndrome (ACS) refers to a set of clinical disorders that result from an imbalance between myocardial oxygen demand and supply. This imbalance primarily results from diminished myocardial blood flow due to occlusive or partially occlusive clots in the artery (atherosclerotic plaque). This reduction in blood flow, or ischemia, compromises the proper functioning of the cardiac cells and can lead to myocardial cell death (infarction). When infarction occurs, a detectable amount of biochemical markers are released into the bloodstream, mainly troponins I or T and creatine kinase (CK) myocardial band (MB).

Acute coronary syndrome encompasses the clinical conditions of unstable angina, non-ST segment elevation myocardial infarction, and ST segment elevation myocardial infarction. With non-ST segment elevation myocardial infarction (NSTEMI), there can be ST-segment depression, T-wave inversion, or no changes at all seen on the electrocardiogram (ECG).

Coronary heart disease is the leading cause of death in men and women in the United States.

CLASSIC SIGNS AND SYMPTOMS OF ACS

- Severe chest pain (substernal, crushing) that may radiate to the left shoulder, arm, jaw, back or neck, diaphoresis, N/V, numbness/tingling sensation, shortness of breath, or dyspnea

- Precipitating factors include: exercise, cold weather, extreme emotions, stress, and sexual intercourse

- Pain is usually not relieved by NTG (SL or spray) or rest

DIAGNOSIS

- UA: chest pain; cardiac enzymes are negative; no ECG changes (or transient)

- NSTEMI: chest pain + positive cardiac enzymes (troponins, CK-MB)

- STEMI: chest pain + positive cardiac enzymes + ST segment changes on ECG (1 mm of ST segment elevation in 2 or more contiguous ECG leads)

RISK FACTORS
Age (men > 45 years of age, women > 55 years of age or had early hysterectomy)
Family history of coronary event before age 55 years of age (men) or 65 years of age (women)
Smoking
Hypertension
Hyperlipidemia
Diabetes
Chronic angina
Known coronary artery disease

Treatment for Unstable Angina/Non-ST segment Elevation Myocardial Infarction (UA/NSTEMI)

Treatment is MONA + GAP-BA (see chart below)

SUMMARY OF DRUGS USED DURING HOSPITAL STAY FOR ACS

DRUG	MOA	CLINICAL COMMENTS
MONA (acronym)		
<u>M</u>orphine	Produces arteriolar and venous dilation; prompts a ↓ in myocardial O_2 demand; pain relief	Morphine sulfate IV can be used in patients with ongoing chest discomfort despite NTG therapy. Generally dosed 2-5 mg IV PRN. Side effects: hypotension, bradycardia, N/V, sedation, and respiratory depression. Antidote: naloxone *(Narcan)*. More clinical pearls in pain chapter.
<u>O</u>xygen		Oxygen if cyanosis or respiratory distress; finger pulse oximetry or ABG to confirm sufficient $SaO_2 > 90\%$

Summary of Drugs Used During Hospital Stay for ACS Continued

DRUG	MOA	CLINICAL COMMENTS
Nitrates	Dilates coronary arteries and improves collateral blood flow; ↓ cardiac oxygen demand by ↓ preload	NTG (SL or spray) followed by IV for immediate relief of ischemia and associated chest pain. If at home and feel chest pain after 1 dose of NTG, call 911. Do not use if patient's SBP < 90 mmHg or HR < 50 BPM. NTG or other nitrates should not be administered to patients receiving PDE-5 Is for ED within 24 hrs of sildenafil or 48 hrs of tadalafil use. The suitable time for the administration of nitrates after vardenafil has not been established. More information on nitrates in chronic angina chapter.
ASA	Inhibits platelet aggregation by inhibiting TxA_2	ASA immediately and continued indefinitely (162-325 mg initially followed by 75-162 mg daily). Take 162-325 mg of non-enteric coated and chew the ASA for the initial dose. If intolerant to ASA, take clopidogrel loading dose and then 75 mg daily indefinitely.

GAP-BA (acronym)

DRUG	MOA	CLINICAL COMMENTS
GP IIb/IIIa receptor antagonists	Blocks fibrinogen binding to the GPIIb/IIIa receptors on platelets, preventing PLT aggregation	Can be used in medical management or for those going for an intervention (PCI +/- stent). Agents include abciximab, eptifibatide, or tirofiban.
Anti-coagulants	Clotting factor inhibitors (see anticoagulant chapter for more specifics)	Used to prevent further clotting. Agents include heparin, LMWH (enoxaparin, dalteparin), fondaparinux, bivalirudin. More information in anticoagulant chapter.
P2Y12 inhibitors	Inhibitor of the P2Y12 receptor on platelets	Clopidogrel or prasugrel (or ticagrelor) for all patients (loading dose followed by a maintenance dose) unless patient is going for CABG surgery.
Beta-Blockers	Blocks beta receptors on the heart; cardioprotective	Oral beta-blocker therapy should be initiated within the first 24 hours for patients who do not have 1 or more of the following: 1) signs of HF, 2) evidence of a low-output state 3) increased risk for cardiogenic shock, 4) other relative contraindications to beta blockade (e.g. PR interval > 0.24 sec, 2nd or 3rd degree heart block, etc.). See hypertension lecture for more information.
ACE-Inhibitors	Inhibits Angiotensin Converting Enzyme and blocks the production of Angiotensin II; prevents cardiac remodeling; ↓ preload and afterload	Oral ACE-Is should be administered within first 24 hours to patients with pulmonary congestion or LV ejection fraction ≤ 0.40, in the absence of hypotension or other contraindications. If patient has a contraindication, use an ARB. Do not use IV ACE-I within first 24 hours due to risk of hypotension. See hypertension lecture for more information.

Medications to avoid

- Discontinue all NSAIDs (including COX-2 inhibitors) due to their ↑ risk of mortality, reinfarction, hypertension, and heart failure in these patients.

- Immediate release form of DHP calcium channel blocker (e.g. nifedipine) should not be used in absence of a beta-blocker.

- IV fibrinolytic therapy is not indicated in patients without acute ST-segment elevation or left bundle branch block.

GP IIB/IIIA RECEPTOR ANTAGONISTS

Block the platelet glycoprotein IIb/IIIa receptor, the binding site for fibrinogen, von Wille-brand factor, and other ligands. These agents reversibly block platelet aggregation, preventing thrombosis.

DRUG	DOSING	SIDE EFFECTS/CONTRAINDICATIONS/MONITORING
Abciximab *(ReoPro)*	LD: 0.25 mg/kg IV bolus MD: 0.125 mcg/kg/min (max 10 mcg/min) IV infusion	**CONTRAINDICATIONS** Thrombocytopenia (platelets < 100,000/mm^3) History of bleeding diathesis (predisposition) Active internal bleeding Recent (within 6 weeks) of major surgery ↑ prothrombin time History of CVA within 2 years (abciximab); History of stroke with 30 days or any history of hemorrhagic stroke (eptifibatide/tirofiban) Severe uncontrolled HTN Hypersensitivity to murine proteins (abciximab) Renal dysfunction (for eptifibatide and tirofiban)
Eptifibatide *(Integrilin)*	LD:180 mcg/kg IV bolus (max 22.6 mg) followed 10 min later by second IV bolus of 180 mcg/kg MD: 2 mcg/kg/min (max 15 mg/hour) IV infusion started after the first bolus Reduce infusion rate by 50% in patients with CrCl < 50 mL/min	**SIDE EFFECTS** Bleeding, thrombocytopenia (esp. abciximab), hypotension **MONITORING** Hgb, Hct, platelets, signs and symptoms of bleeding Administration Notes: Do not shake vials upon reconstitution Must filter abciximab with administration Platelet function returns in 24-48 hrs after discontinuing abciximab and 4-8 hrs after stopping eptifibatide and tirofiban
Tirofiban *(Aggrastat)*	LD: 25 mcg/kg IV bolus MD: 0.15 mcg/kg/min IV infusion Reduce infusion rate by 50% in patients with CrCl < 30 mL/min	

P2Y$_{12}$ INHIBITORS

Inhibitors of platelet activation and aggregation through the binding to the P2Y$_{12}$ class on the ADP receptors on platelets. Clopidogrel and prasugrel are prodrugs and have irreversible binding to the receptor. Ticagrelor is not a prodrug (therefore faster onset) and has reversible binding to the receptor (therefore faster offset).

DRUG	DOSING	CONTRAINDICATIONS/SIDE EFFECTS/MONITORING
Clopidogrel *(Plavix)*	LD: 300-600 mg MD: 75 mg PO daily Alternative dosing per guidelines: Give LD of 600 mg, followed by 150 mg daily for 6 days, then 75 mg daily (if not high risk for bleeding)	**BLACK BOX WARNING → DIMINISHED EFFECTIVENESS IN POOR METABOLIZERS** Effectiveness depends on the activation to an active metabolite mainly by 2C19. Poor metabolizers exhibit higher cardiovascular events than patients with normal 2C19 function. Tests to check CYP 2C19 genotype can be used as an aid in determining a therapeutic strategy. Consider alternative treatment strategies in patients identified as 2C19 poor metabolizers. The CYP2C19*1 allele corresponds to fully functional metabolism while the CYP2C19*2 and *3 alleles are nonfunctional. **CONTRAINDICATIONS** Active pathological bleed (e.g. PUD, ICH) **SIDE EFFECTS** Bleeding, bruising, rash, TTP (rare) Thrombotic thrombocytopenic purpura (TTP) – rare but serious - have patients report fever, weakness, extreme skin paleness, purple skin patches, yellowing of the skin or eyes, or neurological changes. **MONITORING** Signs of bleeding. Hgb/Hct as necessary Do not start in patients likely to undergo CABG surgery and discontinue 5 days prior to any major surgery.
Prasugrel *(Effient)* Indicated for the reduction of thrombotic events in patients with ACS who are to be managed with PCI	LD: 60 mg MD: 10 mg PO daily [5 mg daily if patient < 60 kg]	**BLACK BOX WARNING → BLEEDING RISK** Can cause significant, sometimes fatal, bleeding **CONTRAINDICATIONS** Active pathological bleed, patients with a history of TIA or stroke **SIDE EFFECTS** Bleeding (more than clopidogrel), TTP (rare) In patients ≥ 75 years, prasugrel is generally not recommended due to ↑ risk of fatal and intracranial bleeding and uncertain benefit, except in high risk patients (DM and prior MI). Do not start in patients likely to undergo CABG surgery and discontinue 7 days prior to any major surgery. Once PCI is planned, give the dose promptly and no later than 1 hour after the PCI
Ticagrelor *(Brilinta)* Indicated for reduction of thrombotic events in patients with ACS	LD: 180 mg MD: 90 mg PO BID (use with a daily ASA dose of 75-100 mg)	**BLACK BOX WARNING → BLEEDING RISK** Can cause significant, sometimes fatal, bleeding **CONTRAINDICATIONS** Active pathological bleed , history of ICH, severe hepatic impairment **SIDE EFFECTS** Bleeding, dyspnea Do not start in patients likely to undergo CABG surgery and discontinue 5 days prior to any major surgery. Maintenance doses of ASA above 100 mg reduce the effectiveness of ticagrelor and should be avoided. After any initial dose, use with ASA 75-100 mg daily.

DRUG INTERACTIONS

- Avoid use, if possible, with other agents that ↑ bleeding risk, including other antiplatelets (although clopidogrel is used with low-dose aspirin), NSAIDs, anticoagulants, SSRIs, ginkgo and others. See drug interactions chapter for drugs that can increase bleeding risk.

- Clopidogrel is a prodrug metabolized mainly by CYP2C19. Avoid concomitant use with strong or moderate 2C19 inhibitors (cimetidine, fluconazole, ketoconazole, voriconazole, fluoxetine, fluvoxamine and others). Omeprazole, a moderate 2C19 inhibitor, has been shown to reduce the pharmacological activity of clopidogrel if given concomitantly or if given 12 hours apart. Consider using another PPI with less 2C19 inhibitory activity.

- Prasugrel can ↑ bleeding risk in patients on chronic NSAIDS, anticoagulants, SSRIs, ginkgo, and other agents that can increase bleeding risk. See drug interactions chapter for drugs that can increase bleeding risk.

- .Ticagrelor - avoid use with strong 3A4 inhibitors and inducers. See drug interactions chapter for more information. Patients receiving > 40 mg/d of simvastatin or lovastatin may be at ↑ risk for statin-related adverse effects (myopathy). Monitor digoxin levels with initiation of or any change in ticagrelor dose.

Treatment for ST Segment Elevation Myocardial Infarction (STEMI)

DIAGNOSIS

- Chest pain > 20 min (even after NTG administration)

- ECG shows ST elevation (> 0.1mV in 2 or more contiguous leads)

- Troponin T or I elevation/CK-MB elevation

TREATMENT

- MONA + GAP-BA + the option of giving thrombolytics

THROMBOLYTICS

These agents cause fibrinolysis by binding to fibrin in a thrombus (clot) and converting entrapped plasminogen to plasmin. Most patients receive PCI without the use of thrombolytics. Thrombolytic use is recommended when a hospital cannot perform PCI within 90 minutes (door-to-balloon time) and should be initiated within 30 minutes from time of arrival to the hospital (door-to-needle time) if hospital is a STEMI receiving center. The STEMI guidelines find thrombolytic use still beneficial when given out to 12 hours from symptom onset for STEMI.

DRUG	SIDE EFFECTS/CONTRAINDICATIONS/MONITORING
Alteplase (t-PA, rt-PA, Activase)	**CONTRAINDICATIONS** Active internal bleeding or bleeding diathesis History of CVA Recent intracranial or intraspinal surgery or trauma Intracranial neoplasm Arteriovenous malformation or aneurysm Aortic dissection Severe uncontrolled hypertension
Reteplase (r-PA) (Retevase)	**Relative Contraindications** Severe uncontrolled HTN (SBP > 185 mmHg or DBP > 110 mmHg) For streptokinase/anistreplase: prior exposure (past year) or prior allergic reaction to these agents; uncommonly used due to allergy risk in ACS, (and streptokinase not used for stroke due to hemorrhage risk) Pregnancy Active peptic ulcer Current use of anticoagulants
Tenecteplase (TNK-tPA) (TNKase)	**SIDE EFFECTS** <u>Bleeding, hypotension, intracranial hemorrhage, fever</u> **MONITORING** Hgb, Hct, signs and symptoms of bleeding Door-to-needle time should be < 30 minutes (for thrombolytics) Door-to-balloon time should be < 90 minutes (for PCI)
Streptokinase (Streptase)	

WHAT MEDICATIONS TO STOP/CONTINUE WHEN PATIENT GOES FOR CABG SURGERY

- Continue ASA

- Discontinue clopidogrel and ticagrelor 5 days before elective CAGB. Discontinue prasugrel 7 days before elective CABG. More urgent surgery, if necessary, may be performed by experienced surgeons if the incremental bleeding risk is considered acceptable.

- Discontinue IV GP IIb/IIIa inhibitor (eptifibatide/tirofiban) 4 hours before CABG

- Continue UFH

  - If on enoxaparin, discontinue enoxaparin 12-24 hrs before CABG and dose with UFH

  - If on fondaparinux, discontinue fondaparinux 24 hrs before CABG and dose with UFH

  - If on bivalirudin, discontinue bivalirudin 3 hrs before CABG and dose with UFH

LONG-TERM MEDICAL MANAGEMENT IN PATIENTS S/P MI (SECONDARY PREVENTION)

- ASA therapy will be used indefinitely unless there is a contraindication or allergy

- For patients who receive a stent and do not have an ASA contraindication (bleeding, allergy, etc.), use <u>ASA 162 mg – 325 mg daily for:</u>

    - 1 month with bare metal stent

    - 3 months with sirolimus-eluting stent

    - 6 months with paclitaxel-eluting stent;

Then ASA therapy at 75-162 mg daily indefinitely (use this dose if no stent was placed)

- $P2Y_{12}$ inhibitor - clopidogrel 75 mg daily or prasugrel 10 mg daily for at least 1 month and ideally up to 1 year if patients are not at high risk of bleeding. Continuation of clopidogrel or prasugrel beyond 15 months may be considered in patients following drug eluting stent placement.

- Nitroglycerin SL or spray PRN

- Beta-blocker therapy daily

- ACE-I therapy daily, particularly if EF < 40%

- Statin therapy daily if LDL is > 100 mg/dL. May want to treat to LDL goal < 70 mg/dL.

- Anticoagulation in patients with persistent AF and patients with LV thrombus (INR 2.0-3.0). In patients requiring warfarin, clopidogrel, and ASA therapy, an INR of 2.0-2.5 is recommended with low dose ASA (75-81 mg) and 75 mg daily of clopidogrel.

- Control other conditions (HTN, DM, smoking cessation)

- Physical activity (30 minutes, 5-7 days/wk)

- Weight management (BMI < 25 kg/m^2); waist circumference: men < 40″ and women < 35″

- For pain relief, use APAP, ASA, tramadol, or short-term narcotic analgesics. Also, non-acetylated salicylates can be used. NSAIDs are not recommended.

Patient Counseling for Clopidogrel

- Take this medication once daily. Clopidogrel can be taken with or without food

- Clopidogrel helps prevent platelets from sticking together and forming a clot that can block an artery.

- It is important to take this medication every day. Do not stop taking clopidogrel without talking to your doctor who prescribed it for you. If you stop taking this medication, you can put yourself at risk of developing a clot which can be life-threatening.

- If you miss a dose, take as soon as you remember. If it is almost time for your next dose, skip the missed dose. Take the next dose at your regular scheduled time. Do not take 2 doses at the same time unless instructed by your doctor.

- You may bleed and bruise more easily, even from a minor scrape. It may take longer for you to stop bleeding.

- Call your doctor at once if you have black or bloody stools, or if you cough up blood or vomit that looks like coffee grounds. These could be signs of bleeding in your digestive tract.

- One rare but serious side effect is thrombotic thrombocytopenic purpura (TTP). Seek prompt medical attention if you experience any of these symptoms that cannot otherwise be explained: fever, weakness, extreme skin paleness, purplish spots or skin patches (called purpura), yellowing of the skin or eyes (jaundice), or mental status changes.

- Avoid drinking alcohol while taking clopidogrel. Alcohol may increase your risk of bleeding in your stomach or intestines.

- If you need to have any type of surgery or dental work, tell the surgeon or dentist ahead of time that you are using clopidogrel. You may need to stop using the medicine for at least 5 days before having surgery, to prevent excessive bleeding.

- While you are taking clopidogrel, do not take aspirin or other NSAIDs (non-steroidal anti-inflammatory drugs) without your doctor's advice.

ANTIARRHYTHMICS

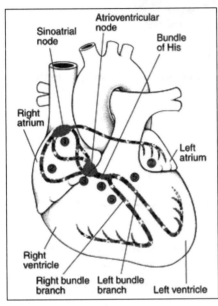

Background

A normal heart beats in a regular, coordinated way because electrical impulses trigger a sequence of organized contractions. Arrhythmias and conduction disorders are caused by abnormalities in the generation or conduction pathway of these electrical impulses, or both. With arrhythmias, the heart rate can be slow or fast. An arrhythmia with a slow heart rate is called a bradyarrhythmia and one with a rapid heart rate is called a tachyarrhythmia. The resting sinus heart rate in adults is normally 60-100 beats/min.

An arrhythmia can be silent and only detected during a physical. Other patients are symptomatic and can experience palpitations, such as feeling like the heart skipped a beat, is fluttering or is beating too fast. They may also feel dizzy, faint, short of breath, chest pain and/or fatigued.

Heart Rhythm

If the heart is beating to the normal rhythm of a healthy heart, the rhythm is referred to as normal sinus rhythm (NSR). The diagram above traces the normal electrical conduction pathway in the heart. The sinoatrial node (1) initiates an electrical impulse that flows through the right and left atria (2), making them contract. When the electrical impulse reaches the atrioventricular node (3), it is delayed slightly. The impulse then travels down the bundle of His (4), which divides into the right bundle branch for the right ventricle (5) and the left bundle branch for the left ventricle (5). The impulse then spreads through the ventricles via the Purkinje system, making them contract.

In an arrhythmia, the heart rhythm is disrupted. The most common cause of an arrhythmia is coronary heart disease, and other conditions that damage cardiac tissue, including heart valve disorders, heart failure and/or damage from a heart attack. Electrolyte imbalances (po-

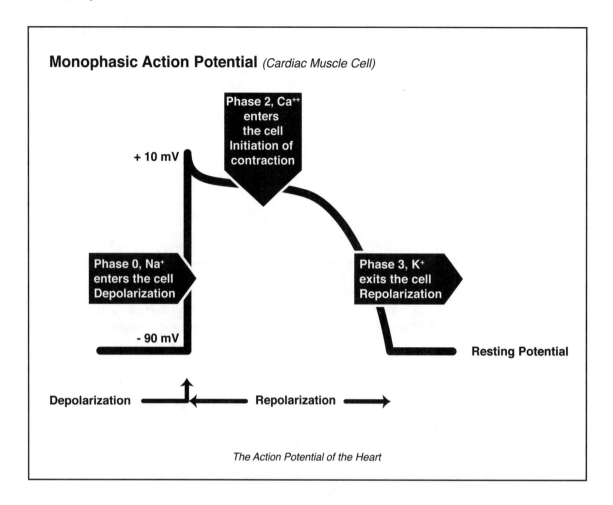

Monophasic Action Potential *(Cardiac Muscle Cell)*

Phase 2, Ca++ enters the cell Initiation of contraction

+ 10 mV

Phase 0, Na+ enters the cell Depolarization

Phase 3, K+ exits the cell Repolarization

- 90 mV

Resting Potential

Depolarization ——— Repolarization ———→

The Action Potential of the Heart

tassium, magnesium, sodium and calcium – these are important in conduction) can result in an arrhythmia. Drugs can cause or worsen arrhythmias; this includes the drugs used to treat arrhythmias. Many drugs can lengthen a segment of the conduction pathway, including the QT interval, and cause a particularly dangerous arrhythmia called torsade de pointes, a type of ventricular tachyarrhythmia.

ARRHYTHMIA TYPES

- Atrial fibrillation (A. Fib) is a very common irregular heart rhythm that causes the atria to contract abnormally. A. Fib carries a high risk of clot formation. Chronic A. Fib requires anticoagulation therapy; see anticoagulation chapter.

- Atrial flutter is caused by one or more rapid circuits in the atrium. Atrial flutter is usually more organized and regular than atrial fibrillation. This arrhythmia occurs most often with heart disease, and in the first week after heart surgery. A. Flutter often converts to atrial fibrillation.

- Premature atrial contractions are early, extra beats that originate in the atria. They are harmless and do not require treatment.

- Premature ventricular contractions (PVCs) are among the most common arrhythmias and occur in people with and without heart disease. This is a "skipped heartbeat" everyone will occasionally experience. In some people, it can be related to stress, too much caffeine or nicotine, or too much exercise. PVCs can also be caused by heart disease, or an electrolyte imbalance, or drugs.

- Paroxysmal supraventricular tachycardia (PSVT) is a rapid heart rate, usually with a regular rhythm, originating from above the ventricles.

QT PROLONGATION & TORSADE DE POINTES

A prolonged QT interval is a marker for ventricular tachyarrhythmias, including torsades de pointes, a particularly lethal arrhythmia which is often caused by drugs and can result in sudden death.

The QT interval is measured from the beginning of the QRS complex to the end of the T wave. It reflects ventricular depolarization and repolarization. A prolonged QT interval is a risk factor for ventricular tachyarrhythmias (e.g. torsades de pointes) and sudden cardiac death.

Use the following QT-prolonging drugs with caution in patients with any arrhythmia risk (including those with existing arrhythmias, or if you see them on an antiarrhythmic). QT prolongation risk depends on the dose and duration. If a patient is using low dose amitriptyline for neuropathic pain, this should not be considered a particularly risky agent due to the low dose, although the risk may be additive with other agents.

ADDITIVE QT PROLONGATION

- Any pre-existing cardiac condition (or history of arrhythmia)

- Class Ia and Class III antiarrhythmics (amiodarone, disopyramide, dronedarone, procainamide, quinidine, sotalol, and others)

- Antibiotics including quinolones (ciprofloxacin, levofloxacin, moxifloxacin, norfloxacin, gemifloxacin, and sparfloxacin), macrolides (azithromycin, erythromycin, clarithromycin and telithromycin), amantadine, foscarnet and others

- Azole antifungals (fluconazole, itraconazole, ketoconazole, posiconazole and voriconazole)

- Anticancer agents (arsenic, dasatinib, lapatinib, nilotinib, sunitinib, tamoxifen)

- Protease inhibitors (saquinavir/ritonavir, atazanavir, lopinavir/ritonavir)

- Antidepressants including tricyclics (amitriptyline, nortriptyline, doxepin, desipramine, and others), SSRIs (citalopram, escitalopram, fluoxetine, paroxetine, sertraline) and SNRIs (venlafaxine and desvenlafaxine) and trazodone

- Antiemetic agents including the 5-HT3 blockers (dolasetron, ondansetron, granisetron, palonosetron) and droperidol

- Antipsychotics (chlorpromazine, thioridazine, pimozide, haloperidol, ziprasidone, risperidone, paliperidone, iloperidone, asenapine and lurasidone)

- Other agents: alfuzosin, apomorphine, chloroquine, galantamine, methadone and pentamidine

PHARMACOLOGICAL TREATMENT

Medications can be used to convert the patient from the arrhythmia to normal sinus rhythm (NSR), or used to maintain NSR, or to reduce the heart rate. Recent trials have shown that ventricular rate control is as effective as rhythm control with cardio-version and antiarrhythmic drugs. Therefore, rate control is often used first-line. The drugs used for rate control in atrial fibrillation, or A. Fib are beta-blockers, non-dihydropyridine calcium channel blockers (diltiazem and verapamil) and digoxin, all of which reduce heart rate.

Antiarrhythmics work by affecting the electrical conduction in the heart – and occasionally, can worsen the existing arrhythmia or cause other arrhythmias. All patients should be instructed to be seen if they suspect they have "worse heartbeat problems" or have an increase in their symptoms.

Prior to starting any medication for a non-life-threatening arrhythmia, be sure to always check the patient's electrolytes and run a toxicology screen.

VAUGHAN-WILLIAMS CLASSIFICATION OF ANTIARRHYTHMICS

The Vaughan Williams classification system is the most commonly used classification system for antiarrhythmic drugs. Here the drugs are split into categories based on their dominant electro-physiologic effect. It has the virtue of simplicity, although many drugs overlap into more than one category.

CLASS	DRUGS
Ia	Quinidine, Procainamide, Disopyramide → SLE
Ib	Lidocaine, Mexiletine
Ic	Flecainide, Propafenone
II	Beta-blockers (e.g. esmolol, propranolol)
III	Amiodarone, Dofetilide, Dronedarone, Ibutilide, Sotalol
IV	Verapamil, Diltiazem

CLASS IA ANTIARRHYTHMIC AGENTS

Class Ia antiarrhythmic drugs block Na^+ channels; ↓ conduction velocity, ↑ refractory period, ↓ automaticity

DRUG	DOSING	SIDE EFFECTS/CONTRAINDICATIONS/MONITORING
Quinidine	Different salt forms are not interchangeable (gluconate, sulfate) Take with food or milk to ↓ GI upset Avoid changes in Na+ intake. ↓ Na+ intake can ↑ quinidine serum concentrations	**BLACK BOX WARNING** Quinidine may ↑ mortality in treatment of A.Fib/A.flutter **SIDE EFFECTS** Diarrhea (35%), stomach cramping (22%), cinchonism (tinnitus, blurred vision, headache, nausea, hearing loss) QT prolongation, hypotension, hemolytic anemia, thrombocytopenia **CONTRAINDICATIONS** Concurrent use of quinolones that prolong the QT interval, amprenavir, ritonavir; 2nd/3rd degree heart block, thrombocytopenia **MONITORING** ECG (QT interval, QRS duration), electrolytes, BP, CBC, LFTs, renal
Procainamide	Has active metabolite, N-acetyl procainamide (NAPA) which is renally cleared Therapeutic levels: Procainamide: 4-10 mcg/mL NAPA: 15-25 mcg/mL Combined: 10-30 mcg/mL Take on an empty stomach	**BLACK BOX WARNINGS (2)** Can cause potentially fatal blood dyscrasias (e.g., agranulocytosis) → monitor patient closely in the first 3 months of therapy and periodically thereafter. Long-term use leads to positive antibody (ANA) test in 50% of patients which may result in drug-induced lupus erythematosus-like syndrome (in 20-30% of patients) **SIDE EFFECTS** Lupus-like syndrome, QT prolongation, hypotension, agranulocytosis **CONTRAINDICATIONS** 2nd/3rd degree heart block, SLE **MONITORING** ECG (QT interval, QRS duration), electrolytes, BP, renal function, signs of lupus (butterfly rash, stabbing chest pain, joint pain), procainamide and NAPA levels, CBC
Disopyramide (*Norpace*, *Norpace CR*)	Take on an empty stomach	**SIDE EFFECTS** Anticholinergic effects (xerostomia, constipation, urinary retention), hypotension, QT prolongation, CHF exacerbation and others **CONTRAINDICATIONS** 2nd/3rd degree heart block, heart failure **MONITORING** ECG (QT interval, QRS duration), electrolytes, BP, signs of heart failure Due to strong anticholinergic effects, do not use in patients with urinary retention, BPH, glaucoma, or myasthenia gravis.

Drug Interactions

- Quinidine is a substrate of 3A4 (major) and inhibits 2C9 (weak), 2D6 (strong), and 3A4 (strong) and P-glycoprotein. Avoid concurrent use with alfuzosin, azole antifungals, dronedarone, eplerenone, PIs, pimozide, nilotinib, ranolazine, salmeterol, silodosin, tamoxifen, etc. Some major drug interactions with quinidine include digoxin (↓ digoxin dose by 50%), warfarin (↑ INR), grapefruit juice, verapamil, diltiazem, erythromycin and others. See drug interactions chapter.

- Procainamide is a substrate of 2D6 (major). Moderate and strong 2D6 inhibitors will ↑ levels of procainamide (see drug interactions section).

- Disopyramide is a substrate of 3A4 (major). Inhibitors of 3A4 and anticholinergics may ↑ risk of side effects. 3A4 inducers may ↓ effects.

- All agents can have additive QT prolongation with other agents that also prolong the QT interval.

CLASS IB ANTIARRHYTHMIC AGENTS

Class Ib antiarrhythmic drugs block Na^+ channels; little effect on conduction velocity, ↓ refractory period, ↓ automaticity

DRUG	DOSING	SIDE EFFECTS/CONTRAINDICATIONS/MONITORING
Lidocaine *(Xylocaine, others)*	Given IV. Reduce dose in patients with CHF, shock, or hepatic dysfunction Can be given via endotracheal tube (need higher dose)	**SIDE EFFECTS** CNS (hallucinations, disorientation, confusion, seizures), hypotension , dizziness, sedation, and slurred speech **CONTRAINDICATION** 2nd/3rd degree heart block and others **MONITORING** ECG, BP, liver function Caution in patients with severe hepatic dysfunction
Mexiletine *(Mexitil)*	Given orally. Take with food. Reduce dose in hepatic impairment	

Drug Interactions

- Lidocaine is a 3A4 and 2D6 (major) substrate; inhibits 1A2 (strong), 2D6 and 3A4 (moderate). Amiodarone, beta-blockers, 2D6 inhibitors, 3A4 inhibitors (e.g., diltiazem, verapamil, grapefruit juice, erythromycin, clarithromycin, itraconazole, ketoconazole, PIs, etc.) will ↑ lidocaine levels.

- Mexiletine is a 1A2 and 2D6 (major) substrate; inhibits 1A2 (strong).

CLASS IC ANTIARRHYTHMIC AGENTS

Class Ic antiarrhythmic drugs block Na^+ channels; significantly ↓ conduction velocity, little effect on refractory period, ↓ automaticity

DRUG	DOSING	SIDE EFFECTS/CONTRAINDICATIONS/MONITORING
Flecainide *(Tambocor)*	These agents are not commonly used	**BLACK BOX WARNING** Pro-arrhythmic effects **SIDE EFFECTS** Dizziness, visual disturbances, dyspnea, worsening HF **CONTRAINDICATIONS** 2nd/3rd degree heart block, cardiogenic shock, coronary artery disease, concurrent use of amprenavir or ritonavir **MONITORING** ECG, BP, HR, electrolytes
Propafenone *(Rythmol, Rythmol SR)*	These agents are not commonly used	**BLACK BOX WARNING** Pro-arrhythmic effects **SIDE EFFECTS** Taste disturbance, bradycardia, AV block (first degree), dyspnea, dizziness, bronchospasm, worsening HF **CONTRAINDICATIONS** 2nd/3rd degree heart block, sinus bradycardia, cardiogenic shock, decompensated heart failure, hypotension, coronary artery disease, bronchospastic disorders, concurrent use of ritonavir **MONITORING** ECG, BP, HR, electrolytes

Drug Interactions

- Flecainide is a 2D6 (major) substrate; inhibits 2D6 (weak).

- Propafenone is a 2D6 (major) substrate; inhibits 1A2 and 2D6 (weak).

CLASS II ANTIARRHYTHMIC AGENTS

Class II antiarrhythmic drugs block beta receptors and indirectly block calcium channels.

DRUG	DOSING	SIDE EFFECTS/CONTRAINDICATIONS/MONITORING
Esmolol *(Brevibloc)*	Beta-1 selective	**SIDE EFFECTS** Hypotension, diaphoresis, bradycardia **CONTRAINDICATIONS** 2nd/3rd degree heart block, sinus bradycardia, cardiogenic shock, decompensated heart failure, asthma/COPD (with propranolol) **MONITORING** ECG, BP, HR, electrolytes
Propranolol *(Inderal LA, InnoPran XL)*	Beta non-specific; lipophilic	

CLASS III ANTIARRHYTHMIC AGENTS

Class III antiarrhythmic drugs block mainly K$^+$ channels; no change on conduction velocity, significant $\uparrow$ in refractory period, no change in automaticity

DRUG	DOSING	SIDE EFFECTS/CONTRAINDICATIONS/MONITORING
Amiodarone (Cordarone, Pacerone, Nexterone)	A. Fibrillation Loading Dose: 10 grams Maintenance Dose: 100-400 mg daily Infusions longer than 2 hours must be administered in a <u>non-polyvinyl chloride (PVC) container such as polyolefin or glass.</u> t½ = 40-55 days	**BLACK BOX WARNINGS (4)** Patients should be hospitalized when therapy is initiated Lung damage may occur without symptoms Liver toxicity Exacerbation of arrhythmias, making them more difficult to tolerate or reverse **SIDE EFFECTS** Hypotension (IV), bradycardia, hypothyroidism/hyperthyroidism (more hypo), $\uparrow$LFTs, corneal microdeposits, optic neuritis, pulmonary fibrosis, ataxia, dizziness, tremor, photosensitivity, slate blue skin discoloration, insomnia **CONTRAINDICATIONS** Severe sinus-node dysfunction, 2nd/3rd degree heart block, bradycardia causing syncope, cardiogenic shock **MONITORING** Pulmonary (including chest X-ray), thyroid, and liver function tests at baseline and periodically thereafter; ECG, BP, HR, electrolytes, regular ophthalmic exams Pregnancy Category D
Dronedarone (Multaq)	400 mg BID with meals t½ = 13-19 hrs (less lipophilic than amiodarone)	**BLACK BOX WARNING** HF (Class IV or any class with recent hospitalization) and use is CI in patients with permanent AF **CONTRAINDICATIONS** 2nd/3rd degree heart block, HR < 50, concomitant use of strong 3A4 inhibitors, concomitant use of drugs that prolong the QT interval, QTc $\geq$ 500 msec, severe hepatic impairment, pregnancy, nursing mothers **SIDE EFFECTS** New cases of hepatic failure (especially within the first 6 months) and renal failure, diarrhea, nausea, hypokalemia, hypomagnesemia, mild $\uparrow$ in SCr (and possibly BUN), abdominal pain, asthenia **MONITORING** LFTs (especially in the first 6 months), ECG, K$^+$, Mg^{2+}, SCr, BUN, HR Pregnancy Category X Only used in patients who can be converted into normal sinus rhythm

Class III Antiarrhythmic Agents Continued

DRUG	DOSING	SIDE EFFECTS/CONTRAINDICATIONS/MONITORING
Sotalol *(Betapace, Betapace AF, Sorine)*	Non-selective beta-blocker *Betapace* should not be substituted for *Betapace AF*	**BLACK BOX WARNINGS** Initiation (or reinitiation) and dosage increase should be done in a hospital, adjust dosing interval based on creatinine clearance to decrease risk of pro-arrhythmia, do not use in patients with QTc > 450 msec **CONTRAINDICATIONS** 2nd/3rd degree heart block, sinus bradycardia, uncompensated HF, cardiogenic shock, asthma, (QTc > 450 msec, CrCl < 40 mL/min, K+ < 4 mEq/L, sick sinus syndrome for *Betapace* AF) **SIDE EFFECTS** Bradycardia, hypotension, torsades, HF, dizziness, fatigue, bronchospasm **MONITORING** ECG (QTc interval), K+, Mg2+, HR, BP, SCr, BUN
Ibutilide *(Corvert)*	Available only as IV	**BLACK BOX WARNINGS (2)** Potentially fatal arrhythmias can occur Patients with chronic A. Fib may not be the best candidates since they often revert back **SIDE EFFECTS** Ventricular tachycardias (e.g. torsades), hypotension
Dofetilide *(Tikosyn)*	500 mcg BID if CrCl > 60 mL/min; reduce dose in renal impairment REMS program - available to prescribers and hospitals through *Tikosyn* Education Program. This program provides comprehensive education about the importance of in-hospital treatment initiation and individualized dosing. T.I.P.S. *(Tikosyn* In Pharmacy System) – designated to allow retail pharmacies to stock and dispense *Tikosyn*; must be enrolled and staff must be educated. Pharmacists must verify that the hospital/ prescriber is a confirmed participant before drug is dispensed.	**BLACK BOX WARNING** Must be initiated (or reinitiated) in a setting with continuous ECG monitoring for a minimum of 3 days or 12 hrs after cardioversion, whichever is greater **CONTRAINDICATIONS** Concurrent use of major 3A4 inhibitors and HCTZ, HR < 50, CrCl < 20 mL/min, QTc > 440 msec, hypokalemia, hypomagnesemia **SIDE EFFECTS** Ventricular tachycardias (e.g. torsades), dizziness, headache **MONITORING** ECG, renal function, K+, Mg2+, HR, BP in the first few days. Then monitor QTc interval and CrCl every 3 months (discontinue if QTc > 500 msec)

Amiodarone Drug Interactions

- Amiodarone is a moderate inhibitor of 2C9, 2D6, and 3A4 and a substrate of 3A4 and 2C8 and a P-gp inhibitor.

- The following medications must have the doses $\downarrow$ 30-50% when starting amiodarone: digoxin, warfarin, quinidine and procainamide. Use lower doses of simvastatin, lovastatin and atorvastatin.

- Avoid the use of co-administration of drugs that prolong the QT interval (e.g., tricyclic antidepressants, erythromycin, and other antiarrhythmics) due to risk of Torsade de Pointes.

- Use extreme caution with other negative chronotropes (e.g., beta-blockers, verapamil, diltiazem) can $\uparrow$ risk of bradycardia.

- Electrolyte abnormalities (K^+, Na^+, Ca^{2+}, Mg^{2+}, etc.) should be corrected before any antiarrhythmic therapy is initiated or the risk of arrhythmia is increased (true for all antiarrhythmics).

- Do not use grapefruit juice/products when using amiodarone.

- Avoid ephedra and St. John's wort.

Dronedarone Drug Interactions

- Dronedarone is a moderate inhibitor of 2D6 and 3A4 and substrate of 3A4. Avoid use with strong inhibitors and inducers of 3A4 and other antiarrhythmics. If using digoxin, reduce dose of digoxin by 50%. Caution with the use of statins at higher doses (see above).

- Avoid the use of co-administration of drugs that prolong the QT interval (e.g., tricyclic antidepressants, erythromycin, and other antiarrhythmics) due to risk of torsades de pointes.

- Use extreme caution with other negative chronotropes (e.g., beta-blockers, verapamil, diltiazem) can $\uparrow$ risk of bradycardia.

- Do not use grapefruit juice/products when using dronedarone.

- Monitor INR after initiating dronedarone in patients taking warfarin.

- Avoid ephedra and St. John's wort.

Dofetilide Drug Interactions

- Dofetilide is a 3A4 substrate. Avoid concomitant use with azole antifungals, nilotinib, thiazide diuretics, trimethoprim, verapamil, others.

- Avoid the use of co-administration of drugs that prolong the QT interval (e.g., tricyclic antidepressants, erythromycin, and other antiarrhythmics) due to risk of Torsade de Pointes.

- Avoid ephedra and St. John's wort.

CLASS IV ANTIARRHYTHMIC AGENTS

Class IV antiarrhythmic drugs block calcium channels.

DRUG	DOSING	SIDE EFFECTS/CONTRAINDICATIONS/MONITORING
Diltiazem *(Cardizem, Cardizem CD, Cardizem LA, Dilacor XR, Dilt-CD, Dilt-XR, Cartia XT, Tiazac, Taztia XT)* **Verapamil** *(Calan, Calan SR, Isoptin SR, Verelan, Verelan PM, Covera HS)*	May be preferred over beta blockers if co-existing asthma/COPD	**SIDE EFFECTS** Hypotension, bradycardia, edema, exacerbation of HF, AV block, constipation (more with verapamil), gingival hyperplasia **CONTRAINDICATIONS** $2^{nd}/3^{rd}$ degree heart block, sick sinus syndrome, severe hypotension (systolic < 90 mmHg), cardiogenic shock, decompensated HF, acute MI **MONITORING** ECG, BP, HR, electrolytes Only non-dihydropyridine CCBs are used as antiarrhythmics

AGENTS NOT IN VAUGHAN WILLIAMS CLASSIFICATION

- Adenosine decreases conduction through the AV node restoring normal sinus rhythm (NSR).

- Digoxin causes direct AV node suppression, ↑ increasing refractory period and decreasing conduction velocity. Digoxin has a positive inotropic effect, enhanced vagal tone, and decreased ventricular rate to fast atrial arrhythmias.

DRUG	DOSING	SIDE EFFECTS/CONTRAINDICATIONS/MONITORING
Adenosine *(Adenocard)*	Used in paroxysmal supraventricular tachycardia (PSVTs) and not for converting A.Fib/A.flutter or ventricular tachycardia 6 mg IV push (may increase to 12 mg if not responding) t½: less than 10 sec	**SIDE EFFECTS** Transient new arrhythmia, facial flushing, headache, chest pain/pressure
Digoxin *(Lanoxin, Digitek)* – tabs, solution, inj	0.125-0.25 mg daily Loading dose [AKA total digitalizing dose (TDD)] is 1.0-1.5 mg. Give ½ of the TDD as the initial dose, followed by ¼ of the TDD in 2 subsequent doses at 6-8 hour intervals. Therapeutic range for A. Fib = 0.8 – 2.0 ng/mL Watch for renal impairment ↓ in renal dysfunction; can be given 0.125 mg every other day or less frequently ↓ 20-25% when going from oral tabs to IV Antidote: *Digibind* or *DigiFab*	**SIDE EFFECTS** Dizziness, headache, diarrhea, nausea, vomiting, rash, mental changes **CONTRAINDICATIONS** 2nd or 3rd degree heart block without a pacemaker, Wolff-Parkinson-White syndrome (WPW) with A Fib, and others **MONITORING** HR, BP, electrolytes (K^+, Ca^{2+}, Mg^{2+}), renal function. ECG and drug level (if suspect toxicity) **Toxicity** First signs of toxicity are nausea/vomiting, loss of appetite and bradycardia. Other signs of toxicity include blurred or "yellow" vision, ab pain, confusion, delirium, prolonged PR interval, accelerated junctional rhythm, bidirectional ventricular tachycardia Pregnancy Category C

Digoxin Drug Interactions

- Beta-blockers and non-DHP calcium channel blockers may have additive effects on ↓ HR.

- Digoxin is mostly renally cleared and partially cleared hepatically. Decreased renal function requires a ↓ digoxin dose, or, if acute renal failure, the digoxin should be held.

- Digoxin levels may ↑ with amiodarone, quinidine, verapamil, erythromycin, clarithromycin, azole antifungals, cyclosporine, propafenone, PIs, and a few others: a dose reduction is likely required.

- Digoxin levels may ↓ with bile acid resins, St. John's wort and others.

- Hypokalemia (K^+ < 3.5 mEq/L) may ↑ risk of digoxin toxicity. Hypercalcemia may also ↑ risk of digoxin toxicity.

PATIENT COUNSELING

Amiodarone Patient Counseling

- Dispense Medication Guide.

- This medication is used to treat certain types of serious (possibly fatal) irregular heartbeat. It is used to restore the normal heart rhythm and maintain a regular, steady heartbeat. Amiodarone works by blocking certain electrical signals in the heart that can cause an irregular heartbeat.

- Take this medication by mouth, usually once or twice daily or as directed by your doctor. You may take this medication with or without food, but it is important to choose one way and take the same way with every dose.

- Severe (sometimes fatal) lung or liver problems have infrequently occurred in patients using this drug. Tell your doctor immediately if you experience any of these serious side effects: cough, fever, chills, chest pain, difficult or painful breathing, coughing up blood, severe stomach pain, fatigue, yellowing eyes or skin, or dark urine.

- Like other medications used to treat irregular heartbeats, amiodarone can infrequently cause them to become worse. Seek immediate medical attention if your heart continues to pound or skips a beat.

- This drug may infrequently cause serious vision changes. Tell your doctor immediately if you develop any vision changes (such as seeing halos or blurred vision).

- This drug can change how your thyroid gland works, and may cause your metabolism to speed up or slow down. Tell your doctor if you develop any symptoms of low or overactive thyroid including cold or heat intolerance, unexplained weight loss/gain, thinning hair, unusual sweating, nervousness, irritability, or restlessness. Please discuss this with your doctor and tests can be ordered to check your thyroid function.

- This drug may cause your skin to be more sensitive to the sun. Infrequently, this medication has caused the skin to become a blue-gray color. This effect is not harmful and usually goes away after the drug is stopped.

- You should have regular check-ups, blood tests, chest x-rays, and eye exams before and during treatment with amiodarone.

- Do not consume grapefruit or drink grapefruit juice while using this medication. Grapefruit juice can increase the amount of medication in your blood.

- This drug can interact with other medicines. Before starting a new medicine, discuss with your pharmacist if it is safe to use with amiodarone.

Digoxin Patient Counseling

- This medicine helps make the heart beat stronger and with a more regular rhythm. Keep taking as directed, even if you feel well.

- Do not stop taking this medicine without talking to your doctor. Stopping suddenly may make your condition worse.

- Avoid becoming overheated or dehydrated as an overdose can more easily occur if you are dehydrated.

- Symptoms of overdose may include nausea, vomiting, diarrhea, loss of appetite, vision changes (such as blurred or yellow/green vision), uneven heartbeats, and feeling like you might pass out. If any of these occur, see a doctor right away.

- There are many medications that can interact with digoxin. Check with your physician or pharmacist before starting any new medicines, including over the counter, vitamin, and/or herbal products.

- If your doctor has asked you to monitor heart rate, please do so as directed. A lower heart rate can indicate that the drug level in your body has become too high.

- To be sure that this medication is not causing harmful effects, your blood may need to be tested on a regular basis. Your kidney function will also need to be tested.

Practice Case

Arnie is a 57 year-old male who comes into your pharmacy with a new prescription for amiodarone 200 mg po daily. He tells you that he went to the doctor because his heart felt like it was racing and he was feeling dizzy. The doctor told him he has atrial fibrillation. He is concerned that this will affect his life span.

CATEGORY	
PMH	Smoker CHF – NYHA Class 3 HTN – Stage 2
Current medications	Digoxin 0.25 mg po daily *Lasix* 40 mg po daily Spironolactone 12.5 mg po daily *Coreg CR* 20 mg po daily Lisinopril 40 mg po daily
Labs	K$^+$ = 5.2 mEq/L SCr = 1.4 mg/dL BUN = 43 mg/dL

QUESTIONS

1. Before the prescription for amiodarone is filled, the pharmacist should call the doctor to decrease the dose of which of the following medications?

    a. Digoxin
    b. *Lasix*
    c. Spironolactone
    d. *Coreg CR*
    e. Lisinopril

2. When counseling Arnie on the use of amiodarone, he should be told to expect periodic monitoring of these organ systems:

    a. Liver, kidney, and eyes
    b. Liver, colon, and kidney
    c. Kidney, gall bladder, and CNS
    d. Thyroid, kidney, and liver
    e. Thyroid, liver, and lungs

3. Which of the following is <u>not</u> a side effect of amiodarone?

    a. Skin discoloration
    b. Corneal deposits
    c. Lung damage
    d. Taste perversions
    e. Hypothyroidism

4. Arnie develops thyroid dysfunction. His doctor switches him to *Multaq* to try and alleviate the problem. Choose the correct therapeutic equivalent for *Multaq*:

    a. Mexiletine
    b. Flecainide
    c. Lidocaine
    d. Dronedarone
    e. Dofetilide

Questions 5-10 do not apply to the above case.

5. A patient is beginning digoxin 0.125 mg daily. The patient has mild renal insufficiency. After a few weeks, the patient develops an infection with nausea and vomiting. She is weak and dehydrated. The patient is admitted to the hospital to treat the infection and to check for digoxin toxicity. Choose the correct statement:

   a. The digoxin may have become toxic due to decreased renal function.
   b. An elevated digoxin level can worsen nausea and vomiting.
   c. Mental confusion may be due to an elevated digoxin level.
   d. A and B.
   e. All of the above.

6. A patient was using furosemide 40 mg twice daily (at 8 am and 12 noon) for heart failure. The doctor forgot to call in a prescription for potassium when he called the pharmacy to order the furosemide. The patient's other medications include carvedilol, digoxin and aspirin. What is likely to occur?

   a. Digoxin toxicity
   b. Carvedilol toxicity
   c. Aspirin toxicity
   d. Furosemide toxicity
   e. None of the above

7. What class of antiarrhythmic is disopyramide in the Vaughn-Williams classification system?

   a. IA
   b. IB
   c. IC
   d. III
   e. IV

8. A patient has a long QT interval. She is at risk for fatal arrhythmias. Which of the following medications will increase her risk of further QT prolongation?

   a. Quinidine
   b. Procainamide
   c. Dronedarone
   d. Amiodarone
   e. All of the above

9. A patient has a bradyarrhythmia. The physician does not wish to further lower the heart rate. Choose the agent that will not cause the patient's heart rate to drop any lower:

   a. Verapamil
   b. Sotalol
   c. Digoxin
   d. Amlodipine
   e. Diltiazem

10. A patient is using digoxin. The doctor must make sure that the potassium level stays within safe range. This safe range is defined as:

    a. 0.8-2 ng/mL
    b. 2-5-5 ng/dL
    c. 3.5-5 mEq/L
    d. 3-5-5 mEq/mL
    e. 7.8-10 mEq/mL

ANSWERS

1-a, 2-e, 3-d, 4-d, 5-e, 6-a, 7-a, 8-e, 9-d, 10-c

35

PULMONARY ARTERIAL HYPERTENSION (PAH)

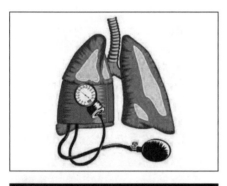

GUIDELINE

ACCF/AHA 2009 Expert Consensus
Document on Pulmonary Hypertension.
J Am Coll Cardiol. 2009;53:1573-1619.

Background

Pulmonary Arterial Hypertension (PAH) is characterized by continuous high blood pressure in the pulmonary artery. The average blood pressure in a normal pulmonary artery (called pulmonary artery pressure) is about 14 mmHg when a person is resting. In PAH, the pulmonary artery pressure (PAP) is greater than 25 mmHg. Other hemodynamic parameters are affected as well.

The pathology of PAH stems from an imbalance of vasoconstrictor/vasodilator substances and an imbalance of proliferation and apoptosis. The vasoconstrictor substances such as endothelin-1 and thromboxane A_2 (TxA_2) are increased in PAH, whereas, the vasodilators (e.g. prostacyclins, others) are decreased. The vasoconstriction results in reduced blood flow and high pressure within the pulmonary vasculature. The walls of the pulmonary arteries thicken as the amount of muscle increases and scar tissue can form on the artery walls (proliferation). As the walls thicken and scar, the arteries become increasingly narrower. These changes make it hard for the right ventricle to pump blood through the pulmonary artery and into the lungs due to the increased pressure. As a result of the heart working harder, the right ventricle becomes enlarged and right heart failure can result. Heart failure is the most common cause of death in people who have PAH.

The biochemical changes mentioned above ($\uparrow TxA_2$, $\downarrow$ prostacyclin), along with other altered pathways, lead to a pro-thrombotic state and patients will require anticoagulation to prevent blood clots from forming. Warfarin, titrated to an INR of 1.5 - 2.5, is recommended.

Pulmonary hypertension can be caused by diseases of the heart and the lungs, including COPD, emphysema, left ventricular failure, recurrent pulmonary embolism, advanced liver disease, among many others. Some patients have no identifiable cause of the disease – this is primary, or idiopathic, PAH (versus secondary, which has a known cause). Less commonly, medications can be the causative factor, including the diet drugs dexfenfluramine *(Redux)* and Fen/Phen or from the chronic use of cocaine and methamphetamine. Recently, <u>dasatinib *(Sprycel)* has been linked to causing PAH</u>.

Symptoms of PAH include dyspnea, chest pain, syncope, edema, tachycardia and/or Raynaud's phenomenon. In Raynaud's, the reduced blood supply causes discoloration and coldness in the fingers, toes, and occasionally other areas.

There is no cure for PAH, but in the last decade, the knowledge of PAH has increased significantly and many more treatment options have become available. In some cases, a lung or heart-lung transplant may be an option, at least for younger patients.

Non-Pharmacologic Treatment

Patients with PAH should follow a sodium restricted diet (< 2.4 grams/day) and manage fluid volume status, especially if they have right ventricle failure. Routine immunizations against influenza and pneumococcal pneumonia are advised. Exposure to high altitudes may contribute to hypoxic pulmonary vasoconstriction and may not be tolerated by patients. Oxygen is used to maintain oxygen saturation above 90%.

Pharmacologic Treatment

Some patients respond to and are candidates for calcium channel blocker therapy. The calcium channel blockers used most frequently are long acting nifedipine, diltiazem, and amlodipine. The use of verapamil is not recommended due to its negative inotropic effects.

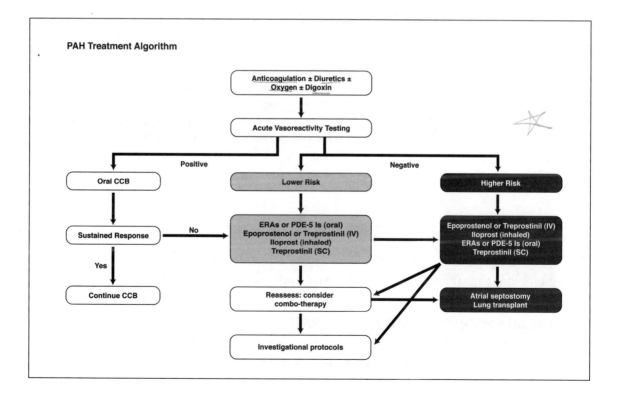

Digoxin is sometimes used in patients with right heart failure and a low cardiac output and in patients with atrial arrhythmias.

For most cases, drug therapy will reduce symptoms and prolong life. Medications include prostacyclin analogues which cause vasodilation. These drugs may be given by continuous IV infusion, infusion under the skin, or as inhaled therapy. Endothelin receptor antagonists block endothelin, a vasoconstrictor. Phosphodiesterase-5 inhibitors (the same drugs used for erectile dysfunction – but with different brand names and doses) relax the blood vessels in the lungs. Some patients may benefit from combination therapy.

PROSTACYCLIN ANALOGUES (OR PROSTANOIDS)

Prostacyclin analogues act as potent vasodilators (on both pulmonary and systemic vascular beds). They are also inhibitors of platelet aggregation. Prostacyclin synthase is reduced in PAH resulting in inadequate production of prostacyclin I_2, a vasodilator with antiproliferative effects.

DRUG	DOSING	SIDE EFFECTS/CONTRAINDICATIONS/MONITORING
Epoprostenol (*Flolan, Veletri*) AKA prostacyclin and PGI_2	20-40 ng/kg/min continuous IV infusion	**SIDE EFFECTS** During Dose Titration – diarrhea, nausea, vomiting (dose-limiting; if this happens, reduce the dose of the drug), flushing, headache, hypotension, anxiety, chest pain/palpitations, tachycardia and edema
		With Chronic Use - Anxiety, flu-like symptoms, and jaw pain
		Iloprost: Lockjaw (trismus), cough
		Avoid interruptions in therapy. Immediate access to back up pump, infusion sets and medication is essential to prevent treatment interruptions.
Treprostinil (*Remodulin* is IV, *Tyvaso* is inhaled)	*Remodulin:* 40-160 ng/kg/min continuous SC or IV infusion	Avoid large, sudden reductions in dose
		Flolan: pump needs to be on ice packs for proper cooling
	Inhalation form (*Tyvaso*) is given 4 times/day	*Veletri:* Thermostable (no need for ice packs)
		Remodulin: SC very painful (85% of patients), may need analgesic to tolerate. Also thermostable – no ice packs needed
Iloprost (*Ventavis*)	2.5-5 mcg/inhalation given 6-9 times/day	The IV agents are considered the most potent of all PAH medications.
		Patients must be instructed on central catheter maintenance to reduce infections and to avoid interruption of therapy – both which can be fatal.

(handwritten annotations: "ice pack")

Prostacyclin Analogue Drug Interactions

- May increase the effects of antihypertensive and antiplatelet agents.

ENDOTHELIN RECEPTOR ANTAGONISTS (ERAs)

These agents block endothelin receptors on vascular endothelium and smooth muscle. Endothelin is a vasoconstrictor with cellular proliferative effects.

DRUG	DOSING	SIDE EFFECTS/CONTRAINDICATIONS/MONITORING
Bosentan *(Tracleer)* This is one of the REMS drugs (Risk Evaluation and Mitigation Strategies)	62.5 mg BID (for 4 wks) then 125 mg BID	**BLACK BOX WARNING** Use in pregnancy is contraindicated (Pregnancy Category X) Because of the risks of hepatic impairment and possible teratogenic effects, bosentan is only available through the *Tracleer* Access Program (T.A.P.). Prescribers and pharmacists must be certified and enroll patients in TAP. Avoid use in moderate-to-severe hepatic impairment **SIDE EFFECTS** Headache, ↓ Hgb (usually in first 6 weeks of therapy), anemia, ↑ LFTs (dose related), upper respiratory tract infections, edema (all > 10%) Spermatogenesis inhibition (25%) leading to male infertility (with bosentan only) **CONTRAINDICATIONS** Pregnancy; concurrent use of cyclosporine or glyburide **MONITORING** Monitor LFTs and bilirubin at baseline and every month thereafter. Monitor hemoglobin and hematocrit at baseline and at 1 month and 3 months, then every 3 months thereafter. Women of childbearing potential must have a negative pregnancy test prior to initiation of therapy and monthly thereafter (prior to shipment of the monthly refill). Barrier techniques of contraception are recommended.
Ambrisentan *(Letairis)* This is one of the REMS drugs (Risk Evaluation and Mitigation Strategies)	5 or 10 mg daily	**Black Box Warning** Use in pregnancy is contraindicated (Pregnancy Category X) Because of the risk of possible teratogenic effects, ambrisentan is only available through the *Letairis* Education and Access Program (LEAP) restricted distribution program. Prescribers and pharmacists must be certified and enroll patients in LEAP. **SIDE EFFECTS** Peripheral edema, headache, ↓ Hgb, flushing, palpitations, and nasal congestion **CONTRAINDICATIONS** Pregnancy **MONITORING** Monitor hemoglobin and hematocrit at baseline and at 1 month, then periodically thereafter. Women of childbearing potential must have a negative pregnancy test prior to initiation of therapy and monthly thereafter (prior to shipment of the monthly refill). Monitoring of LFTs was removed from the package insert on March 4, 2011 (FDA)

Endothelin Receptor Antagonist Drug Interactions

- Both drugs should not be used with St. John's wort or grapefruit juice.

- Bosentan is contraindicated with glyburide and cyclosporine. Levels of bosentan may ↑ with CYP450 2C8/9 and 3A4 inhibitors.

- Ambrisentan dose should not exceed 5 mg/d when given concomitantly with cyclosporine.

PHOSPHODIESTERASE-5 INHIBITORS (PDE-5 Is)

These agents inhibit phosphodiesterase type 5 (PDE-5) in smooth muscle of pulmonary vasculature. PDE-5 is responsible for the degradation of cyclic guanosine monophosphate (cGMP). Increased cGMP concentrations lead to pulmonary vasculature relaxation and vasodilation.

DRUG	DOSING	SIDE EFFECTS/CONTRAINDICATIONS/MONITORING
Sildenafil *(Revatio)*	IV: 10 mg IV 3 times/day Oral: 20 mg TID, taken 4-6 hours apart	**SIDE EFFECTS** Dizziness, sudden drop in blood pressure, headache, flushing, dyspepsia, back pain *(Adcirca)*, and epistaxis. Priapism (< 2%) – if erection lasts for > 4 hours, get medical help right away. Sudden vision loss in one or both eyes – seek medical help right away. May cause permanent vision loss. Other visual problems (blurred vision, increased sensitivity to light, bluish haze, or temporary difficulty distinguishing between blue and green) may occur. Sudden decrease or loss of hearing has been reported, usually in one ear. Tinnitus is another rare, but possible, side effect. **CONTRAINDICATIONS** Concurrent use of nitrates. With sildenafil used for PAH, avoid in patients taking PIs regimens. Avoid use in severe hepatic impairment. With tadalafil, avoid use when CrCl < 30 mL/min.
Tadalafil *(Adcirca)*	40 mg daily (20 mg daily if mild to moderate renal/ hepatic impairment) Take 2, 20 mg tabs once a day	

PDE-5 Is Drug Interactions

■ Do not give with PDE-5 Is used for erectile dysfunction. Avoid concurrent use of nitrates, itraconazole, and ketoconazole. Avoid grapefruit juice.

PDE-5 Is are Contraindicated With Nitrates!

■ Concurrent use of nitrate medications (for example, nitroglycerin [*NitroQuick, Nitro-Bid, Nitro-DUR, Nitroderm, Nitrogard, Nitrolingual, Nitrostat*], isosorbide mononitrate [*ISMO*], or isosorbide dinitrate [*Isordil, ISDN, Sorbitrate*]) increases the potential for excessively low blood pressure. Taking nitrates is an absolute contraindication to the use of these medicines. These include the illicit drugs such as amyl nitrate and butyl nitrate ("poppers").

- If a patient with ED has taken a PDE-5 inhibitor and then develops angina, nitroglycerin should not be used until after 24 h for sildenafil or vardenafil and after 48 h for tadalafil. Of course, other anti-anginal and anti-ischemic therapies may be used - such as beta blockers, calcium channel blockers, aspirin, morphine, statins and percutaneous coronary intervention. (Sometimes nitrates are used in an acute emergency, despite this warning, with careful monitoring.)

Caution with PDE-5 Is and Concurrent Alpha Blocker Therapy

[tamsulosin *(Flomax)*, doxazosin *(Cardura)*, others]

- Caution is advised when PDE-5 inhibitors are co-administered with alpha blockers. PDE-5 inhibitors and alpha-adrenergic blocking agents are both vasodilators with BP lowering effects. When vasodilators are used in combination, an additive effect on BP may be anticipated. In some patients, concomitant use of these two drug classes can lower BP significantly leading to symptomatic hypotension (e.g. dizziness, light headedness, fainting).

- The precaution goes on to suggest that patients should be on stable alpha-blocker therapy before PDE-5 inhibition and that lowest doses of the PDE-5 inhibitors be used to initiate therapy. Conversely, if a patient is already taking an optimal dose of PDE-5 inhibitor and an alpha blocker needs to be started, the alpha blocker should be started at the lowest dose, and preferably the alpha-1a selective agents are chosen (tamsulosin, silodosin, others).

36

ASTHMA

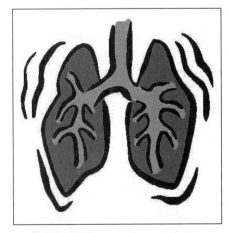

GUIDELINES

Expert Panel Report 3. Guidelines for the Diagnosis and Management of Asthma. National Heart, Lung and Blood Institute, August 2007. Available at http://www.nhlbi.nih.gov/guidelines/asthma

Background

Asthma is characterized by a predisposition to chronic inflammation of the lungs in which the airways (bronchi) are reversibly narrowed. Asthma affects 5-7% of the population of the United States. During asthma attacks (exacerbations of asthma), the smooth muscle cells in the bronchi constrict, the airways become inflamed and swollen, and breathing becomes difficult.

The National Heart, Lung and Blood Institute defines asthma as a common chronic disorder of the airways characterized by variable and recurring symptoms, airflow obstruction, bronchial hyperresponsiveness (bronchospasm), and underlying inflammation. Asthma is a chronic inflammatory disorder of the airways in which many cells and cellular elements play a role, in particular, mast cells, eosinophils, neutrophils, T lymphocytes, macrophages, and epithelial cells. This inflammation causes recurrent episodes of the classic signs and symptoms of asthma: <u>wheezing, breathlessness, chest tightness, and coughing</u>; particularly at night or early in the morning. Airway remodeling can occur consisting of fibrosis and increased goblet cells.

COMMON TRIGGERS OF ASTHMA

TRIGGERS	EXAMPLES
Allergens	Airborne pollens (grass, trees, weeds), house-dust mites, animal dander (cats, dogs, horses, rabbits, rats, mice), cockroaches, fungal spores
Drugs	Aspirin, NSAIDs, sulfites, β-Blockers

Common Triggers of Asthma Continued

TRIGGERS	EXAMPLES
Environmental	Cold air, fog, ozone, sulfur dioxide, nitrogen dioxide, tobacco smoke, wood smoke
Exercise	Cold air or humid, hot air
Occupational	Bakers (flour dust), farmers (hay mold), spice and enzyme workers; painters (arabic gum), chemical workers (azo dyes, toluene diisocyanates, polyvinyl chloride); plastics, rubber, and wood workers (formaldehyde, dimethyethanolamine)
Respiratory Infections	Respiratory syncytial virus (RSV), rhinovirus, influenza, parainfluenza, *Mycoplasma pneumonia*

GOALS OF ASTHMA THERAPY

- Prevent chronic and troublesome symptoms (e.g. coughing, breathlessness)

- Require infrequent use of inhaled short-acting β_2 agonist for quick relief of symptoms (not including EIB)

- Maintain (near) normal pulmonary function

- Maintain normal activity levels (including exercise and other physical activity and attendance at work or school)

- Prevent recurrent exacerbations of asthma and minimize the need for hospital visits

- Provide optimal pharmacological therapy with minimal or no adverse effects of therapy

- Meet patients' and families' expectations of satisfaction with asthma care

SPECIAL POPULATIONS

Exercise-induced bronchospasm (EIB)

- Pretreatment before exercise with short-acting β_2 agonists, leukotriene receptor antagonists, or mast cell stabilizers, is recommended. Short-acting β_2 agonists are the drugs of choice generally.

- Short-acting β_2 agonists (SABAs) can be taken right before exercise and last up to 2-3 hours.

- If you need longer duration, can take long-acting β_2 agonists (LABAs) but need to take 15 minutes prior to exercise (for formoterol) and 30 minutes prior to exercise (for salmeterol). Remember LABAs should not be used as monotherapy in patients with persistent asthma.

- Montelukast must be taken 2 hours prior to exercise and it lasts up to 24 hours. However, it only works in 50% of patients.

Pregnancy

- Albuterol is the preferred short-acting β_2 agonist.

- Budesonide is the preferred inhaled corticosteroid due to more data in pregnancy.

- Monitor asthma as it may get worse. Safer to be treated with asthma medications than to have poorly controlled asthma to ensure oxygen supply to the fetus.

Pharmacologic Therapy

BETA-2 AGONISTS

Bind to beta-2 receptors causing relaxation of bronchial smooth muscle resulting in bronchodilation – inhaled route is the preferred route of administration

DRUG	DOSING	SIDE EFFECTS/CONTRAINDICATIONS/MONITORING

Short-Acting Beta-2 Agonists (SABAs)

DRUG	DOSING	SIDE EFFECTS/CONTRAINDICATIONS/MONITORING
Epinephrine *(Primatene Mist)* Metaproterenol *(Alupent)*	Agents should not be used due to non- beta-2 selective	**SIDE EFFECTS** Tremor, shakiness, lightheadedness, cough, palpitations, hypokalemia, tachycardia, hyperglycemia **MDI** Shake well before use. Prime prior to first use (3-4 sprays into the air away from face) and again if inhaler has not been used for > 2 weeks
Albuterol *(Ventolin HFA, Proventil HFA, ProAir HFA, AccuNeb)*	1-2 inhalations Q4-6H (MDI) 2.5 mg Q4-8H (NEB) 2-4 mg Q4-6H (PO), others	Prefer a beta-2 selective agent and the inhaled route. These are rescue medications used PRN in asthma. HFA inhalers have softer, less forceful sprays. Patients may experience a different taste and feel a warmer spray than with CFC inhalers (which have been discontinued due to environmental concerns). HFA inhalers need to be cleaned more often as they can clog. If using SABA > 2 days/week, then need to ↑ maintenance therapy
Levalbuterol *(Xopenex, Xopenex HFA)*	1-2 inhalations Q4-6H (MDI) 0.63 mg or 1.25 mg Q6-8H (NEB)	Short acting beta-2 agonists are the drugs of choice for exercise-induced bronchospasm (EIB) Levalbuterol contains R-isomer of albuterol **MONITORING** Number of days of use of SABA, symptom frequency, FEV1, peak flow, BP, HR, blood glucose, and K⁺
Pirbuterol *(Maxair Autohaler)*	1-2 inhalations Q4-6H (MDI)	

Pharmacologic Therapy Continued

DRUG	DOSING	SIDE EFFECTS/CONTRAINDICATIONS/ MONITORING

Long-Acting Beta-2 Agonists (LABAs)

DRUG	DOSING	SIDE EFFECTS/CONTRAINDICATIONS/MONITORING
Salmeterol *(Serevent Diskus)* **+ fluticasone propionate (Advair Diskus, Advair HFA)**	Usual dose is 1 inhalation BID, except the HFA is 2 inhalations BID	**BLACK BOX WARNING** ↑ risk of asthma-related deaths. Do not use LABA as monotherapy; need to have persistent asthma patients on long-term control therapy
Formoterol *(Foradil Aerolizer)* **+ budesonide (Symbicort)**	1 capsule via Aerolizer BID 2 inhalations BID	*Foradil* Place 1 capsule in aerolizer and puncture with the device only once. DO NOT swallow the capsule. Capsules are stable at room temp for 4 months.

MAST CELL STABILIZERS

Prevent mast cell release of histamine and leukotrienes by inhibiting degranulation after contact with allergens/antigens

DRUG	DOSING	SIDE EFFECTS/CONTRAINDICATIONS/MONITORING
Cromolyn sodium *(Intal)*	2-4 inhalations Q6-8H (MDI) 20 mg Q6-8H (NEB)	**SIDE EFFECTS** Unpleasant taste, cough, nausea, etc. EIB – Give 10-15 min prior to exercise; not found to be as effective as SABAs OTC cromolyn nasal spray–used for nasal allergies *(NasalCrom)*

CORTICOSTEROIDS

Inhibit the inflammatory response, depresses migration of polymorphonuclear (PMN) leukocytes, fibroblasts and others. to prevent inflammation

SIDE EFFECTS OF SYSTEMIC STEROIDS

Long-term adverse effects of systemic corticosteroids are listed below (if used for < 1 month, short-term systemic side effects can include ↑ appetite/weight gain, fluid retention, emotional instability (euphoria, mood swings, irritability), insomnia, GI upset; and with higher doses, can see blood pressure elevations and ↑ blood glucose).

Hypothalamic-pituitary-adrenal suppression	Hyperglycemia/diabetes	Hirsutism
Cushing's syndrome	Impaired wound healing	Acne
Growth retardation	Dermal thinning/bruising	Hyperpigmentation
Osteoporosis/fractures	Inhibition of leukocyte and monocyte function	Insomnia/nervousness
Pancreatitis	Glaucoma	Amenorrhea
Psychiatric disturbances (mood swings, delirium, psychoses)	Cataracts	Peptic ulcers
Sodium and water retention/ hypertension	Moon facies	Abdominal distention
Hypokalemia	Central redistribution of fat	Nausea/vomiting
	Increased appetite/weight gain	Muscle wasting

DRUG	DOSING	SIDE EFFECTS/CONTRAINDICATIONS/MONITORING
Beclomethasone HFA (QVAR HFA) – solution, do not need to shake	Low dose: 80-240 mcg/d Medium dose: > 240-480 mcg/d High dose: > 480 mcg/d	**SIDE EFFECTS (INHALED)** Dysphonia, oral candidiasis (thrush), cough, hoarseness, URTI's, hyperglycemia, increase risk of fractures and pneumonia (with high dose, long-term use) To prevent oral candidiasis, rinse mouth and throat with warm water and spit out or use a spacer device
Budesonide (Pulmicort Flexhaler, Pulmicort Respules) **+ formoterol (Symbicort HFA)**	Low dose: 180-600 mcg/d Medium dose: > 600-1,200 mcg/d High dose: > 1,200 mcg/d	Inhaled steroids <u>are first-line</u> for long term control of all ages with persistent asthma Systemic steroids have a rapid onset of action and are used as "pulse" therapy – for up to 15 days after an asthma attack *QVAR* and *Alvesco* –do not have to shake before use
Ciclesonide (Alvesco) -prodrug	80-320 mcg BID	**Pulmicort Respules** – indicated for 1-8 years of age **Advair Diskus** – 100, 250, 500 mcg fluticasone + 50 mcg salmeterol/inh. Take <u>1 inhalation BID</u> (indicated for ages ≥ 4 years) *Advair HFA* – 45, 115, 230 mcg fluticasone + 21 mcg salmeterol/inh. Take <u>2 inhalations BID</u> (ages ≥ 12 years)
Flunisolide HFA (Aerospan HFA) – has built-in spacer	Low dose: 320 mcg/d Medium dose: > 320-640 mcg/d High dose: > 640 mcg/d	**Symbicort HFA** – 80, 160 mcg budesonide + 4.5 mcg formoterol/inh. Take <u>2 inhalations BID</u> (ages ≥ 12 years) *Dulera* – 100, 200 mcg mometasone + 5 mcg formoterol/inh. Take <u>2 inhalations BID</u> (ages ≥ 12 years)
Fluticasone (Flovent HFA, Flovent Diskus) **+ salmeterol (Advair Diskus, Advair HFA)**	For MDI: Low dose: 88-264 mcg/d Medium dose: 264-440 mcg/d High dose: > 440 mcg/d For Diskus: Low dose: 100-300 mcg/d Medium dose: > 300-500 mcg/d High dose: > 500 mcg/d	
Mometasone (Asmanex Twisthaler) **+ formoterol (Dulera)**	Low dose: 220 mcg/d Medium dose: 440 mcg/d High dose: > 440 mcg/d	

ORAL STEROIDS - DOSE EQUIVALENTS

DRUG	DOSE EQUIVALENT	COMMENTS
Prednisone/Prednisolone	5 mg	Maintenance prednisone therapy: use 5-60 mg daily or every other day (for severe asthma)
Methylprednisolone/Triamcinolone	4 mg	
Betamethasone	0.6 mg	
Dexamethasone	0.75 mg	
Hydrocortisone	20 mg	
Cortisone	25 mg	

LEUKOTRIENE MODIFYING AGENTS

Zafirlukast and montelukast are leukotriene-receptor antagonists (LTRA) of leukotriene D4 (LTD4 - both) and E4 (LTE4 – just zafirlukast). Zileuton is a 5-lipoxygenase inhibitor which inhibits leukotriene formation. All agents help ↓ airway edema, constriction and inflammation.

DRUG	DOSING	SIDE EFFECTS/CONTRAINDICATIONS/MONITORING
Zafirlukast (*Accolate*)	20 mg BID (empty stomach) Children 5-11 years: 10 mg BID	**CAUTION** Neuropsychiatric events have been reported. Patients should notify doctor if develop signs of aggressive behavior, hostility, agitation, depression, suicidal thinking **SIDE EFFECTS** Headache , dizziness, abdominal pain, ↑ LFTs, upper respiratory tract infections, pharyngitis, sinusitis, and Churg-Strauss syndrome (rare) **CONTRAINDICATIONS** Active liver disease – zileuton
Montelukast (***Singulair***)	10 mg daily: take in the evening Age 6 mos - 5 years: take 4 mg daily; Age 5-14 years: take 5 mg daily	**MONITORING** Zileuton - need to monitor LFTs every month for first 3 months, every 2-3 months for the rest of the first year of therapy
Zileuton (*Zyflo CR*)	1,200 mg (2 tabs) BID within 1 hour of morning and evening meals Children: not recommended	

Drug Interactions

- Zafirlukast – substrate of 2C9 (major), inhibitor of 2C9 (moderate) – may ↑ levels of warfarin and 2C9 substrates. Levels of zafirlukast may be ↓ by erythromycin, theophylline, and food (↓ bioavailability by 40%) – take 1 hour before or 2 hrs after meals

- Montelukast – substrate of 2C9 (major)

- Zileuton – inhibitor of 1A2 (moderate) – may ↑ levels of propranolol, theophylline, and warfarin

THEOPHYLLINE

Blocks phosphodiesterase causing ↑ cyclic AMP (cAMP) which promotes release of epinephrine from adrenal cells. This results in bronchodilation, diuresis, CNS and cardiac stimulation.

DRUG	DOSING	SIDE EFFECTS/CONTRAINDICATIONS/MONITORING
Theophylline Immediate Release *(Elixophyllin)* Extended Release *(TheoCap, Theo-24, Uniphyl, Theochron)*	200-600 mg daily Therapeutic range: 5-15 mcg/mL (measure peak level)	**SIDE EFFECTS** Nausea, headache, tachycardia, insomnia, tremor, and nervousness Avoid excessive amounts of caffeine, extreme amounts of dietary protein and carbohydrates and charbroiled beef – can alter theophylline levels Signs of toxicity - persistent and repetitive vomiting, ventricular tachycardias, seizures LD = (Cp-Co)(Vd)(Wt) Vd = 0.5 L/kg; Cp = desired theo concentration; Co = initial theo concentration; Wt – use IBW in kg If using IV aminophylline, then divide by 0.8 (aminophylline contains 80% theophylline) **MONITORING** Theophylline levels, symptoms of asthma, use of SABA, lung function tests

Drug Interactions

Theophylline is a substrate of 1A2 and 3A4 (both major) and an inhibitor of 1A2 (weak). It has first order kinetics, followed by Michaelis-Menten (or saturable) kinetics (similar to phenytoin and voriconazole). A small increase in dose can result in a large increase in the theophylline concentration.

- Drugs that may ↑ theophylline levels due to 1A2 inhibition: oral contraceptives, zafirlukast, zileuton, acyclovir, cimetidine, ciprofloxacin, ethinyl estradiol, fluvoxamine, isoniazid

- Drugs that may ↑ theophylline levels due to 3A4 inhibition: amiodarone, azole antifungals, clarithromycin, cyclosporine, erythromycin, diltiazem, verapamil, lovastatin, simvastatin, atorvastatin, PIs, and others

- Drugs that may ↑ theophylline levels due to other mechanisms: allopurinol, erythromycin, propranolol, ephedrine, and possibly with other systemic bronchodilators (and possibly phenylephrine, pseudoephedrine). Also conditions such as CHF, cirrhosis, or hypothyroidism can ↓ clearance.

- Drugs that may ↓ theophylline levels: carbamazepine, phenobarbital, phenytoin, primidone, rifampin, ritonavir, tobacco/marijuana smoking, St. John's wort, tipranavir/ritonavir, thyroid hormones (levothyroxine), high protein diet, low carbohydrate diet, and charbroiled foods

- Theophylline will ↓ lithium (theophylline ↑ renal excretion of lithium) and will ↓ zafirlukast

ANTICHOLINERGICS

Mainly used in the emergency department for acute attacks. See COPD section for more detail.

OMALIZUMAB *(XOLAIR)*

IgG monoclonal antibody that inhibits IgE binding to the IgE receptor on mast cells and basophils. Omalizumab is indicated for moderate to severe persistent asthma in patients with a positive skin test to perennial aeroallergen and inadequately controlled symptoms on inhaled steroids (Step 5 or 6 per guidelines)

DRUG	DOSING	SIDE EFFECTS/CONTRAINDICATIONS/MONITORING
Omalizumab *(Xolair)*	Based on pretreatment serum IgE levels and body wt – given SC every 2 or 4 wks Drug should always be given in the doctor's office	**BLACK BOX WARNING** Anaphylaxis, including delayed-onset, can occur. Reactions usually occur within 2 hours of administration but can be delayed up to 24 hours. Observe patients after *Xolair* administration. **SIDE EFFECTS** Headache, injection site reactions, upper respiratory tract infections, sinusitis, viral infection, arthralgia, and pain. Possible malignancies. **MONITORING** Baseline IgE, FEV1, peak flow, and body weight.

"RESCUERS" – THESE AGENTS ARE COMMONLY USED IN ASTHMA EXACERBATIONS	"CONTROLLERS" – OR LONG-TERM, MAINTENANCE THERAPY
Short-acting β_2 agonists Systemic (IV) steroids Anticholinergics	Inhaled steroids Leukotriene Modifying Agents Theophylline Long-acting β_2 agonists Cromolyn Omalizumab *(Xolair)*

CLASSIFYING ASTHMA SEVERITY & INITIATING TREATMENT
IN YOUTHS ≥ 12 YEARS OF AGE AND ADULTS

Components of Severity		Classification of Asthma Severity ≥12 years of age			
			Persistent		
		Intermittent	Mild	Moderate	Severe
Impairment Normal FEV₁/FVC: 8–19 yr 85% 20–39 yr 80% 40–59 yr 75% 60–80 yr 70%	Symptoms	≤2 days/week	>2 days/week but not daily	Daily	Throughout the day
	Nighttime awakenings	≤2x/month	3–4x/month	>1x/week but not nightly	Often 7x/week
	Short-acting beta₂-agonist use for symptom control (not prevention of EIB)	≤2 days/week	>2 days/week but not daily, and not more than 1x on any day	Daily	Several times per day
	Interference with normal activity	None	Minor limitation	Some limitation	Extremely limited
	Lung function	• Normal FEV₁ between exacerbations • FEV₁ >80% predicted • FEV₁/FVC normal	• FEV₁ >80% predicted • FEV₁/FVC normal	• FEV₁ >60% but <80% predicted • FEV₁/FVC reduced 5%	• FEV₁ <60% predicted • FEV₁/FVC reduced >5%
Risk	Exacerbations requiring oral systemic corticosteroids	0–1/year (see note)	≥2/year (see note) →→→→→		
		←—— Consider severity and interval since last exacerbation. ——→ Frequency and severity may fluctuate over time for patients in any severity category. Relative annual risk of exacerbations may be related to FEV₁.			
Recommended Step for Initiating Treatment (See figure 4–5 for treatment steps.)		Step 1	Step 2	**Step 3** and consider short course of oral systemic corticosteroids	**Step 4 or 5**
		In 2–6 weeks, evaluate level of asthma control that is achieved and adjust therapy accordingly.			

—

Key: FEV₁, forced expiratory volume in 1 second; FVC, forced vital capacity; ICU, intensive care unit

Notes:

■ The stepwise approach is meant to assist, not replace, the clinical decisionmaking required to meet individual patient needs.

■ Level of severity is determined by assessment of both impairment and risk. Assess impairment domain by patient's/caregiver's recall of previous 2–4 weeks and spirometry. Assign severity to the most severe category in which any feature occurs.

■ At present, there are inadequate data to correspond frequencies of exacerbations with different levels of asthma severity. In general, more frequent and intense exacerbations (e.g., requiring urgent, unscheduled care, hospitalization, or ICU admission) indicate greater underlying disease severity. For treatment purposes, patients who had ≥2 exacerbations requiring oral systemic corticosteroids in the past year may be considered the same as patients who have persistent asthma, even in the absence of impairment levels consistent with persistent asthma.

ASSESSING ASTHMA CONTROL & ADJUSTING THERAPY
IN YOUTHS ≥ 12 YEARS OF AGE AND ADULTS

Components of Control		Classification of Asthma Control (≥12 years of age)		
		Well Controlled	**Not Well Controlled**	**Very Poorly Controlled**
Impairment	Symptoms	≤2 days/week	>2 days/week	Throughout the day
	Nighttime awakenings	≤2x/month	1–3x/week	≥4x/week
	Interference with normal activity	None	Some limitation	Extremely limited
	Short-acting beta$_2$-agonist use for symptom control (not prevention of EIB)	≤2 days/week	>2 days/week	Several times per day
	FEV$_1$ or peak flow	>80% predicted/ personal best	60–80% predicted/ personal best	<60% predicted/ personal best
	Validated questionnaires ATAQ ACQ ACT	0 ≤0.75* ≥20	1–2 ≥1.5 16–19	3–4 N/A ≤15
Risk	Exacerbations requiring oral systemic corticosteroids	0–1/year	≥2/year (see note)	
		Consider severity and interval since last exacerbation		
	Progressive loss of lung function	Evaluation requires long-term followup care		
	Treatment-related adverse effects	Medication side effects can vary in intensity from none to very troublesome and worrisome. The level of intensity does not correlate to specific levels of control but should be considered in the overall assessment of risk.		
Recommended Action for Treatment (see figure 4–5 for treatment steps)		• Maintain current step. • Regular followups every 1–6 months to maintain control. • Consider step down if well controlled for at least 3 months.	• Step up 1 step and • Reevaluate in 2–6 weeks. • For side effects, consider alternative treatment options.	• Consider short course of oral systemic corticosteroids. • Step up 1–2 steps, and • Reevaluate in 2 weeks. • For side effects, consider alternative treatment options.

— *ACQ values of 0.76–1.4 are indeterminate regarding well-controlled asthma.
— Key: EIB, exercise-induced bronchospasm; ICU, intensive care unit

Notes:

■ The stepwise approach is meant to assist, not replace, the clinical decisionmaking required to meet individual patient needs.

■ The level of control is based on the most severe impairment or risk category. Assess impairment domain by patient's recall of previous 2–4 weeks and by spirometry/or peak flow measures. Symptom assessment for longer periods should reflect a global assessment, such as inquiring whether the patient's asthma is better or worse since the last visit.

■ At present, there are inadequate data to correspond frequencies of exacerbations with different levels of asthma control. In general, more frequent and intense exacerbations (e.g., requiring urgent, unscheduled care, hospitalization, or ICU admission) indicate poorer disease control. For treatment purposes, patients who had ≥2 exacerbations requiring oral systemic corticosteroids in the past year may be considered the same as patients who have not-well-controlled asthma, even in the absence of impairment levels consistent with not-well-controlled asthma.

■ Validated Questionnaires for the impairment domain (the questionnaires do not assess lung function or the risk domain)
    ATAQ = Asthma Therapy Assessment Questionnaire© (See sample in "Component 1: Measures of Asthma Assessment and Monitoring.")
    ACQ = Asthma Control Questionnaire© (user package may be obtained at www.qoltech.co.uk or juniper@qoltech.co.uk)
    ACT = Asthma Control Test™ (See sample in "Component 1: Measures of Asthma Assessment and Monitoring.")
    Minimal Important Difference: 1.0 for the ATAQ; 0.5 for the ACQ; not determined for the ACT.

■ Before step up in therapy:
— Review adherence to medication, inhaler technique, environmental control, and comorbid conditions.
— If an alternative treatment option was used in a step, discontinue and use the preferred treatment for that step.

STEPWISE APPROACH FOR MANAGING ASTHMA IN YOUTHS ≥ 12 YEARS OF AGE AND ADULTS

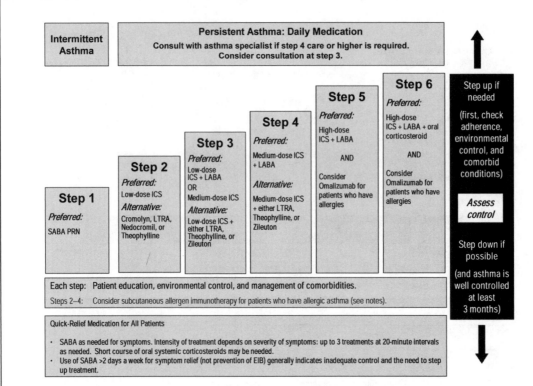

—   Key: **Alphabetical order is used when more than one treatment option is listed within either preferred or alternative therapy.** EIB, exercise-induced bronchospasm; ICS, inhaled corticosteroid; LABA, long-acting inhaled beta$_2$-agonist; LTRA, leukotriene receptor antagonist; SABA, inhaled short-acting beta$_2$-agonist

Notes:

■   The stepwise approach is meant to assist, not replace, the clinical decisionmaking required to meet individual patient needs.

■   If alternative treatment is used and response is inadequate, discontinue it and use the preferred treatment before stepping up.

■   Zileuton is a less desirable alternative due to limited studies as adjunctive therapy and the need to monitor liver function. Theophylline requires monitoring of serum concentration levels.

■   In step 6, before oral systemic corticosteroids are introduced, a trial of high-dose ICS + LABA + either LTRA, theophylline, or zileuton may be considered, although this approach has not been studied in clinical trials.

■   Step 1, 2, and 3 preferred therapies are based on Evidence A; step 3 alternative therapy is based on Evidence A for LTRA, Evidence B for theophylline, and Evidence D for zileuton. Step 4 preferred therapy is based on Evidence B, and alternative therapy is based on Evidence B for LTRA and theophylline and Evidence D for zileuton. Step 5 preferred therapy is based on Evidence B. Step 6 preferred therapy is based on (EPR—2 1997) and Evidence B for omalizumab.

■   Immunotherapy for steps 2–4 is based on Evidence B for house-dust mites, animal danders, and pollens; evidence is weak or lacking for molds and cockroaches. Evidence is strongest for immunotherapy with single allergens. The role of allergy in asthma is greater in children than in adults.

■   Clinicians who administer immunotherapy or omalizumab should be prepared and equipped to identify and treat anaphylaxis that may occur.

SAMPLE ASTHMA ACTION PLAN (ADULT)

ENGLISH

My Asthma Action Plan

Patient Name: _____

Medical Record #: _____

Physician's Name: _____ DOB: _____

Physician's Phone #: _____ Completed by: _____ Date: _____

Long-Term-Control Medicines	How Much To Take	How Often	Other Instructions
		_____ times per day **EVERY DAY!**	
		_____ times per day **EVERY DAY!**	
		_____ times per day **EVERY DAY!**	
		_____ times per day **EVERY DAY!**	

Quick-Relief Medicines	How Much To Take	How Often	Other Instructions
		Take ONLY as needed	NOTE: If this medicine is needed frequently, call physician to consider increasing long-term-control medications.

Special instructions when I feel ● *good,* ○ *not good,* and ● *awful.*

I feel *good.*
(My peak flow is in the GREEN zone.)

GREEN ZONE

My Personal Best Peak Flow

I do *not* feel *good.*
(My peak flow is in the YELLOW zone.)

80% Personal Best

My symptoms may include one or more of the following:
• Wheeze
• Tight chest
• Cough
• Shortness of breath
• Waking up at night with asthma symptoms
• Decreased ability to do usual activities
• _____
_____

YELLOW ZONE

I feel *awful.*
(My peak flow is in the RED zone.)

50% Personal Best

Warning signs may include one or more of the following:
• It's getting harder and harder to breathe
• Unable to sleep or do usual activities because of trouble breathing

Liters/Min.

Peak Flow Meter

RED ZONE

Danger! Get help immediately!

PREVENT asthma symptoms everyday:

☐ Take my long-term-control medicines (above) every day.

☐ Before exercise, take _____ puffs of _____

☐ Avoid things that make my asthma worse like:
_____

CAUTION. I should continue taking my long-term-control asthma medicines every day AND:

☐ Take _____
_____

If I still do not feel good, or my peak flow is not back in the *Green Zone* within 1 hour, then I should:

☐ Increase _____

☐ Add _____
_____

☐ Call _____

MEDICAL ALERT! *Get help!*

☐ Take _____
until I get help immediately.

☐ Take _____

☐ Call _____

Call 9–1–1 if you have trouble walking or talking due to shortness of breath or lips or fingernails are gray or blue.

Peak Flow Meters

INTRODUCTION
- Peak expiratory flow rate (PEFR) – the greatest velocity attained during a forced expiration starting from fully inflated lungs

- Determined by height, gender, and age

- PEFR is effort dependent

PURPOSE
- Identifies exacerbations early allowing patient to initiate treatment sooner

- Peak flow may show changes before patient can feel the symptoms

- Physician can adjust treatment to prevent emergency room visits and hospitalizations

- Proper technique and best effort are essential. Less than best effort can lead to false 'exacerbation' and unnecessary medication treatment

ZONES

Green zone (80-100% of personal best)
- Indicates "all clear" – good control

- Patients are instructed to follow routine maintenance plan

Yellow zone (50-80% of personal best)
- Indicates "caution" – indicative of worsening lung function

- Patient-specific intervention required (action plan) – usually an increase in beta$_2$-agonist use and the addition or increase in other medications

Red zone (< 50% of personal best)
- Indicates medical alert and patient needs to seek medical attention

- Patient-specific intervention required (action plan) – usually patients increase use of beta$_2$-agonist, take steroids, and are sent to the emergency room

PERSONAL BEST/PREDICTED PEFR OBTAINED BY PEAK FLOW METER
- To obtain your personal best, use your peak flow meter several times each day for 2-3 weeks

- Take a reading between noon and 2:00 pm each day

- Write down each number you get and the highest number over this time period will be your personal best number

- Your personal best can change over time so it is wise to obtain your personal best annually

TECHNIQUE

- Move the indicator to bottom of numbered scale. Stand up straight. Exhale comfortably.

- Inhale as deeply as you can. Place lips firmly around mouthpiece, creating a tight seal.

- Blow out as <u>hard</u> and as <u>fast</u> as possible. Write down the PEFR.

- Repeat steps two more times. Record the highest value.

PEAK FLOW METER USE TO MONITOR ASTHMA

- Use the peak flow meter every morning you wake up, before you take medicine.

- Always use the same brand of peak flow meters.

- Peak flow meters should be cleaned once a week at least; if patient has an infection, they should clean more frequently. Wash peak flow meters in warm water with <u>mild soap.</u> Rinse gently but thoroughly.

- Do not use brushes to clean inside the peak flow meters. Do not place peak flow meters in boiling water.

- Allow to air dry before taking next reading.

SPACERS

- Some spacer devices and chambers greatly enhance the coordination necessary to administer inhaled medication from a MDI.

- Spacer devices help <u>prevent thrush</u> from inhaled corticosteroids and can reduce cough associated with some inhalers.

- Need to clean at least <u>once a week</u> in warm, <u>soapy water.</u>

- Do not share spacer devices with anyone.

PATIENT COUNSELING

Albuterol MDI (e.g. *ProAir HFA)*

- Check each time to make sure the canister fits firmly in the plastic actuator. Remove the cap off the mouthpiece. Look into mouthpiece to make sure there are no foreign objects there, especially if the cap is not being used to cover the mouthpiece.

- Prime the inhaler before you use it for the first time or if you have not used it for > 14 days. To prime, spray it into the air away from your face. Shake and spray the inhaler 2 more times to finish priming it.

- <u>Shake the inhaler well before each spray.</u>

- Hold the inhaler with the mouthpiece down. <u>Breathe out fully through your mouth</u>. Put the mouthpiece in your mouth and close your lips around it.

- <u>Push the top of the canister all the way down while you breathe in deeply and slowly through your mouth</u>. Right after the spray comes out, take your finger off the canister. After you have inhaled in all the way, take the inhaler out of your mouth and close your mouth.

- <u>Hold your breath as long as you can</u>, up to 10 seconds, then breathe normally.

- If your doctor has prescribed more sprays, wait 1 minute and <u>shake</u> the inhaler again. Repeat.

- Put the cap back on the mouthpiece after every time you use the inhaler.

- <u>Throw the inhaler away</u> when you have used 200 sprays. You should not keep using the inhaler after 200 sprays even though the canister may not be completely empty because you cannot be sure you will receive any medicine.

- <u>Do not use the inhaler</u> after the expiration date, which is on the packaging it comes in.

- The inhaler should be stored at room temperature. Do not leave it in extreme temperatures.

Advair Diskus

- Take *ADVAIR DISKUS* out of the box and foil pouch. Write the "Pouch opened" and "Use by" dates on the label on top of the *DISKUS*. The "Use by" date is 1 month from date of opening the pouch. The *DISKUS* will be in the closed position when the pouch is opened.

- The dose indicator on the top of the *DISKUS* tells you how many doses are left. The dose indicator number will decrease each time you use the *DISKUS*. After you have used 55 doses from the *DISKUS*, the numbers 5 to 0 will appear in red to warn you that there are only a few doses left

- Hold the *DISKUS* in one hand and put the thumb of your other hand on the thumbgrip. Push your thumb away from you as far as it will go until the mouthpiece appears and snaps into position.

- Hold the *DISKUS* in a level, flat position with the mouthpiece towards you. Slide the lever away from you as far as it will go until it clicks. The *DISKUS* is now ready to use.

- To avoid releasing or wasting doses once the *DISKUS* is ready: do not close the *DISKUS*, do not tilt the *DISKUS*, do not play with the lever, and do not move the lever more than once.

- Before inhaling your dose from the *DISKUS*, breathe out (exhale) fully while holding the *DISKUS* level and away from your mouth. <u>Remember, never breathe out into the *DISKUS* mouthpiece</u>.

- Put the mouthpiece to your lips. Breathe in quickly and deeply through the *DISKUS*. Do not breathe in through your nose.

- Remove the *DISKUS* from your mouth. Hold your breath for about 10 seconds, or for as long as is comfortable. Breathe out slowly.

- The *DISKUS* delivers your dose of medicine as a very fine powder. Most patients can taste or feel the powder. Do not use another dose from the *DISKUS* if you do not feel or taste the medicine.

- Rinse your mouth with water after breathing-in the medicine. Spit the water out. Do not swallow.

- Close the *DISKUS* when you are finished taking a dose so that the *DISKUS* will be ready for you to take your next dose. Put your thumb on the thumbgrip and slide the thumbgrip back towards you as far as it will go. The *DISKUS* will click shut. The lever will automatically return to its original position. The *DISKUS* is now ready for you to take your next scheduled dose, due in about 12 hours.

- Never breathe into the *DISKUS*.

- Never take the *DISKUS* apart.

- Always ready and use the *DISKUS* in a level, flat position.

- Do not use the *DISKUS* with a spacer device.

- After each dose, rinse your mouth with water and spit the water out. Do not swallow.

- Never wash the mouthpiece or any part of the *DISKUS*. Keep it dry.

- Always keep the *DISKUS* in a dry place.

- Never take an extra dose, even if you did not taste or feel the medicine.

Flovent HFA

- Take your *FLOVENT HFA* inhaler out of the moisture-protective foil pouch just before you use it for the first time. Safely throw away the foil pouch and the drying packet that comes inside the pouch.

- Before you use *FLOVENT HFA* for the first time, you must prime the inhaler so that you will get the right amount of medicine when you use it. To prime the inhaler, take the cap off the mouthpiece and shake the inhaler well for 5 seconds. Then spray the inhaler into the air away from your face. Avoid spraying in eyes. Shake and spray the inhaler like this 3 more times to finish priming it. The counter should now read 120.

- You must prime the inhaler again if you have not used it in more than 7 days or if you drop it. Take the cap off the mouthpiece and shake the inhaler well for 5 seconds. Then spray it 1 time into the air away from your face.

- An adult should watch a child use the inhaler to be sure it is used correctly. If a child needs help using the inhaler, an adult should help the child use the inhaler with or without a holding chamber attached to a facemask. The adult should follow the instructions that came with the holding chamber.

- Take the cap off the mouthpiece of the actuator.

- Look inside the mouthpiece for foreign objects. Make sure the mouthpiece is clean and free of debris. Make sure the canister fits firmly in the actuator.

- Shake the inhaler well for 5 seconds.

- Hold the inhaler with the mouthpiece down. Breathe out through your mouth and push as much air from your lungs as you can. Put the mouthpiece in your mouth and close your lips around it.

- Push the top of the canister all the way down while you breathe in deeply and slowly through your mouth

- Right after the spray comes out, take your finger off the canister. After you have breathed in all the way, take the inhaler out of your mouth and close your mouth.

- Hold your breath as long as you can, up to 10 seconds. Then breathe normally.

- After you finish taking this medicine, rinse your mouth with water. Spit out the water. Do not swallow it.

- Put the cap back on the mouthpiece after each time you use the inhaler. Make sure it snaps firmly into place.

- Clean the inhaler at least once a week after your evening dose. It is important to keep the canister and plastic actuator clean so the medicine will not build-up and block the spray.

- Take the cap off the mouthpiece. The strap on the cap will stay attached to the actuator. Do not take the canister out of the plastic actuator.

- Use a clean cotton swab dampened with water to clean the small circular opening where the medicine sprays out of the canister. Gently twist the swab in a circular motion to take off any medicine. Repeat with a new swab dampened with water to take off any medicine still at the opening.

- Wipe the inside of the mouthpiece with a clean tissue dampened with water. Let the actuator air-dry overnight.

- Put the cap back on the mouthpiece after the actuator has dried.

- Store at room temperature with the mouthpiece down.

- Do not use the inhaler after the expiration date, which is on the packaging it comes in.

Symbicort HFA

- Take 2 puffs in the morning and 2 puffs in the evening every day.

- Rinse your mouth with water and spit the water our after each dose (2 puffs) of *Symbicort*. Do not swallow the water. This will help lessen the chance of getting a fungus infection (thrush) in your mouth.

- *Symbicort* does not relieve sudden symptoms and should never be used as a rescue inhaler. Always have a rescue inhaler with you to treat sudden symptoms.

- Throw away *Symbicort* when the counter reaches zero or 3 months after you take *Symbicort* out if its foil pouch, whichever comes first.

- A counter is attached to the top of the metal canister. This counter will count down each time you release a puff of *Symbicort*. The arrow points to the number of inhalations left in the canister.

- Shake your *Symbicort* inhaler well for 5 seconds right before each use. Remove mouthpiece cover and check for foreign objects.

- Prime your inhaler before you use it. Shake for 5 seconds and release a test spray, Shake again for 5 seconds and release another test spray. Your inhaler is now ready to use.

- If you do not use your *Symbicort* inhaler for more than 7 days or if you drop it, you will need to prime again.

- Do proper inhaler technique (mentioned under *Flovent HFA).*

- Clean the inhaler every 7 days. To clean, remove mouthpiece cover, wipe inside and outside the mouthpiece with a clean, dry cloth. Replace mouthpiece cover. Do NOT put *Symbicort* inhaler into water.

Singulair

For adults and children 12 months of age and older with asthma:

- Take *SINGULAIR* once a day in the evening.

- Take *SINGULAIR* every day for as long as your doctor prescribes it, even if you have no asthma symptoms.

- You may take *SINGULAIR* with food or without food.

- If your asthma symptoms get worse, or if you need to increase the use of your inhaled rescue medicine for asthma attacks, call your doctor right away.

- Do not take *SINGULAIR* for the immediate relief of an asthma attack. If you get an asthma attack, you should follow the instructions your doctor gave you for treating asthma attacks.

- Always have your inhaled rescue medicine for asthma attacks with you.

- Do not stop taking or lower the dose of your other asthma medicines unless your doctor tells you to.

- The most common side effects with *SINGULAIR* include: stomach pain, heartburn, tiredness, fever, stuffy nose, cough, flu, etc.

For patients 15 years of age and older for the prevention of exercise-induced asthma:

- Take *SINGULAIR* at least 2 hours before exercise.

- Always have your inhaled rescue medicine for asthma attacks with you.

- If you are taking *SINGULAIR* daily for chronic asthma or allergic rhinitis, do not take an additional dose to prevent exercise-induced asthma. Speak to your doctor about your treatment of exercise-induced asthma.

- Do not take an additional dose of *SINGULAIR* within 24 hours of a previous dose.

For adults and children 2 years of age and older with seasonal allergic rhinitis, or for adults and children 6 months of age and older with perennial allergic rhinitis:

- Take *SINGULAIR* once a day, at about the same time each day.

- Take *SINGULAIR* every day for as long as your doctor prescribes it.

- You may take *SINGULAIR* with food or without food.

How should I give *SINGULAIR* oral granules to my child?

- Do not open the packet until ready to use.

- *SINGULAIR* 4-mg oral granules can be given:

  - directly in the mouth;

  - dissolved in 1 teaspoonful (5 mL) of cold or room temperature baby formula or breast milk;

  - mixed with a spoonful of one of the following soft foods at cold or room temperature:

applesauce, mashed carrots, rice, or ice cream. Be sure that the entire dose is mixed with the food, baby formula, or breast milk and that the child is given the entire spoonful of the food, baby formula, or breast milk mixture right away (within 15 minutes).

- <u>Important:</u> Never store any oral granules mixed with food, baby formula, or breast milk for use at a later time. Throw away any unused portion. Do not put *SINGULAIR* oral granules in any liquid drink other than baby formula or breast milk.

Practice Case

Terri is a 22 year-old female patient who comes to your pharmacy and asks for a refill on all her asthma medications. You ask her how she is doing and see states that she has been using her *Maxair* inhaler 4 times/week for chest tightness and shortness of breath. She asks you to recommend a good sleep agent to help her fall back asleep. You notice that she is also picking up ferrous sulfate tablets, aspirin, *Dexatrim*, *Sucrets* lozenges, and *Maalox*. Terri is a college student who lives with her parents.

CATEGORY	
Medications	*Maxair* 1-2 puffs Q4-6H PRN (last refilled 18 days ago)
	Flovent Diskus 100 mcg/inh - take 2 inh BID (last refilled 27 days ago)
	Singulair 10 mg daily (last refilled 27 days ago)
	Aciphex 20 mg daily (last refilled 27 days ago)
	Advil 200 mg TID PRN headaches
	Ferrous Sulfate 325 mg daily

QUESTIONS

1. Terri seems to be exhibiting signs of uncontrolled asthma. Which of the following would be the <u>best</u> recommendation for better control?

    a. Take *Maxair* on a scheduled basis.

    b. Change the *Flovent Diskus* to 3 inhalations BID.

    c. Take *Singulair* 10 mg BID.

    d. Go to the emergency room as she is having an acute asthma attack.

    e. Elevate the head of the bed by 30 degrees when she sleeps.

2. Terri states that she doesn't understand why her asthma is worsening. Which of the following could be a trigger for her symptoms?

    a. Living in the same place for many years

    b. NSAID use

    c. Ferrous sulfate use

    d. *Aciphex* use

    e. She could be sleeping on her stomach more

3. Terri asks you if the *Sucrets* lozenges will help the sore throat she has. She was told by her doctor that she has signs of thrush. You should recommend the following to prevent this from happening in the future:

    a. Take the *Sucrets* lozenges because they will help with her sore throat and cure thrush.

    b. Recommend that she gargle with warm salt water instead.

    c. Recommend that she rinse her mouth after her *Flovent Diskus*, if not already doing so.

    d. Tell her to save her money; *Sucrets* do not work.

    e. Tell her to purchase a spacer device for the *Flovent Diskus*.

4. Terri comes back to your pharmacy with a prescription for *Foradil*. Which of the following statements is correct?

    a. The medication can be stored at room temperature by Terri.

    b. This medication needs to be taken with 8 oz of water.

    c. This medication needs to be stored in a refrigerator when not in use.

    d. This medication is taken once daily.

    e. This medication will interact with *Aciphex*.

5. Which of the following side effects is most likely to occur when using *Foradil* therapy?

   a. Neuropsychiatric behavior

   b. Palpitations

   c. Stomach upset

   d. Enuresis

   e. Depression

6. Terri comes to you 2 months later after a severe asthma exacerbation. She is currently taking dexamethasone 3 mg po daily. Convert her to an equivalent dose of prednisone. This dose would be:

   a. 20 mg

   b. 12 mg

   c. 3.75 mg

   d. 2 mg

   e. 0.75 mg

7. Terri is placed on theophylline therapy for treatment of her asthma. Which of the following can decrease theophylline levels?

   a. Ciprofloxacin

   b. Carbamazepine

   c. Erythromycin

   d. Cirrhosis

   e. None of the above

Questions 8-10 do not relate to the above case.

8. Omalizumab has a black box warning for:

   a. Anaphylaxis

   b. Stevens-Johnson syndrome

   c. Thrombocytopenia

   d. GI ulcers

   e. Increased risk of MI

9. A patient with asthma has been prescribed the *Advair Diskus*. Which of the following statements is correct?

   a. *Advair Diskus* contains fluticasone, a long-acting beta$_2$ agonist.

   b. *Advair Diskus* contains formoterol, an inhaled corticosteroid.

   c. *Advair Diskus* is usually dosed 2 inhalations once daily.

   d. *Advair Diskus* treats both airway constriction and inflammation.

   e. All of the above.

10. Carla is a 10 year old girl with asthma. The physician wants to give her montelukast, but is not sure of the correct dose. Choose the correct dose of montelukast for a 10-year old child:

   a. A 5 mg chewable tablet taken BID

   b. A 5 mg tablet chewable taken once daily

   c. A 10 mg chewable tablet taken once daily

   d. A 10 mg chewable tablet taken BID

   e. A 4 mg packet of granules mixed with milk

11. The therapeutic range for theophylline is:

   a. 10-20 mcg/mL

   b. 5-10 mcg/mL

   c. 5-15 mg/mL

   d. 8-12 mg/mL

   e. 5-15 mcg/mL

ANSWERS

1-b, 2-b, 3-c, 4-a, 5-b, 6-a, 7-b, 8-a, 9-d, 10-b, 11-e

COPD

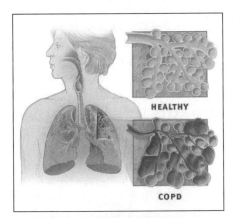

GUIDELINE

Global Strategy for the Diagnosis, Management and Prevention of COPD, Global Initiative for Chronic Obstructive Lung Disease (GOLD) 2010 update. Available at: http://www.goldcopd.org/uploads/users/files/GOLDReport_April112011.pdf

Background

Chronic obstructive pulmonary disease (COPD), which encompasses chronic bronchitis and emphysema, is a preventable and somewhat treatable disease characterized by chronic, progressive airflow limitation. In contrast to asthma, the limitation of airflow is not fully reversible and generally worsens over time. COPD is the 4th leading cause of death in the United States and its incidence is on the rise.

COPD is caused by noxious particles or gas, <u>most commonly from tobacco smoking</u>, which triggers an abnormal inflammatory response in the lung. The inflammatory response in the larger airways is known as chronic bronchitis, which is diagnosed clinically when symptoms of chronic cough and sputum production are present. In the alveoli, the inflammatory response causes destruction of the tissues of the lung, a process known as emphysema. Therefore, the pathological changes include chronic inflammation and structural changes resulting from repeated injury and repair. The natural course of COPD is characterized by occasional, sudden worsening of symptoms called acute exacerbations, most of which are caused by infections or air pollution.

A clinical diagnosis of COPD should be considered in any patient who has <u>dyspnea</u> (particularly persistent and progressive), <u>chronic cough or sputum production</u>, and/or a history of exposure to risk factors for the disease. The diagnosis should be confirmed by spirometry. <u>Smoking cessation</u> is the only management strategy proven to slow progression of disease. Other important management strategies include <u>vaccinations</u>, pulmonary rehabilitation programs, and <u>drug therapy (often using inhalers)</u>. Some patients go on to requiring long-term <u>oxygen</u> therapy or lung transplantation.

RISK FACTORS

The major risk factors for developing COPD include <u>smoking</u>, alpha-1 antitrypsin deficiency, occupational dusts and chemicals (chemical agents and fumes), and indoor and outdoor air pollution.

PHARMACOLOGICAL MANAGEMENT

No medication used in COPD has been shown to modify the long-term decline in lung function that is the hallmark of COPD. Therefore, pharmacotherapy is used to decrease symptoms and/or complications. Bronchodilators (beta$_2$-agonists, anticholinergics) are used as-needed or on a regular basis, depending on symptom severity. If used on a regular basis, long-acting bronchodilators are more effective and more convenient than treatment with short-acting bronchodilators. <u>The combination of a short-acting beta$_2$ agonist and an anticholinergic produces greater improvements in lung function that either drug given alone. The addition of an inhaled corticosteroid to bronchodilators is appropriate for symptomatic COPD patients with more severe disease</u> (Stage III and Stage IV disease). However, chronic treatment with systemic (oral) corticosteroids should be avoided due to an unfavorable benefit-risk ratio in most patients.

<u>Influenza (each fall) and pneumococcal vaccines</u> (x 1, repeat if > 65 years old and received vaccine more than 5 years ago) should be given to patients with COPD, unless contraindications exist. Vaccines are used to prevent infections and reduce the risk of acute exacerbations.

Treatment Algorithm for COPD

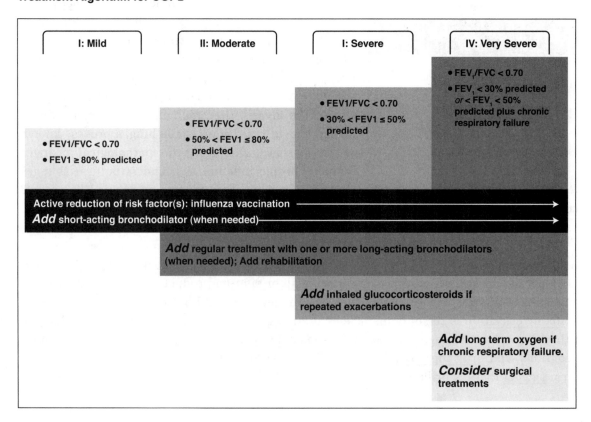

If patients have severe hereditary alpha-1 antitrypsin deficiency, they may be placed on an alpha-1 proteinase inhibitor *(Prolastin, Aralast, or Zemaira)* for chronic augmentation therapy. These agents are given as weekly IV infusions and are associated with many side effects, including anaphylaxis.

For treatment of acute COPD exacerbations, see the infectious disease section. Outside of antibiotics, an inhaled anticholinergic bronchodilator plus oral steroids (tapered over 2 weeks) are effective treatments. The use of azithromycin 250 mg/d reduces the risk of acute exacerbations due to its anti-inflammatory and immunomodulatory properties. Caution with use as it may decrease hearing.

Pharmacological Agents

DRUG	DOSING	SIDE EFFECTS/CONTRAINDICATIONS/MONITORING

Anticholinergics – block the action of acetylcholine [and ↓ cyclic guanosine monophosphate (cGMP)] at parasympathetic sites in bronchial smooth muscle causing bronchodilation.

Short-acting anticholinergics		Precaution: use with caution in patients with myasthenia gravis, narrow-angle glaucoma, benign prostatic hyperplasia, or bladder neck obstruction
Ipratropium bromide *(Atrovent HFA)*	1-2 inhalations TID-QID (MDI)	
	0.5 mg TID-QID (NEB)	**SIDE EFFECTS** Dry mouth (much more common with tiotropium), upper respiratory tract infections, pharyngeal irritation, sinusitis, and bitter taste
+ albuterol *(Combivent, Combivent Respimat, DuoNeb)*	2 inhalations QID	
	0.5 mg TID-QID (NEB)	Avoid spraying in the eyes
		Do NOT swallow capsules of tiotropium
Long-acting anticholinergic		*Combivent* contains soya lecithin – caution in patients with a soybean or peanut allergy
Tiotropium *(Spiriva HandiHaler)*	1 capsule inhaled daily via the HandiHaler device (requires 2 puffs)	Unlike *Combivent, Combivent Respimat* does not contain CFCs. *Combivent* will be phased out by Dec. 31, 2013.

Beta$_2$-agonists – bind to beta$_2$ receptors causing relaxation of bronchial smooth muscle, resulting in bronchodilation – inhaled route is the preferred route of administration. For short-acting beta$_2$-agonists, see asthma section

Long-acting Beta$_2$ agonists		**SIDE EFFECTS** Tremor, shakiness, lightheadedness, cough, palpitations, hypokalemia, tachycardia, and hyperglycemia
Salmeterol *(Serevent Diskus)*	1 inhalation BID	
+ fluticasone *(Advair Diskus)*	1 inhalation BID	Bronchodilators are used on a PRN or scheduled basis to reduce symptoms
+ fluticasone *(Advair HFA)*	2 inhalations BID	
Formoterol *(Foradil Aerolizer, Perforomist)*	12 mcg capsule via Aerolizer BID	Long-acting inhaled bronchodilators are more effective and convenient
	20 mcg BID (NEB)	Combination therapy with inhaled steroids can ↑ the risk of pneumonia, however, the combination showed a ↓ in exacerbations and improvement in lung function when compared to the individual components
+ budesonide *(Symbicort)*	2 inhalations BID	
+ mometasone *(Dulera)*	2 inhalations BID	
Arformoterol *(Brovana)*	15 mcg BID (NEB)	Arformoterol contains R-isomer of formoterol
Indacaterol *(Arcapta)*	75 mcg capsule via Neohaler device daily	

DRUG	DOSING	SIDE EFFECTS/CONTRAINDICATIONS/ MONITORING

Phosphodiesterase 4 inhibitor - PDE-4 inhibitor that ↑ cAMP levels, leading to a reduction in lung inflammation

Roflumilast *(Daliresp)*	500 mcg PO daily	**SIDE EFFECTS** Weight loss, ↓ appetite, diarrhea, insomnia, depression and psychiatric events including suicidality **CONTRAINDICATIONS** Moderate to severe liver impairment Use only in severe COPD due to modest benefit

See asthma section for details on theophylline and inhaled corticosteroids

DRUG INTERACTIONS WITH ROFLUMILAST

Roflumilast is a substrate of 3A4 and 1A2. Use with strong enzyme inducers (carbamazepine, phenobarbital, phenytoin, rifampin) is not recommended. Use with 3A4 inhibitors or dual 3A4 and 1A2 inhibitors (erythromycin, ketoconazole, fluvoxamine, cimetidine) will ↑ roflumilast levels.

PATIENT COUNSELING FOR *ATROVENT HFA*

- Insert the metal canister into the clear end of the mouthpiece. Make sure the canister is fully and firmly inserted into the mouthpiece.

- The *ATROVENT HFA* canister is to be used only with the *ATROVENT HFA* mouthpiece.

- Do not use the *ATROVENT HFA* mouthpiece with other inhaled medicines.

- Remove the green protective dust cap. If the cap is not on the mouthpiece, make sure there is nothing in the mouthpiece before use. For best results, the canister should be at room temperature before use.

- Breathe out (exhale) deeply through your mouth. Put the mouthpiece in your mouth and close your lips. Keep your eyes closed so that no medicine will be sprayed into your eyes. If sprayed into the eyes, *ATROVENT HFA* can cause blurry vision and other vision abnormalities, eye pain or discomfort, dilated pupils, or narrow-angle glaucoma or worsening of this condition. If any combination of these symptoms develops, you should consult your physician immediately.

- Breathe in (inhale) slowly through your mouth and at the same time spray the *ATROVENT HFA* into your mouth.

- Hold your breath for ten seconds and then take the mouthpiece out of your mouth and breathe out slowly.

- Replace the green protective dust cap after use.

- Keep the mouthpiece clean. At least once a week, wash the mouthpiece, shake it to remove excess water and let it air dry all the way.

- There are approximately 40 actuations (sprays) left when the dose indicator displays "40," where the background changes from green to red. This is when you need to refill your prescription or ask your doctor if you need another prescription for *ATROVENT HFA* inhalation aerosol. Discard the inhaler once the dose indicator displays "0".

PATIENT COUNSELING FOR *COMBIVENT*

COMBIVENT Inhalation Aerosol should not be used in patients who:

- Are allergic to soya lecithin or related food products such as soybeans and peanuts

- Are allergic to any of the ingredients in *COMBIVENT* Inhalation Aerosol or to atropine or other similar drugs

COMBIVENT Inhalation Aerosol can cause the narrowing of the airways to get worse (paradoxical bronchospasm) in some patients, which may be life threatening. If this happens, stop taking *COMBIVENT* Inhalation Aerosol at once and call your doctor or get emergency help.

1. Insert metal canister into clear end of mouthpiece. Make sure the canister is fully and firmly inserted into the mouthpiece. The *COMBIVENT* (ipratropium bromide and albuterol sulfate) Inhalation Aerosol canister is to be used only with the *COMBIVENT* (ipratropium bromide and albuterol sulfate) Inhalation Aerosol mouthpiece. This mouthpiece should not be used with other inhaled medicines.

2. Remove orange protective dust cap. If the cap is not on the mouthpiece, make sure there is nothing in the mouthpiece before use.

3. Shake and Test Spray. Perform this step before using for the first time, and whenever the aerosol has not been used for more than 24 hours; otherwise, proceed directly to Step 4. After vigorously shaking the canister for at least 10 seconds (see step 4 for instructions on shaking), "test-spray" into the air 3 times. <u>Avoid spraying in eyes.</u>

4. Shake the canister vigorously for at least 10 seconds. Vigorous shaking for at least 10 seconds before each spray is very important for proper product performance. For best results, perform Steps 5 and 6 within 30 seconds of shaking the canister.

5. Breathe out (exhale) deeply through your mouth. Holding the canister upright, put the mouthpiece in your mouth and close your lips. Keep your eyes closed so that no medicine will be sprayed into your eyes. *COMBIVENT* (ipratropium bromide and albuterol sulfate) can cause blurry vision, narrow-angle glaucoma or worsening of this condition or eye pain if the medicine is sprayed into your eyes.

6. Breathe in (inhale) slowly through your mouth and at the same time spray the product into your mouth.

7. Hold your breath for 10 seconds, remove the mouthpiece from your mouth and breathe out slowly.

8. Wait approximately 2 minutes, shake the inhaler vigorously for at least 10 seconds again (as described in Step 4), and repeat Steps 5 to 7.

9. Replace the orange protective dust cap after use.

10. Keep the mouthpiece clean. Wash with hot water. If soap is used, rinse thoroughly with plain water. Dry thoroughly before use. When dry, replace cap on the mouthpiece when not using the drug product.

11. Keep track of the number of sprays used and discard after 200 sprays. Even though the canister is not empty, you cannot be sure of the amount of medicine in each spray after 200 sprays.

If your prescribed dose does not provide relief or your breathing symptoms become worse, get medical help right away

PATIENT COUNSELING FOR *SPIRIVA*

- Do not swallow *SPIRIVA* capsules. *SPIRIVA* capsules should only be used with the HandiHaler device. *SPIRIVA* HandiHaler should only be inhaled through your mouth (oral inhalation).

- Do not open the *SPIRIVA* capsule before you insert it into the HandiHaler device.

- Open the dust cap by pressing the green piercing button.

- Pull the dust cap upwards to expose the mouthpiece.

- Open the mouthpiece by pulling the mouthpiece ridge upwards away from the base.

- Always store *SPIRIVA* capsules in the sealed blisters. Remove only one *SPIRIVA* capsule from the blister right before use. Do not store *SPIRIVA* capsules in the HandiHaler device. Inhale the contents of the *SPIRIVA* capsule using the HandiHaler device right away after the blister packaging of an individual *SPIRIVA* capsule is opened, or else it may not work as well.

- If more *SPIRIVA* capsules are opened to air, they should not be used and should be thrown away

- Insert the *SPIRIVA* capsule in the center chamber of the HandiHaler device. It does not matter which end of the *SPIRIVA* capsule you put in the chamber.

- Close the mouthpiece until you hear a click, but leave the dust cap open.

- Be sure that you have the mouthpiece sitting firmly against the gray base.

- Hold the HandiHaler device with the mouthpiece upright. It is important that you hold the HandiHaler device in an upright position when pressing the green piercing button.

- Press the green piercing button until it is flat against the base and release. This is how you make holes in the *SPIRIVA* capsule so that you get the medicine when you breathe in.

- Do not press the green button more than once.

- Breathe out completely. Do not breathe into the mouthpiece of the HandiHaler device at any time. Hold the HandiHaler device by the gray base. Do not block the air intake vents.

- Raise the HandiHaler device to your mouth and close your lips tightly around the mouthpiece.

- Keep your head in an upright position. The HandiHaler device should be in a horizontal position.

- Breathe in slowly and deeply so that you hear or feel the *SPIRIVA* capsule vibrate.

- Breathe in until your lungs are full.

- Hold your breath as long as is comfortable and at the same time take the HandiHaler device out of your mouth. Breathe normally again.

- To make sure you get the full dose, you must breathe out completely, and inhale again.

- If you do not hear or feel the *SPIRIVA* capsule vibrate, do not press the green piercing button again. Instead, hold the HandiHaler device in an upright position and tap the HandiHaler device gently on a table. Check to see that the mouthpiece is completely closed. Then, breathe in again.

- After you finish taking your daily dose of *SPIRIVA* HandiHaler, open the mouthpiece again. Tip out the used *SPIRIVA* capsule and throw it away.

- Close the mouthpiece and dust cap for storage of your HandiHaler device.

- Do not store used or unused *SPIRIVA* capsules in the HandiHaler device.

- Clean the HandiHaler device one time each month or as needed.

  - Open the dust cap and mouthpiece. Open the base by lifting the green piercing button.

  - Look at the center chamber for *SPIRIVA* capsule fragments or powder residue.

  - Rinse the HandiHaler device with warm water. Check that any powder buildup.

  - Do not use cleaning agents or detergents.

  - Do not place the HandiHaler device in the dishwasher for cleaning.

  - Dry the HandiHaler device well by tipping the excess water out on a paper towel. Air-dry afterwards, leaving the dust cap, mouthpiece, and base open.

  - Do not use a hair dryer to dry the HandiHaler device.

  - It takes 24 hours to air dry, so clean the HandiHaler device right after you use it so that it will be ready for your next dose.

  - Do not use the HandiHaler device when it is wet. If needed, you may clean the outside of the mouthpiece with a clean damp cloth.

38

SMOKING CESSATION

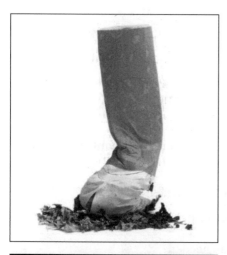

GUIDELINES/REFERENCES

Treating Tobacco Use and Dependence. 2008 Update. April 2009. U.S. Public Health Service. Agency for Healthcare Research and Quality. Available at http://www.ahrq.gov/clinic/

Galanti LM. Tobacco Smoking Cessation Management: Integrating Vareni-cline in Current Practice. Vasc Health Risk Manag 2009;4:837-45.

FDA Drug Safety Communication: Safety review update of Chantix (varenicline) and risk of neuropsychiatric adverse events, Available at: http://www.fda.gov/Drugs/DrugSafety/ucm276737.htm

Ashwin CA and Watts K. Women's use of Nicotine Replacement Therapy in Pregnancy-A Structured Review of the Literature. *Midwifery* 2010;26:304-10

Background

Tobacco dependence is a chronic disease that often requires repeated intervention and multiple attempts to quit. Effective treatments exist that can significantly increase rates of long-term abstinence. It is essential that clinicians and healthcare delivery systems <u>consistently identify and document tobacco use status</u> and treat every tobacco user seen in a healthcare setting.

<u>Counseling and medication</u> are more effective when used <u>together</u> than either modality used alone. Two counseling components that are especially effective are practical counseling (problem-solving/skills training) and social support delivered as part of treatment. <u>There is a strong correlation between counseling intensity and quitting success</u> (counseling sessions should be > 10 minutes in length and number of sessions should be ≥ 4).

Smoking accounts for more than 435,000 deaths per year in the U.S. It is a known cause of multiple cancers, heart disease, stroke, complications of pregnancy, COPD, and many other diseases. Still, roughly 21% of adult Americans smoke representing ~45 million current adult smokers.

<u>Nicotine replacement products are considered first-line</u> and there are 2 agents (5 nicotine and 2 non-nicotine) drugs that increase long-term smoking abstinence: Nicotine gum, inhaler, lozenge, nasal spray, patch and bupropion SR and varenicline. <u>Use combination</u> nicotine products (use extreme caution if any cardiovascular

condition because the side effects are additive) or combo with bupoprion, if a single agent is not enough (e.g., patch + gum or nasal spray or inhaler or bupropion SR + patch). Bupropion plus a nicotine product is used, but there is less evidence of benefit with this combination versus nicotine combinations. There is benefit (and increased side effects) with the use of bupropion and two nicotine products. Do not use varenicline with nicotine due to increased side effects.

Smoking causes an induction of some isoforms of the P450 system. Therefore, smokers who quit can experience side effects from supratherapeutic drug levels of caffeine, theophylline, fluvoxamine, olanzapine, and clozapine. High levels of clozapine have increased risk for agranulocytosis. Ensure that smokers get required vaccines, including pneumococcal (Pneumovax23) and an annual (fall) influenza vaccine. If no local programs are available smokers can get free assistance by calling the U.S. national quit-line network at 1-800-QUIT-NOW (1-800-784-8669) or 1-800-NO-BUTTS (1-800-258-9090). The help line has services available in 7 languages.

SMOKING IN PREGNANCY

Smoking in pregnancy can cause adverse outcomes for the child, including spontaneous abortion, low birth weight and sudden infant death. If women smoke 5 or less cigarettes daily (occasional, "nervous" type smokers) they should be encouraged to quit with behavioral support. If they smoke more than 5 cigarettes daily, ACOG recommends bupropion (pregnancy category C), and other sources recommend nicotine replacement in pregnancy, however the efficacy is not as high as it is in non-pregnant patients. All nicotine products are pregnancy category D, except the gum is pregnancy category C.

The "5 A's" model for treating tobacco use and dependence

ASK ABOUT TOBACCO USE
- Identify and document tobacco use status for every patient at every visit.

ADVISE TO QUIT
- In a clear, strong, and personalized manner, urge every tobacco user to quit.

ASSESS
- For current tobacco user, is the tobacco user willing to make a quit attempt at this time?

- For the ex-tobacco user, how recent did you quit and are there any challenges to remaining abstinent?

ASSIST
- For the patient willing to make a quit attempt, offer medication and provide or refer for counseling or additional behavioral treatment to help the patient quit.

- For patients unwilling to quit at this time, provide motivational interventions designed to increase future quit attempts.

- For the recent quitter and any with remaining challenges, provide relapse prevention.

ARRANGE

- All those receiving the previous A's should receive follow up.

NICOTINE REPLACEMENT THERAPY (NRT)

DRUG	DOSING	SIDE EFFECTS	CAUTIONS/NOTES
Nicotine gum (*Nicorette, etc.*) OTC	If < 25 cigs/d, use 2 mg gum If ≥ 25 cigs/d, use 4 mg gum 1 gum Q1-2H x 6 wks, then 1 gum Q2-4H x 3 wks, then 1 gum Q4-8H hrs x 3 wks; max 24 pieces/day Use up to 12 weeks	Dyspepsia, mouth soreness, hiccups, jaw ache	Nicotine replacement products are pregnancy category C (nicotine gum) and category D (transdermal patches, inhalers, and spray nicotine products) Cautions: recent MI (within 2 weeks), serious arrhythmias, serious or worsening angina
Nicotine Inhaler (*Nicotrol Inhaler*) Rx	6-16 cartridges daily; taper frequency of use over the last 6-12 weeks Use up to 6 months	Local irritation in the mouth and throat (40%), coughing (32%), rhinitis (23%)	Patients must show identification for proof of age prior to purchase of nicotine products since the FDA prohibits sale of nicotine products to individuals younger than 18 years of age (REMS)
Nicotine nasal spray (*Nicotrol NS*) Rx	1 dose = 2 sprays (1 spray in each nostril), give 1-2 doses per hour, ↑ PRN for symptom relief; 8- 40 doses/day Use 3-6 months	Nasal irritation (94% in 1st 2 days, ↓ to 81% afterwards), nasal congestion, transient changes in taste and smell	Gum has been shown to reduce or delay weight gain – review gum counseling at end of this section Inhaler has a hand to mouth use; mimics smoking action, providing a coping mechanism
Nicotine patch (*NicoDerm CQ, Habitrol*) OTC or Rx Highest adherence rate May need something else for acute cravings	7 mg/hr, 14 mg/hr, 21 mg/hr; apply upon waking on quit date If > 10 cigs/d, use 21 mg/24 hr x 6wk, then 14 mg/24 hr x 2 wk, then 7 mg/24 hr x 2wk If ≤ 10 cigs/d, use 14 mg/24 hr x 6 wk, then 7 mg/24 hr x 2 wk	Local skin reaction (50%), insomnia, vivid dreams	Nasal spray has the fastest delivery system; useful for rapid relief of withdrawal; highest dependence potential among NRT's. Avoid in severe reactive airway disease Patch is worn for 24 hrs, or for 16 hrs to avoid insomnia
Nicotine Lozenge (*Commit*) OTC	1st cigarette smoked > 30 min after waking up: use 2 mg lozenge 1st cigarette smoked within 30 min of waking up: use 4 mg lozenge Do not exceed 20 lozenges/day Minimum of 9 lozenges/day 1 lozenge Q1-2H x 6 wks, then 1 lozenge Q2-4H x 3 wks, then 1 lozenge Q4-8H x 3 wks.	Nausea, hiccups, heartburn	Lozenge has not been shown to be effective in pregnant smokers

ORAL PRESCRIPTION AGENTS

DRUG	DOSING	SIDE EFFECTS/CONTRAINDICATIONS/MONITORING
Bupropion SR *(Zyban)* Blocks neural re-uptake of dopamine and/or norepinephrine and blocks nicotinic acetylcholinergic receptors. Can be used in combo with NRT. Beneficial for smokers with history of depression – do not use in patients taking any other form of bupropion. Helpful to prevent weight gain when quitting. Counseling should include recomendations for diet and physical activity.	150 mg QAM for 3 days, then 150 mg BID. Start 1-2 weeks before quit date	**BLACK BOX WARNING** Not approved for use in children, not approved for bipolar, ↑ risk of suicidal thinking and behavior in young adults with depression or other psychiatric disorders **SIDE EFFECTS** Dry mouth, insomnia, headache/migraine, nausea/vomiting, constipation, and tremors/seizures (dose-related), possible blood pressure changes (more hypertension than hypotension – monitor), weight loss No effects on 5HT and therefore no sexual dysfunction **CONTRAINDICATIONS** History of seizures, eating disorder, use of MAO-I within the previous 14 days – 2 week washout required. Delays weight gain, can be used with CVD risk Do not exceed 450 mg/day due to seizure risk Preg Categ C (but used in pregnancy) MedGuide required because it is an antidepressant
Varenicline *(Chantix)* is a partial neuronal alpha4-beta2 nicotinic receptor agonist. Also stimulates dopamine activity to a small degree, resulting in reduced cravings and other withdrawal symptoms. Combo with NRTs not recommended due to nicotine antagonist properties.	Start one week before the quit date Days 1-3: 0.5 mg daily Days 4-7: 0.5 mg BID Days 8 (quit date) and beyond: 1 mg BID (use lower dosage to ↓ nausea and vomiting) Take with food and full glass of water to ↓ nausea Take 2nd pill at dinner rather than bedtime to ↓ insomnia	**BLACK BOX WARNING** Serious neuropsychiatric events including depression, suicidal ideation, suicide attempt and completed suicide have been reported in patients taking *Chantix*. Stop taking this medication if patients become hostile, agitated, depressed, or have changes in behavior or thinking that are not typical for the patient. **SIDE EFFECTS** Nausea (~30% and dose dependent), abnormal dreams, constipation, flatulence, vomiting Angioedema, hypersensitivity rxns, and serious skin reactions have occurred Reduce dose in patients with significant renal impairment (CrCl < 30 mL/min) Use with caution in pts with underlying psychiatric disorders and while driving or operating machinery, traffic accidents have occurred. Avoid use in pilots, air traffic controllers, commercial truckers, bus drivers. If patient has cardiovascular disease they can use if stable but need to STOP smoking-varenicline may exacerbate CVD, but at this point it is thought that risk may be worth the benefit. Preg Categ C MedGuide required

NICOTINE REPLACEMENT COUNSELING

Counseling with the nicotine gum

- Gum should be chewed slowly until a "peppery" or "flavored" taste emerges, then "parked" between cheek and gum to facilitate nicotine absorption through the oral mucosa. Gum should be slowly and intermittently chewed and parked for about 30 minutes or until the taste dissipates.

- Acidic beverages (e.g., coffee, juices, soft drinks) interfere with the buccal absorption of nicotine, so eating and drinking anything except water should be avoided for 15 minutes before or during chewing.

- Patients often do not use enough gum to obtain optimal clinical effects. Instruct to use at least 1 piece q1-2 hours.

Counseling with inhaler

- Frequent, continuous puffing for 20 minutes is advised with each cartridge. Once a cartridge is opened, it is only good for one day. Peak effect is achieved within 15 minutes. After your dose is established, it is generally maintained for 3 months and then gradually tapered during the following 3 months. Clean mouthpiece with soap and water regularly. Delivery of nicotine from the inhaler declines significantly below 40°F. In cold weather, the inhaler and cartridge should be kept in an inside pocket or other warm area.

- Acidic beverages (i.e. coffee, juices, soft drinks) interfere with the buccal absorption of nicotine, so eating and drinking anything except water should be avoided for 15 minutes before or during the use of the nicotine inhaler.

Counseling with the lozenge

- The lozenge should be allowed to dissolve in the mouth rather than chewing or swallowing it.

- Acidic beverages (i.e. coffee, juices, soft drinks) interfere with the buccal absorption of nicotine, so eating and drinking anything except water should be avoided for 15 minutes before or during use of the nicotine lozenge.

- Patients often do not use enough PRN nicotine replacement medications to obtain optimal clinical effects. Generally, patients should use 1 lozenge every 1-2 hours during the first 6 weeks of treatment, using a minimum of 9 lozenges/day, then decrease over time.

Counseling with nasal spray

- Patients should not sniff, swallow, or inhale through the nose while administering doses, as this increases irritating effects. The spray is best delivered with the head tilted slightly back.

Counseling with the nicotine patch

- At the start of each day, place the patch on a relatively hairless location, typically between the neck and waist, rotating the site to reduce local skin irritation.

- Patches should be applied <u>as soon as the patient wakes on the quit day.</u> With patients who experience <u>sleep disruption, have the patient remove the 24-hour patch prior to bedtime, or use the 16 hour patch.</u>

- Up to 50% of patients using the nicotine patch will experience a <u>local skin reaction.</u> Skin reactions usually are mild and self-limiting, but occasionally worsen over the course of therapy. Local treatment with hydrocortisone cream (1%) or triamcinolone cream (0.5%) and rotating patch sites may ameliorate the reaction. Fewer than 5% of patients discontinue patch treatment due to skin reactions.

Bupropion Counseling

- <u>It takes about 1 week for the medication to start working. For your best chance of quitting, you should not stop smoking until you have been taking for 1 week. Set a date to stop smoking during the second week of starting this medication.</u>

- The most common side effects are dry mouth and trouble sleeping. These side effects are generally mild and often disappear after a few weeks.

- Some people have severe allergic reactions to bupropion. Stop taking and call your doctor right away if you get a rash, itching, hives, fever, swollen lymph glands, painful sores in your mouth or around your eyes, swelling of your lips or tongue, chest pain, or have trouble breathing. These could be signs of a serious allergic reaction.

- <u>Do not take if have a seizure disorder, are taking *Wellbutrin* (IR, SR, or XL), or have taken an MAO-I within the last 14 days or had an eating disorder.</u>

- Do not chew, cut, or crush the tablets. If you do, the medicine will be released into your body too quickly. If this happens you may be more likely to get side effects including seizures. Tablets must be swallowed whole. Do not exceed 450 mg daily, or 150 mg at each dose if using the IR formulation, due to seizure risk.

- Take the doses at least 8 hours apart.

- <u>If you, your family, or caregiver notice agitation, hostility, depression or changes in behavior or thinking</u> that are not typical for you, or you develop any of the following symptoms, stop taking the medication and call your healthcare provider right away:

  - ❏ thoughts about suicide or dying, or attempts to commit suicide

  - ❏ new or worse depression, anxiety or panic attacks

  - ❏ feeling very agitated or restless

  - ❏ acting aggressive, being angry, or violent

  - ❏ acting on dangerous impulses

  - ❏ an extreme increase in activity and talking (mania)

  - ❏ abnormal thoughts or sensations

  - ❏ seeing or hearing things that are not there (hallucinations)

□ feeling people are against you (paranoia)

□ feeling confused

□ other unusual changes in behavior or mood

Varenicline Counseling

■ Choose a <u>quit date to stop smoking</u>.

■ <u>Start taking the medication 1 week (7 days) before the quit date</u>. This allows the medication to build up in the body. May continue to smoke during this time. Try to stop smoking on the quit date. If it doesn't happen, try again. Some people need to take the medication for a few weeks to work best.

■ Take the medication <u>after eating and with a full glass (8 ounces) of water</u>.

■ Most people will take this medicine for up to 12 weeks. If quit smoking by 12 weeks, another 12 weeks of therapy may helpful to stay cigarette-free.

■ Symptoms of nicotine withdrawal include the urge to smoke, depressed mood, trouble sleeping, irritability, frustration, anger, feeling anxious, difficulty concentrating, restlessness, decreased heart rate, and increased appetite or weight gain.

■ <u>Before taking this medication, tell your doctor if you have ever had depression or other mental health problems</u>.

■ <u>If you, your family, or caregiver notice agitation, hostility, depression or changes in behavior or thinking</u> that are not typical for you, or you develop any of the following symptoms, stop taking the medication and call your healthcare provider right away:

□ thoughts about suicide or dying, or attempts to commit suicide

□ new or worse depression, anxiety or panic attacks

□ feeling very agitated or restless

□ acting aggressive, being angry, or violent

□ acting on dangerous impulses

□ an extreme increase in activity and talking (mania)

□ abnormal thoughts or sensations

□ seeing or hearing things that are not there (hallucinations)

□ feeling people are against you (paranoia)

□ feeling confused

□ other unusual changes in behavior or mood

- Some people can have allergic reactions to this medication. Some of these allergic reactions can be life-threatening and include: swelling of the face, mouth, and throat that can cause trouble breathing. If these symptoms occur, stop taking the medication and get medical attention right away.

- Some people can have <u>serious skin reactions</u> while taking this medication. These can include rash, swelling, redness, and peeling of the skin. Some of these reactions can become life-threatening. If a rash with peeling skin or blisters in your mouth occurs, stop taking the medication and get medical attention right away.

- Tell your pharmacist about all your other medicines including prescription and nonprescription medicines, vitamins and herbal supplements. Especially, tell your pharmacist if you take: insulin, asthma medicines, or blood thinners.

- <u>Use caution driving or operating machinery</u> until you know how this medication may affect you. Some people may become sleepy, dizzy, or have trouble concentrating, that can make it hard to drive or perform other activities safely.

39

ALLERGIC RHINITIS, COUGH & COLD

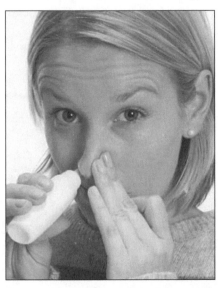

Background

Allergic Rhinitis (sometimes known as "hay fever") is the 6th most prevalent chronic disease and one where pharmacists can really assist patients in therapeutic options. Allergic rhinitis is a major reason for decreased work productivity, lost work or school days each year. Rhinitis is an inflammation of the membrane linings in the nose. Symptoms include sneezing, nasal itch, rhinorrhea, nasal congestion, and postnasal drip.

Following allergic rhinitis this chapter includes common cough and cold products and a discussion of safe options for children.

Non-Pharmacologic Management

This includes environmental control which means avoiding exposure to allergens, if possible. Neti pots, described later in this section, can be useful for some patients. Not overly sanitizing infants is important: children need to build a healthy immune system and over-worry about cleanliness ends up causing more illness.

Pharmacologic Management

Agents for itchy eyes are in the ophthalmic section. Intranasal corticosteroids are first line for moderate-to-severe rhinitis. Milder, intermittent symptoms can be treated with oral antihistamines. Decongestants are used for congestion, and come in nasal and oral formulations. A variety of other agents can be modestly useful.

INTRANASAL CORTICOSTEROIDS

The most effective medication class in controlling symptoms of allergic rhinitis and are considered 1st line treatment for moderate-severe rhinitis. NOTE that these steroids come as different names and in different delivery vehicles when used for asthma. Do not mix up the brand names. There is a table with a blank column at the end of this chapter where you can test yourself on the asthma drug names. For example, fluticasone for nasal allergy relief is *Flonase* (nase for nose) and for asthma is *Flovent*.

INTRANASAL CORTICOSTEROIDS

DRUG	ADULT DOSE	PEDIATRIC DOSE	SIDE EFFECTS
Beclomethasone (*Beconase, Beconase AQ, Vancenase Pockethaler, Vancenase AQ*)	1 to 2 sprays in each nostril daily or BID	Ages 6 to 12 years: 1 to 2 sprays in each nostril BID	Local irritation; burning or stinging (more with glycol-containing solutions) Nasal bleeding Nasal septal perforation (rare)
Budesonide (*Rhinocort Aqua*)	1 to 4 sprays in each nostril daily	Ages 6 to 12 years: 1 to 2 sprays in each nostril daily	
Ciclesonide (*Omnaris*)	2 sprays in each nostril daily	NA (Manufacturer seeking approval for > 2 years of age)	
Flunisolide (*Nasarel, Nasalide*)	2 sprays in each nostril BID to TID	Ages 6 to 14 years: 2 sprays in each nostril BID - or - 1 spray in each nostril TID	
Fluticasone furoate (***Veramyst***)	2 sprays in each nostril daily	Ages 2 to 11 years: 1 spray in each nostril daily	
Fluticasone propionate (***Flonase***)	2 sprays in each nostril daily	Ages 4 to 12 years: 1 spray in each nostril daily	
Mometasone (***Nasonex***)	2 sprays in each nostril daily	Ages 2 to 11 years: 1 spray in each nostril daily	
Triamcinolone (***Nasacort AQ***)	1 to 2 sprays in each nostril daily	Ages 2 to 12 years: 1 to 2 sprays in each nostril daily	

ORAL ANTIHISTAMINES

- Are considered first line for patients with mild-moderate disease

- They are effective in reducing symptoms of itching, sneezing, and rhinorrhea. They have little effect on nasal congestion.

- They help with allergic conjunctivitis.

- MOA – antagonists of histamine at the H1 receptor site; competitive binding.

- Second-generation agents have less side effects, including less sedation; see chart.

ORAL & INTRANASAL ANTIHISTAMINES: BLOCK HISTAMINE AT THE H1-RECEPTOR

DRUG	ADULT DOSE	SIDE EFFECTS/MONITORING/CONTRAINDICATIONS

First Generation

DRUG	ADULT DOSE	SIDE EFFECTS/MONITORING/CONTRAINDICATIONS
Chlorpheniramine (*Chlor-Trimeton*)	4 mg Q4-6H or 8-12 mg SR Q6-8H (max: 24 mg/d)	CNS effects include sedation and cognitive impairment
Clemastine –do not use in pregnancy (*Tavist*)	1.34-2.68 mg Q8-12H (max: 8.04mg/d)	Anticholinergic effects include dry mouth, blurred vision, urinary retention, and constipation
Diphenhydramine (Benadryl)	**25-50 mg Q4-6H (max: 300 mg/d)**	Caution with use of 1st generation agents with prostate enlargement (will make it much more difficult to urinate), glaucoma (can elevate IOP), constipation (will worsen), urinary retention (will worsen).

Second Generation

DRUG	ADULT DOSE	SIDE EFFECTS/MONITORING/CONTRAINDICATIONS
Cetirizine (*Zyrtec*)	5-10 mg daily (max: 10 mg/d)	Sedation can still be seen occasionally with the 2nd generation agents (more with cetirizine and levocetirizine)
Desloratadine (*Clarinex*)	5 mg daily (max: 5 mg/d)	Onset: cetirizine and levocetirizine work faster than other 2nd generation agents – onset in ~1 hour.
Fexofenadine (*Allegra D12H, D24H*)	60 mg BID or 180 daily (max: 180 mg/d)	Orange, grapefruit and apple juice ↓ GI absorption of fexofenadine (*Allegra*), separate by 4 hours.
Levocetirizine (*Xyzal*)	5 mg QHS	
Loratadine (*Claritin, Claritin-D 24 hour, Claritin RediTabs, Alavert*)	10 mg daily or 5 mg Q12H (max: 10mg/d)	

Intranasal Antihistamines

DRUG	ADULT DOSE	SIDE EFFECTS/MONITORING/CONTRAINDICATIONS
Azelastine (*Astelin, Astepro*)	1-2 sprays each nostril BID	Side effects include bitter taste
Olopatadine (*Patanase*)	2 sprays each nostril BID	Helps with nasal congestion as well

DECONGESTANTS

- Effective in reducing nasal congestion.

- MOA – alpha adrenergic agonists that cause nasal vasoconstriction.

- Side effects (more so with pseudoephedrine) are nervousness, restlessness, excitability, dizziness, headache, fear, anxiety, tremors, hallucinations, and possible seizures. See the next "use caution" warning for possible effects on certain conditions.

- Use caution with hypertension (raises BP), tachycardia and any cardiovascular condition (speeds up heart rate), hyperthyroidism (worsens), glaucoma (can worsen IOP control), diabetes (may raise blood glucose), prostate enlargement (will make it much more difficult to urinate). It is difficult to use antihistamines and decongestants in BPH – both classes will make urination more difficult.

- Do not use with MAO Is. Both agents pregnancy category C.

- If a product contains a D after the name (such as *Mucinex D* or *Robitussin D*, it usually contains a decongestant, which is either pseudoephedrine or phenylephrine.

Oral Agents

- Pseudoephedrine *(Sudafed)* 30 mg 1-2 tablets, Q 12 hours

- Phenylephrine *(Sudafed PE)* – (much less effective than pseudoephedrine) 5 mg, 1-2 tablets, Q 4-6 hours, max 8/day

Topical Agents

- Naphazoline *(Privine)*

- Phenylephrine *(Neo-Synephrine 4-Hour)*

- Oxymetazoline *(Afrin, Neo-Synephrine 12-Hour)*

- Tetrahydrozoline *(Tyzine)*

- Xylometazoline *(Otrivin)*

The topical agents are effective. Similar to the oral agents they are alpha agonists (and cause localized vasoconstriction) and have similar side effects if used excessively; if used to a limited extent they are better tolerated. Oxymetazoline generally causes less side effects than phenylephrine and lasts 12 hours. This product *(Afrin* and store brands) is a popular pharmacist recommendation.

A large caveat with the use of these agents is whether or not the patient will use them very short term or not: if used longer than 3 days they worsen congestion. Limit use to < 3 days to prevent rebound congestion, or rhinitis medicamentosa. If this occurs the patient will need to stop the drug, with worsened congestion, which is difficult.

ADDITIONAL ALLERGY AGENTS

Intranasal cromolyn *(Nasalcrom)*

- Takes 4-7 days to see symptom relief; up to 2 weeks for maximal effect

- Not as effective as other agents

- Due to its safety profile, consider for young children and pregnancy

COMBAT METHAMPHETAMINE EPIDEMIC ACT 2005

Pseudoephedrine (PSE) is located behind pharmacy counters as part of the "Combat Meth Act" under the Patriot Act to crack down on the methamphetamine epidemic. In order to sell this product, stores must keep a logbook of sales (exception is the single dose package that contains a maximum of 60 mg—this is 2 of the 30 mg tablets.)

For any sale above this amount, customer must show photo ID issued by the State (e.g. license, ID card) or Federal Govt (e.g. passport).

Customer records their name, date and time of sale—you verify the name matches the photo ID and that the date and time are correct. Record the address. (Some stores can swipe the drivers license to get the name and address recorded.) The store staff must record what the person received [max 3.6 grams or 120 of the 30 mg tablets, and 9 grams (300 tablets) in a 30-d period.] The customer has to sign the logbook. Keep log for at least 2 years. The logbook has to be kept secured and the information in it cannot be shared with the public. (Inspectors, law enforcement only.)

This includes combo products with PSE, such as cough/cold tablets and syrups. Any product containing PSE must be kept behind the counter or in a locked cabinet. They often are, but do not need to be, located in the pharmacy.

Intranasal ipratropium bromide *(Atrovent Nasal Spray)*

- Effective in reducing rhinorrhea but no effect on other nasal symptoms (can cause nasal dryness)

- Usually used in combination with other agents when rhinorrhea is the predominant symptom

Oral antileukotrienes (Montelukast - *Singulair)*

- Not any more effective than antihistamines or pseudoephedrine

- Dose: 10 mg daily (15 years and up), 5 mg chewable tablet (ages 6-14 years), 4 mg chewable tablet (ages 2-5 years), or one packet of 4 mg oral granules (ages 6 months- 5 years).

Neti-Pot

A neti pot looks like a small genie lamp or teapot. It is used to hold salt water (saline solution) that is poured into one nostril and allowed to drain out of the other nostril. This technique may help with sinus symptoms. It can clear out your nasal passages and reduce swelling. Neti pots are safe for children and pregnant women. The most common side effects are burning or stinging in the nose.

Additional Cough And Cold Agents

BACKGROUND

Refer to the Medication safety chapter for hand washing techniques. Most colds, as well as influenza, are transmitted primarily by mucus secretions via patient's hands. It is essential to wash surfaces such as telephones and keyboards, and to wash hands often. Viruses are also transmitted through the air by coughing or sneezing. Coughing or sneezing into the elbow or into a tissue is preferable over coughing into a hand, which can then touch surfaces and spread illness. About half of all colds are caused by rhinoviruses. Other viruses (coronavirus, others) cause the rest.

Distinguishing between Influenza and a Cold

- Colds do not cause body aches; the flu does.

- Colds generally do not cause fever; the flu does.

- Coughs are worse with the flu. With colds the cough is more like an annoying drip in the back of the throat, which may require a decongestant.

- Colds cause much more nasal symptoms (dripping or clogged nose).

Natural Products used for Colds

Zinc, in various formulations including lozenges, is used for cold prevention and treatment. There is little efficacy data for cold prevention, but zinc lozenges may slightly decrease cold duration if used correctly (taken every 2 hours while awake, starting within 48 hours of symptom onset.) For this purpose zinc supplements are rated as "possibly effective" by the

Natural Medicines Database. Do not recommend zinc nasal swabs or sprays due to the risk of loss of smell.

Vitamin C supplements are commonly used, with little efficacy for cold prevention. They might decrease the duration of the cold by 1-1.5 days and are rated as "possibly effective" for cold treatment by the Natural Medicines Database.

Echinacea is also rated as possibly effective for cold treatment. With any of these products it is important to use the correct dose in a reputable formulation. Drugs, including mild natural products, have dose-response relationships.

Airborne is a popular product that contains a variety of ingredients, including vitamins C, E, zinc and echinacea. It is costly and has no known benefit in the combinations provided.

Dextromethorphan (DM)

Dextromethorphan is the most commonly used cough suppressant. It is in a multitude of cough and cold preparations in a variety of formulations (syrup, tablets, gel caps and others). The most common brand name is *Delsym*. If a product contains DM at the end of the name, such as *Robitussin DM*, it contains dextromethorphan.

DM has several mechanisms. For coughs it blocks the cough reflex center in the brain. DM acts as a serotonin reuptake inhibitor, and there is a risk of serotonergic syndrome if taken in high doses along with other serotonergic medications. Cases of serotonergic syndrome are due to an additive effect. A dose of fluoxetine and normal dosing of DM should not pose a problem, but DM is also a drug of abuse when taken in large quantities. It acts as an NMDA-receptor blocker, which gives it euphoric, hallucinogenic properties similar to PCP. DM is used in some of the recipes for the illicit drug "purple drank."

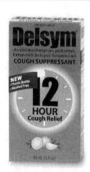

Delsym contains dextromethorphan (DM), which provides benefit. It is also a drug of abuse (hallucinogenic) if taken in very high doses. Generics (or store brands) of any of these products saves the patient $$.

Guaifenesin

Guaifenesin is an expectorant used to decrease the viscosity (thickness) of phlegm in the lower respiratory tract and may possibly increase secretions in the upward respiratory tract to help move the phlegm upwards and out (so that the patient can cough out the phlegm). The most common brand name is *Mucinex,* which comes in various formulations, including pills and liquid. It is also present in some of the cough and cold combination products. It is unclear if guaifenesin provides a useful benefit, however some patients feel that it is useful and singers sometimes use guaifenesin to help preserve their voice during long performances or in dry weather.

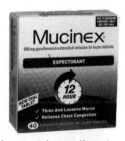

Mucinex contains guaifenesin, an expectorant, which has very mild, if any, benefit. Drinking liquids such as warm tea can also provide a mild benefit.

COUGH AND COLD PRODUCTS IN CHILDREN

OTC cough and cold products should NOT be used in children under age 4.

The FDA recommendation includes a warning not to use antihistamines (such as diphenhydramine, etc.) to make children sleepy. Promethazine is used and is prescription only. Do not use promethazine in any form in children. The FDA advises against the use of promethazine with codeine cough syrups in children less than 6 years of age, due to the risk of respiratory depression, cardiac arrest and neurological problems.

If a young child has a cold it is safe and useful to recommend nasal bulbs for gentle suctioning, saline drops/sprays *(Ocean* and generics) and tell parents that the medicines have not been shown to work in young children, they can be dangerous, and symptoms usually resolve in a few days or up to 2 weeks. If symptoms worsen or don't go away, the child should be seen by a pediatrician. Do not use aspirin in children due to the risk of Reyes; ibuprofen and acetaminophen are safe to use, if kept to safe doses, in young children.

Tips

- If you are dispensing any liquid to a child (or adult), always dispense a calibrated oral syringe (if the package does not contain one) and counsel parents not to use "teaspoons" used for eating because they come in different sizes.

- Do not use aspirin in children due to risk of Reyes – see NSAID pain section for details.

- Keep well hydrated!

- Menthol and camphor used topically, such as in *Vick's VapoRub,* do not work well and should not be used in children less than 2 years. The risk with these agents is ingestion – do not apply to nostrils or leave out where young children can ingest. (Menthol can result in aspiration and cardiac and CNS toxicity if ingested, and camphor may rarely be unsafe – this is being debated.) *Vick's BabyRub* contains petrolatum and is not thought to be potentially harmful but there is no evidence of efficacy.

- Humidifiers and vaporizers, on the other hand, are useful. The hot water types can cause burns in children if spilled, otherwise they work just as well. Keep them clean – dirty mist can worsen colds, allergies or asthma.

Acetaminophen & Ibuprofen in Children

If a parent purchases OTC infant drops for acetaminophen or ibuprofen (let pediatrician recommend if under age 4), remind them to use the dropper that came with the bottle.

- Acetaminophen infant drops: 80 mg/0.8 mL (15 mg/kg) (concentrated strength to be discontinued due to many cases of accidental poisoning)

- Acetaminophen children's liquid suspensions: 160 mg/5 mL (both Q 4-6 hrs)

- Ibuprofen infant drops: 50 mg/1.25 mL (10-15 mg/kg)

- Ibuprofen children's liquid suspensions: 100 mg/5 mL (both Q 6-8 hrs)

- Some doctors recommend alternating so as not to risk acetaminophen toxicity (and sometimes, due to feared stomach upset from ibuprofen).

PATIENT COUNSELING FOR *VERAMYST* (FLUTICASONE)

from website - www.veramyst.com

Priming your VERAMYST Nasal Spray

You need to prime your bottle of VERAMYST Nasal Spray before using it for the first time, not every time.

You ONLY need to reprime your bottle of VERAMYST Nasal Spray if:

- Device has not been used for 30 days or more.

- Cap has been left off the bottle for 5 days or longer

- With the cap on, shake the device well.

- Take the cap off by squeezing the finger grips and pulling it straight off. Do not press the button while you take off the cap.

- Hold the bottle with the nozzle pointing up and away from you. Place your thumb on the button. Then firmly press and release the button 6 times or until a fine mist is sprayed from the nozzle.

How to use VERAMYST Nasal Spray

Follow the instructions below. If you have any questions, ask your doctor or pharmacist.

- Before taking a dose of VERAMYST Nasal Spray, gently blow your nose to clear your nostrils. Shake VERAMYST Nasal Spray before each use. Then do these 3 simple steps: Place, Press, Repeat.

- Place – Tilt you head forward a little bit. Hold the device upright. Place the nozzle in one of your nostrils. Point the end of the nozzle toward the side of your nose, away from the center of your nose (sputum).

- Press – Firmly press the button 1 time to spray the medicine in your nose while you are breathing in. Do not get any spray in your eyes. If you do, rinse your eyes well with water. Take the nozzle out of your nose. Breathe out through your mouth.

- Repeat – Follow these steps in the other nostril.

- Put the cap back on the device after you have finished taking you dose.

DO...

- Spray in the nose ONLY.

- Use once daily for best results.

- Take VERAMYST exactly as your doctor tells you. If VERAMYST is prescribed for a child, an adult should help administer VERAMYST

DON'T...

- Get any spray in your eyes. If you do, rinse your eyes well with water.

- Spray into your mouth.

- Change the dose or stop usage before talking to your doctor.

- Give this medicine to someone else.

USING NASAL SPRAYS CORRECTLY

Types of nasal sprays

- Nasal sprays come in two kinds of containers: pressurized canisters and pump bottles.

Steps for using a pressurized canister

- Gently blow your nose to clear it of mucus before using the medicine.

- Make sure the canister fits snugly in its holder. Shake the canister several times just before using it.

- Keep your head upright. Breathe out slowly.

- Hold your nasal spray canister in one nostril. Use your finger to close the nostril on the side not receiving the medicine.

- Press down on the canister as you begin to breathe in slowly through your nose. Repeat these steps for the other nostril. If you are using more than one spray in each nostril, follow steps 2 through 5 again.

- Try not to sneeze or blow your nose just after using the spray.

Steps for using a pump bottle

- Gently blow your nose to clear it of mucus before using the medicine.

- Remove the cap. Shake the bottle. The first time you use the pump spray each day, you may have to "prime" it, squirting a few times into the air until a fine mist comes out.

- Tilt your head forward slightly. Breathe out slowly.

- Hold the pump bottle with your thumb at the bottom and your index and middle fingers on top. Use a finger on your other hand to close nostril on the side not receiving the medicine.

- Squeeze the pump as you begin to breathe in slowly through your nose. Repeat these steps for the other nostril. If you are using more than one spray in each nostril, follow steps 2 through 5 again.

- Try not to sneeze or blow your nose just after using the spray.

Memory Practice

DRUG	FILL IN THE NAME OF THE ASTHMA DRUG HERE FOR PRACTICE
Beclomethasone (*Beconase, Beconase AQ, Vancenase Pockethaler, Vancenase AQ*)	Qvar
Budesonide (*Rhinocort Aqua*)	
Ciclesonide (*Omnaris*)	
Flunisolide (*Nasarel, Nasalide*)	Aerobid
Fluticasone furoate (*Veramyst*)	
Fluticasone propionate (*Flonase*)	Flovent
Mometasone (*Nasonex*)	Asmanex
Triamcinolone (*Nasacort AQ*)	Asmacor

40

CYSTIC FIBROSIS

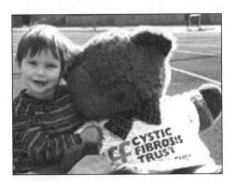

Background

Cystic fibrosis (CF) is an inherited disease that causes thick, sticky mucus to form in the lungs, pancreas and other organs. In the lungs, this mucus blocks the airways, causing lung damage and making it hard to breathe. In the pancreas, it clogs the pathways leading to the digestive system, interfering with proper digestion.

CF is an autosomal recessive disease caused by a mutation of the cystic fibrosis transmembrane receptor (CFTR) gene. Gene mutations cause an abnormality in the cystic fibrosis transmembrane conductance regulator, a cyclic AMP regulated chloride ion channel found in the apical membranes of secretory epithelial cells. Mutations of the CTFR gene disrupt epithelial ion transport of chloride and can lead to respiratory failure, pancreatic insufficiency, infertility, as well as a range of other defects. There is, at present, no cure for the disease.

Clinical Presentation

Patients with CF experience shortness of breath due to reduced forced expiratory volume, air trapping and other pulmonary defects, cough with sputum production, and digital clubbing due to chronic hypoxia. If the digestive system is involved, patients can experience steatorrhea, malnutrition and a failure to thrive if not treated.

Pharmacological Treatment

An early diagnosis of CF and a comprehensive treatment plan can improve both survival and quality of life. Specialty clinics for cystic fibrosis are helpful and can be found in many communities.

TREATMENT FOR LUNG PROBLEMS INCLUDES:

- Inhaled bronchodilators to help open the airways.

- Hypertonic saline *(HyperSal)* for hydrating the airway mucus secretions and facilitating mucociliary function.

- DNAse enzyme replacement therapy to thin mucus and make it easier to cough up.

- Inhaled antibiotics to prevent and treat lung and sinus infections.

- Lung transplant, in some cases.

TREATMENT FOR INTESTINAL AND NUTRITIONAL PROBLEMS MAY INCLUDE:

- A special diet to help with nutrition.

- Pancreatic enzymes to replace those that are missing which will optimize growth and nutritional status and promote healthy bowels.

- Vitamin supplements, especially the fat-soluble vitamins A, D, E, and K.

CONTROLLING INFECTIONS IN THE LUNGS

- *Staphylococcus aureus* (early on), *Haemophilus influenzae* and *Pseudomonas aeruginosa* (later on) are the 3 most common organisms that cause lung infections in CF patients.

- Productive cough with a change in sputum color (greenish) is usually the first respiratory symptom of an infection. An extended course of antibiotics (2-4 weeks) is generally given.

- If the patient has a *Pseudomonas aeruginosa* infection, 2 drugs given IV are generally required to prevent resistance. These could be aminoglycosides, beta lactams, quinolones, and others that cover *Pseudomonas*. See infectious diseases chapter for a complete discussion on treatment of *Pseudomonas aeruginosa*. Doses tend to be larger than normal due to a large volume of distribution (Vd) and the need to obtain a therapeutic concentration in lung tissue.

- Inhaled antibiotics may be used to prevent infections in the lungs (namely *Pseudomonas)*. See agents below. If patient is using a bronchodilator and/or mucolytic, make sure these are given prior to the antibiotic inhalation.

INHALED ANTIBIOTIC	DOSE/INDICATION	SIDE EFFECTS/NOTES
Tobramycin Inhaled Solution *(TOBI)* Ready to use ampules Recommended to store in fridge; can be kept at room temperature up to 28 days	300 mg via nebulizer Q12H x 28 days, followed by 28 days off cycle Indicated in CF patients ≥ 6 years who are colonized with *Pseudomonas* to reduce infection/ hospitalization	**SIDE EFFECTS** Ototoxicity, tinnitus, dizziness, bronchospasm Little systemic absorption Use with *PARI LC Plus* reusable nebulizer and *DeVilbiss Pulmo-Aide* air compressor
Aztreonam Lysine Inhalation Solution *(Cayston)* Need to reconstitute with 1 mL of sterile diluent (provided); give immediately	75 mg TID x 28 days, followed by 28 days off cycle Indicated in CF patients ≥ 7 years with *Pseudomonas* in the lungs	**SIDE EFFECTS** Allergic reactions (may be severe), bronchospasm, fever Doses should be taken at least 4 hours apart Use with *Altera* nebulizer system

Select Patient Instructions on Using *TOBI*

- TOBI should be taken using only the PARI LC® PLUS Reusable Nebulizer and DeVilbiss® Pulmo-Aide® air compressor.

- Make sure to finish the whole dose of TOBI. Do not leave any in the nebulizer.

- One dose takes 15-20 minutes to administer with a clean nebulizer and air compressor.

- TOBI comes in a plastic vial called an ampule. Each foil pouch contains 4 ampules (2 days worth). These should be stored in the refrigerator; however, they can be stored at room temperature for up to 28 days. If it is not refrigerated, the product may darken with age. Color change does not indicate change in the quality of the product.

- Do not use TOBI if it is cloudy, if there are particles in solution, if it has been stored at room temperature beyond 28 days, or it is past the expiration date on the ampule.

- Do not expose to intense light.

- Take doses as close to 12 hours apart (and not less than 6 hours apart).

- If you are taking several medications, the recommended order is as follows: bronchodilator first, chest physiotherapy next, then other inhaled medications, and finally, TOBI.

- Sit or stand in an upright position during your treatment. Place mouthpiece between your teeth and on top of your tongue and breathe normally only through your mouth (use nose clips if you have difficulty breathing through your mouth).

- To reduce the risk of infection, illness or injury from contamination, thoroughly clean all parts of the nebulizer after each treatment. Wash with warm water and liquid dish soap. Can also wash parts in a dishwasher (except for tubing).

- Every other treatment day, you must disinfect the nebulizer parts (except tubing) by boiling them in water for a full 10 minutes.

- Do not share your nebulizer.

PROMOTING CLEARANCE OF MUCUS

Albuterol helps to open the airways and improve lung function in patients who demonstrate a bronchodilator response. The dose is two puffs prior to therapy 2-4 times per day.

Hypertonic saline *(HyerSal)* is used to improve lung function ($\uparrow$ FEV$_1$, $\uparrow$ FVC), sustain mucus clearance, and decrease exacerbations. *HyperSal* is dosed 4 mL via a nebulizer 2-4 times per day.

Acetylcysteine *(Mucomyst)* is a mucolytic that is also used for APAP toxicity. As a mucolytic, it is given in a nebulizer. It has questionable benefit in CF as it may damage lung tissue and promote bronchitis, whereas *Pulmozyme* does not and is the preferred mucolytic agent.

Dornase alfa *(Pulmozyme)* is a DNA enzyme produced from Chinese Hamster Ovary (CHO) cells by recombinant gene therapy. It selectively cleaves DNA, thus reducing mucous viscosity and therefore, improving airflow in the lung and the risk of infections may be decreased. The most common side effects are <u>chest pain, voice alteration and throat irritation</u> (the latter 2 are mild and transient). A <u>2.5 mg dose is given in a nebulizer once daily for 6 months</u> by a recommended nebulizer. Store the ampules in the refrigerator and protect from light. Do not mix this medicine with any other drug in the nebulizer. It works best in patients with a FVC ≥ 40%.

Bronchodilators (albuterol or other short-acting beta-2 agonists) are given prior to chest percussion, which clears mucus. Inhaled antibiotics are always given last.

Adequate Nutrition

Dietary measures must ensure adequate nutrition and include high calorie, high protein, high-fat diets with liberal use of salt to encourage normal weight and growth. The needs are high due to the extra work involved with breathing and a hyper-metabolic state associated with bronchial infection. Due to poor fat absorption, patients use 1-2 multivitamins daily, and some require additional doses.

PANCREATIC ENZYME PRODUCTS (PEPS): CREON, PANCREAZE, ZENPEP – THESE ARE FDA APPROVED

The thick mucus obstructs pancreatic enzyme flow, resulting in a paucity of these enzymes reaching the gastrointestinal tract. Frequently, greasy, foul-smelling stools are manifestations of this pancreatic insufficiency. Most CF patients need to supplement their diet with appropriate amounts of pancreatic enzyme supplements.

Pancrelipase is a natural product harvested from the porcine pancreatic glands and contains a combination of lipase, amylase, and protease. They are formulated to dissolve in the more basic pH of the duodenum so they can act locally to break down fats, protein and starch. The dose is individualized for each patient and can range from 2,000 to 48,000 units of lipase with meals and with snacks. Once enzyme therapy is started, the dose is adjusted every 3-4 days until stools are normalized. Do not use doses > 6,000 units/kg/meal due to colonic stricture risk.

<u>Enzymes are given prior to meals and snacks: full doses are given before meals and 50% of the mealtime dose is given with snacks. Meals with high fat content require higher doses.</u> Microencapsulated formulations are generally given as 1-3 capsules per meal. Counsel patients not to chew or crush the capsules. If a patient cannot swallow them whole, the microsphere-contents can be sprinkled on soft food with a low pH that does not require chewing (such as applesauce, gelatin, baby food, etc). Do not mix with milk-based foods, such as yogurt or pudding since these have a higher pH. There is also a powder formulation. <u>Take the entire dose at the beginning of each meal or snack. Take with a generous amount of liquid.</u> Retention in the mouth before swallowing may cause mucosal irritation and stomatitis.

<u>Do not substitute pancreatic enzyme products. This is a FDA recommendation. They do not require refrigeration.</u> They do degrade; check the expiration date. If infants spit them out, immediately follow with liquid until they are swallowed. Older formulations are being removed from the market as they were never approved and had variations between batches. Recommend FDA approved products listed above.

41

ONCOLOGY

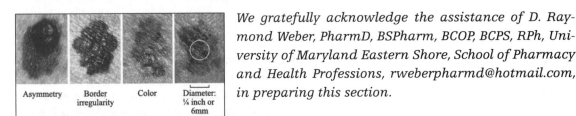

| Asymmetry | Border irregularity | Color | Diameter: ¼ inch or 6mm |

We gratefully acknowledge the assistance of D. Raymond Weber, PharmD, BSPharm, BCOP, BCPS, RPh, University of Maryland Eastern Shore, School of Pharmacy and Health Professions, rweberpharmd@hotmail.com, in preparing this section.

GUIDELINES

National Comprehensive Cancer Network (NCCN) website (www.nccn.org – by cancer type) and through the American Society of Clinical Oncology (ASCO) website (www.asco.org).

WARNING SIGNS

The American Cancer Society lists seven warning signs of cancer in an adult. Any of these warning signs should warrant referral to a physician:

Change in bowel or bladder habits

A sore that does not heal

Unusual bleeding or discharge

Thickening or lump in breast or elsewhere

Indigestion or difficulty swallowing

Obvious change in wart or mole

Nagging cough or hoarseness

Background

Cancer is a group of diseases characterized by uncontrolled growth and spread of abnormal cells. If the spread is not controlled, it can result in death. Cancer is caused by both external factors (such as chemicals, radiation and infectious organisms – including viruses) and internal factors (heredity, hormones, immune disorders, and genetic mutations). Growing older is certainly contributory. Sunlight exposure, tobacco use, excessive alcohol intake, obesity, a poor diet and low physical activity level increase the risk for certain types of cancer.

Classification

Malignancies are classified based on the tissue type as epithelial, connective, lymphoid or nerve. A sample of tissue should be taken for diagnosis along with X-rays, CT scans, MRIs and other diagnostic tools to evaluate the cancer's stage. Lab work is required for blood chemistries and tumor markers.

Cancer Screening Recommendations (American Cancer Society*)

BREAST CANCER

- Yearly <u>mammograms</u> are recommended starting at age 40 and continuing for as long as a woman is in good health.

- <u>Clinical breast exam</u> (CBE) about every 3 years for women in their 20s and 30s and every year for women 40 and over.

- Women should know how their breasts normally look and feel and report any breast change promptly to their health care provider. <u>Breast self-exam</u> (BSE) is an option for women starting in their 20s.

- The American Cancer Society recommends that some women – because of their family history, a genetic tendency, or certain other factors – be screened with MRI in addition to or that mammogram screening begins earlier than age 40.

COLORECTAL CANCER AND POLYPS

- Beginning at age 50, both men and women should follow a schedule that includes various combinations of <u>sigmoidoscopy, colonoscopy</u>, barium enema or CT scan <u>and</u> a yearly fecal occult blood test (<u>FOBT</u>), or fecal immunochemical test (FIT), to screen for colon cancer.

CERVICAL CANCER

- All women should begin cervical cancer screening about 3 years after they begin having vaginal intercourse, but no later than 21 years old.

- Screening should be done every year with the regular <u>Pap test</u> or every 2 years using the newer liquid-based Pap test. Women over 70 with normal results can stop testing.

PROSTATE CANCER

- Research has not yet proven that the potential benefits of testing outweigh the harms of testing, diagnostic procedures and treatment.

- Screening information should be provided to men 50 years and over so an informed decision can be made. If a family history or if an African American man then screening should begin at an earlier age (45 years).

- The <u>PSA blood test with or without a digital rectal exam</u> is standard if screening for prostate cancer.

Everyone should be encouraged to control their health to reduce cancer risk:

- Stay away from tobacco.

- Stay at a healthy weight.

- Get moving with regular physical activity.

- Eat healthy with plenty of fruits and vegetables.

---

* *Recommendations by other agencies may vary from these.*

- Limit how much alcohol you drink (if you drink at all).

- Protect your skin.

- Know yourself, your family history, and your risks.

- Have regular check-ups and cancer screening tests.

Treatment Overview

Cancer is treated with surgery, radiation, chemotherapy, hormone therapy, biological therapy, targeted therapy, immunotherapy and now vaccines. Treatment decisions are based on the cancer type and stage. For most cancers (such as breast, lung, prostate and colon cancer), the stage is based on the size of the tumor and whether the cancer has spread to lymph nodes or elsewhere. The treatment decisions also consider patient characteristics, such as age, performance status, tumor markers and ethnicity. Goals depend on prognosis. The plan may attempt to achieve remission (with curative intent) or be palliative (to reduce tumor size and symptoms). Most cancers will not relapse if a patient remains cancer free for 5 years. These patients may be "cured" but are really considered cancer free survivors. Response to treatment is classified as complete (no evidence of disease for at least 1 month) or partial ($\geq$ 50% tumor size decrease). Stable disease means less than a 25% decrease or increase in tumor size, and progression is $\geq$ 25% tumor growth or new tumor growth.

Often the primary treatment is surgery, followed by chemotherapy. Neoadjuvant, or induction therapy, may be used prior to the start of the primary treatment regimen to shrink the tumor initially (e.g., radiation). Adjuvant therapy is given after the primary treatment in an attempt to eradicate residual disease (e.g., radiation, hormonal therapy – for example, using the drug trastuzumab (Herceptin) for breast cancer, or a combination of therapies).

Sometimes, surgery is not an option for initial treatment and the treatment regimen begins with chemotherapy. This is called primary induction chemotherapy.

Chemotherapeutic regimens are usually designed for synergism. Drugs with different mechanisms of action that complement each other should be chosen. Synergy will not work unless each drug is active on the tumor independently. Most drugs work on rapidly dividing DNA since they work by damaging the DNA. They may work on different phases of the cell cycle (described below) or are phase non-specific. The success or failure of previous treatments is an important consideration.

Chemotherapeutic regimens can be highly toxic and preventing adverse events is part of the treatment plan. The goal is to maintain a high quality of life for the patient. The majority of adverse effects are due to damaging effects on cells that divide more rapidly than others, but are not cancerous. This is why chemotherapy affects fast growing cells in the GI tract, hair follicles and bone marrow (blood cells). Patient specific factors affect treatment choice, and can include the patient's age, co-morbidities, renal clearance, etc. Sometimes, a patient's condition will lead the clinician and family to recommend palliative measures (to reduce the symptoms) over a more aggressive treatment plan that might have a chance to prolong life – but with side effects that could be prohibitive for the patient. Since chemotherapy can have severe side effects, the patient's well-being must be assessed. Common rating systems for monitoring well-being include the Karnofsky and Zubrod scales.

Chemotherapeutics

DANGER DURING PREGNANCY & BREASTFEEDING

Chemotherapy should be avoided during pregnancy and breastfeeding, although some patients treated while pregnant have delivered normal healthy children. Counsel both the male and female to avoid conceiving during treatment. Some of the medications can cause sterility long-term.

CHEMOTHERAPY DOSING

Most chemotherapeutics are dosed using the Body Surface Area calculations. A common method to calculate BSA is the Dubois and Dubois Equation:

$$BSA(m^2) = 0.007184 \times [weight\ (kg)^{0.425}] \times [height\ (cm)^{0.725}]$$

The weight is usually <u>actual</u>, and sometimes <u>adjusted</u> if the patient is overweight. Use the actual weight (unless instructed to use another weight) and keep in mind that a patient > 130% of IBW is generally dosed on their adjusted body weight. You must mark the weight used, since the weight changes the dose. Check the weight with the prescriber or directly with the patient or caregiver.

There is a practice BSA problem in the case at the end of this chapter. Remember to convert pounds to kg by dividing the pounds by 2.2, and convert inches to cm by multiplying the inches by 2.54.

PHASES OF THE CELL CYCLE
M Mitosis – cell divides into 2 daughter cells
G₀ Resting phase post mitosis - no cell division occurs
G₁ Post-mitotic phase – where enzymes and proteins are synthesized
S DNA synthesis and duplication occurs
G₂ Pre-mitotic phase – RNA and topoisomerase I and II are produced to prepare for cell division
Cell death and cell differentiation are cell cycle independent processes

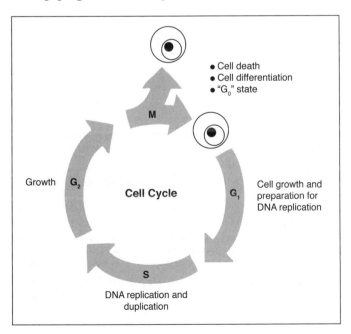

CHEMOTHERAPY AGENTS

DRUG	SIDE EFFECTS/MONITORING/CONTRAINDICATIONS

Alkylators

Cross link DNA - preventing cell replication

Altretamine *(Hexalen)*	Myelosuppression, nausea/vomiting, alopecia
Bendamustine *(Treanda)*	Pulmonary toxicity (busulfan, carmustine, lomustine)
Busulfan *(Myleran)*	Neurologic toxicity (seizures, encephalopathy - chlorambucil, ifosfamide, temazolamide, thiotepa)
Carmustine *(BiCNU, Gliadel –* wafer for brain CA)	Skin pigmentation changes (busulfan, carmustine)
Chlorambucil *(Leukeran)* – requires refrigeration	Dacarbazine causes flu-like symptoms
Cyclophosphamide *(Cytoxan)*	<u>Bladder toxicity with high-dose cyclophosphamide and ALL doses of ifosfamide give MESNA *(Mesnex)* to protect against hemorrhagic cystitis and also ensure adequate hydration</u>
Dacarbazine *(DTIC)*	Procarbazine is a Monoamine Oxidase Inhibitor (MAOI) with neurologic and cardiovascular (hypertensive crisis) toxicity. Avoid sympathomimetic amines or foods with high tyramine content.
Ifosfamide *(Ifex)*	
Lomustine *(CeeNU)*	Lomustine PO, dosed QHS with antiemetic
Mechlorethamine *(Mustargen)*	
Melphalan *(Alkeran)* – tablets require refrigeration	
Procarbazine *(Matulane)*	
Streptozocin *(Zanosar)*	
Temozolomide *(Temodar)*	
Thiotepa *(Thioplex)*	

Antiandrogens

Block androgens at the receptor site. Given PO daily, usually with LHRH agonists for prostate CA

Bicalutamide *(Casodex)*	Diarrhea/nausea/vomiting, gynecomastia, hepatotoxicity, hot flashes, ↓ libido, impotence. More GI toxicity with flutamide and visual disturbances – night blindness with nilutamide.
Flutamide *(Eulexin)*	
Nilutamide *(Nilandron)*	

Antiandrogen – Androgen Production Inhibitor

Abiraterone acetate *(Zytiga)*	A pregnenolone analog that irreversibly inhibits CYP450 c17, the rate limiting enzyme in androgen production in the testes, adrenal gland and prostate without causing adrenal insufficiency.
	Mineralocorticoid elevation with fluid retention, hypertension, hypokalemia.

Antiandrogen – GRH antagonist

Gonadotropin Releasing Hormone Antagonist used in Prostate Cancer

Degarelix *(Firmagon)*	Similar net result (efficacy/toxicity) to LHRH agonists (below) but true blockade of GRH and as a result does NOT cause an initial outpouring of testosterone with tumor flare.

Chemotherapy Agents Continued

DRUG	SIDE EFFECTS/MONITORING/CONTRAINDICATIONS

Antiandrogen-Antiestrogen – LHRH agonists (Luteinizing-hormone-releasing hormone)

Used for prostate CA in males and for endometriosis, fibroids and breast cancer in females: initially increase the production of androgens and estrogens; followed by down regulation through a negative feedback loop resulting in suppressed gonadotropin release, LH, and FSH, resulting in a chemical castration/oophorectomy.
These are given monthly to every six months in a medical office.

Drug	Side Effects/Monitoring/Contraindications
Goserelin *(Zoladex)*	Hot flashes, bone pain, impotence, injection site pain/swelling, dyslipidemia, QT prolongation, gynecomastia (men), peripheral edema
Histrelin *(Vantos)*	↓ bone density and increased risk for osteoporosis: consider calcium and vitamin D supplementation, weight bearing exercise and DEXA screening.
Leuprolide *(Lupron)*	An initial surge in LH, FSH, and testosterone – estrogen can cause a disease flare (manifested as metastatic bone pain or paralysis if spinal cord compression). In patients at risk, start a blocker of androgen or estrogen receptors prior to the LHRH agonist.
Triptorelin *(Trelstar)*	

Antiandrogen-Antiestrogen – Aromatase Inhibitors: ALL PO

Prevent conversion to active estrogen / androgen / corticosteroid / mineralocorticoid to reduce cell growth in breast, prostate and/or adrenal CA

Drug	Side Effects/Monitoring/Contraindications
Aminoglutethimide *(Cytadren)* non-selective	Lethargy/fatigue, rash, menopause symptoms, hot flashes, nausea, vomiting
Anastrozole *(Arimidex)* estrogens – breast CA	↓ bone density and risk for osteoporosis: consider calcium and vitamin D supplementation, weight bearing exercise, DEXA screening.
	Increased cardiovascular disease risk compared to SERMs.
Exemestane *(Aromasin)* estrogens – breast CA	Aminoglutethimide and mitotane are non-selective aromatase inhibitors requiring glucocorticoid and mineralocorticoid supplementation.
Letrozole *(Femara)* estrogens – breast CA	
Mitotane *(Lysodren)* non-selective	

Antiestrogens/SERMs – Most PO, fulvestrant is IM

Selectively block estrogen at the receptor site. For breast CA in hormone receptor + tumors (estrogen/progesterone)

Drug	Side Effects/Monitoring/Contraindications
Fulvestrant *(Faslodex)*	Menopausal symptoms, hot flashes, flushing, N/V, edema, weight gain, HTN, mood changes, amenorrhea, vaginal bleeding/discharge, skin changes
	Tamoxifen increases risk of endometrial cancers – others decrease risk.
Raloxifene *(Evista)* Used for osteoporosis in women at risk of breast CA	Tamoxifen CYP 2D6 polymorphism *4 / *5 results in shorter disease free survival. Consider alternative therapy (Aromatase Inhibitor)
	Fulvestrant osteoporosis, hyperlipidemia – others improve these.
Tamoxifen *(Nolvadex)*	**BLACK BOX WARNING** ↑ Risk of thromboembolic events (DVT, PE, MI, stroke) with all SERMs (these are Selective Estrogen Receptor Modulators, or "Designer Estrogens"–they block estrogen in breast tumors, but act as estrogen agonists in some other tissues.)
Toremifene *(Fareston)*	

Chemotherapy Agents Continued

DRUG	SIDE EFFECTS/MONITORING/CONTRAINDICATIONS

Anthracyclines

Work by several mechanisms, including intercalation into DNA, inhibiting topoisomerase II, and creating oxygen-free radicals that damage cells

Daunorubicin *(Cerubidine)*	Very effective but use limited by cardiac toxicity and N/V.
Daunorubicin liposomal *(DaunoXome)*	Myelosuppression, alopecia, mucositis, hyperpigmentation, red urine and body secretions.
	High risk of severe tissue damage with extravasation – antidote is dexrazoxane *(Totect)* OR dimethyl sulfoxide. (Do NOT use both.)
Doxorubicin *(Adriamycin)*	Radiation recall reactions occur.
	The liposomal products are associated with a higher incidence of hand-foot syndrome and allergic reactions.
Doxorubicin liposomal *(Doxil)*	Cardiotoxicity – ↓ risk by not exceeding max lifetime dose:
Epirubicin *(Ellence)*	Serial monitoring of cardiac output is necessary at baseline and with anthracycline doses exceeding: 250 mg/m² doxorubicin; 320 mg/m² daunorubicin
	Doxorubicin max lifetime dose = 400-500 mg/m²
Idarubicin *(Idamycin)*	Daunorubicin max lifetime dose = 550 mg/m² (400 mg/m² with chest radiation)
	Epirubicin max lifetime dose = 900 mg/m²
Mitoxantrone *(Novantrone)*	Idarubicin cardiotoxicity risk above 150 mg/m²
Valrubicin *(Valstar)*	The cardioprotective dexrazoxane *(Zinecard)* should be considered when doxorubicin doses are anticipated to continue beyond 300mg/m².
	Mitoxantrone is an anthracenedione similar to anthracyclines in toxicity but a three rather than four membered ring structure and turns body fluids blue rather than red.
	Valrubicin is instilled in the bladder for refractory bladder cancer.

Epothilone

Microtubule stabilizer enhancing polymerization of tubules halting cell division at metaphase in mitosis.

Ixabepilone *(Ixempra)*	Similar mechanism to taxanes but still efficacy in taxane resistant breast CA.
	Myelosuppression, N/V/D, mucositis, alopecia, neuropathy
	Hypersensitivity due to Cremophor EL – polyoxyethylated castor oil solvent system requiring H1-and H2- antihistamines. Add steroids and acetaminophen as needed.

Folate Antimetabolites

Prevents DNA synthesis

Methotrexate (MTX, *Trexall*, *Mexate, Folex*)	Myelosuppression, mucositis, hepatic and renal toxicity (renal is dose-related). Pulmonary toxicity – monitor.
Lower doses used in RA and psoriasis (7.5-22.5 mg Q weekly)	Red-tender palms and feet (hand-foot syndrome)
	High-Dose MTX provides a dose increase 10-100 fold higher increasing the amount of MTX that penetrates the blood-brain barrier and overcomes relative resistance in malignancies (osteosarcoma). High Dose MTX requires leucovorin (or levoleucovorin) rescue to ↓ MTX toxicity. Leucovorin is the active form of folic acid bypassing the enzyme block of dihydrofolate reductase by MTX.
	Active transport elimination ↓ by aspirin, penicillins, probenecid, and NSAIDs, resulting in toxicity (avoid concurrent use).
	Maintain hydration. Drink fluids.

Chemotherapy Agents Continued

DRUG	SIDE EFFECTS/MONITORING/CONTRAINDICATIONS
Pemetrexed *(Alimta)*	Requires regular folic acid supplements (PO) and vitamin B12 (cyanocobalamin) injections before and during treatment plus dexamethasone pre-medication to reduce toxicities (hematologic, mucositis, diarrhea, dermatologic).
Pralatrexate *(Fotolyn)*	Myelosuppression, mucositis, esophagitis, gastritis, N/V/D, anorexia, fatigue, fever, edema, skin rashes.
	Requires regular folic acid supplements (PO) and vitamin B12 (cyanocobalamin) injections before and during treatment.
	Active transport elimination ↓ by NSAIDs, probenecid, and TMP/SMX, resulting in toxicity (avoid concurrent use).

Halichondrin

Microtubule destabilizer inhibiting polymerization of tubules halting cell division at metaphase in mitosis.

Eribulin mesylate *(Halaven)*	Similar mechanism to vinca alkaloids. Has shown efficacy in heavily treated or recurrent metastatic breast cancer.
	Neutropenia, anemia, febrile neutropenia, alopecia, mucositis, N/V/D, peripheral neuropathy, gastroparesis, fatigue, QT prolongation (correct K^+, Mg^{2+}).

Hypomethylating agents

Restore normal function to genes (DNA) that are critical for differentiation and proliferation

Azacitidine (5AZC, *Vidaza*)	Myelosuppression, nephrotoxicity (renally cleared), N/V, cough, dyspnea. "Azacitidine syndrome" includes: fever, fatigue, rigors, skin rash, neurologic symptoms (headache, dizziness, confusion) and/or pain (bone, back, muscle and chest pain)
Decitabine *(Dacogen)*	Myelosuppression, pyrexia, nausea, cough, petechiae, constipation, diarrhea, and hyperglycemia, peripheral edema, cardiac murmur, hypoxia, pulmonary edema. "Decitabine syndrome" includes: fever, fatigue, rigors, skin rash, neurologic symptoms (headache, dizziness, confusion, and pain)
Nelarabine *(Arranon)*	Fatigue, somnolence, neuropathy, weakness, N/V/D, constipation, myelosuppression, elevated LFTs, hypokalemia
Romidepsin *(Istodax)*	Fatigue, N/V/D, myelosuppression, dermatitis, pruritus, elevated LFTs, electrolyte anomalies, QT prolongation (correct K^+, Mg^{2+})
	Substrate/Inhibitor for CYP 3A4, 3A5, 1A1, 2B6, 2C19, p-glycoprotein
Vorinostat *(Zolinza)*	Clotting (DVT/PE) peripheral edema, thrombocytopenia, anemia, N/V/D, xerostomia, fatigue, QT prolongation. Uniquely increases SCr from muscle production but renal function actually remains stable.

Immuno-modulators

↓ angiogenesis

Lenalidomide *(Revlimid)* – PO	**PREGNANCY CATEGORY X**
	Severe birth defects (similar to thalidomide in animal studies). Only available under restricted distribution program RevAssist – patient, prescriber and pharmacist must be registered with RevAssist. Used for multiple myeloma and myelodysplastic syndrome (MDS)
	Neutropenia, thrombocytopenia – monitor CBC weekly during treatment and monthly afterward. Constipation or diarrhea, fatigue, fever, cough, pruritus, rash, arthralgias, back pain. DVT and PE – seek medical care if develop shortness of breath, chest pain, or arm or leg swelling!

Chemotherapy Agents Continued

DRUG	SIDE EFFECTS/MONITORING/CONTRAINDICATIONS
Thalidomide *(Thalomid)* – PO – take at least 1 hr after a meal	**PREGNANCY CATEGORY X** <u>Severe birth defects (limb defects, cardiac, GI, ear, eye, GU). All pharmacies and prescribers must be enrolled in the System for Thalidomide Education and Prescribing Safety (STEPS) program to dispense.</u> Used for multiple myeloma and myelodysplastic syndrome (MDS). Somnolence, constipation, dizziness, orthostatic hypotension, rash, peripheral neuropathy, constipation, neutropenia, DVT/PE. Consider prophylactic anticoagulation.

Interferons

Multiple actions not fully understood: Inhibit tumor growth, increase tumor antigenicity, down regulate oncogenes, induce differentiation, inhibits angiogenesis and inhibits cell proliferation

Interferons - alfa alfa-2a *(Roferon)* alfa-2b *(Intron-A)* **Peginterferon** alfa-2a *(Pegasys)* alfa-2b *(PEG-Intron, Sylatron)*	<u>Depression, suicidal ideation</u>, suicide, somnolence, sleep disturbances, paresthesias, seizures, mild myelosuppression, N/V/D, anorexia, alopecia, dry skin, hypothyroidism, weight loss, <u>flu-like syndrome</u> with fever, chills, diaphoresis, rigors, myalgias, arthralgias, headache.
Interferons - beta beta-1a *(Avonex)* beta-1b *(Betaseron)*	Fatigue, <u>depression, suicidal ideation</u>, sleep disturbances, N/V/D, anorexia, elevated transaminases, mild myelosuppression, <u>flu-like syndrome</u> with fever, chills, diaphoresis, rigors, myalgias, arthralgias, headache.

Interleukins

Stimulates immune system to target cancer cells.

Aldesleukin (IL-2, *Proleukin*)	Use restricted to patients with normal cardiac and pulmonary functions as defined by thallium stress testing and pulmonary function testing. At the FDA approved dose to give only in hospital in an intensive care setting. Can cause capillary leak syndrome (hypotension, ↓ organ perfusion, possible death). Induces a sepsis-like state. High incidence of bacterial endocarditis, if indwelling catheter then provide Gm+ antibiotic prophylaxis prior to therapy. May also require meperidine (for chills), antihistamines and acetaminophen/NSAIDs. Corticosteroids ↓ effectiveness of drug and cannot be used.
Denileukin diftitox *(Ontak)* Fusion protein of interleukin-2 (IL-2) and diphtheria toxin fragments A and B	Unique MOA: Binds to IL-2 receptors (CD-25) on T-lymphocytes. Then internalized into the cell releasing fragment A of the diphtheria toxin which, inhibits protein synthesis resulting in death of the T-lymphocyte. Acute hypersensitivity reactions during infusion (hypotension, rash, etc) – stop, or ↓ infusion rate. Capillary leak syndrome, N/V, hepatotoxicity. Pre-treat with acetaminophen, diphenhydramine, and steroids.

Monoclonal Antibody – Angiogenesis Inhibitor

Limit tumor's blood supply

Bevacizumab *(Avastin)* Binds to VEGF-A Vascular endothelial growth factor A but not VEGF-B, C or D	Used with other agents in numerous types of cancer but a high cost for modest benefit resulting in debate on the benefit-cost ratio. Patients have to report GI pain due to risk of GI perforation, which can be fatal. Impairs wound healing – stop at least 28 days before elective surgery. Bleeding, hypertension, thrombosis (including DVT, PE and stroke), nephrotic syndrome, proteinuria.

Chemotherapy Agents Continued

DRUG	SIDE EFFECTS/MONITORING/CONTRAINDICATIONS

Monoclonal Antibodies – Cell Surface Marker Target

Alemtuzumab *(Campath)* Targets CD-52 on lymphocytes	Cytokine release syndrome – premedication with acetaminophen and diphenhydramine. Severe-prolonged myelosuppression (2-12 months) requiring prophylactic antibiotics (SMZ/TMP and famciclovir) for a minimum of 2 months or until CD4 counts are > 200 cells/liter .
Brentuximab vedotin *(Adcetris)* Targets CD-30 on lymphocytes releasing monomethyl auristatin E (MAE) which is conjugated to the antibody. The MAE disrupts microtubules.	Peripheral neuropathy, neutropenia, anemia; thrombocytopenia, fever, fatigue, nausea/vomiting, diarrhea, upper respiratory tract infections, rash, cough, pain. Monomethyl auristatin E is primarily metabolized by CYP450 isoenzyme 3A with possibility of increased toxicity in the presence of a strong inhibitor. Store in refrigerator (2-8°C) prior to use.
Gemtuzumab *(Mylotarg)* Targets CD-33 on leukocytes where it is internalized and releases Calicheamicin which binds to DNA	Cytokine release syndrome – premedication with acetaminophen and H1-blocker. Prolonged myelosuppression leading to secondary infections, N/V/D, hepatotoxicity, Tumor Lysis Syndrome. Very light sensitive – must prepare in the dark.
Ibritumomab *(Zevalin)* Targets CD-20 but radiolabeled	Yttrium^{90} induces cellular damage by the formation of free radicals in the target and neighboring cells. Pure beta-emitter penetrates ~ 5mm. Cytokine release syndrome – premedication with acetaminophen and diphenhydramine. Other side effects similar to Rituximab but more prolonged thrombocytopenia/neutropenia.
Ofatumumab *(Arzerra)* Targets CD-20 but in a different configuration from Rituximab.	Human monoclonal antibody so less a risk of type 1 allergic reactions compared to rituximab but still risk of severe cytokine release syndrome requiring upward titration of dosage and pre-medication with acetaminophen, H1-blocker and corticosteroids. Prolonged immune suppression increases the risk of opportunistic infections and reactivation of hepatitis B. Tumor lysis syndrome, rash, pruritus, toxic epidermal necrolysis.
Rituximab *(Rituxan)* CD-20 target on lymphocytes kills the cancer but also releases cytokines	Rituximab-induced cytokine release infusion reactions and sequelae include urticaria, hypotension, angioedema, hypoxia, bronchospasm, pulmonary infiltrates, acute respiratory distress syndrome, myocardial infarction, ventricular fibrillation, cardiogenic shock, anaphylaxis, and/or death. Infusions must be given in hospital or clinic since they can be fatal . Severe reactions typically occur during the first infusion with time to onset of 30-120 minutes. Administer diphenhydramine and acetaminophen prior to infusion. Myelosuppression with prolonged immune suppression increases the risk of opportunistic infections and reactivation of hepatitis B. Tumor lysis syndrome, rash, pruritus, toxic epidermal necrolysis.
Tositumomab *(Bexxar)* Also targets CD-20 but radiolabeled	Iodine^{131} induces cellular damage by the formation of free radicals in the target and neighboring cells. Both Gamma emitter and beta-emitter with radiation leaving the patient's body. Cytokine release syndrome – premedication with acetaminophen and diphenhydramine. Thyroid-protective iodine regimen needed prior to tositumomab. Other side effects similar to Rituximab but more prolonged thrombocytopenia/neutropenia.

Chemotherapy Agents Continued

DRUG	SIDE EFFECTS/MONITORING/CONTRAINDICATIONS

Monoclonal Antibody – Immunotherapy
Stimulates the patient's immune system

Ipilimumab *(Yervoy)* Blocks the Cytotoxic T-lymphocyte antigen-4 (CTL4) receptor, which effectively takes the brake off T-cell activation. Activated T-cells then can recognize melanoma cells for removal but at a risk of autoimmune activity.	Primarily autoimmune system unchecked: dermatologic (rashes, pruritus), gastrointestinal (diarrhea, colitis, esophagitis, gastritis, jejunitis, ulcers), endocrine (hypophysitis, hypothyroidism, hypoadrenalism, hyponatremia, pancreatitis), hepatitis, uveitis, and nephritis Expensive ~$120,000 per course of therapy

Monoclonal antibodies - Over Expression Targeted
Inhibit growth factors that are promoting cancer cell growth

Cetuximab *(Erbitux)* EGFR positive expression correlates with better response rates. K-ras mutation indicates poor response	Severe infusion reactions (3%), cardiopulmonary arrest (2%), give diphenhydramine prior to infusion. N/V/D, fatigue. Magnesium and calcium wasting. Acne-like rash onset in 1st few weeks of treatment, severe rash possible. Presence of rash correlates with a higher survival rate. Pharmacogenomics: Colorectal cancer does NOT respond to cetuximab/panitumumab if patients have a K-ras mutation (~40% of pts) Wild-type (or normal) K-ras colorectal cancer has double the overall survival. Must test for K-ras mutations before treatment.
Panitumumab *(Vectibix)* Same EGFR and K-ras issues as cetuximab	Dermatologic toxicities (89%): acne-like lesions, itching, redness, rash, skin exfoliation, etc.; infusion reactions (1%) – can be fatal; N/V/D, fatigue. Presence of rash correlates with a higher survival rate. Magnesium and calcium wasting
Trastuzumab *(Herceptin)* **HER2/neu over-expression required for use**	Pharmacogenomics: trastuzumab binds to and reverses effects of overactive HER2 receptors; HER2 gene is over-expressed in ~25% of early-stage breast tumors. Must be > 2+ by Immunohistochemical (IHC) testing to respond/use this. Allergic infusion reactions – premedicate with acetaminophen and H1-blocker, pulmonary toxicity, N/V/D, joint pain, lethargy. Cardiomyopathy (CHF, ↓ LVEF), Added efficacy with some chemotherapeutics but avoid use with anthracyclines due to additive cardiotoxicity.

mTOR inhibitors
Inhibit downstream regulation of VEGF reducing cell growth, metabolism, proliferation and angiogenesis

Everolimus *(Afinitor)* – PO daily with or without food	Dyslipidemia, hyperglycemia, myelosuppression, rashes, pruritus, hand-foot syndrome, stomatitis, fatigue, N/V/D, peripheral edema, interstitial lung disease, elevated creatinine with decreased renal function, elevated LFTs. Cytochrome P-450 3A4 inhibitor/substrate
Temsirolimus *(Torisel)*	Dyslipidemia, hyperglycemia, myelosuppression, rashes, acne, acute hypersensitivity reactions (polysorbate 80 solvent system), N/V/D, peripheral edema, pain, dyspnea, cough, fever, asthenia, interstitial lung disease. Cytochrome P-450 3A4 inhibitor/substrate

Chemotherapy Agents Continued

DRUG	SIDE EFFECTS/MONITORING/CONTRAINDICATIONS

Platinum-Based Compounds
X-links DNA, leading to apoptosis

DRUG	SIDE EFFECTS/MONITORING/CONTRAINDICATIONS
Carboplatin *(Paraplatin-AQ)* **Cisplatin** *(Platinol)*	Cisplatin: Nephrotoxicity-vigorous hydration and sometimes mannitol used to avoid renal failure; electrolyte wasting requiring magnesium and potassium supplementation. Amifostine *(Ethyol)* may also be used prophylactically. Severe N/V, acute and delayed. Both agents: hypersensitivity reactions (including anaphylaxis) may respond to pretreatment with steroids and antihistamines. Myelosuppression, neuropathy (cumulative, dose-dependent). Carboplatin Dose (total in mg) = Target AUC X (GFR + 25). Target AUC ranges from 1 to 7 with 1-2 as a radiosensitizer; 4-6 in combination therapy and 7 as a single agent.
Oxaliplatin *(Eloxatin)*	Anaphylaxis, pancreatitis, pulmonary toxicity, hepatotoxicity. Neuropathy exacerbated by exposure to cold; infusion of calcium and magnesium (1 gm each) prior to oxaliplatin reduces neuropathy by ~ 50%. Usually given with 5-FU/leucovorin in GI malignancy.

Purine Analog Antimetabolites
Inhibit purine synthesis

DRUG	SIDE EFFECTS/MONITORING/CONTRAINDICATIONS
Azathioprine *(Imuran)* – pro-drug of Mercaptopurine (6-MP) see below	See mercaptopurine. Used as immune suppressant but not in the oncology setting.
Cladribine *(Leustatin)*	Myelosuppression, primarily lymphopenia, requiring trimethoprim-sulfamethoxazole prophylaxis against *Pneumocystis jiroveci*.
Fludarabine *(Fludara IV)*	Myelosuppression – severe prolonged leukopenia, lymphopenia requiring prophylactic antibiotics for opportunistic infections (fluconazole, co-trimoxazole, anti-virals).
Mercaptopurine (6-MP, *Purinethol)* – PO dose is 1 hr before, 2 hrs after meals	Myelosuppression, nausea, hepatotoxicity. 6-MP undergoes extensive first pass metabolism in the liver by xanthine oxidase which can be inhibited by allopurinol and can raise 6-MP bioavailability by 400 to 500%. Requires dosage reduction. Pharmacogenetic testing for TPMP and ITPA deficiency required before starting therapy to properly dose/ avoid toxicity.
Pentostatin *(Nipent)*	Myelosuppression, nausea, neurologic and pulmonary toxicities.
Thioguanine *(6-TG, 6-thioguanine Tabloid)*	Myelosuppression, nausea, vomiting, hepatotoxicity, rash, Veno-Occlusive Disease (VOD), neurotoxicity.

Pyrimidine Analog Antimetabolites
Inhibit pyrimidine synthesis

DRUG	SIDE EFFECTS/MONITORING/CONTRAINDICATIONS
Capecitabine *(Xeloda)* – **prodrug of 5-FU – PO take with meal**	Pharmacogenomic testing for dihydropyrimidine dehydrogenase (DPD) deficiency (increases risk of severe toxicity) Myelosuppression, mucositis, dermatitis, diarrhea, cardiotoxicity, edema, dermatitis, more hand-foot syndrome than 5-FU Capecitabine ↑ INR up to 91% due to 2C9 inhibition; requires ↓ warfarin dosage/ INR monitoring.

Chemotherapy Agents Continued

DRUG	SIDE EFFECTS/MONITORING/CONTRAINDICATIONS
Cytarabine (Ara-C, *Cytosar*) Cytarabine liposomal *(DepoCyt)* For intrathecal administration	Mucositis, myelosuppression, hepatotoxicity, pulmonary toxicity, encephalopathy, etc. "Ara-C syndrome" includes fever, general weakness, skin rash, reddened eyes, bone, muscle, joint and/or chest pain - responds to corticosteroids.
Fluorouracil (5-FU, *Adrucil)* *Efudex* is topical formulation for wrinkles, *Carac* and *Fluoroplex* are topical for actinic keratosis – for chemo, it is given with leucovorin to increase efficacy of 5-FU	Pharmacogenomic testing for dihydropyrimidine dehydrogenase (DPD) deficiency (increases risk of severe toxicity) Myelosuppression, mucositis, dermatitis, diarrhea, cardiotoxicity, hand-foot syndrome (with continuous infusions).
Floxuridine *(FUDR)*	Analog of 5-FU given via intra-hepatic artery or portal vein infusion for isolated hepatic metastases. Less than 10% reaches systemic circulation so less toxicity with more of a targeted effect on the metastases.
Gemcitabine *(Gemzar)* – IV	Myelosuppression, hepatotoxicity, pulmonary toxicity, encephalopathy, nausea, flu-like syndrome during first 24 hours – use acetaminophen treatment.

Retinoids (vitamin A analogues)
Decreases cell proliferation and promotes apoptosis.

| Alitretinoin *(Panretin)*

Bexarotene *(Targretin)*

Tretinoin (ATRA, **All-trans Retinoic Acid,** *Vesanoid)* | Pregnancy Category X. Lots of SEs and patients do get them: headache, chills, peripheral edema, dyslipidemia, hypothyroidism, leukopenia, skin/mucous membrane dryness, bone pain, nausea/vomiting, rash, mucositis, pruritus, increased sweating, visual disturbances, ocular disorders, alopecia, changed visual acuity, bone inflammation. "Acute Promyelocytic Leukemia (APL) Differentiation Syndrome": fever, dyspnea, weight gain, pulmonary infiltrates, pericardial or pleural effusions, leukocytosis, respiratory distress, renal failure, cardiac failure, hypotension - Management: dexamethasone 10 mg IV Q12H. |

Taxanes
Inhibit microtubule function and angiogenesis (dysfunctional microtubule bundling). Elimination of taxanes is reduced when given immediately after administration of cisplatin or carboplatin. Give taxanes first.

Carbazitaxel *(Jevtana)*	Hypersensitivity rxn (40-50%) due to polysorbate 80 solvent system, severe anaphylaxis rxn rare. Premedicate with H1-, H2- antihistamines and corticosteroids. Peripheral edema, fatigue, alopecia, N/V/D, myelosuppression, myalgia/arthralgia, neuropathy, stomatitis.
Docetaxel *(Taxotere)*	Hypersensitivity rxn (40-50%) due to polysorbate 80 solvent system, severe anaphylaxis rxn rare – symptoms include dyspnea, hypotension, angioedema, and generalized urticaria. Cardio-Pulmonary: Fluid retention, pericardial effusion, pleural effusion and edema (41-70%). Pretreatment with dexamethasone 8mg BID x 3 days starting the day prior to docetaxel retards the development of fluid retention. Myelosuppression, N/V, mucositis, alopecia, peripheral neuropathy, fatigue, arthralgia/myalgia. Will ↑ INR; ↓ warfarin dose and monitor.
Paclitaxel *(Taxol)* Paclitaxel albumin-bound *(Abraxane)* – less hypersensitivity rxns, does not require pre-medication	Anaphylaxis, hypersensitivity rxn (78%) due to polyoxyethylated castor oil solvent system, can be severe in 2-4% of patients. Symptoms include dyspnea, hypotension, angioedema, and generalized urticaria. Pre-treat with dexamethasone, diphenhydramine and H2-blocker (not needed with *Abraxane).* Myelosuppression, cardiotoxicity, hepatotoxicity, myalgia/arthralgias, alopecia (can be entire body), N/V, peripheral neuropathy. Monitor bilirubin, transaminases. Will ↑ INR; ↓ warfarin dose and monitor.

DRUG	SIDE EFFECTS/MONITORING/CONTRAINDICATIONS

Topoisomerase I Inhibitors

Block the coiling and uncoiling of the DNA helix. Topoisomerase I facilitates single stand breaks followed by religation.

Irinotecan *(Camptosar)*	Acute diarrhea is a cholinergic symptom including tearing, etc. – treat with atropine. Delayed diarrhea treat with loperamide (up to 24 mg daily).
	Pharmacogenomic testing: Those who are homozygous for the UGT1A1*28 allele are at an increased risk for neutropenia and other toxicities.
	Myelosuppression, N/V/D, alopecia; dyspnea, elevated LFTs.
Topotecan *(Hycamtin)*	Myelosuppression, N/V/D, alopecia; dyspnea, flu-like symptoms.

Topoisomerase II Inhibitors

Block the coiling and uncoiling of the DNA helix by facilitating single stand breaks followed by religation.

Etoposide *(VePesid, VP-16)* – *VePesid* capsules require refrigeration	Myelosuppression, neurotoxicity/neuropathy (cumulative), hepatotoxicity, alopecia, N/V, mucositis.
	Hypotension if infusion rate too fast.
Teniposide *(Vumon)*	

Tyrosine Kinase Inhibitors (TKIs)

All the TKIs have significant drug interactions with the CYP 450 system especially 3A4 – avoid grapefruit juice.
They are arranged in the following sections by their specific targets:

Tyrosine Kinase Inhibitors (TKIs) targeting ALK Anaplastic Lymphoma Kinase (ALK) regulates cell growth in ~1-7% of Non-Small Cell Lung Cancer.	
Crizotinib *(Xalkori)*	Must be ALK positive to use this (pharmacogenomic testing).
Primary target is ALK but also inhibits cMET (Mesenchymal Epithelial Transition Factor)	Vision disturbances (visual impairment, flashes of light, blurred vision, floaters, double vision, sensitivity to light, visual field defects), nausea, diarrhea, vomiting, swelling (edema), constipation, interstitial pneumonitis.
PO BID with or without food	Expensive ~ $9,600 per month.

Tyrosine Kinase Inhibitors (TKIs) targeting BCR-ABL

A fusion gene is created when the ABL1 gene on chromosome 9 is translocated to the Breakpoint Cluster Region (BCR) gene on chromosome 22 resulting in cancer cell growth, replication and immortality. Blocking this results in a halt to cancer cell growth and likely apoptosis.

Dasatinib *(Sprycel)* PO with or without food	Maintains clinical activity in CML resistant to imatinib but more expensive as first line therapy.
Needs acid for absorption; avoid PPIs and H2 blockers.	Leukopenia, thrombocytopenia, N/V/D, fluid retention, edema, pleural effusions, skin rashes, headache, musculoskeletal pain , PAH.
	Also inhibits cKit, PDGFR, SCF, SRC tyrosine kinases.
Imatinib *(Gleevec)* PO, with water and full meal	Philadelphia-chromosome positive (Ph+) Chronic Myelogenous Leukemia (CML) or cKIT (CD117)-positive gastrointestinal stromal tumors (GIST).
	Leukopenia, thrombocytopenia, N/V/D, fluid retention, edema, CHF, skin rashes, muscle spasms.
	Also inhibits cKit, PDGFR, SCF, SRC tyrosine kinases.
Nilotinib *(Tasigna)* PO, 1 hr before, 2 hr after meal	Maintains clinical activity in CML resistant to imatinib but more expensive as first line therapy.
	Leukopenia, thrombocytopenia, N/V/D, fluid retention, edema, skin rashes, pruritus, and alopecia. Prolongs the QT interval (torsades de pointe); correct potassium/magnesium.

DRUG	SIDE EFFECTS/MONITORING/CONTRAINDICATIONS

Tyrosine Kinase Inhibitors (TKIs) targeting BRAF

BRAF protein kinase mutation

Vemurafenib *(Zelboraf)* PO BID	Only BRAF positive melanoma with the V600E mutation (~50% of patients) Nausea, arthralgias, fatigue, dermatologic disorders (rashes, photosensitivity, alopecia, pruritus, Stevens Johnson Syndrome, Toxic Epidermal Necrolysis), prolonged QT syndrome, elevated liver enzymes, and secondary squamous cell CA. Expensive ~ $9,400 per month.

Tyrosine Kinase Inhibitors (TKIs) targeting EGFR

Epidermal Growth Factor Receptors (1, 2, 3 and 4) control cell growth, angiogenesis, invasion, metastasis and resistance to apoptosis. Blocking this results in a halt to cancer cell growth and possibly apoptosis.

Erlotinib *(Tarceva)* – PO, 1 hr before, 2 hr after meal	EGFR Inhibitor – Hepatotoxicity, GI perforation, diarrhea, acneiform rash, severe skin reactions, eye damage, nephrotoxicity, stomatitis, interstitial lung disease. Monitor bilirubin, transaminases
Gefitinib *(Iressa)* – PO with or without food	EGFR Inhibitor – Facial rash, acneiform rash correlated with response to treatment, diarrhea, elevated LFTs, fatigue, interstitial lung disease (~ 1/3 fatal) No survival benefit in NSCLC overall. Responses in EGFR positive K-ras wild type lung cancer. Higher incidence of K-ras wild type in Asians and light smokers or non-smokers

Tyrosine Kinase Inhibitors (TKIs) targeting HER-2 neu

HER-2 neu is a tyrosine kinase regulating cell proliferation and survival in over-expressed cancers (~25% of breast cancer). Blocking this results in a halt to cancer cell growth and possibly apoptosis.

Lapatinib *(Tykerb)* – PO, on empty stomach	Inhibits HER-2/neu (ErbB2) and EGFR (Erb1) tyrosine kinases. Used in metastatic breast cancer in patients who failed trastuzumab and chemotherapy. Myelosuppression, hand-foot syndrome, acneform rash, N/V/D, fatigue, elevated LFTs, interstitial lung disease hepatotoxicity, CHF, decreased LVEF and QT-prolongation.

Tyrosine Kinase Inhibitors (TKIs) targeting MULTIPLE proteins

Pazopanib *(Votrient)* – PO with food, do not crush	Inhibits: PDGF-R alpha and beta; VEGF R 1/2/3; FGFR 1/3, cKit; and others Elevated LFTs, hyperglycemia, hypothyroidism, electrolyte loss (phosphorus, sodium, magnesium)
Sorafenib *(Nexavar)*	Inhibits: Raf-mek pathway kinases (CRAF, BRAF); PDGF; EGFR; VEGF R 2/3; SCF R; cKIT; FLT-3. N/V/D, mucositis/stomatitis, dyspepsia, GI bleed, acneform rash, hand-foot syndrome, alopecia, neutropenia, anemia, thrombocytopenia, lymphopenia, elevated blood pressure, electrolyte imbalance, elevated LFTs, elevated lipase/amylase, impaired wound healing (dehiscence), interstitial pneumonitis, hair color changes.
Sunitinib *(Sutent)* – PO not affected by food.	Inhibits multiple Tyrosine Kinases: PDGF; VEGF R 1/2; SCF R; cKIT and others. N/V/D, mucositis/stomatitis, dyspepsia, anorexia, taste disturbance, skin discoloration, acneform rash, hand-foot syndrome, alopecia, neutropenia, anemia, thrombocytopenia, lymphopenia, elevated blood pressure, edema, CHF, decreased LVEF, QT prolongation, fatigue, electrolyte imbalance, elevated LFTs, elevated lipase, hypothyroidism.

DRUG	SIDE EFFECTS/MONITORING/CONTRAINDICATIONS

Tyrosine Kinase Inhibitors (TKIs) targeting RET

Vandetanib *(Zactima)* Primary target is RET, the main target in Medullary Thyroid Cancer	Nausea, diarrhea, interstitial pneumonitis. hypertension, headache, skin disorders from rash to Stevens Johnson Syndrome, prolonged QT syndrome.

Vaccine, Therapeutic
Customized cellular immunotherapy

Sipuleucel-T *(Provenge)*	Infusion of autologous CD 54+ antigen presenting cells obtained through leukapheresis and primed to target prostate cells in the treatment of advanced prostate CA. These cells are activated with the conjugate PAP-GM-CSF (prostatic acid phosphatase antigen – granulocyte-macrophage colony stimulating factor). The goal is for T-cell immunity against the prostate cells.
	Premedicate with acetaminophen and antihistamine due to acute infusion reactions: flu-like symptoms, chills, fatigue, fever, backache, nausea, joint/muscle ache, pain, headache and stroke.
	Limited availability and very expensive (> $90,000).

Vinca Alkaloids
Inhibit microtubule function (destabilizers)

Vinblastine *(Velban)*	Myelosuppression, cumulative (dose-dependent) nerve damage (paresthesias, gastroparesis, paralytic ileus, risk falls, etc.)
Vincristine *(Vincasar)*	Vesication occurs when extravasated, treat with injections of hyaluronidase and moderate heat.
	IV only; Do not administer intrathecally – fatal
Vinorelbine *(Navelbine)*	Alopecia is common with vincristine

Miscellaneous Agents

Arsenic trioxide *(Trisenox)* Induces terminal differentiation of cells or apoptosis	QT-prolongation: monitor ECG, avoid concurrent QT prolonging agents, keep Mg^{2+} and K^+ within normal range. Neuropathy, pain, dry skin, etc.
	Anemia, thrombocytopenia, N/V/D, constipation, fatigue
	"APL Differentiation Syndrome" (Retinoic acid syndrome): fever, dyspnea, weight gain, pulmonary infiltrates, pericardial or pleural effusions, leukocytosis – treat with high-dose steroids
Asparaginase *(Elspar)* – PEG- (polyethylene glycol) modified form – *(Oncospar)*	Deprives leukemia cells of asparagine – essential amino acid in leukemia
	Hepatotoxicity, N/V, encephalopathy, pancreatitis, hyperglycemia, anaphylaxis – requires test dose. Prolonged prothrombin time (PT/INR) and thrombin time (TT)
Bleomycin *(Blenoxane)* – intercalcating agent blocking topoisomerase II	Pulmonary reactions (10%), most common presentation is pneumonitis, which may progress to pulmonary fibrosis, mucositis, hyperpigmentation, hypersensitivity reactions, scleroderma-like skin changes, anemia, N/V
	Bleomycin max lifetime dose = 400 units (well established)
Bortezomib *(Velcade)* 26S proteasome inhibitor	Peripheral neuropathy, psychiatric disturbances, insomnia, weakness, paresthesias, arthralgias/myalgias, cardiotoxicity, pulmonary toxicity, hypotension, thrombocytopenia, neutropenia, N/V/D, tumor lysis syndrome. Interactions: Substrate/Inhibitor of CYP 1A2, 2C9, 2C19, 2D6, 3A4

DRUG	SIDE EFFECTS/MONITORING/CONTRAINDICATIONS
Dactinomycin *(Cosmegen)* Intercalating agent and blocks DNA directed RNA synthesis	Leukopenia, thrombocytopenia, N/V, mucositis, stomatitis, rashes, alopecia, vesicant, radiation recall
Estramustine *(Emcyt)* PO – 1 hr before, 2 hrs after meal – requires refrigeration	Inhibits microtubule assembly and weak estrogenic activity Edema, nausea and vomiting, diarrhea, thromboembolism, gynecomastia, sodium retention. Uptake enhanced in cells containing "estramustine binding proteins" i.e. prostate carcinoma
Hydroxyurea *(Hydrea)* Inhibits ribonucleoside diphosphate reductase, which converts ribonucleotides to deoxyribonucleotides.	Used as a debulking agent in leukemias and in sickle cell disease Myelosuppression, anorexia, N/V, diarrhea, constipation, dermatological rxns, including maculopapular rash, skin ulceration, erythema, hyperpigmentation, skin/nail atrophy, scaling, violet papules and/or skin cancer
Mitomycin *(Mutamycin)* Free radical formation and alkylator	Leukopenia, thrombocytopenia, N/V, fatigue, vesicant

MANAGEMENT OF SIDE EFFECTS & COMORBIDITIES

Chemotherapeutic agents are toxic – to the tumor and to the rest of the patient. Many pharmacists are directly involved with cancer treatment and assist patients with the complications of chemotherapy. ALL pharmacists should be able to assist with the related therapies while specialists are required to help manage the chemotherapeutic regimen.

This section discusses the treatment of myelosuppression (primarily anemia, neutropenia and thrombocytopenia), nausea/vomiting, mucositis and hypercalcemia of malignancy. Weight loss/gain and tumor lysis syndrome are in separate sections.

MYELOSUPPRESSION OVERVIEW

Myelosuppression (↓ in bone marrow activity resulting in fewer red blood cells, white blood cells, and platelets) is a complication with the use of most chemotherapic agents. Neutrophils and platelets are often affected since these cells have a short lifespan and consequently have rapid turnover. If white blood cells decrease, the patient is at increased risk of infection and will have trouble fighting an infection. If red blood cells decrease, the patient becomes anemic – with weakness and fatigue. If platelets decrease, there is an increased risk of serious bleeding.

The lowest point that the cells reach (the nadir) occurs about 10-14 days after chemotherapy, although some agents have a delayed effect. The cell lines generally recover 3-4 weeks post treatment. The next dose of chemotherapy is given after the patient's cells have returned to a safe level. It may be necessary to help restore safe blood cell counts with medications. Severe cases might require a transfusion (providing the missing cell line directly, such as giving packed red blood cells for severe anemia). All agents used for myelosuppression discussed here are usually given by SC (subcutaneous) injection, either by the patient, caregiver or medical provider.

Anemia

Until recently, anemia was routinely treated with an erythropoiesis stimulating agent (ESA). However, most anemias are not life-threatening and, there is now awareness that the ESAs can shorten survival and increase tumor progression in some cancers. This has resulted in much less frequent use of the ESAs. To make sure that patients are aware of the risks, MedGuides are dispensed with each prescription/filling. For cancer, the use of ESAs must fulfill the requirements of the ESA APPRISE Oncology program. This is a program whose purpose is to make sure the healthcare providers are trained and that the patient has received proper counseling on risks and benefits.

ANEMIA ASSESSMENT

Hemoglobin levels are used to assess anemia. Normal levels are within 12-16 g/dL for females and 13-18 g/dL for males (hematocrit is 36-46% females; 37-49% males). Ferritin, serum iron and a total iron binding capacity (TIBC) may be ordered since the ESAs cannot work well to correct anemia if iron levels are inadequate. Levels of folate and vitamin B-12 may also be appraised, especially if there is a poor response to the ESA.

ANEMIA TREATMENT WITH AN ESA

Epoetin alpha *(Procrit, Epogen)* SC usually Q weekly OR

Darbepoetin *(Aranesp)* SC usually Q 2-3 weeks (less frequent dosing)

- In order to be able to prescribe ESAs for cancer, the prescriber must be enrolled and certified by the ESA APPRISE Oncology Program. The patient must sign a form that states they have received counseling about risks and benefits.

- The patient MUST receive the ESA's MedGuide when ESA therapy begins and at least monthly, if continuing.

- The goal of therapy is now redefined as giving the lowest dose necessary to avoid the need for RBC transfusions. ESAs should only be used if the hemoglobin level is < 10 g/dL prior to therapy and the patient should be symptomatic.

- ESA use is associated with CHF, chest pain, thrombosis, arrhythmias, cardiovascular death and in some cases acceleration of tumor growth.

- Common side effects may include hypertension, hypotension, arthralgias/myalgias/back pain, injection site pain, edema, fatigue and headache.

Neutropenia

Low neutrophils increase infection risk and make it difficult to fight infection.

NEUTROPENIA ASSESSMENT

An absolute neutrophil count (ANC) of < 500 mm^3 places the patient at a high risk for a poor outcome. An ANC of < 100 mm^3 is a severe risk for infection.

NEUTROPENIA PREVENTION WITH A CSF

The colony stimulating factors (CSFs):

■ Sargramostim (GM-CSF, *Leukine)* ✓

■ Filgrastim (G-CSF, *Neupogen)* ✓

■ Pegfilgrastim (Pegylated G-CSF, *Neulasta)* ✓

■ These are expensive and do not improve overall survival outcomes. They do shorten the time that a patient is at risk due to neutropenia and reduces infectious mortality when given prophylactically in patients at a high risk of febrile neutropenia. Consequently, their use is usually limited to conditions outlined in an institution's protocol to define those patients at a high risk of febrile neutropenia. The GM-CSF is limited to use in stem cell transplantation whereas both forms of G-CSF are indicated in febrile neutropenia.

■ The primary side effect is bone pain.

Thrombocytopenia

Low platelets (thrombocytes) can result in spontaneous, uncontrolled bleeding.

THROMBOCYTOPENIA ASSESSMENT

The normal range for platelets is 150,000-450,000/mm^3.

Platelet transfusions are generally indicated when the count falls below 10,000/mm^3.

THROMBOCYTOPENIA PREVENTION WITH OPRELVEKIN

■ Oprelvekin (IL-11, *Neumega)*

■ Side effects are significant which has limited use in the clinical setting. These include hypersensitivity reactions, anaphylaxis, fluid retention, peripheral edema (may need diuretics), tachycardia, atrial fibrillation, pleural effusions and dyspnea.

Nausea and Vomiting: Prevention is essential.

Nausea and vomiting are common with chemotherapy. Certain agents, such as cisplatin, have increased risk (higher emetogenicity). Agents with high risk require prophylaxis with multiple antiemetic agents. Patient factors which increase risk include female gender, < 50 years of age, dehydration, history of motion sickness, and history of nausea and vomiting with prior regimens.

Anthracyclines, carboplatin and oxaliplatin are considered moderate risk, but if used in high dose or in combination with another moderately emetogenic agent, they are considered high emetogenic risk.

To prevent acute nausea and vomiting, three drugs are used in combination:

- Dexamethasone

- Ondansetron or other 5-HT3 receptor blocker

- Aprepitant, a neurokinin-1 receptor blocker

Delayed emesis can be prevented by either one of these agents alone or in combinations depending on the risk and severity. At any point, an adjunct of lorazepam *(Ativan)* may be added for anxiety/amnestic response or an H2 blocker or PPI if upper GI symptoms similar to GERD are present. An agent that is low emetogenic risk may require a single agent such as dexamethasone, prochlorperazine or metoclopramide.

Prochlorperazine or similar phenothiazines-like agents, antihistamines (diphenhydramine, etc), or metoclopramide *(Reglan)* are sometimes used, however each has safety concerns. Phenothiazines and metoclopramide are dopamine-blocking agents and could cause or worsen movement disorders. Both classes are sedating and can cause cognitive dysfunction. Metoclopramide requires a reduced dose with renal dysfunction, which may not be considered. When overdosed, the side effect profile is worsened. Centrally-acting antihistamines such as diphenhydramine cause central and peripheral anticholinergic side effects, which can be intolerable in elderly patients.

Dronabinol *(Marinol)* and nabilone *(Cesamet)* can be used as 2nd line agents. These are synthetic delta-9- tetrahydrocannabinol, a naturally occurring component of Cannabis sativa (marijuana).

ANTIEMETIC AGENTS

DRUG	SIDE EFFECTS
5-HT3 serotonin receptor antagonists	
Ondansetron *(Zofran)* – IV, PO, ODT, solution 4-24 mg	Headache, fatigue, dizziness, constipation or diarrhea
	Elevated liver enzymes (~1%)
	Contraindicated with Parkinson's drug apomorphine (*Apokyn*)
Granisetron *(Kytril, Sancuso transdermal patch)* IV/PO 1-2 mg	***Zofran ODT***: With dry hands, peel back the foil backing of 1 blister and gently remove the tablet and immediately place on top of the tongue where it will dissolve in seconds, then swallow with saliva.
	Sancuso patch: useful if sores in mouth (mucositis), dysphagia or if expected to need up to 5 days nausea prevention (apply on the upper arm the day before chemo and leave on at least 24 hr after last session – lasts up to 7 days). Avoid sunlight near patch site.
Dolasetron *(Anzemet)* IV/PO 100-200 mg – do not use for CINV due to risk of QT prolongation	Risk of prolonged QT interval (torsades de pointes) with all 5-HT3 antagonists; correct Mg^{2+} and K^+ and monitor ECG.
Palonosetron *(Aloxi)*, IV/PO	

Antiemetic Agents Continued

DRUG	SIDE EFFECTS
Phenothiazines	
Prochlorperazine (Compazine) 5-10 mg Q4H	<u>Do not use in children < 2 years old</u> and use dosing guidelines for older children. Sedation, lethargy, hypotension, neuroleptic malignant syndrome (NMS), QT prolongation, acute EPS (common in children – antidote is diphenhydramine or benztropine)
Chlorpromazine *(Thorazine)*	
Promethazine (Phenergan)	

DRUG	SIDE EFFECTS
Corticosteroid	
Dexamethasone (Decadron) – PO, IV	Anxiety, insomnia, GI upset, acute psychosis (if high doses + lack of sleep, etc.)

DRUG	SIDE EFFECTS
Cannabinoids	
Dronabinol (Marinol) TID-QID Refrigerate capsules, CIII	Drowsiness, euphoria, increased appetite, orthostatic hypotension
Nabilone *(Cesamet)* BID CII – No refrigeration needed	

DRUG	SIDE EFFECTS
Substance P/Neurokinin-1 receptor antagonist	
Aprepitant (Emend) Injectable *Emend* is the prodrug fosaprepitant	Dizziness, fatigue, constipation, hiccups PO: 125 mg 1 hr before chemo, then 80 mg daily x 2 days IV: 115 mg pre chemo

Mucositis

Inflammation and sores in the mouth, esophagus and lower GI tract can cause considerable suffering. There are many agents used to try and prevent and treat mucositis ("Magic Mouthwash", chlorhexidine rinse, etc) but only one FDA approved agent: palifermin *(Kepivance)* which is restricted to high dose chemo prior to stem cell transplant. Patients at risk for mucositis should be counseled to use a saline rinse several times daily.

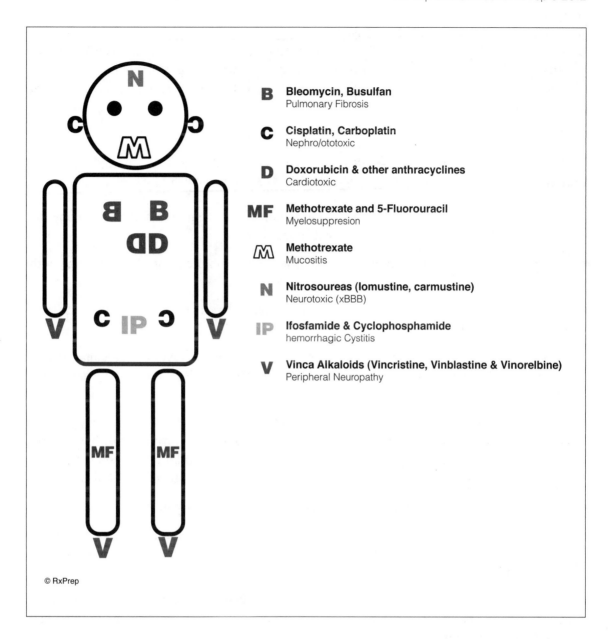

B	**Bleomycin, Busulfan**	Pulmonary Fibrosis
C	**Cisplatin, Carboplatin**	Nephro/ototoxic
D	**Doxorubicin & other anthracyclines**	Cardiotoxic
MF	**Methotrexate and 5-Fluorouracil**	Myelosuppresion
M	**Methotrexate**	Mucositis
N	**Nitrosoureas (lomustine, carmustine)**	Neurotoxic (xBBB)
IP	**Ifosfamide & Cyclophosphamide**	hemorrhagic Cystitis
V	**Vinca Alkaloids (Vincristine, Vinblastine & Vinorelbine)**	Peripheral Neuropathy

© RxPrep

Hypercalcemia of Malignancy

Prior to the therapeutic use of bisphosphonates in metastatic bone cancer, hypercalcemia occurred in ~25% of cancer patients and was the most common metabolic complication of breast cancer. It also occurs commonly with lung cancer and multiple myeloma. The bone destruction that results in hypercalcemia causes significant symptoms for the patient, including nausea, vomiting, fatigue, dehydration and mental status changes. Bone pain can be significant, and the complication carries a high risk of long-term skeletal damage (fractures, spinal cord compression, etc.) which is why bisphosphonates or denosumab *(Xgeva)* are used early in metastatic disease to prevent skeletal related events. Hypercalcemia is generally treated with aggressive hydration, forced diuresis (loop diuretics) and IV bisphosphonates. IV bisphosphonates are routinely used in oncology indications, although oral formulations are sometimes used. The IV agents indicated for hypercalcemia of malignancy include zoledronic acid *(Zometa)* and pamidronate *(Aredia)*. Zoledronic acid as *Reclast* is indicated for osteoporosis – this is an injection only – but the dose is different. The usual dose is 5 mg/year with *Reclast* compared to 4 mg monthly with *Zometa*. The bisphosphonates require adjustment for renal insufficiency whereas the denosumab as a monoclonal antibody does not. All these have a risk of osteonecrosis of the jaw (ONJ) for which discontinuation of therapy is required.

PATIENT COUNSELING EXAMPLES

Patient Counseling for SERMs [using tamoxifen *(Nolvadex)* as an example]

- This medication can be used to prevent your chance of getting breast cancer, reduce the spread of breast cancer or be used to treat breast cancer.

- Swallow the tablet whole, with water or another non-alcoholic liquid. You can take with or without food.

- Take your medicine every day. It may be easier to remember if you take it at the same time each day.

- If you forget a dose, take it when you remember, then take the next dose as usual. If it is almost time for your next dose or you remember at your next dose, do not take extra tablets to make up the missed dose.

- Do not become pregnant while taking this medication or for 2 months after you stop. This medication can stop hormonal birth control methods from working (i.e. birth control pills, patches, injections, rings and implants). Therefore, while taking this medication, another method of contraception such as condoms, diaphragms with spermicide, or IUD's.

- If you get pregnant, stop taking this medication right away and call your doctor.

- Be sure to have regular gynecology check-ups ("female exams"), breast exams and mammograms. Your doctor will tell you how often. These will check for signs of breast cancer and cancer of the endometrium (lining of the uterus).

- This medication can cause some serious, but rare, adverse effects such as endometrial cancer, strokes, or blood clot in the lungs (or pulmonary embolism). This medication can also increase the risk of getting cataracts.

- The most common side effects include hot flashes, hypertension, peripheral edema, mood changes, depression, skin changes, and vaginal discharge.

- You should call your doctor right away if you develop:

  - vaginal bleeding or bloody discharge that could be a rusty or brown color, change in your monthly bleeding, such as in the amount or timing of bleeding or increased clotting, or pain or pressure in your pelvis (below your belly button).

  - sudden chest pain, shortness of breath, coughing up blood, pain, tenderness, or swelling in one or both of your legs.

❏ sudden weakness, tingling, or numbness in your face, arm or leg, especially on one side of your body; sudden confusion, trouble speaking or sudden trouble seeing in one or both eyes, sudden trouble walking, dizziness, loss of balance or coordination, or sudden severe headache with no known cause.

❏ signs of liver problems like lack of appetite and yellowing of your skin or whites of your eyes.

For *Evista* – discontinue at least 72 hours prior to and during prolonged immobilization (e.g., post- surgical recovery, prolonged bed rest), and patients should be advised to avoid prolonged restrictions of movement during travel because of the increased risk of venous thromboembolic event.

Aromatase Inhibitors

■ This medication is to treat breast cancer in patients who have finished menopause. This medication does not work in women who have not finished menopause.

■ Take exactly as prescribed by your doctor.

■ Can be taken with or without food.

■ If you miss a dose, take it as soon as you remember. If it is almost time for your next dose, skip the missed dose. Take your next regularly scheduled dose. Do not take two doses at the same time.

■ Common side effects include hot flashes, weakness, joint pain, bone pain, osteoporosis, mood changes, high blood pressure, depression, and rash.

■ This medication can cause rare, but serious, adverse effects such as heart disease, increased cholesterol, skin reactions, allergic reactions, and liver problems.

■ Call your doctor right away if you develop:

❏ chest pain, shortness of breath.

❏ any skin lesions, ulcers, or blisters.

❏ swelling of the face, lips, tongue, or throat, trouble swallowing, or trouble breathing.

❏ a general feeling of not being well with yellowing of the skin or whites of the eyes or pain on the right side of your abdomen.

❏ Tell your doctor or pharmacist about all the medicines you take, including prescription and non-prescription medicines, vitamins, and herbal supplements. This medication should not be taken with tamoxifen or any medicines containing estrogen including pills, patches, creams, rings, or suppositories.

Lupron

■ This medication will lower sex hormones (testosterone and estrogen) produced by the body.

- <u>In men (prostate CA):</u> common side effects include hot flashes and impotence. During the first few weeks of treatment you may experience increased bone pain, increased difficulty in urinating, and less commonly but most importantly, you may experience the onset or aggravation of nerve symptoms. In any of these events, discuss the symptoms with your doctor.

Promethazine

- This medication may cause marked drowsiness or impair the mental and/or physical abilities required for the performance of potentially hazardous tasks, such as driving a vehicle or operating machinery.

- The use of alcohol or other central-nervous-system depressants such as sedatives/hypnotics (including barbiturates), narcotics, narcotic analgesics, general anesthetics, tricyclic antidepressants, and tranquilizers, may worsen mental impairment. These drugs should be avoided.

- IV administration is not recommended due to risk of severe tissue injury, including gangrene and hypotension if rapid administration. Do not administer SC either. Only IM, PO, or rectal. If IV administration is deemed necessary, dilute further and administer as an infusion over 20-30 minutes through a patent IV site.

Practice Case

Tommy is a 53 year old male (height 5'10", weight 200 lbs.) who is receiving the following medication regimen for the treatment of non-Hodgkin lymphoma. His past medical history is significant for mild stage 1 CHF. He is to receive 6 cycles of "CHOP" chemotherapy.

CATEGORY	
Chemotherapy Regimen	Cyclophosphamide 750 mg/m² IV on day 1
	Doxorubicin 50 mg/m² IV on day 1
	Vincristine 1.4 mg/m² IV on day 1
	Prednisone 100 mg PO on days 1-5 given first

Questions

Questions 1-5 refer to the above case.

1. The pharmacist must first calculate the patient's BSA and will use the Dubois and Dubois Equation: BSA(m²) = 0.007184 x [weight (kg)$^{0.425}$] x [height (cm)$^{0.725}$] The patient's BSA is:

   a. 1.15 m²
   b. 1.03 m²
   c. 2.09 m²
   d. 2.18 m²
   e. 3.15 m²

2. What is the correct milligram dose of doxorubicin that the patient should receive on Day 1?

   a. 104.5 mg
   b. 510 mg
   c. 949.5 mg
   d. 948.5 mg
   e. 300 mg

3. The physician wants to know if there are any medications that can reduce the likelihood of cardiotoxicity with doxorubicin therapy. Which of the following would you suggest?

   a. Totect
   b. Zinecard
   c. Lasix
   d. Epogen
   e. Mesna

4. The physician is worried about Tommy developing acute nausea and vomiting from this chemotherapeutic regimen. Which of the following regimens would you recommend for prevention?

   a. Metoclopramide + lorazepam
   b. Aprepitant + chlorpromazine
   c. Ondansetron + aprepitant
   d. Dexamethasone + Aprepitant
   e. None of the above

5. What is the dose limiting toxicity of vincristine?

   a. Neuropathy
   b. Nephrotoxicity
   c. Hypersensitivity reaction
   d. Ototoxicity
   e. Pulmonary toxicity

Questions 6-14 do not relate to the above case.

6. A patient is using apomorphine (Apokyn) injections for advanced Parkinson's disease. The patient has been suffering from nausea. Which of the following antiemetics is contraindicated with apomorphine?

   a. Lorazepam
   b. Metoclopramide
   c. Prochlorperazine
   d. Granisetron
   e. All of the above

7. A patient will begin raloxifene therapy. Choose the correct counseling points:

    a. This drug can increase your risk of breast cancer.

    b. Avoid long periods of immobility, such as during long airplane flights – get up and move when you can.

    c. This medication can cause weakened bones and fractures.

    d. A and B

    e. A, B, and C

8. Which of the following medications should be taken <u>with food</u>?

    a. Gleevec

    b. Xeloda

    c. Rituxan

    d. A and B

    e. All of the above

9. The antidote for toxicity from high-dose methotrexate is:

    a. Folic acid supplements (OTC or Rx)

    b. Leucovorin

    c. Vitamin B12

    d. Cholestyramine

    e. Vitamin D

10. A pharmacist received a prescription for *Gleevec*. An appropriate generic interchange is:

    a. Aprepitant

    b. Imatinib

    c. Temozolomide

    d. Anastrozole

    e. Capecitabine

11. A pharmacist received a prescription for *Temodar*. An appropriate generic interchange is:

    a. Temozolomide

    b. Tamoxifen

    c. Raloxifene

    d. Capecitabine

    e. Metoclopramide

12. A pharmacist received a prescription for *Arimidex*. An appropriate generic interchange is:

    a. Aprepitant

    b. Anastrozole

    c. Exemestane

    d. Letrozole

    e. Tamoxifen

13. A patient is receiving dronabinol for nausea. Appropriate counseling points should include:

    a. The capsules should be kept in the refrigerator.

    b. Your appetite may increase.

    c. This medication cannot be shared with others.

    d. A and B only.

    e. All of the above.

14. A patient has chemotherapy-induced anemia. She states she is weak. The pharmacist has access to her labs and finds that <u>the current hemoglobin level is 11 g/dL</u>. Ferritin, serum iron, TIBC, folate and vitamin B12 are all at acceptable levels. Her oncologist has prescribed *Procrit*. The patient has brought the *Procrit* prescription to the pharmacy. Choose the correct statement:

    a. The prescription can be filled after the pharmacist confirms that the patient is registered with the ESA APPRISE program.

    b. The generic name of *Procrit* is darbepoetin.

    c. The patient should be aware that they may experience euphoria and increased appetite.

    d. A and B only.

    e. The prescription should not be filled; the pharmacist should contact the prescriber.

ANSWERS

1-c, 2-a, 3-b, 4-c, 5-a, 6-d, 7-b, 8-d, 9-b, 10-b, 11-a, 12-b, 13-e, 14-e

ANEMIA

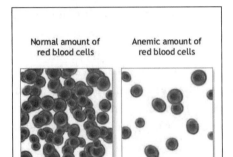

Normal amount of red blood cells

Anemic amount of red blood cells

GUIDELINES/REFERENCES

KDOQI Clinical Practice Guideline and Clinical Practice Recommendations for Anemia in Chronic Kidney Disease: 2007 Update of Hemoglobin Target, Available at: http://www.kidney.org/professionals/kdoqi/guidelines_anemia/cpr21.htm and FDA warning update June, 2011.

Note: Iron requirements for infants, per the American Pediatric Association, are in the Natural Products and Vitamins section.

Background

Anemia is a disease characterized by a decrease in hemoglobin or red blood cells (RBCs). This can happen when a patient is bleeding, when the RBCs are not functional (such as in sickle cell anemia), when the bone marrow cannot produce enough RBCs to equal the destruction or loss, or (most commonly) when there is a lack of nutrients to provide optimal RBC functioning (such as with iron, vitamin B12 and/or folate deficiency).

Red blood cells (erythrocytes) are the most common type of blood cell. They carry oxygen in the blood and through the circulatory system to the body's tissues. Oxygen enters the RBCs in the lungs and is delivered through the capillaries. Oxygen-poor blood is sent back to the lungs, where carbon dioxide is released and more oxygen is received. Normally, a red blood cell has a lifespan of about 120 days. If the red blood cells are not working properly or are deficient, anemia will result.

Signs and Symptoms

In anemia, the tissues are not getting enough oxygen-rich blood and most of the signs and symptoms are due to tissue hypoxia. Most patients with mild anemia or in the beginning stages are generally asymptomatic. As the anemia worsens, the patient may experience some of the classic symptoms such as fatigue, malaise, weakness, shortness of breath, dizziness, and/or pale skin. More severe symptoms, usually due to acute blood loss, may include chest pain, angina, fainting, palpitations and tachycardia. Glossitis (an inflamed, sore tongue), koilonychias (thin, concave, spoon-shaped nails) or pica (craving and eating non-foods such as chalk or clay) may develop.

A decreased oxygen supply can cause ischemic damage to many organs. Anemia is most notable in causing heart damage if it persists long-term – the heart will try to compensate for low oxygen levels by pumping faster (tachycardia) and by increasing the mass of the ventricular wall; this can eventually lead to heart failure.

LABORATORY VALUES

Anemia is defined by low hemoglobin (Hgb) and low hematocrit (Hct) levels. Anemias are usually diagnosed by measuring the hemoglobin level.

The most common way to classify the type of anemia is by the mean corpuscular volume (MCV), or the red blood cell volume. While the symptoms may be similar for both macrocytic or microcytic anemia, the MCV, will differ. The MCV is small (< 80) in microcytic anemia due to a small cell size from a lack of iron. The MCV is large (> 100) in macrocytic (AKA megaloblastic) anemia due to folate or vitamin B12 deficiency. Anemias can also have a normal MVC (80-100) and are therefore called normocytic anemia. These anemias can result from acute blood loss (surgery or trauma), hemolysis, bone marrow failure, or anemia of chronic disease. Certain genetic conditions cause dysfunctional RBCs resulting in anemia, such as sickle cell anemia.

Patients with chronic kidney disease generally lack erythropoietin, a hormone secreted by the kidneys that increases the rate of production of red blood cells in response to falling levels of oxygen in the tissues. In addition, iron stores can be low. Iron is essential for hemoglobin formation. The iron values are important to assess prior to the initiation of erythropoietin therapy. If the iron stores are low, the drug will not be able to work. Patients with chronic kidney disease may have poor iron absorption and may be receiving iron by injection. The majority of patients who need iron replacement are able to use oral supplementation. The majority of patients who receive iron by injection are on hemodialysis.

Hemoglobin (Hgb)

- 13-18 g/dL – normal for males; 12-16 g/dL – normal for females

Hematocrit (Hct)

- 37-49% – normal for males; 36-46% – normal for females

Mean Corpuscular Volume (MCV)

- Normal values are 80-100 micrometers^3; defined as the average volume of RBCs

Total Iron-Binding Capacity (TIBC)

- Normal values are 250-400 mcg/dL; indirectly measures iron-binding capacity of transferrin; high TIBC may be indicative of iron deficiency anemia

Serum Ferritin

- 30-300 ng/mL – normal for males; 10-200 ng/mL – normal for females; decreased in iron-deficiency anemia

Microcytic Anemia

The most common type of anemia is <u>microcytic, or iron-deficiency, anemia</u>. Iron deficiency results when iron demand by the body is not met by iron absorption from the diet. Dietary iron is available in two forms; heme iron (found in meat) and nonheme iron (found in plant and dairy foods). Absorption of heme iron is minimally affected by dietary factors but non-heme iron makes up the majority of consumed iron. The bioavailability of nonheme iron requires gastric acid and varies by an order of magnitude depending on the concentration of enhancers (e.g. meat, ascorbate) and inhibitors (e.g. calcium, fiber, tea, coffee, wine) in the diet. <u>Microcytic anemia is diagnosed by a low hemoglobin and a low mean corpuscular volume (MCV) < 80</u>. Serum ferritin levels may also be measured and these levels would be low. Microcytic anemia is generally treated with OTC iron and takes months to adequately treat.

AT-RISK PATIENTS

Pregnant women, pre-term and low birth weight infants, older infants and toddlers, teenage girls, women with heavy menstrual periods, and renal failure patients are the most common cases with iron deficiency. Gastrointestinal diseases, including Crohn's and celiac disease, can reduce absorption and require replacement therapy. Total dietary iron intake in vegetarian diets may meet recommended levels; however, that iron is less available (non-heme iron) for absorption than in diets that include meat (heme-containing iron). Occasionally vegetarians need iron replacement.

Women taking hormone contraception experience less bleeding during their periods and therefore have a lower risk of developing an iron deficiency. A pharmacist will occasionally dispense contraception to a female (mostly younger – since younger women tend to have heavier blood loss) that is being used to reduce anemia.

Treatment of Microcytic Anemia

ORAL IRON THERAPY

- <u>Oral iron therapy (ferrous sulfate) is usually used first-line for patients with iron-deficiency anemia, except those patients on hemodialysis (discussed in parental iron therapy section below)</u>.

- Ferrous iron is absorbed more readily than the ferric form.

- An increase in Hgb level by 1 g/dL should occur every 2-3 weeks on iron therapy; however, it may <u>take up to 4 months for the iron stores to return to normal after the Hgb level is corrected</u>.

- <u>Sustained-release formulations of iron are not recommended as initial therapy</u> because they reduce the amount of iron that is present for absorption in the duodenum.

- <u>Absorption of iron is enhanced in an acidic gastric environment</u>. Ascorbic acid (vitamin C 200 mg), taken concurrently, may enhance absorption, to a minimal extent.

- <u>Food will decrease the absorption of iron</u>. It is best to take iron at least 1 hour before meals. However, many patients must take iron with food because they experience GI upset (nausea) when iron is administered on an empty stomach.

ORAL IRON THERAPY

DRUG	DOSING	SIDE EFFECTS/CONTRAINDICATIONS/ MONITORING
Ferrous sulfate (*Feosol with Ferrous Sulfate, FeroSul*) **Infant Drops** *Fer-In-Sol* Iron Supplement Drops *Poly-Vi-Sol* Vitamin Drops With Iron use if they need the vitamin D <u>and</u> iron **Children** *Flintstones* Children's Chewable Multivitamin, Tablets, plus Iron *Pokemon* Children's Multiple Vitamin with Iron, Chewable Tablets	<u>325 mg PO daily to TID</u> <u>(65 mg elemental iron)</u> <u>1st line therapy</u>	Ferrous sulfate – 20% elemental iron Ferrous sulfate, exsiccated – 30% elemental iron Ferrous fumarate – 33% elemental iron Ferrous gluconate – 12% elemental iron **BLACK BOX WARNING** Accidental overdose of <u>iron-containing</u> products is a leading cause of fatal poisoning in children under 6. Keep iron out of reach of children. In case of accidental overdose, go to ER or call poison control center immediately. **SIDE EFFECTS** <u>Stomach upset, nausea, constipation (dose related), dark and tarry stools</u>
Ferrous fumarate (*Ferretts, Hemocyte*, generic)	324 mg PO daily to TID (other doses available) (106 mg elemental iron)	**MONITORING** Hgb, serum iron, TIBC, ferritin **NOTES** <u>Enteric coated and delayed-release products are not recommended due to decrease in iron absorption</u> by delaying time of release [Less iron is absorbed since it passes the duodenum (site of maximal absorption) and is released into the ileum of the small intestine]
Ferrous gluconate (*Fergon*, generic)	324 mg PO daily to TID (38 mg elemental iron)	Although fiber is 1st line treatment for constipation, a stool softener such as <u>docusate</u> is often recommended for iron-induced constipation
Ferrous sulfate, dried (exsiccated) **Controlled Release (*Slow Fe*)**	160 mg PO daily to TID	
Carbonyl iron (*Feosol with Carbonyl Iron, Ferracap, Ferralet 90*)	varies	<u>Highest amount of iron (100 % elemental iron)</u>

IRON DRUG INTERACTIONS

- Antacids and agents that raise pH (H_2RAs, PPIs) decrease iron absorption by increasing pH.

- Antibiotics, mainly tetracycline and quinolones, can decrease iron absorption through chelation. Take iron 2 hours before or 4 hours after.

- Vitamin C increases acidity thus increases the absorption of iron; little benefit with low doses (need ~200 mg of ascorbic acid).

- Food decreases absorption as much as 50%; try to take on an empty stomach. If unable to tolerate, take with a small amount of food.

- Iron can interact and decrease the levels of the following medications: levodopa, methyldopa, levothyroxine, and mycophenolate. Separate the doses by 2 hours.

IRON: TOXIC IN OVERDOSE!

Accidental iron poisoning is the <u>leading cause of poisoning deaths among young children</u>. As little as 15 tablets can lead to overdose. The child can appear asymptomatic (initially) or have already developed severe nausea, vomiting, gastrointestinal bleeding (most often vomiting blood), and diarrhea. <u>If a parent suspects their child took iron pills or liquid, they should be directed to the nearest emergency room immediately</u> – whether symptomatic or not. Left untreated, iron overdose will damage most organs, including the brain, and can be fatal. <u>The antidote for iron overdose is deferoxamine</u>. Iron pills are now routinely packaged in unit-dose blister packs to reduce the risk of accidental childhood ingestion.

PARENTERAL IRON THERAPY

Parenteral iron therapy is as effective but can be more dangerous and is much more expensive than oral therapy. The following clinical situations may warrant IV administration:

- <u>Hemodialysis (most common use of IV iron)</u> – the National Kidney Foundation (NKF) guidelines state that to achieve and maintain a hemoglobin level of 11 g/dL (and hematocrit 33-36%), most hemodialysis patients will require IV iron on a regular basis.

- Unable to tolerate iron given orally; or losing iron too fast for oral replacement.

- Intestinal malabsorption, such as Crohn's.

- Patients donating large amounts of blood for autoinfusion.

INTRAVENOUS (PARENTERAL) IRON SUPPLEMENTATION

DRUG	SIDE EFFECTS/CONTRAINDICATIONS/MONITORING
Iron Dextran (INFeD, Dexferrum)	**Black Box Warning with Iron Dextran only** Risk of anaphylactic reactions. A test dose should be given to all patients prior to first therapeutic dose. Fatal reactions have occurred even in patients who tolerated the test dose. History of drug allergy and/or concomitant use of ACE inhibitor may ↑ risk.
Sodium Ferric Gluconate (Ferrlecit, Nulecit)	**SIDE EFFECTS** Hypotension, chest tightness, peripheral edema, risk of anaphylaxis with all agents (greatest risk with iron dextran – test dose required only for iron dextran)
Iron Sucrose (Venofer)	**MONITORING** Hgb, Hct, serum ferritin, serum iron, TIBC, vital signs, electrolytes, anaphylaxis
Ferumoxytol (Feraheme)	

Macrocytic Anemia

Macrocytic anemia is due to either a vitamin B12 or folate deficiency, or both. Pernicious anemia is a type of macrocytic anemia that results in low B12 levels due to a lack of intrinsic factor, which is required for adequate B12 absorption in the small intestine. Since gut absorption is impaired in those who lack intrinsic factor, pernicious anemia requires life-long vitamin B12 replacement therapy. Some patients can get enough supplementation with high-dose tablets of oral vitamin B12, but many clinicians prefer injections since macrocytic anemia can lead to neurological complications.

If macrocytic anemia continues long-term, the patient is at risk for serious neurological consequences – including cognitive dysfunction (dementia) and peripheral nerve damage.

Alcoholism, Crohn's disease and celiac disease are other causes of macrocytic anemia. Macrocytic anemia is diagnosed by a low hemoglobin and a high mean corpuscular volume (MCV) > 100. Vitamin B12 and/or serum folate levels will be low. The Schilling test can diagnose vitamin B12 deficiency due to lack of intrinsic factor.

TREATMENT OF MACROCYTIC ANEMIA

Treatment may start with vitamin B12 injections and follow with oral supplements. Injections are used for anyone with a severe deficiency or with neurological symptoms due to the high risk of more severe neurological complications. Also, recommend the injectable for patients who cannot take or adhere to oral medications or those who cannot absorb oral medications (diarrhea, vomiting, IBD).

DRUG	DOSING	SIDE EFFECTS/CONTRAINDICATIONS/ MONITORING
Cyanocobalamin (Vitamin B12)	IM or deep SC: 30-1,000 mcg/ day (depending on the regimen followed); can be given monthly	**SIDE EFFECTS** Itching, diarrhea, edema
	Oral/Sublingual: 1,000-2,000 mcg/day for mild-moderate deficiencies	**CONTRAINDICATIONS** Cobalt allergy
	Intranasal: 500 mcg in one nostril once weekly (*Nascobal*) or each nostril daily (*CaloMist*)	**MONITORING** Hgb, Hct, vitamin B12, folate, iron Do not use sustained-release B12 supplements as the absorption is not adequate.
Folic Acid (folate)	1 tab daily 0.4, 0.8 mg tabs (OTC) 1 mg tabs (Rx)	**SIDE EFFECTS** Bronchospasm, flushing, rash, pruritus **MONITORING** Hgb, Hct, folate, vitamin B12, iron

DRUG INTERACTIONS

Vitamin B12

Colchicine, ethanol and long-term treatment with metformin may ↓ B12 absorption.

Folic acid

Drugs that ↓ folic acid absorption include phenobarbital, phenytoin, primidone, oral contraceptives, cholestyramine, azathioprine, 6-mercaptopurine, methotrexate, and thioguanine.

Anemia of Chronic Kidney Disease

Renal disease causes anemia due to a lack of erythropoietin, or EPO, a hormone produced by healthy kidneys. Erythropoietin stimulates the bone marrow to produce RBCs. In renal disease, the deficiency results in the bone marrow making fewer red blood cells. Erythropoietin can be given by injection (generally subcutaneous); however, it is important to check that the anemia warrants the use. In recent years, the use of erythropoietin has narrowed due to safety concerns but it is still used frequently.

ANEMIA TREATMENT WITH ERYTHROPOIESIS-STIMULATING AGENTS (ESAs)

Until recently, anemia due to CRF and cancer was routinely treated with an erythropoiesis stimulating agent (ESA). However, most anemias are not life-threatening and there is now awareness that the ESAs can be dangerous in certain situations.

The black box warnings for the use of ESAs include:

- Chronic Kidney Disease: Patients experienced greater risks for death, serious cardiovascular events, and stroke when administered ESAs to target a hemoglobin level > 11 g/dL. No trial has identified a Hgb target level, ESA dose, or dosing strategy that does not increase these risks. Use the lowest dose sufficient to reduce the need for RBC transfusions.

- Cancer: ESAs shortened overall survival and/or increased the risk of tumor progression or recurrence in clinical studies of patients with breast, head and neck, non-small-cell lung, lymphoid, and cervical cancers. Prescribers and hospitals must enroll in and comply with the ESA APPRISE Oncology Program to prescribe and/or dispense to patients with cancer. ESAs should only be used if the hemoglobin level is < 10 g/dL. Use the lowest dose to avoid RBC transfusions. ESAs are not indicated when the anticipated outcome is cure. Discontinue following completion of a chemotherapy course.

- Perisurgery: Due to increased risk of deep venous thrombosis (DVT), DVT prophylaxis is recommended.

For chronic renal failure, ESAs should be used at the lowest possible dose that reduce the need for blood transfusions. Start when hemoglobin is < 10 g/dL and reduce or stop therapy when hemoglobin is near 11 g/dL. Transferrin saturation should be at least 20%, and ferritin should be at least 100 ng/mL prior to starting ESA treatment. Levels of folate and vitamin B-12 may also be assessed, especially if there is a poor response to the ESA.

DRUG	DOSING	SIDE EFFECTS/CONTRAINDICATIONS/MONITORING
Epoetin alfa (Epogen, Procrit)	IV/SC: 50-100 units/kg 3 times weekly initial, then individualize maintenance dose (CKD dose)	**BLACK BOX WARNINGS (SEE ABOVE)** **SIDE EFFECTS** Hypertension, arthralgia, back pain, inject site pain, muscle spasm, pyrexia, vascular occlusion, upper respiratory tract infections, thrombosis **CONTRAINDICATIONS** Uncontrolled HTN, pure red cell aplasia (PRCA) that begins after treatment
Darbepoetin (Aranesp)	IV/SC: 0.45 mcg/kg weekly or 0.75 mcg/kg every 2 weeks	**MONITORING** Hgb, Hct, iron stores, BP IV route is recommended for patients on hemodialysis. Store in refrigerator

IRON PATIENT COUNSELING

- This medication is best taken on an empty stomach 1 hour before or 2 hours after meals. If stomach upset occurs, you may take this medication with food.

- Avoid taking antacids, dairy products, tea, coffee or wine within 2 hours before or after this medication because they will decrease its effectiveness.

- This medication needs to be taken for at least a few months after your anemia symptoms have improved; do not stop until directed by your doctor.

- Iron can cause your stool to become dark. This is expected.

- If you develop constipation, ask your pharmacist for a recommendation for a stool softener, such as docusate (if you are not pregnant). If pregnant, use fiber products such as psyllium.

ESA PATIENT COUNSELING

- This drug can increase your risk of life-threatening heart or circulation problems, including heart attack or stroke. This risk will increase the longer you use this drug. Seek emergency medical help if you have symptoms of heart or circulation problems, such as: chest pain or heavy feeling, pain spreading to the arm or shoulder, nausea, sweating, general ill feeling, feeling short of breath, even with mild exertion.

- Less serious side effects may include dizziness, mild headache, fever, sore throat, body aches, nausea, vomiting, diarrhea, or pain or tenderness where you injected the medication.

- This drug may shorten remission time in patients with breast cancer, non-small cell lung cancer, head and neck cancer, cervical cancer, or lymphoid cancer. Talk with your doctor about your individual risk.

- Your doctor may occasionally change your dose to make sure you get the best results from this medication.

- Do not shake the medication vial (bottle). Vigorous shaking will ruin the medicine. Do not draw up the drug dose into a syringe until you are ready to give yourself an injection. Do not use the medication if it has changed colors or has any particles in it. Use each disposable needle only one time. Throw away used needles in a puncture-proof container (ask your pharmacist where you can get one and how to dispose of it). Keep this container out of the reach of children and pets.

- Do not inject into an area that is tender, red, bruised, hard, or has scars or stretch marks. Recommended sites for injection are the outer area of the upper arms, the abdomen (except for 2 inches around the navel), the front of the middle thighs, and the upper outer area of the buttocks. See shaded areas for injection below.

- Store this drug in the refrigerator and do not allow it to freeze.

- To be sure this medication is helping your body produce red blood cells, your blood will need to be tested on a regular basis. You may also need to check your blood pressure during treatment. Do not miss any scheduled appointments.

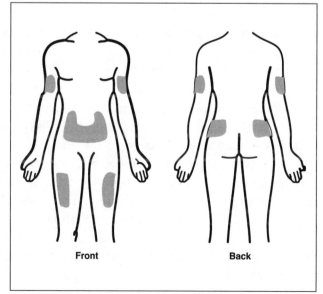

Front   Back

TRANSPLANT/
IMMUNOSUPPRESSION

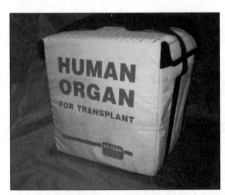

We gratefully acknowledge the assistance of Morgan R. Comee, PharmD, Assistant Professor of Pharmacy Practice at MPCHS-Worcester and solid organ liver transplant pharmacist at UMass University Campus.

Background

Transplantation medicine is one of the most challenging and complex areas of modern medicine. Some of the key areas for medical management are the problems of transplant rejection, during which the body has an immune response to the transplanted organ, possibly leading to transplant failure and the need to immediately remove the organ from the recipient. When possible, transplant rejection can be reduced through serotyping to determine the most appropriate donor-recipient match and through the use of immunosuppressant drugs.

An allograft is the transplant of an organ or tissue from one individual to another of the same species with a different genotype. This can also be called an allergenic transplant or homograft. A transplanted organ from a genetically identical donor (i.e. identical twin) is called an isograft. An autograft is when a tissue is a transplant from one site to another on the same patient, also termed autologous transplant (or autologous stem cell transplant).

Rejection is the process of the host mounting an immune response against an allograft. There are different types of rejection depending on when they occur from the time of transplantation. Hyperacute rejection is when the onset of rejection is within minutes to hours from the transplant surgery. Accelerated rejection is within 24 hours to 4 days post transplant, acute rejection is days to months after transplant and chronic rejection is defined as several months to years after transplantation. Acute rejection is primarily due to the activation of T-lymphocytes (T-cells) which is mediated largely by interleukin-2 (IL-2). A combination of two to four immunosuppressive drugs are used to target different levels of the immune cascade to prevent allograft rejection and to allow lower doses of individual agents to be used to minimize toxicity.

Different immunosuppressive regimens are used to prevent the different types of rejection. For example, induction agents (antibodies, IL-2 receptor antagonists) are used to induce immunity and prevent hyperacute, accelerated and acute rejection. Maintenance regimens are used to maintain immunity and prevent chronic rejection of the organ. A typical maintenance regimen includes 3 drug classes (steroids, calcineurin inhibitors, and anti-proliferative agents) to achieve proper immune suppression. By attacking the immune system via multiple mechanisms through different drug classes, the risk of graft rejection is reduced. All immunosuppressive agents require intense monitoring to minimize toxicities and decrease the incidence of rejection.

Chronic immunodeficiency can lead to serious infections and lymphoproliferative disease. Patients are started on sulfamethoxazole/trimethoprim *(Bactrim)* (or atovaquone if they have sulfa allergy or cannot tolerate the drug) to prevent *Pneumocystis carinii* pneumonia and urinary tract infections. Cytomegalovirus (CMV) is prevented with the use of valganciclovir (or acyclovir if both donor and recipient are CMV negative). Nystatin is used for the prevention of oral thrush.

Induction Agents

DRUG	SIDE EFFECTS/CONTRAINDICATIONS/MONITORING

Antibodies – reverse rejection by binding to antigens on T-lymphocytes (killer cells) and interfering with their function

Antithymocyte Globulin *(ATG, Atgam)*	**BLACK BOX WARNING** Should be administered under the supervision of a physician experienced in immunosuppressive therapy. Adequate laboratory and supportive medical resources must be readily available (e.g., epinephrine). **SIDE EFFECTS** Anaphylaxis (intradermal skin testing recommended prior to 1st dose), fever, chills, pruritus, rash, leukopenia, chest pain, hypertension, edema and others **MONITORING** Lymphocyte profile (T-cell count), CBC with differential, vital signs during administration May need to pre-medicate (diphenhydramine, acetaminophen and steroids). Epinephrine and resuscitative equipment should be nearby.
Muromonab-CD3 *(Orthoclone)*	**BLACK BOX WARNING** Anaphylactic reactions may occur after administration of any dose. Should be administered under the supervision of a physician experienced in immunosuppressive therapy. Adequate laboratory and supportive medical resources must be readily available (e.g., epinephrine). **CONTRAINDICATIONS** Patients with a seizure history, uncompensated HF, uncontrolled HTN, those who are fluid overloaded, pregnancy **SIDE EFFECTS** Tachycardia, hyper or hypotension, edema, fever, chills and others May need to pre-medicate (diphenhydramine, acetaminophen and steroids). Epinephrine and resuscitative equipment should be nearby.

Induction Agents Continued

DRUG	SIDE EFFECTS/CONTRAINDICATIONS/MONITORING

Interleukin 2 (IL-2) receptor antagonists - Chimeric (murine/human) monoclonal antibodies that inhibit the IL-2 receptor on the surface of activated T-lymphocytes preventing cell-mediated allograft rejection

Daclizumab *(Zenapax)* Basiliximab *(Simulect)*	**BLACK BOX WARNING** Should only be used by physicians experienced in immunosuppressive therapy. **SIDE EFFECTS** Hypertension, edema, electrolyte abnormalities, severe hypersensitivity **MONITORING** Signs and symptoms of hypersensitivity and infection

Maintenance Medications

DRUG	SIDE EFFECTS/CONTRAINDICATIONS/MONITORING

Corticosteroids – naturally occurring hormones that prevent or suppress inflammation and humoral immune responses

Prednisone, others	**SHORT-TERM SIDE EFFECTS** Fluid retention, stomach upset, emotional instability (euphoria, mood swings, irritability), insomnia, ↑ appetite, weight gain. If high dose, then acute rise in blood glucose, possible rise in blood pressure **LONG-TERM SIDE EFFECTS** Adrenal suppression/Cushing's syndrome, impaired wound healing, hypertension, hyperglycemia, cataracts, osteoporosis, hypokalemia, growth suppression in children, muscle wasting, dermal thinning, bruising, acne, menstrual irregularities and others **MONITORING** BP, glucose, CBC, renal, weight, signs of infection, bone density Must taper slowly to avoid adrenal crisis if used greater than 7-10 days

Antiproliferative Agents – inhibit T-lymphocyte proliferation by altering purine synthesis

Mycophenolate Mofetil (*CellCept*) **Mycophenolic Acid (*Myfortic*)** 1-1.5 g BID, depending on transplant type 	**BLACK BOX WARNINGS (3)** ↑ risk of infection; ↑ development of lymphoma and skin malignancies; ↑ risk of congenital malformations and spontaneous abortions when used during pregnancy **SIDE EFFECTS** Diarrhea, GI upset, vomiting, hyper- and hypotension, edema, tachycardia, pain, hyperglycemia, hypo and hyperkalemia, hypomagnesemia, hypocalcemia, hypercholesterolemia, leukopenia and others **MONITORING** CBC, renal, liver, signs of infection *CellCept* and *Myfortic* should not be used interchangeably due to differences in absorption. *Myfortic* is enteric coated which helps to ↓ diarrhea. Should be taken on an empty stomach to avoid variability in absorption. Take exactly as prescribed. Pregnancy Category D

Maintenance Medications Continued

DRUG	SIDE EFFECTS/CONTRAINDICATIONS/MONITORING
Azathioprine (*Azasan, Imuran*)	**BLACK BOX WARNINGS (2)** ↑ risk of neoplasia and serious infections; should be prescribed by physicians familiar with the risks, including hematologic toxicities and mutagenic potential **SIDE EFFECTS** Myelosuppression (dose dependent), hepatotoxicity, nausea, vomiting, diarrhea **MONITORING** Monitor for thiopurine methyltransferase (TPMT). Patients with genetic deficiency of TPMT may have ↑ risk of myelosuppressive effects; those patients with low or absent TPMT activity are at risk for developing severe myelotoxicity

Calcineurin antagonists - suppresses cellular immunity by inhibiting T-lymphocyte activation

DRUG	SIDE EFFECTS/CONTRAINDICATIONS/MONITORING
Tacrolimus (*Prograf*)	**BLACK BOX WARNINGS (2)** ↑ susceptibility to infection and possible development of lymphoma **SIDE EFFECTS** Tremor, headache, hyperglycemia (including diabetes), hyperkalemia, hypomagnesemia, hypophosphatemia, hair loss, nephrotoxicity, tremor, hypokalemia, hyperlipidemia, QT prolongation, diarrhea, hypertension, neurotoxicity and others **MONITORING** Renal, hepatic, electrolytes (especially K+), glucose, BP, CBC, signs of infection Should be taken on an empty stomach to avoid variability in absorption. Take exactly as prescribed.
Cyclosporine (*Neoral, Gengraf, Sandimmune*)	**BLACK BOX WARNINGS (7)** Renal impairment (with high doses); ↑ risk of lymphoma and other malignancies; ↑ risk of skin cancer; ↑ risk of infection, may cause hypertension; dose adjustments should only be made under the direct supervision of an experienced physician; **cyclosporine (modified – Gengraf/Neoral) has ↑ bioavailability compared to cyclosporine (non-modified - Sandimmune) and cannot be used interchangeably.** **SIDE EFFECTS** Hypertension, hirsutism, gingival hyperplasia, hypertriglyceridemia, nephropathy, hypertrichosis, edema, tremor, hyperkalemia, hyperuricemia, hypo/hyperglycemia and others **MONITORING** BP, renal, electrolytes, uric acid, lipids, CBC, signs of infection

Mammalian target of rapamycin (mTOR) kinase inhibitor which inhibits T-lymphocyte activation and proliferation

DRUG	SIDE EFFECTS/CONTRAINDICATIONS/MONITORING
Sirolimus (*Rapamune*)	**BLACK BOX WARNINGS (2)** ↑ risk of infection and development of lymphoma; not recommended in lung or liver transplant patients **SIDE EFFECTS** Delayed wound healing, pneumonitis, hyperlipidemia, thrombocytopenia, anemia, hypertension, peripheral edema and others **MONITORING** Liver, renal, lipids, BP, CBC, signs of infection Tablets and oral solution are not bioequivalent due to differences in absorption Take consistently each day

Maintenance Medications Continued

DRUG	SIDE EFFECTS/CONTRAINDICATIONS/MONITORING
Everolimus (*Zortress*)	**BLACK BOX WARNINGS (4)** ↑ risk of infection; ↑ risk of lymphoma and skin cancer; <u>reduced doses of cyclosporine are recommended when used concomitantly</u>; ↑ risk of renal thrombosis may result in graft loss **SIDE EFFECTS** <u>Peripheral edema</u>, <u>constipation</u>, <u>hypertension</u>, <u>hyperlipidemia</u>, <u>delayed wound healing</u>, <u>pneumonitis</u>, nausea, anemia, and UTI **MONITORING** Liver, renal, lipids, glucose, BP, CBC, signs of infection Take consistently each day

DRUG INTERACTIONS

- Azathioprine – allopurinol, aspirin, ACEIs and sulfamethoxazole/trimethoprim may ↑ levels of azathioprine

- Mycophenolate - can ↓ levels of OCs; mycophenolate levels can be ↓ by antacids and multivitamins, cyclosporine, metronidazole, proton pump inhibitors, fluoroquinolones, sevelamer, bile acid resins, and rifamycin derivatives.

- Tacrolimus, everolimus, and sirolimus are 3A4 substrates and 3A4 (weak) inhibitors (except everolimus). Avoid grapefruit juice and strong 3A4 inhibitors. Inhibitors of 3A4 can ↑ levels of tacrolimus/sirolimus/everolimus and inducers of 3A4 can ↓ levels of tacrolimus/sirolimus/everolimus. Doses of cyclosporine need to be reduced when everolimus is started. See drug interactions chapter for more information.

- Cyclosporine is a substrate of 3A4 and moderate 3A4 inhibitor. Avoid grapefruit juice. Inhibitors of 3A4 can ↑ levels of cyclosporine and inducers of 3A4 can ↓ levels of cyclosporine. See drug interactions chapter for more information. Also, caution against the use of other agents that can cause nephrotoxicity and agents that can ↑ blood pressure.

PATIENT COUNSELING FOR ALL IMMUNOSUPPRESSANTS

- Take the medication <u>exactly</u> as prescribed by your doctor. It is important that you take your medication at the same time every day. Also, <u>stay consistent</u> on how you take your medication.

- Never change or skip a dose of medication. Remember, if you stop taking your immunosuppressive medications, your body will reject your transplanted organ.

- Monitor your health at home and keep <u>daily</u> records of your <u>temperature, weight, blood pressure</u>, and glucose (if diabetes is present).

- Do <u>not</u> take any NSAIDs (e.g., *Advil, Naprosyn, Aleve)* as these drugs could cause harm to your kidneys.

- Do <u>not</u> take any over-the-count, herbal, or alternative medications without consulting with your doctor.

- Protect and cover your skin from the sun. Be sure to use sunscreen with a SPF of 30 or higher. Avoid using tanning beds or sunlamps. People who take immunosuppressive agents have a higher risk of getting skin cancer.

- Do not get immunizations/vaccinations without the consent of your doctor. The use of <u>live vaccines should definitely be avoided</u>. Avoid contact with people who have recently received oral polio vaccine or nasal flu vaccine.

- Patients are vulnerable to developing infections (severe infections) due to their suppressed immune system. Avoid contact with people who have the flu or other contagious illness. Practice infection control techniques such as good hand washing.

- Chronic immunosuppression has been associated with an increased risk of cancer, particularly lymphoma and skin cancer.

- If getting a blood test to measure the drug level, take your medication <u>after</u> you had your blood drawn (not before). We want to measure the lowest (trough) level of drug in your blood.

PATIENT COUNSELING FOR MYCOPHENOLATE

- Take <u>exactly</u> as prescribed, every 12 hours (8am and 8pm). It is important that you take your medication at the same time every day.

- If you miss a dose and it is <u>less than 4 hours after the scheduled dose, take the missed dose</u> and continue on your regular schedule. If you miss a dose and it is <u>more than 4 hours after your scheduled dose</u>, <u>SKIP the missed dose</u>, and return to your regular dosing schedule. Never take 2 doses at the same time. Record any missed doses. Call your healthcare provider if you are not sure what to do.

- Take capsules, tablets and oral suspension <u>on an empty stomach</u>, either 1 hour before or 2 hours after a meal, unless your healthcare provider tells you otherwise.

- Do not open or crush tablets or capsules. If you are not able to swallow tablets or capsules, your healthcare provider may prescribe an oral suspension. Your pharmacist will mix the medicine before giving it to you.

- Do not mix the oral suspension with any other medicine.

- This medication can cause <u>diarrhea</u>. Call your healthcare provider right away if you have diarrhea. Do not stop the medication without first talking with your healthcare provider. Other side effects include nausea, vomiting, abdominal pain/cramping, headache, and decreased white blood cells and platelets.

- Do not get pregnant while taking this medication. Women who take this medication during pregnancy have a higher risk of losing a pregnancy (miscarriage) during the first 3 months (first trimester), and a higher risk that their baby will be born with birth defects.

- <u>Do not take with antacids or multivitamins concurrently. Separate the doses by 2 hours. Avoid use with bile acid resins.</u>

- <u>Limit the amount of time you spend in sunlight.</u> Avoid using tanning beds or sunlamps. Use sunscreen with a SPF of 30 or higher. People who take this medicine have a higher risk of getting skin cancer.

- <u>Mycophenolic acid *(Myfortic)* and mycophenolate mofetil *(CellCept)* are not interchangeable. Do not switch between products unless directed by your healthcare provider. These medicines are absorbed differently. This may affect the amount of medicine in your blood.</u>

PATIENT COUNSELING FOR CYCLOSPORINE (USING NEORAL AS AN EXAMPLE)

- Because different brands deliver different amounts of medication, <u>do not switch brands of cyclosporine without your doctor's permission and directions.</u>

- Take this medication by mouth, usually twice daily at the same times each day, or take as directed by your doctor. Swallow this medication whole. Do not crush or chew the capsules. Dosage is based on your medical condition, cyclosporine blood level, kidney function, and response to therapy. Follow the dosing schedule for this medication carefully.

- Patients should be advised to take *Neoral* on a consistent schedule with regard to time of day and relation to meals. <u>Grapefruit and grapefruit juice affect metabolism</u>, increasing blood concentration of cyclosporine, thus <u>should be avoided.</u>

- If you miss a dose and it is <u>less than 4 hours after the scheduled dose, take the missed dose</u> and continue on your regular schedule. If you miss a dose and it is <u>more than 4 hours after your scheduled dose, SKIP the missed dose</u>, and return to your regular dosing schedule. Never take 2 doses at the same time. Record any missed doses. Call your healthcare provider if you are not sure what to do.

- Patients should be informed of the necessity of repeated laboratory tests while they are receiving cyclosporine. Laboratory tests (e.g., kidney function tests, blood tests) may be performed to monitor your progress. If getting a blood test to measure the drug level, take your medication <u>after</u> you had your blood drawn.

- Patients should be given careful dosage instructions. *Neoral* Oral Solution (cyclosporine oral solution, USP) MODIFIED should be diluted, preferably with orange or apple juice that is at room temperature. Do not administer oral liquid from plastic or Styrofoam cup. The combination of *Neoral* Oral Solution (cyclosporine oral solution, USP) MODIFIED with milk can be unpalatable. *(Sandimmune* may be diluted with milk, chocolate milk, or orange juice). Avoid changing diluents frequently. Mix thoroughly and drink at once. Use syringe provided to measure dose, mix in glass container and rinse container with more diluent to ensure total dose was taken.

- Cyclosporine can also cause <u>high blood pressure</u> and <u>kidney problems</u>. The risk of both problems increases with higher doses and longer treatment with this drug.

- Side effects of cyclosporine also include increased cholesterol, headache, nausea, vomiting, diarrhea, stomach upset, increased hair growth on the face/body, tremor, swollen/red/painful gums, and acne. If any of these effects persist or worsen, notify your doctor or pharmacist promptly.

- This drug may increase your risk for developing skin cancer. Avoid prolonged sun exposure, tanning booths and sunlamps. Use a sunscreen, SPF 30 or higher, and wear protective clothing when outdoors.

- This medication <u>may cause swelling and growth of the gums (gingival hyperplasia).</u> Brush your teeth and floss daily to minimize this problem. See your dentist regularly.

PATIENT COUNSELING FOR TACROLIMUS

- Take this medication as directed by your doctor, usually every 12 hours. Take on an empty stomach for best absorption. You must be consistent (with food or without food) and take this medication the same way everyday so that your body always absorbs the same amount of drug.

- It is important to take all doses on time to keep the amount of medicine in your body at a constant level. Remember to take it at the same times each day. Patients should be informed of the need for repeated appropriate laboratory tests while they are receiving tacrolimus. They should be given complete dosage instructions, advised of the potential risks during pregnancy, and informed of the increased risk of neoplasia. Patients should be informed that changes in dosage should not be undertaken without first consulting their physician.

- If you miss a dose and it is <u>less than 4 hours after the scheduled dose, take the missed dose</u> and continue on your regular schedule. If you miss a dose and it is <u>more than 4 hours after your scheduled dose, SKIP the missed dose</u>, and return to your regular dosing schedule. Never take 2 doses at the same time. Record any missed doses. Call your healthcare provider if you are not sure what to do.

- As with other immunosuppressive agents, owing to the potential risk of malignant skin changes, exposure to sunlight and ultraviolet (UV) light should be limited by wearing protective clothing and using a sunscreen with a SPF of 30 or higher.

- <u>Avoid eating grapefruit or drinking grapefruit juice</u> while being treated with tacrolimus. Grapefruit can increase the amount of tacrolimus in your bloodstream.

- Tacrolimus may cause your blood pressure to increase. You may be required to check your blood pressure periodically and/or take another medication to control your blood pressure.

- Side effects of tacrolimus also include tremors/shaking, headache, diarrhea, nausea/vomiting, upset stomach, loss of appetite, tingling of the hands/feet, increased blood pressure, increased cholesterol, increased blood sugar, and increase in potassium levels.

- <u>Tacrolimus may cause diabetes.</u> Tell your doctor or pharmacist if you experience any of the following symptoms of high blood sugar: increased thirst/hunger or frequent urination.

- Tacrolimus may cause a condition that affects the heart rhythm (QT prolongation). QT prolongation can infrequently result in serious fast/irregular heartbeat and other symptoms (such as severe dizziness, fainting) that require immediate medical attention. The risk of QT prolongation may be increased if you have certain medical conditions or are taking other drugs that may affect the heart rhythm. Before using tacrolimus, tell your doctor or pharmacist if you have any of the following conditions: certain heart problems (heart failure, slow heartbeat, QT prolongation in the EKG), family history of certain heart problems (QT prolongation or sudden cardiac death).

- High (or low) levels of potassium or magnesium in the blood may also increase your risk of QT prolongation. This risk may increase if you use certain drugs (such as diuretics/"water pills") or if you have conditions such as severe sweating, diarrhea, or vomiting. This drug may increase your potassium levels.

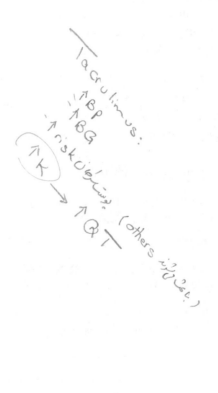

INTRAVENOUS DRUGS, FLUIDS & ANTIDOTES

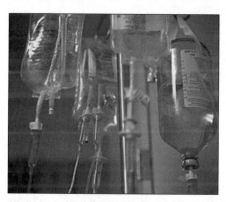

Background

Intravenous therapy, or IV therapy, is the giving of liquid substances directly into a vein. The word intravenous simply means "within a vein". It is commonly referred to as a drip because many systems of administration employ a drip chamber, which prevents air entering the blood stream (and causing an air embolism) and allows an estimate of flow rate. Compared with other routes of administration, the intravenous route is the fastest way to deliver fluids and medications throughout the body. This may be needed given the patient severity's of illness (e.g. code blue) or status (nothing by mouth or NPO). Some medications may only be formulated for intravenous administration.

Many intravenous medications may be needed for a patient, particularly if a patient is in the intensive care unit (ICU) on a ventilator and cannot swallow medications. Several IV lines may be going at once and pharmacists are commonly asked about IV compatibilities of medications. Patients can also receive total parental nutrition (TPN) through the intravenous route. TPN is discussed further in the calculations chapter.

There are 2 main types of intravenous lines, a peripheral IV line and a central IV line. A peripheral IV line consists of a short catheter (a few centimeters long) inserted through the skin into a peripheral vein, usually in the hand or arm. Central IV lines flow through a catheter with its tip placed in a large vein (e.g. subclavian, internal jugular, inferior vena cava) located in the chest or abdomen area.

A central IV line has several advantages over a peripheral line:

- It can deliver fluids/medications that are overly irritating to peripheral veins (e.g. some chemotherapy drugs, TPN, higher concentrations of potassium)

- They can contain multiple parallel compartments (or lumens) within the catheter so multiple medications can be given at once even if they would not be chemically compatible within a single catheter.

- Some central lines can measure central venous pressure and other hemodynamics (cardiac output, etc.) through a central line

Central lines do have some disadvantages such as higher risks of bleeding, infection, and thromboembolism and they are more difficult to insert correctly (requires expertise and may be placed by a physician or other trained staff). One commonly used central line is the peripherally inserted central catheter, or PICC line. PICC lines are used when access to the vein is required for a prolonged period of time or when the infused substance would damage a peripheral vein. The PICC line is inserted into a peripheral vein, typically in the upper arm, and advanced until the catheter tip terminates in a large vein in the chest near the heart.

Intravenous medications require the use of an infusion pump for administration. Infusion pumps can administer fluids in ways that would be impractical, expensive or unreliable if performed manually by nursing staff. For example, they can administer as little as 0.1 mL per hour injections (too small for a drip), injections every minute, injections with repeated boluses as requested by the patient, up to maximum number per hour (e.g. in patient-controlled analgesia or PCA), or fluids whose volumes vary by the time of day. They offer another "safety mechanism" to make sure the correct drug, correct dose and correct rate are given to the patient. See Medication Errors, Patient Safety, and the Joint Commission chapter for more information.

Types of Fluids

When patients enter a hospital, they are generally started on IV fluids to maintain their fluid status. Fluids can also be used to treat the initial stages of hypoperfusion, or shock. There are 2 categories of fluids: crystalloids and colloids.

Crystalloids are based on a solution of sterile water with added electrolytes to approximate 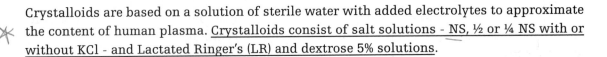 the content of human plasma. Crystalloids consist of salt solutions - NS, ½ or ¼ NS with or without KCl - and Lactated Ringer's (LR) and dextrose 5% solutions.

Colloids do not freely diffuse across a semi-permeable membrane, hence, keeping the fluid within the intravascular space. Colloids are used to increase the osmotic pressure in patients and are substantially more expensive than crystalloids. Colloids include albumin 5% and 25%, hetastarch 6%, pentastarch 10%, dextran and others.

Crystalloids or colloids can be used for fluid resuscitation. Crystalloids are used for maintaining fluid status and keeping IV lines open (patent).

Septic Shock and Shock Syndromes

Shock results from a lack of oxygen due to hypoperfusion and low blood pressure (SBP < 90 mmHg). Fluid resuscitation with crystalloids or colloids is generally recommended as first-line therapy. If the patient does not respond to this fluid challenge, then vasopressor/inotropic therapy should be initiated.

Inotropes work by increasing contractility either through β-adrenergic stimulation or through inhibition of phosphodiesterase. These mechanisms lead to an increase in cardiac output (CO). Vasopressors work via vasoconstriction (think "pressing down on the vasculature") and thereby increasing BP and CO.

INOTROPES AND VASOPRESSORS USED IN SHOCK SYNDROMES

DRUG	MOA	SIDE EFFECTS/CONTRAINDICATIONS/MONITORING
Dobutamine (*Dobutrex*)	Primarily β_1-agonist causing ↑ contractility, ↑ CO, ↑ HR Used in cardiogenic shock	**SIDE EFFECTS** ↑ BP, ↑ HR, tachyarrhythmias, ventricular arrhythmias, ventricular ectopy, tachyphylaxis, others
Milrinone (*Primacor*)	Selective phosphodiesterase inhibitor in cardiac and vascular tissue, resulting in vasodilation and inotropic effects with little chronotropic effects	**MONITORING** Requires continuous BP monitoring, HR, ECG, CVP, MAP, urine output Amrinone (*Inocor*) is no longer used due to significant thrombocytopenia
Dopamine	Endogenous precursor of norepinephrine (NE) that stimulates different receptors at different doses Low dose - stimulates D_1 receptors Medium dose - stimulates β_1 receptors High dose - stimulates α_1 receptors	**SIDE EFFECTS** Arrhythmias, bradycardia, tachyphylaxis, peripheral ischemia, tissue necrosis (gangrene), others **MONITORING** Requires continuous BP monitoring, HR, MAP, urine output, infusion site for extravasation
Epinephrine (*Adrenalin*)	β-agonist activity at low doses. At high doses, more α-agonist effects	*EpiPen, Twinject* - pre-filled auto injectors used for anaphylactic allergic reactions. Epinephrine used for IV route is 0.1 mg/mL or 1:10,000 ratio strength. Epinephrine used for the IM route is 1:1,000 ratio strength
Norepinephrine (*Levophed*)	Stimulates β_1 receptors and α receptors causing ↑ contractility and heart rate as well as vasoconstriction. α effects are greater than β effects Used in septic shock	Solutions should not be used if they are discolored (brown) or contain a precipitate
Phenylephrine (*Neo-Synephrine*)	Pure α-agonist	

TREATMENT OF EXTRAVASATION WITH VASOPRESSORS

- Extravasation, or leakage of IV into surrounding tissue, of vasopressors/inotropes can cause tissue damage and necrosis. Treat immediately.

- With norepinephrine, use phentolamine *(Regitine)*, an α-adrenergic blocker that antagonizes the effects of norepinephrine. Dilute 5-10 mg of phentolamine in 10 mL of NS and give SC to infiltrated area. Blanching should reverse immediately.

ICU Sedation and Analgesia

Sedation/analgesia is commonly used for patients in the intensive care unit, particularly if the patient is on mechanical ventilation. It is often necessary to provide sedation/analgesia to limit the anxiety and agitation experienced by patients, to maintain synchronized breathing if on a ventilator (prevent "bucking" the ventilator), prevent ICU delirium, and keep patients free of pain and suffering in the harsh ICU environment. Patients in the ICU can quickly become disoriented, agitated, and delirious given the amount of interventions they experience, the constant noise of monitors and alarms, and the frequent interruptions from hospital personnel disrupting their normal sleep cycle. This, combined with fear and anxiety associated with their environment and current critical condition, can invoke an aggressive, agitated, disoriented and confused patient.

Agents used for ICU sedation and analgesia can include a varied combination of opioids (morphine, fentanyl), benzodiazepines (midazolam, lorazepam), antipsychotics (haloperidol, quetiapine, risperidone) and/or hypnotics (propofol, dexmedetomidine). A full discussion and review on opioids can be found in the pain chapter, benzodiazepines are discussed in the anxiety chapter, and antipsychotics can be found in the schizophrenia chapter. A brief review of several of these agents is found below.

A tested and validated sedation scale should be used to frequent assess patient response to therapy and needs for continued therapy since requirements for treating agitation fluctuate over time. Some commonly used sedation scales include the Richmond Agitation Sedation Scale (RASS), the Ramsay Agitation Scale (RAS), the Riker Sedation-Agitation Scale (SAS), and the Minnesota Sedation Assessment Tool (MSAT). Patients are monitored generally every 2-3 hours while receiving a sedation protocol to make sure patients are receiving the minimal amount of drug(s) to keep them calm and pain-free.

AGENTS USED FOR ICU SEDATION AND AGITATION

DRUG	DOSING	SIDE EFFECTS/CONTRAINDICATIONS/MONITORING
Lorazepam *(Ativan)*	LD: 2-4 mg IV push MD: 2-6 mg IV Q4-6H or an infusion 1-10 mg/h Mixed in D5W only	**SIDE EFFECTS** Respiratory depression, oversedation, hypotension, propylene glycol poisoning at high doses and prolonged infusions (look for metabolic acidosis and renal insufficiency) **MONITORING** BP, HR, sedation scale Inexpensive, used for long-term sedation (> 48 hours), no active metabolite, longer t½ than midazolam
Midazolam *(Versed)*	LD: 2-5 mg IV push MD: 1-20 mg/h	**SIDE EFFECTS** Respiratory depression, oversedation, hypotension **CONTRAINDICATIONS** Use small, initial doses in elderly (e.g. 1 mg, not to exceed 2.5 mg) Contains benzyl alcohol, avoid rapid injection or prolonged infusions **MONITORING** BP, HR, sedation scale Many drug interactions (major 3A4 substrate), ↑ levels with 3A4 inhibitors; active metabolite accumulates in renal failure Used for short-term sedation (< 48 hours), shorter acting than lorazepam if patient has preserved organ function (no hepatic or renal impairment or CHF), has active metabolite that accumulates in renal dysfunction

Agents Used for ICU Sedation and Agitation Continued

DRUG	DOSING	SIDE EFFECTS/CONTRAINDICATIONS/MONITORING
Propofol *(Diprivan)* (C IV expected)	MD: 5-80 mcg/kg/min	**SIDE EFFECTS** Hypotension, apnea, hypertriglyceridemia, green urine, propofol-related infusion syndrome (PRIS – rare but can be fatal), zinc depletion **MONITORING** BP, respiration, triglycerides (if on longer than 2 days), signs and symptoms of pancreatitis, zinc, sedation scale Shake well before use. Use strict aseptic technique due to potential for bacterial growth. Discard vial and tubing within 12 hours of use. If transferred to a syringe prior to administration, must discard syringe within 6 hours. Do not use if there is separation of phases in the emulsion. Do not use filter of < 5 micron for administration Formulated in 10% lipid emulsion (provides 1.1 kcal/mL)
Fospropofol *(Lusedra)* C IV	5.0-6.5 mg/kg initially and titrate to effect	**SIDE EFFECTS** Paresthesias, pruritus, hypotension **MONITORING** BP, respiration, patient responsiveness Prodrug of propofol; delayed onset due to need for conversion to active metabolite
Dexmedetomidine *(Precedex)* Alpha$_2$-adrenergic agonist	LD: 0.5-1 mcg/kg over 10 minutes (may be omitted) MD: 0.2-0.7 mcg/kg/hr for 24 hours Mix with normal saline (NS) only	**SIDE EFFECTS** Transient hypertension during loading dose (may need to ↓ infusion rate), hypotension, bradycardia, dry mouth **MONITORING** BP, HR, sedation scale Used for sedation in intubated and non-intubated patients. Duration of infusion should not exceed 24 hours. Patients are arousable and alert when stimulated; does not cause respiratory depression
Morphine	LD: 2-4 mg IV push MD: 2-30 mg/hr	**SIDE EFFECTS** Respiratory depression, hypotension, oversedation, bradycardia, pruritus, xerostomia, constipation, others **MONITORING** BP, HR, respiratory status, sedation/pain scale Has an active metabolite (morphine-6-glucuronide) which can accumulate in renal impairment; causes a histamine release, preferred agent in patients who are hemodynamically stable
Fentanyl	LD: 25-50 mcg IV push MD: 0.7-10 mcg/kg/h	**SIDE EFFECTS** Respiratory depression, bradycardia, oversedation, constipation, rigidity with high doses **MONITORING** BP, HR, respiratory status, sedation/pain scale Less hypotension than morphine due to no histamine release. Fast onset of action and short duration of action. 100 times more potent than morphine. Preferred agent in patients with unstable hemodynamics

DRUG	DOSING	SIDE EFFECTS/CONTRAINDICATIONS/MONITORING
Hydromorphone *(Dilaudid)*	LD: 0.2-0.6 mg IV push MD: 0.5-3 mg/hr	**SIDE EFFECTS** Respiratory depression, oversedation, high potential for abuse **MONITORING** BR, HR, respiratory status, sedation/pain scale No active metabolites; not commonly used for ICU sedation
Remifentanil *(Ultiva)*	LD: 1 mcg/kg over 1 min MD: 0.6-15 mcg/kg/hr	**SIDE EFFECTS** Nausea, vomiting, bradycardia, hypotension, respiratory depression, oversedation **MONITORING** BR, HR, respiratory status, sedation/pain scale Metabolized by tissue esterases, no accumulation
Haloperidol *(Haldol)*	2-10 mg IV push; may repeat Q15-30 minutes until calm, then administer 25% of last dose Q6H	**SIDE EFFECTS** Hypotension, QT prolongation, tachycardia, extrapyramidal symptoms (EPS), anticholinergic effects, neuroleptic malignant syndrome, others **MONITORING** QT interval and ECG, extrapyramidal symptoms (EPS), abnormal involuntary movements, vital signs Not to be given via continuous infusion

ANESTHETICS

Anesthetics are used for a variety of effects including numbing of an area (local anesthesia), to block pain (regional anesthesia), or to cause a reversible loss of consciousness and sleepiness during surgery (general anesthesia). Anesthetics can be given via several routes of administration: topical, inhaled, intravenously, epidural or spinal. More increasingly, anesthetics are being used concomitantly with opioids to reduce the amount of opiates a patient requires for pain control. They work by blocking the initiation and conduction of nerve impulses by decreasing the neuronal permeability to sodium ions. Patients receiving anesthetics must be continuously monitored to make sure the body is functioning properly (continuous vital sign monitoring, respiratory monitoring, and others).

The main side effects of anesthetics include hypotension, bradycardia, nausea and vomiting, and a mild drop in body temperature that can cause shivering. Some patients may have allergic reactions to anesthesia. These drugs, if given too much or too high of a dose, can cause respiratory depression and cardiac arrest. Below are some commonly used anesthetics.

- Topical, local – Lidocaine *(Xylocaine)*, benzocaine

- Inhaled – Desflurane *(Suprane)*, sevoflurane *(Ultane)*, isoflurane *(Forane)*, nitrous oxide, others

- Injectable – bupivacaine *(Marcaine, Sensorcaine)*, lidocaine *(Xylocaine)*, ropivacaine *(Naropin)*, others

NEUROMUSCULAR BLOCKING AGENTS (NMBAs)

These agents cause paralysis. Patients may require the use of a paralytic agent in certain scenarios such as to facilitate mechanical intubation, manage increased intracranial pressure, treat muscle spasms (tetany), and others. These agents do not provide sedation nor analgesia. Therefore, patients should receive adequate sedation and analgesia PRIOR to starting a NMBA. Patients must be mechanical ventilated as these agents paralyze the diaphragm. These are considered high risk medications by ISMP. All NMBAs should be labeled with bright red auxiliary labels stating "WARNING, PARALYZING AGENT".

There are 2 types of NMBAs - depolarizing and non-depolarizing. Succinylcholine is the only available depolarizing agent. Resembling acetylcholine, it binds to and activates the acetylcholine receptors. The non-depolarizing NMBAs work by binding to the acetylcholine receptor and blocking the actions of endogenous acetylcholine.

DRUG	SIDE EFFECTS/CONTRAINDICATIONS/MONITORING
Non-depolarizing NMBAs	**SIDE EFFECTS** Flushing, bradycardia, hypotension, tachyphylaxis, acute quadriplegic myopathy syndrome (AQMS) with long-term use **MONITORING** Peripheral nerve stimulator to assess depth of paralysis [also called train-of-four (TOF)], vital signs (BP, HR, RR)
Atracurium *(Tracrium)*	Short t½; intermediate acting; metabolized by Hofmann elimination
Cisatracurium *(Nimbex)*	Short t½; intermediate acting; metabolized by Hofmann elimination
Pancuronium *(Pavulon)*	Long-acting agent, can accumulate in renal or hepatic dysfunction, ↑ HR (tachycardia)
Rocuronium *(Zemuron)*	Intermediate-acting agent
Vecuronium *(Norcuron)*	Intermediate-acting agent; can accumulate in renal or hepatic dysfunction

Venous Thromboembolism Prophylaxis

Venous thromboembolism (VTE) is a clinical manifestation of a deep vein thrombosis (DVT) and/or a pulmonary embolism (PE). DVTs can travel to the pulmonary arteries and cause a PE. Many patients in the intensive care unit are at high risk of developing a DVT and/or PE.

The CHEST guidelines provide specific recommendations for the prevention of VTE depending on the level of risk and specific indication or type of surgery. Non-pharmacologic therapy consists of intermittent pneumatic compression (IPC) devices, graduated compression stockings (GCS), and/or the use of a venous foot pump (VFP). Drugs and their respective doses for VTE

RISK FACTORS FOR VTE	
Surgery	Thrombophilia
Trauma	Left ventricular dysfunction
Immobility	
Cancer	Acute myocardial infarction
Previous VTE	
Increasing age	Indwelling catheters
Pregnancy/Postpartum	Venous obstruction
Acute medical illness	Estrogen therapy

prophylaxis are below. A complete review of these agents can be found in the anticoagulation chapter.

DRUG	DOSE
Low dose unfractionated heparin (LDUH)	5,000 units SC BID-TID
Low Molecular Weight Heparin (LMWH)	Enoxaparin 30 mg SC BID or 40 mg SC daily
	(If CrCl < 30 mL/min, give 30 mg SC daily)
	Dalteparin 2,500 – 5,000 units SC daily
Factor Xa inhibitor	Fondaparinux 2.5 mg SC daily (Do not use if CrCl < 30 mL/min or patient weighs < 50 kg)
	Rivaroxaban 10 mg PO daily
	(Do not use in patients with CrCl < 30 mL/min)

Stress Ulcer Prophylaxis

Stress ulcers can result from the metabolic stress experienced by a patient in an intensive care unit (ICU). Patients with critical illness have reduced blood flow to the gut as blood flow is diverted to the major organs of the body. This results in a breakdown of gastric mucosal defense mechanisms including prostaglandin synthesis, bicarbonate production, and cell turnover.

RISK FACTORS FOR THE DEVELOPMENT OF STRESS ULCERS

Mechanical ventilation

Coagulopathy

Sepsis

Traumatic brain injury

Burn patients

Acute renal failure

High dose corticosteroids

Histamine$_2$-receptor antagonists (H$_2$RAs) and proton pump inhibitors (PPIs) are the recommended agents to use for prevention of stress-related mucosal damage. H$_2$RAs can cause some adverse events such as thrombocytopenia, mental status changes (in the elderly or those with renal/hepatic impairment), and tachyphylaxis. PPIs have been associated with an increase risk of GI infections *(C. difficile)* and nosocomial pneumonia. These agents are fully discussed in the GERD and PUD chapters.

Acid-Base Homeostasis

An acid is a substance that can <u>donate</u> protons, or H$^+$ ions. A base is a substance that can <u>accept</u> protons. The degree of acidity is expressed as pH, or the negative logarithm (base 10) of the hydrogen ion concentration. Hence, the hydrogen ion concentration and pH are inversely related.

The normal pH of blood is 7.4 (range 7.35-7.45). The primary buffering system of the body is the bicarbonate/carbonic acid system. The kidneys help to maintain a neutral pH by controlling bicarbonate (HCO$_3^-$) resorption and elimination. The normal bicarbonate level is 24 mEq/L (range 22-26 mEq/L). The lungs help maintain a neutral pH by controlling carbonic acid (which is directly proportional to the partial pressure of carbon dioxide - PaCO$_2$) retained or released from the body. The normal partial pressure of carbon dioxide is 40 mmHg (range 35-45 mmHg).

Bicarbonate acts as a buffer and a base, whereas carbon dioxide acts as a buffer and an acid. Alterations from the normal values lead to acid-base disorders. Diet and cellular metabolism lead to a large production of H^+ ions that need to be excreted to maintain acid-base balance. The acid-base status of a patient can be determined by an arterial blood gas (ABG).

ABG: $pH/PaCO_2/ HCO_3^-/PO_2/O_2$ Sat

An acid-base disorder that leads to a pH < 7.35 is called an acidosis. If the disorder leads to a pH > 7.45, it is called an alkalosis. These disorders are classified as either metabolic or respiratory in origin. For example, the primary disturbance in a metabolic acid-base disorder is the plasma HCO_3^- concentration. A metabolic acidosis is characterized by a decrease in plasma HCO_3^- concentration whereas, in a metabolic alkalosis, the plasma HCO_3^- concentration is increased. In respiratory acidosis, the $PaCO_2$ is elevated and in respiratory alkalosis, the $PaCO_2$ is decreased. Each disturbance has a compensatory (secondary) response that attempts to correct the imbalance toward normal and keep the pH neutral.

SOME ETIOLOGIES OF ACID/BASE DISORDERS

- Metabolic acidosis - lactic acidosis, renal tubular acidosis, large doses of propylene glycol (lorazepam IV), others

- Metabolic alkalosis - loop and thiazide diuretics, high dose penicillins, vomiting, diarrhea, cystic fibrosis

- Respiratory acidosis - opioids, sedatives, anesthetics, stroke, asthma/COPD

- Respiratory alkalosis - pain, fever, brain tumors, salicylates, catecholamines, theophylline

Treatment of acid-base disorders is always to stop the offending agent or cause (e.g. stop the drug or stop vomiting). In treating metabolic acidosis, sodium bicarbonate may be used to raise pH to ≥ 7.20, although there is no benefit in morbidity and mortality compared to general supportive care.

Other Intravenous Drugs

The drugs below represent other intravenous drugs used in an intensive care setting. A complete review of these medications can be found in their respective chapters. Here are a few key points when using these IV medications.

DRUG	MOA	NOTES
Amiodarone	Class III antiarrhythmic which inhibits adrenergic stimulation; affects sodium, potassium, and calcium channels	Solution is stable for 24 hours in polyolefin or glass containers, or for 2 hours in PVC. Infusions > 2 hours must be administered in glass or polyolefin containers. PVC tubing sets can be used with amiodarone. Use of an in-line filter is recommended Recommended to be added to D5W Light sensitive.

Other Intravenous Drugs Continued

DRUG	MOA	NOTES
Amphotericin B (conventional)	Antifungal	Dilute with D5W only. Infuse over 2-6 hours Light sensitive.
Furosemide	Inhibits sodium and chloride reabsorption in the ascending loop of Henle and distal renal tubule causing diuresis	Store at room temperature. Refrigeration may result in precipitation or crystallization. Crystals may dissolve upon warming to room temp. Do not use if solution is yellow in color. Light sensitive. IV to oral ratio = 1:2
Levothyroxine IV injection	Thyroid replacement	Give immediately upon reconstitution. Protect from light. IV to oral ratio = 1:2 (IV dose is 50% of oral dose)
Metronidazole	Antibiotic	Refrigeration may result in crystal formation. The crystals may dissolve upon warming to room temp. Protect from light. IV to oral ratio = 1:1
Phenytoin	Sodium neuronal membrane stabilizer to ↓ seizures	Further dilution is controversial (use NS if need to further dilute). Use as soon as possible due to short stability (need to discard after 4 hours). Do not refrigerate as may cause precipitation. Precipitate may dissolve upon warming to room temp. An in-line filter (0.22-5 micron) is recommended for IVPB solutions due to potential for precipitation. Follow with a saline flush to prevent vein irritation. Max infusion rate is 50 mg/min. IV to oral ratio = 1:1
Sulfamethoxazole/ Trimethoprim	Antibiotic	Dilute with D5W only. Infuse over 60-90 minutes; adjust dose for renal impairment Store at room temp. Do not refrigerate. Protect from light. Stability depends on concentration of solution. 5 mL/125 mL D5W – stable for 6 hours 5 mL/75 mL D5W – stable for 2 hours IV to oral ratio = 1:1

Intravenous Compatibilities

Trissel's Handbook on Injectable Drugs is the go-to source for IV drug compatibility.

Instability: occurs when a product/solution is modified because of storage conditions (e.g. time, temperature, light, absorption). A product is considered unstable when it loses more than 10% of its labeled potency from the time of preparation.

Incompatibility: occurs when one product is mixed or combined with another and changes occur that make the product unsuitable for patient use (e.g. degradation, precipitation, a change in pH).

There are 4 different types of tables listed in _Trissel's_ – solution compatibility, additive compatibility, drugs in syringe compatibility, and y-site injection compatibility.

TRISSEL'S HANDBOOK EXAMPLE: USING DOPAMINE AS AN EXAMPLE

Look up Dopamine. You will find different charts depending on how the drugs will be mixed (solution compatibility, additive compatibility, y-site compatibility, etc.). Find the correct chart to reference.

ADDITIVE COMPATIBILITY

DRUG*	MFR*	CON/L*	MFR	CONC/L	TEST SOLN	REMARKS	REF	C/I
Ciprofloxacin	MI	2 g		400 mg	NS	C for 24 hrs at 25°C	888	C

Y-SITE INJECTION COMPATIBILITY (1:1 MIXTURE)

DRUG*	MFR*	CON/L*	MFR	CONC/L	REMARKS	REF	C/I
Cefepime	BMS	20 mg/mL	AST	3.2 mg/mL	Haze and precipitate form in 1 hr	1689	I
	BMS	120 mg/mL		0.4 mg/mL	Physically compatible with < 10% cefepime loss	2513	C
Heparin	ES	100 units/mL	AB	3.2 mg/mL	Visually compatible for 4 hr at 27°C	2062	C

*Info on the test drug (e.g. cipro, cefepime, heparin)

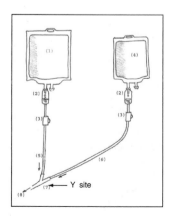
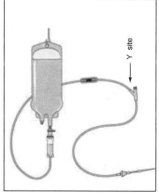

Antidotes

ANTIDOTES FOR SELECT TOXICITIES

DRUG/TOXIC AGENT	ANTIDOTE
Acetaminophen	**N-acetylcysteine**
Anticoagulants	**Phytonadione (AquaMephyton, Mephyton)**
Anticholinesterase insecticides/organophosphates (nerve agents)	**Atropine/Pralidoxime (Protopam)**
Anticholinergic compounds	**Physostigmine (Antilirium)**
Arsenic, Lead	Succimer (Chemet)
Benzodiazepines	**Flumazenil (Romazicon)**
Beta Blockers	Glucagon (GlucaGen)
Botulism	Botulism antitoxin
Calcium channel blockers	Calcium Chloride 10%, Glucagon
Carbon monoxide	Oxygen
Cyanide	Sodium nitrate, sodium thiosulfate
Digoxin	**Digoxin immune Fab (Digibind, DigiFab)**
Ethylene glycol, methanol	**Ethanol or fomepizole (Antizol)**
Heavy metals	Dimercaprol/Penicillamine
Heparin	**Protamine**
Iron	**Deferoxamine (Desferal)**
Isoniazid	**Pyridoxine (Vitamin B6)**
Methemoglobinemia	Methylene Blue
Opioids	**Naloxone (Narcan)**
Salicylate	Sodium Bicarbonate
Snake bites	**Crotalidae polyvalent (Antivenin, Crofab)**
TCA's	Sodium bicarbonate

DEPRESSION

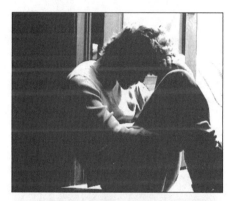

GUIDELINES

APA's Practice Guidelines for the Treatment of Patients With Major Depressive Disorder: Third Edition, 2010, Available at http://www.psych.org/guidelines/mdd2010

Diagnostic and Statistical Manual of Mental Disorders (DSM-IV-TR)

Background

Major Depressive Disorder (MDD, or referred to here as "depression") is one of the most common health conditions in the world. When a person is depressed they suffer greatly from persistent feelings of hopelessness, dejection, constant worry, poor concentration, a lack of energy, an inability to sleep and, sometimes, suicidal tendencies.

Most cases of depression should be viewed as chronic illness that requires long-term treatment, much like diabetes or high blood pressure. Although some people experience only one episode, the majority have recurrent episodes. Recurrent disease generally requires long-term (often life-long) treatment. Effective diagnosis and treatment can help reduce even severe depressive symptoms. And with effective treatment, many people with depression feel better, often within weeks, and can return to the activities they previously enjoyed. A significant treatment problem is patients that do not continue their medication, or, they may continue but do not receive an appropriate response. This is discussed under "Treatment-Resistant Depression" below.

Causes of Depression

The causes of depression are not well understood, but involve some combination of genetic, biologic and environmental factors. We are most concerned with biological factors, since these are treated with medications. Serotonin (5HT) may be the most important neurotransmitter (NT) involved with feelings of well being. Other NTs include acetylcholine (ACh) and catecholamines (including dopamine (DA), norepinephrine (NE), and epinephrine EPI)). The medications used for treating depression affect the levels of these NTs. Since it is not possible at this time to measure deficiencies or excesses in brain chemicals, treatment for mood disorders, including depression, depends on a competent assessment and a trial and error process on the best option for therapy. If a drug does not work, a combination or different set of NTs can be targeted. Patient history is critical in treating any mental illness; what worked in the past, or did not work, should help guide current and future therapy.

Depression Diagnosis

DSM-IV criteria includes presence of at least 5 of the following symptoms during the same two week period (must include symptom 1 or 2):

1. Depressed mood

2. Marked diminished interest/pleasure

3. Significant weight loss or weight gain

4. Insomnia or hypersomnia

5. Psychomotor agitation or retardation

6. Fatigue or loss of energy

7. Feelings of worthlessness

8. Diminished ability to concentrate

9. Recurrent suicidal ideation

Concurrent Bipolar or Anxiety Disorders

It is necessary to rule-out bipolar disorder prior to initiating antidepressant therapy in order to treat the patient properly and avoid rapid-cycling (cycling rapidly from one phase to the other). This is why screening forms for MDD now include questions designed to identify mania symptoms such as "There are times when I get into moods where I feel very speeded up or irritable."

Benzodiazepines (BZDs) are often used adjunctively in depression with concurrent anxiety, although in many cases the BZD is the only "treatment" and the depression itself is left untreated. BZDs can cause and/or mask depression and put the patient at risk for physiological dependence (with withdrawal symptoms when the dose is wearing off (tachycardia, anxiety, etc.) They also require careful selection and monitoring in individuals with co-occurring substance use disorders.

Lag Effect and Suicide Prevention

Patients should be told that the medicine must be used daily, and will take time to work. <u>It is important to inform the patient that physical symptoms such as energy improve within two weeks but psychological symptoms, such as low mood, may take 4-6 weeks or longer.</u> If the medicine does not help, the patient should not despair. If you see a patient who reports they are considering suicide, refer to the ER or elsewhere for help. Do not take these statements

MEDICATIONS THAT CAN CAUSE OR WORSEN DEPRESSION

Beta-blockers
(particularly propranolol)

Clonidine

Corticosteroids

Cyclosporine

Ethanol

Isotretinoin

Indomethacin

Interferons

Low vitamin D levels (possible link)

Methadone

Methyldopa

Methylphenidate/Other ADHD Stimulants/
Atomoxetine: Monitor mood

Procainamide

Reserpine

Varenicline

And…antidepressants require monitoring
for worsening mood, especially among
younger people

In addition to the medications listed, medical conditions such as stroke, Parkinson's disease, dementia, multiple sclerosis, thyroid disorders (particularly hypothyroidism), metabolic conditions (e.g., hypercalcemia), malignancy and infectious diseases can be contributory.

lightly; this is a call for help. If someone has a plan for suicide, it is more likely that the threat is real.

PHARMACOTHERAPY

Treatment in the acute phase should be aimed at inducing remission of the major depressive episode and achieving a full return to the patient's baseline level of functioning. Acute phase treatment may include pharmacotherapy, depression-focused psychotherapy, the combination of medications and psychotherapy, or other somatic therapies such as electroconvulsive therapy (ECT), vagal nerve stimulation (VNS) or light therapy.

The guidelines state that because the effectiveness of the different antidepressant classes is generally comparable, the initial choice of an agent should be based on the side effect profile, safety concerns and the patient-specific symptoms. For most patients an SSRI, SNRI or (with specific concurrent conditions or considerations) mirtazapine or bupropion is preferred.

Due to safety concerns (the risk of drug-drug and drug-food interactions) the use of the oral non-selective monoamine oxidase inhibitors (MAOIs) (phenelzine, tranylcypromine and isocarboxazid) is restricted to patients who do not respond to other treatments. Serotonin syndrome can occur with administration of one or more serotonergic medications (and higher doses increases risk) but it is most severe when an MAO-I is administered with another serotonergic medication.

All drug therapy trials should preferably be given with competent, concurrent psychotherapy, although this is not typically done. If a drug is being discontinued it should be tapered off over several weeks. In some instances a drug with a longer half-life (e.g. fluoxetine) can be used to minimize withdrawal symptoms. Withdrawal symptoms (anxiety, agitation, insomnia, dizziness, flu-like symptoms) can be quite distressing to the patient. Paroxetine and some other agents carry a high risk of withdrawal symptoms and must be tapered upon discontinuation.

TREATMENT-RESISTANT DEPRESSION

<u>Patients should try at least six weeks on a medication before concluding that it is not working well. In addition, the dose should be therapeutic</u>. Even if both conditions are met it is unfortunate that only about half of patients respond to the prescribed antidepressant and just about one-third will reach remission (the elimination of depressive symptoms). The goal of therapy is remission. An incomplete response can necessitate any of the following:

- A dosage increase.

- A combination of antidepressants (which may or may not be appropriate).

- Augmentation with buspirone *(BuSpar)* or a low dose of an atypical antipsychotic. Agents approved as augmentation therapy with antidepressants are aripiprazole *(Abilify)*, olanzapine+fluoxetine *(Symbyax)* and quetiapine ext-rel *(Seroquel XR)*.

Natural Products

St. John's wort or SAMe (S-adenosyl-L- methionine) may be helpful. Both are classified as "likely effective" for treating depression in the *Natural Medicines Database*, however overall there is less evidence of efficacy than with standard treatments. Both agents cannot be used with other serotonergic agents. <u>St. John's wort is a broad-spectrum inducer of CYP 450 enzymes and has many significant drug interactions.</u>

Suicide risk in Adolescents and Young Adults: Antidepressants Require a MedGuide that includes this Statement:

Antidepressants increase the risk (compared to placebo) of suicidal thinking and behavior (suicidality) in children, adolescents, and young adults in short term studies of major depressive disorder (MDD) and other psychiatric disorders. Anyone considering the use of an antidepressant in a child, adolescent or young adult must balance this risk with the clinical need. Monitor appropriately..."

SSRIs: Selective Serotonin Reuptake Inhibitors

DRUG	DOSING	SIDE EFFECTS/MONITORING/ CONTRAINDICATIONS
Fluoxetine (Prozac, Sarafem, Prozac Weekly) + olanzapine (Symbyax) – for resistant depression	10-60 mg/day 90 mg weekly 20 mg/5 mL liquid Premenstrual dysphoric disorder (PMDD): *Sarafem* daily, or weekly and 14 and 7 days prior to menses	All approved for depression and a variety of anxiety disorders except fluvoxamine **SIDE EFFECTS** Fluoxetine can cause activation → take dose in AM, others AM (usually) or PM, if sedating All may cause akathisia (restlessness) Sexual side effects: (20-50%) include ↓ libido, ejaculation difficulties, anorgasmia
Paroxetine (Paxil, Pexeva, Paxil CR)	IR: 10 – 60 mg/day CR: 12.5 – 75 mg/day 10 mg/5mL Each 10 mg IR = 12.5 mg CR	N/V, diarrhea (dose-dependent, generally dissipates) Headache (but may help migraines if used continuously) ↑ weight in some patients (more with paroxetine) SIADH Restless leg syndrome (see if this began when treatment was started)
Fluvoxamine (*Luvox,* Luvox CR)	100-300 mg/day IR form for OCD only, CR for OCD and SAD (social anxiety disorder) – fluvoxamine has more drug interactions	↑ bleeding risk if taken concurrently with warfarin, dabigatran, rivaroxaban, antiplatelets or other agents that increase bleeding risk ↑ fall risk; use extreme caution in frail patients, osteopenia/osteoporosis, use of CNS depressants
Sertraline (Zoloft)	50-200 mg/day 20 mg/mL liquid Premenstrual dysphoric disorder (PMDD): *Zoloft* 150 mg/d continuously or 100 mg/d during the 2 weeks prior to menses	**Contraindication** POTENTIALLY LETHAL DI: SSRIs and MAOIs – see wash-out information. Do not stop suddenly – will get anxiety, insomnia, flu-like withdrawal symptoms. Fluoxetine can be stopped with less of a taper due to long half-life. Note FDA warning regarding QT risk and citalopram at >40 mg/day listed under dosing column.
Citalopram *(Celexa)*	20-40 mg/day 2011 FDA warning not to use > 40 mg/day due to QT risk. Max 20 mg/day with inhibitors.	
Escitalopram (Lexapro – **isomer of citalopram)**	10 mg/day (can ↑ 20 mg/d) 1 mg/mL liquid	
Vilazodone (*Viibryd*) Dosing to the right is in the patient starter kit.	Titrate to 40 mg/d; start at: 10 mg x 7d, then 20 mg x 7d, then 40 mg ALL WITH FOOD	**SIDE EFFECTS** Diarrhea, nausea/vomiting, dizziness, dry mouth, insomnia, ↓ libido (less sexual SEs compared to SSRIs and SNRIs) ↑ bleeding risk if taken concurrently with warfarin, dabigatran, rivaroxaban, antiplatelets or other agents that increase bleeding risk.

SSRI DRUG INTERACTIONS

- MAOIs and hypertensive crisis: 2 weeks either going to an MAO I or from an MAO I to an SSRI <u>except</u> fluoxetine which requires a 5 wk washout period if going from fluoxetine to an MAOI (due to the long half-life of fluoxetine of at least 7 days).

- Fluoxetine: 2D6, 2C19 inhibitor. Fluvoxamine: 1A2, 2D6, 2C9, 2C19, 3A4 inhibitor. Paroxetine: 2D6 inhibitor. Note all three are 2D6 inhibitors and some other psych drugs are 2D6 substrates. Psych drugs are sometimes used in combination.

- Decreased effectiveness of tamoxifen with fluoxetine, paroxetine and sertraline (and duloxetine and bupropion).

- SSRIs and anticoagulants (warfarin, dabigatran, rivaroxaban, etc.) watch for ↑ bleeding risk; INR (if using with warfarin) may be in therapeutic range.

- Caution with drugs that cause orthostasis or CNS depressants due to risk of falls. Caution with QT prolonging agents and inhibitors with citalopram.

SSRI COUNSELING

- Dispense MedGuide & instruct patient to read it. Especially in adolescents and young adults: counsel on risk of suicide – particularly during therapy initiation.

- Fluoxetine is taken in the morning; the others morning or at bedtime.

- To reduce your risk of side effects, your doctor may direct you to start taking this drug at a low dose and gradually increase your dose.

- Use this medication regularly in order to get the most benefit from it. To help you remember, use it at the same time each day. Antidepressants do not work if they are taken as-needed.

- It is important to continue taking this medication even if you feel well. Do not stop taking this medication without consulting your doctor. Some conditions may become worse when the drug is suddenly stopped. Your dose may need to be gradually decreased.

- It may take 1 to 2 weeks to feel a benefit from this drug and 6-8 weeks to feel the full effect on your mood. Tell the doctor if your condition persists or worsens. You can try a medication in a different class. One will work or it may take different tries to find the right medicine that will help you feel better.

- Some patients, but not all, have sexual difficulties when using this medicine. If this happens, talk with the doctor. They can change you to a medicine that does not cause these problems.

SNRIs – Serotonin and Norepinephrine Reuptake Inhibitors

DRUG	DOSING	SIDE EFFECTS/MONITORING/ CONTRAINDICATIONS
Venlafaxine (Effexor, Effexor XR) Depression GAD	37.5, 75, 150 mg XR cap (typical dosing range 150-375 mg) Different generics; check orange book	**SIDE EFFECTS** Similar to SSRIs: N/V, sexual dysfunction SNRIs also have SEs related to ↑ NE uptake, including ↑ pulse, dilated pupils, dry mouth, excessive sweating & constipation All have warning for ↑ BP, but risk is greatest with venlafaxine when dosed > 150 mg/day; yet all have risk especially at higher doses. (↑ BP may respond to dose reduction, use of antihypertensive or change in therapy)
Duloxetine **(Cymbalta)** Depression Peripheral Neuropathy (Pain) Fibromyalgia GAD Chronic Low Back Pain Chronic Osteoarthritis Pain	20, 30, 60 mg (typical dosing 60-120 mg/d) Duloxetine is a good choice if the patient has both pain and depression (no generic)	**CONTRAINDICATIONS** POTENTIALLY LETHAL DI: SNRIs and MAOIs see wash-out information.
Desvenlafaxine ER **(Pristiq)** Depression	50, 100 mg 50 mg daily (typical)	

SNRI DRUG INTERACTIONS

- MAOIs and hypertensive crisis: 2 week washout if going to or from a MAO Inhibitor.

- Duloxetine is a 2D6 inhibitor.

- Decreased effectiveness of tamoxifen with fluoxetine, paroxetine, sertraline, duloxetine and bupropion.

- SNRIs and anticoagulants (warfarin, dabigatran, rivaroxaban, etc.) watch for ↑ bleeding risk (INR may be in therapeutic range).

- If on antihypertensive medications, use caution and monitor (can ↑ BP), especially at higher doses.

SNRI COUNSELING

- Dispense MedGuide & instruct Patient to read it. Especially in adolescents and young adults: counsel on risk of suicide – particularly during therapy initiation.

- This medication may cause nausea and stomach upset (if venlafaxine IR can try change to XR).

- You may experience increased sweating; if so, discuss with your doctor. You should check your blood pressure regularly to make sure it stays in a safe range.

- Desvenlafaxine: When you take this medicine, you may see something in your stool that looks like a tablet. This is the empty shell from the tablet after the medicine has been absorbed by your body.

- To reduce your risk of side effects, your doctor may direct you to start taking this drug at a low dose and gradually increase your dose.

- Do not crush or chew extended-release formulations.

- Use this medication regularly in order to get the most benefit from it. To help you remember, use it at the same time each day. Antidepressants do not work if they are taken as-needed.

- It is important to continue taking this medication even if you feel well. Do not stop taking this medication without consulting your doctor. Some conditions may become worse when the drug is suddenly stopped. Your dose may need to be gradually decreased.

- It may take 1 to 2 weeks to feel a benefit from this drug and 6-8 weeks to feel the full effect on your mood. Tell the doctor if your condition persists or worsens. You can try a medication in a different class. One will work it may take different tries to find the right medicine that will help you feel better.

- Some patients, but not all, have sexual difficulties when using this medicine. If this happens, talk with the doctor. They can change you to a medicine that does not cause these problems.

Tricyclics

NE and 5HT Reuptake Inhibitors (and block ACh and histamine receptors which contributes to the SE profile).

DRUG	DOSING	SIDE EFFECTS/MONITORING/ CONTRAINDICATIONS
TERTIARY AMINES **Amitriptyline** *(Limbitrol, Elavil – brand N/A) – Etrafon* is with perphenazine for depression + severe anxiety **Doxepin** *(Sinequan) – Zonalon* cream is for prurutis Clomipramine *(Anafranil)* Imipramine *(Tofranil)* Trimipramine *(Surmontil)* **SECONDARY AMINES** Amoxapine *(Asendin*-brand N/A) Desipramine *(Norpramine)* Maprotiline *(Ludiomil*-brand N/A) Nortriptyline *(Pamelor)* Protriptyline *(Vivactil)* (Secondary are relatively selective for NE – tertiary may be slightly more effective but have worse SE profile)	**AMITRIPTYLINE** neuropathic pain: migraine prophylaxis: 10-50 mg QHS depression: 100-150 mg BID **NORTRIPTYLINE** depression: 25 mg TID-QID **DOXEPIN** depression: 100-300 mg daily	**SIDE EFFECTS** **Cardiotoxicity** QT-prolongation with overdose – can be used for suicide-counsel carefully; get baseline ECG if cardiac risk factors or age > 50 years old Orthostasis, tachycardia **Anticholinergic** Dry mouth, blurred vision, urinary retention, constipation (taper off to avoid cholinergic rebound) Vivid dreams Weight gain (varies by agent and patient), sedation Myoclonus (muscle twitching-may be symptoms of drug toxicity) ↑ Fall risk – especially in elderly due to combination of orthostasis and sedation

TRICYCLIC DRUG INTERACTIONS

- MAOIs and hypertensive crisis: 2 week washout if going to or from a MAO Inhibitor.

- Additive QT prolongation risk; see Drug Interaction section for other high-risk QT drugs to attempt to avoid additive risk.

- Metabolized by 2D6 (up to 10% of Caucasians are slow metabolizers); check for DIs

TRICYCLIC COUNSELING

- Dispense MedGuide & Instruct Patient to read it. Especially in adolescents and young adults: counsel on risk of suicide – particularly during therapy initiation. TCAs are dangerous if the patient wishes to kill themselves a month's supply can be deadly. Counseling is critical.

- This drug can cause constipation. You may need to use a stool softener or laxative if this becomes a problem.

- This drug may cause dry/blurry vision. You may need to use an eye drop lubricant.

- This drug may make it more difficult to urinate.

- This drug may cause dry mouth. This can contribute to dental decay (cavities) and difficulty chewing food. It is important to use proper dental hygiene when taking any medication that causes dry mouth, including brushing and flossing. Sugar free lozenges may be helpful.

- This drug may cause changes in your blood pressure. Use caution when changing from lying down or sitting to a standing position. Hold onto the bed or rail until you are steady.

- If you experience anxiety, or insomnia (sometimes with vivid dreams), these usually go away. If they do not, contact your doctor.

- Use this medication regularly in order to get the most benefit from it. To help you remember, use it at the same time each day. Antidepressants do not work if they are taken as-needed.

- It is important to continue taking this medication even if you feel well. Do not stop taking this medication without consulting your doctor. Some conditions may become worse when the drug is suddenly stopped. Your dose may need to be gradually decreased.

- It may take 1 to 2 weeks to feel a benefit from this drug and 6-8 weeks to feel the full effect on your mood. Tell the doctor if your condition persists or worsens. You can try a medication in a different class. One will work it may take different tries to find the right medicine that will help you feel better.

MAO-Is: Monoamine Oxidase Inhibitors

Inhibit the enzyme monoamine oxidase, which breaks down catecholamines, including 5HT, NE, EPI, DA. If these NTs ↑ dramatically, hypertensive crisis, and death can result.

DRUG	DOSING	SIDE EFFECTS/MONITORING/ CONTRAINDICATIONS
Isocarboxazid *(Marplan)* Phenelzine *(Nardil)* Tranylcypromine *(Parnate)*		**SIDE EFFECTS** Anticholinergic effects (taper upon discontinuation to avoid cholinergic rebound) Orthostasis Sedation (except tranylcypromine → stimulation) Sexual dysfunction, weight gain, HA, insomnia **CONTRAINDICATIONS** <u>Not commonly used but watch for drug-drug and drug-food interactions – if missed could be fatal</u> Hypertensive crisis can occur when taken with TCAs, SSRIs, SNRIs, many other drugs and tyramine-rich foods (see DIs below)
Selegiline transdermal *(Emsam)* MAO I B Selective Inhibitor	6, 9 or 12 mg/day patch Changed daily	**SIDE EFFECTS** Constipation, gas, dry mouth, loss of appetite, sexual problems **CONTRAINDICATIONS** Avoid tyramine-rich foods and drinks while using 9 mg & 12 mg/d patches and for 2 weeks after stopping. No dietary issues with 6 mg patch.

MAO INHIBITOR DRUG INTERACTIONS

- MAOIs and hypertensive crisis: 2 week washout if going to or from a MAO Inhibitor and an SSRI, SNRI or TCA antidepressant [exception: if going from fluoxetine back to MAOI need to wait 5 weeks.]

- MAOIs CANNOT be used with many other drugs or the drugs will not be broken down and hypertensive crisis, serotonin syndrome or psychosis may result. The interaction could be fatal. These include any drugs with effects on the concentrations of epinephrine, norepinephrine, serotonin or dopamine. This includes bupropion, ephedrine and analogs (pseudoephedrine, etc), levodopa, linezolid, lithium, meperidine, SSRIs, SNRIs, TCAs, tramadol, mirtazapine, dextromethorphan, cyclobenzaprine (and other skeletal muscle relaxants) and St. John's wort.

- MAOIs cannot be used with tyramine-rich foods, including aged cheese, pickled herring, yeast extract, air-dried meats, sauerkraut, soy sauce, fava beans and some red wines and beers (tap beer and any beer that has not been pasteurized – canned and bottled beers contain little or no tyramine). Foods can become high in tyramine when they have been aged, fermented, pickled or smoked.

MAO-I INHIBITOR COUNSELING

- Dispense MedGuide & instruct patient to read it. Especially in adolescents and young adults: counsel on risk of suicide – particularly during therapy initiation.

- Warn patients regarding the need to avoid mixing with any interacting food or drug. See list in above drug interaction section. Stay away from tyramine-rich containing foods.

- Report immediately to your doctor if you have 3 or more of the following: agitation or restlessness, palpitations, diarrhea, hallucinations, feeling hot, loss of coordination, rapid changes in BP, and vomiting. (These are symptoms of serotonin syndrome)

- Use this medication regularly in order to get the most benefit from it. To help you remember, use it at the same time each day. Antidepressants do not work if they are taken as-needed.

- It is important to continue taking this medication even if you feel well. Do not stop taking this medication without consulting your doctor. Some conditions may become worse when the drug is suddenly stopped. Your dose may need to be gradually decreased.

- It may take 1 to 2 weeks to feel a benefit from this drug and 6-8 weeks to feel the full effect on your mood. Tell the doctor if your condition persists or worsens. You can try a medication in a different class. One will work – it may take different tries to find the right medicine that will help you feel better.

- *EMSAM* Patch Application: Change once daily. Pick a time of day you can remember. Apply to either upper chest or back (below the neck and above the waist), upper thigh, or to the outer surface of the upper arm. Rotate site and do not use same site 2 days in a row. Wash hands with soap after applying patch.

ADDITIONAL AGENTS

DRUG	DOSING	SIDE EFFECTS/MONITORING/ CONTRAINDICATIONS
Bupropion (*Wellbutrin*, *Budeprion XL, Aplenzin*) (***Zyban*** for smoking)	Dopamine (DA) and norepinephrine (NE) reuptake Inhibitor 300-450 mg daily Wellbutrin IR is TID Wellbutrin SR is BID (to 200 mg BID) Wellbutrin XL is daily *Aplenzin* dosing: 174 mg (equiv to 150 mg), 348 mg (equiv to 300 – this is the usual target dose)	**SIDE EFFECTS** Dry mouth, insomnia, headache/migraine, nausea/vomiting, constipation, and tremors/seizures (dose-related), possible blood pressure changes (more hypertension than hypotension – monitor), weight loss No effects on 5HT and therefore no sexual dysfunction; can be used if issues with other antidepressants **CONTRAINDICATIONS** Do not use in seizure disorder Do not exceed 450 mg/d due to seizure risk Do not use *Zyban* and other form of bupropion together – same drug

Continued

DRUG	DOSING	SIDE EFFECTS/MONITORING/ CONTRAINDICATIONS
Mirtazapine (*Remeron*, Remeron Soltab) Used commonly in oncology and skilled nursing since it helps with sleep at night (dosed QHS) & increases appetite (good for weight gain in frail elderly)	NE and serotonin (5HT) reuptake Inhibitor 15-45 mg QHS	**SIDE EFFECTS** Sedation and ↑ appetite, weight gain Dry mouth, dizziness Agranulocytosis (rare)
Trazodone (*Desyrel*) 100-150 BID Trazodone ER (*Oleptro*) – 150, 300 mg – may be less sedating and is dosed QHS Rarely used as an antidepressant due to sedation. Used primarily off-label for sleep (dosed 50-100 mg QHS)	Inhibits 5-HT reuptake and is an α1-adrenergic blocker and a histamine blocker 100-150 mg BID	**SIDE EFFECTS** Sedation Orthostasis (risk in elderly for falls) Sexual dysfunction and risk of priapism (medical emergency – requires immediate medical attention if painful erection longer than 4 hrs)
Nefazodone (*Serzone* – brand N/A)	Similar to trazodone but less sedating and increased risk of hepatotoxicity	Similar to trazodone, but less sedating Rarely used due to hepatotoxicity: monitor LFTs, counsel on symptoms of liver damage

BUPROPION DRUG INTERACTIONS

- Do not use with *Zyban* for smoking cessation; same drug.

- Do not use in patients with seizure history; drug ↓ seizure threshold. Do not exceed 450 mg daily in anyone.

KEY COUNSELING POINTS FOR ABOVE AGENTS

- Dispense MedGuide & instruct patient to read it. Especially in adolescents and young adults: counsel on risk of suicide – particularly during therapy initiation.

- Counsel on lag time, need to take daily as with other agents.

- Bupropion: Include not to exceed 450 mg daily, or 150 mg at each dose if using immediate-release formulations due to seizure risk.

- Mirtazapine: Counsel to take at night, drug is sedating, and should increase appetite.

For Treatment Resistance Depression Only

Rule-out bipolar disorder, check if antidepressant is at optimal dose, sometimes use combination standard antidepressants, or augment with various options. The antipsychotics below are approved for treatment-resistant depression.

All antipsychotics require MedGuides with this Warning:

Elderly patients with dementia-related psychosis (having lost touch with reality due to confusion and memory loss) treated with this type of medicine are at an increased risk of death, compared to placebo (sugar pill).

And because it is being used to augment AD therapy:

Antidepressants have increased the risk of suicidal thoughts and actions in some children, teenagers, and young adults.

DRUG	DOSING	SIDE EFFECTS/MONITORING/ CONTRAINDICATIONS
Aripiprazole *(Abilify)*	Start 2-5 mg/day (QAM), can ↑ to 15 mg	**Side Effects** Each of these drugs can cause metabolic issues, including dyslipidemia, weight gain, diabetes Risk of Neuroleptic Malignant Syndrome Risk of Tardive Dyskinesia (TD) Risk of leukopenia, neutropenia, agranulocytosis All can cause orthostasis/dizziness
Olanzapine/fluoxetine *(Symbyax)*	Usually started at 6 mg/25 mg capsule QHS (fluoxetine is activating, but olanzapine is more sedating), can ↑ cautiously. CI with pimozide, thioridazine, & caution with other QT prolongating drugs/conditions	**Abilify** Akathisia/restlessness (esp in younger patients), insomnia, constipation, fatigue, blurred vision **Olanzapine** Cognitive dysfunction, dry mouth, fatigue, sedation, ↑ appetite/weight, peripheral edema, tremor, blurred vision **Quetiapine** Sedation, dry mouth, constipation, dizziness, ↑ appetite/weight, nausea
Quetiapine extended-release *(Seroquel XR)*	Start 50 mg QHS, ↑ nightly to 150-300 mg QHS	

Practice Case

Steve is a thin, anxious-appearing 57 year-old male. He is married with two children. Steve's wife has brought him to the clinic due to his constant worry, anxiety, and feelings of worthlessness. When he was in college, Steve had several bouts of depression and was treated successfully with doxepin. He stopped using the medication when he graduated and moved to California. He felt the sunshine made him feel better. His wife reports, however, that this is the 3rd or 4th time in the past few years that Steve has felt so low that she became concerned he might harm himself. His wife reports that Steve is up all night, with constant worry. She does not think he has had a good night's sleep in months.

Celexa ®

At the last clinic visit (2 months ago) the doctor started Steve on citalopram 40 mg once daily and lorazepam 1 mg QD-TID prn. Steve has been using the medication and states that it helps a little, but not much. He is taking the lorazepam 1 mg TID. His other medications include propranolol for hypertension/nerves and fosinopril for hypertension. He does not smoke and drinks occasional alcohol.

CATEGORY	
Medications	Fosinopril 20 mg daily
	Inderal LA 120 mg daily
	Citalopram 40 mg daily
	Lorazepam 1 mg QD-TID as-needed
Vitals	Height 5'10", weight 155 lbs, BP (in clinic today) 158/102

Questions

1. Steve has depression that has not responded to an adequate trial of fluoxetine or citalopram. Which of the following options represents the best alternative?

    a. Sertraline
    b. Venlafaxine
    c. Fluvoxamine
    d. Escitalopram
    e. Mirtazapine

2. If Steve was started on _Effexor XR_ (he won't be), which of the following parameters should be carefully monitored in this patient?

    a. Blood pressure
    b. Thyroid parameters
    c. White blood cell count
    d. A and B
    e. A and C

3. A pharmacist counseling a patient on the use of any antidepressant should include the following counseling points:

    a. Your energy level may pick up before your mood starts to feels better.
    b. Your mood should improve; this usually takes about a month.
    c. If this medicine does not work, the doctor will try a different agent, which may work better.
    d. This medication needs to be taken every day; it does not work if it is taken occasionally.
    e. All of the above.

4. What is the mechanism of action of venlafaxine?

a. Selective serotonin reuptake inhibitor
b. Serotonin and dopamine reuptake inhibitor
c. Serotonin and norepinephrine reuptake inhibitor
d. Norepinephrine and dopamine reuptake inhibitor
e. Norepinephrine and acetylcholine reuptake inhibitor

5. The doctor takes a thorough medication history and decides that it would be worthwhile to try Doxepin, since the patient had a good history of use with this agent. Which of the following statements is correct?

a. Doxepin is a monoamine oxidase inhibitor.
b. Doxepin can cause excess salivation and has significant food interactions.
c. He should be carefully evaluated for suicide risk.
d. A and C only.
e. All of the above.

Questions 6-10 do not apply to the case.

6. A patient has been started on bupropion for depression. His other medications include *Lopid, Pravachol and Zyban*. Which of the following statement is correct?

a. Bupropion will raise his triglycerides.
b. Bupropion will raise his HDL cholesterol.
c. Bupropion will lower his HDL cholesterol.
d. Bupropion should not be used in this patient.
e. None of the above.

7. A patient has been started on bupropion 200 mg TID for depression. His medical conditions include partial seizures and obsessive compulsive disorder. His medications include fluvoxamine and phenytoin. Which of the following statements is correct?

a. Bupropion will induce the metabolism of phenytoin.
b. The bupropion dose is too high.
c. Bupropion should not be used in this patient.
d. B and C only.
e. All of the above.

8. A patient has been using fluoxetine for depression for four months. He has suffered from sexual dysfunction and feels worse than when he started. Previously, he was well-controlled on tranylcypromine. The physician has decided to stop the fluoxetine and restart the tranylcypromine. Which of the following statements is correct?

a. No wash-out period is required.
b. A 2 week wash-out period is required.
c. A 3 week wash-out period is required.
d. A 5 week wash-out period is required.
e. An 8 week wash-out period is required.

9. Which of the following statements concerning trazodone is correct?

a. Trazodone is activating and can cause insomnia; it should be taken Q AM.
b. Trazodone can (rarely) cause a sustained erection.
c. If priapism is present, the patient must go to the ER right away.
d. B and C only.
e. All of the above.

10. Which of the following statements concerning duloxetine is correct?

a. The brand name is *Pristiq*.
b. Duloxetine can be useful for both neuropathic pain and depression.
c. Duloxetine is a strong 3A4 Inducer.
d. A and B only.
e. All of the above.

ANSWERS

1-e, 2-a, 3-e, 4-c, 5-c, 6-d, 7-d, 8-d, 9-d, 10-b

SCHIZOPHRENIA/ PSYCHOSIS

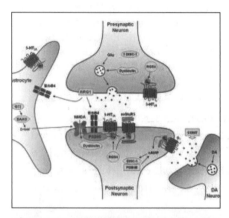

We gratefully acknowledge the assistance of Gollapudi Shankar, BPharm, MS, PharmD, CGP, BCPP, PhC, Western University College of Pharmacy, gshankar@westernu. edu, in reviewing this section.

Background

Schizophrenia is a debilitating brain disorder characterized by chronic, relapsing and remitting episodes. Patients suffer from hallucinations, delusions, disordered thinking and behavior. They withdraw from the world around them and enter a world of psychosis. Schizophrenia ranges from relatively mild to severe. Some people may be able to function adequately in daily life, while others need specialized, intensive care. Treatment adherence is important and often difficult to obtain, which is regrettable to the patient's significant others and to themselves, since the patient with schizophrenia typically lives a life of torment. This condition has one of the highest suicide rates.

The onset of symptoms usually begins in young adulthood. A diagnosis is not based on lab tests, but on the patient's behavior, which should include negative and positive signs and symptoms (described on the following page). Schizophrenia occurs in ~1% in all societies regardless of class, color, religion, culture or national origin.

GUIDELINES

Diagnostic and Statistical Manual of Mental Disorders (DSM-IV-TR). DSM-V expected release date May, 2013.

American Psychiatric Association. Practice guideline for the treatment of patients with schizophrenia. 2nd ed. Arlington (VA): American Psychiatric Association; 2009. Available at: http:// www.psychiatryonline.com/pracGuide/ pracGuideTopic_6.aspx

CAUSES OF SCHIZOPHRENIA

Schizophrenia is a brain disorder, although genetics, environment, stressors and some illicit drugs can be contributing factors. Abnormalities in the role of neurotransmitters is central. There is increased dopamine in the mesolimbic pathway. Antipsychotics are primarily dopamine blockers, although newer agents that block dopamine and target additional receptors have benefit.

SIGNS AND SYMPTOMS	
Negative signs and symptoms (normal behaviors that are missing) Loss of interest in everyday activities Lack of emotion Inability to plan or carry out activities Poor hygiene Social withdrawal Loss of motivation (avolition) Poverty of speech (alogia)	**Positive signs and symptoms** Hallucinations; hearing voices (auditory hallucinations are common) Delusions, which are beliefs the patient has, but are without a basis in reality Thought disorders, or difficulty speaking and organizing thoughts, such as stopping in mid-sentence or jumbling together meaningless words Difficulty paying attention

NATURAL PRODUCTS

Fish oils are being used for psychosis, as well as other psychiatric disorders including ADHD and depression. The evidence is preliminary, but promising. Do not recommend cod liver oil due to risk of vitamin A toxicity. Keep in mind that natural products have dose-response relationships; check the Natural Medicines Database for dosing recommendations that appear to have benefit from clinical trials.

MEDICATIONS THAT CAN CAUSE PSYCHOTIC SYMPTOMS

- Amphetamines
- Methamphetamine, ice, crack
- Cannabis (low risk, but can occur in some cases)
- Cocaine
- Phencyclidine (PCP)
- Lysergic acid diethylamide (LSD) and other hallucinogenics
- Anticholinergics (centrally-acting, high doses)
- Dopamine or dopamine agonists used for Parkinson's disease (*Requip, Mirapex, Sinemet,* etc)
- Interferons
- Steroids (typically with lack of sleep – ICU psychosis)
- Stimulants (esp if already at risk), including ADHD drugs, modafinil etc.

PHARMACOTHERAPY

In general second generation antipsychotic (SGAs) are used first-line due to a lower risk of extrapyramidal side effects (EPS), however, they are not first-line in all patients and some respond better to a first generation antipsychotic (FGA).

In assessing treatment resistance or partial response (reduction in some symptoms) it is important to evaluate whether the patient has had an adequate trial (at least 4-6 weeks) of an antipsychotic, including whether the dose is adequate and whether the patient has been taking the medication as prescribed. A previous positive or negative history with antipsychotics should be used to guide therapy.

Clozapine has superior efficacy, but can cause agranulocytosis, seizures and myocarditis – in addition to having high metabolic risk. A clozapine trial should be considered for a patient who has had no or poor response to two trials of antipsychotics medication (at least one should be a SGA) or for a patient with significant ADRs.

High-potency FGAs such as haloperidol are associated with a high risk of EPS effects, a moderate risk of sedation and a low risk of orthostatic hypotension, tachycardia, and anticholinergic effects. In contrast, low-potency FGAs agents are associated with a lower risk of EPS, a high degree of sedation, a high risk of orthostatic hypotension and tachycardia, and a high risk of anticholinergic effects. Although other side effects also vary with the specific medication, in general, the first-generation antipsychotic medications are associated with a moderate risk of weight gain, a low risk of metabolic effects, and a high risk of sexual side effects. With certain agents (thioridazine particularly), QT risk is present.

Other possible side effects include seizures, allergic reactions, and dermatological, hepatic, ophthalmological, and hematological effects.

With the commonly used SGAs, weight gain and metabolic side effects are common with clozapine, olanzapine, quetiapine, and somewhat with risperidone and paliperidone. It is necessary to have regular monitoring of weight, body mass index, lipids, and glucose levels with these agents.

FORMULATIONS

Long-Acting Injections: Haloperidol is an older agent and comes in various formulations, including an IM injection for acute use, a long-acting decanoate, tablets and a solution. The advantage to a long-acting formulation, such as the *Haldol* decanoate (4 weeks), the *Risperdal Consta* (2 weeks), the *Invega Sustenna* (4 weeks) and a few others is that the patient with resistance to medications or poor "insight" (lack of recognition of the disease) will not need to be forced to take daily pills – which they are not likely to take. They are also used in acute care settings prior to the release of patients to the street (such as with homelessness).

Orally Disintegrating Tablets (ODTs): These are used to help solve the problem of "cheeking" where the patient holds the medication in their cheek and then spits it in the toilet. With ODTs the medicine dissolves rapidly in the mouth, without the need for water. Several of the SGAs come as ODTs (clozapine, olanzapine, risperidone and asenapine).

Acute IM Injections: Intramuscular (IM) injections work "stat" to help calm down an acutely agitated, psychotic patient. They are often mixed with other drugs, such as benzodiazepines. In this way the patient will not need to wait for oral absorption of a drug (which could take up to an hour to start to work). And, they will be sedated and hopefully "sleep off" the the worst of the episode.

Choosing a SGA Based on the Side Effect Profile

Clinicians choose among the various SGAs based on the formulary availability and the following considerations:

- If a patient has <u>cardiovascular risk</u> do not choose an agent that has risk of QT prolongation/arrhythmia (ziprasidone, risperidone, paliperidone, iloperidone, asenapine and lurasidone).

- If a patient is <u>overweight, has little physical activity or has metabolic issues</u> (elevated blood glucose and/or lipids) avoid agents that cause metabolic risk (most notably olanzapine and quetiapine). Clozapine has high metabolic risk but is used in refractive cases and might be required anyway. Several of the newer agents do not carry metabolic risk and do not cause weight gain. Olanzapine has the highest risk of metabolic issues (but does not have a high risk of QT prolongation).

- Increasing <u>prolactin levels</u> causes galactorrhea, or milk production without pregnancy, sexual dysfunction, gynecomastia (painful, swollen breast tissue) and irregular or missed periods (in women). After several years this can contribute to osteoporosis. This is a concern with risperidone and paliperidone, especially with higher doses.

- If the patient has a history of TD, or any type of movement disorder, avoid risperidone and paliperidone. Quetiapine has low risk of movement disorders. Clozapine has very low risk but is not used lightly.

- <u>Adherence Issues</u>: see formulation section above. In addition an agent that comes as once-daily dosing (versus BID or TID) may be preferred.

<u>Cost</u>: The only currently available generic SGA is risperidone. Fortunately, several of the formulations have decent patient assistance programs providing the patient has someone to help them complete the paperwork. Information on the programs can be found at www.rxassist.org, or by contacting the manufacturer directly via the contact information on the drug's website (www.putinbrandnameofdrug.com).

Antipsychotic Mechanism of Action

Antipsychotics, both FGAs and SGAs <u>are primarily dopamine$_2$ (D$_2$) receptor blockers</u> – excess dopamine is a primary factor contributing to psychosis. All SGAs agents block D$_2$ and block 5HT$_{2A}$ receptors, with the exception of aripiprazole which is a D$_2$ and 5HT$_{1A}$ partial agonist and 5HT$_{2A}$ antagonist.

BLACK BOX WARNING

<u>Antipsychotics cause increased risk of mortality in elderly patients with dementia-related psychosis, primarily due to an increased risk of stroke</u>. Note that APs are not particularly helpful to treat dementia-related anger/outbursts, but they are used and we are required to counsel on this risk. See the counseling section for wording suggestion.

NEUROLEPTIC MALIGNANT SYNDROME (NMS)

NMS is rare but is highly lethal. It occurs most commonly with the FGAs and is due to D_2 blockade. NMS occurs less commonly with SGAs and with other dopamine blocking agents including metoclopramide (*Reglan*). The majority of cases occur within two weeks of starting therapy. Occasionally, patients develop NMS even after years of antipsychotic use. (Antipsychotics used to be called neuroleptics; and thus, the name.)

Signs include:

■ Hyperthermia (high fever, with profuse sweating)

■ Extreme muscle rigidity (called "lead pipe" rigidity)

■ Mental status changes

■ Other signs can include tachycardia and tachypnea and blood pressure changes

Treatment:

STOP the antipsychotic.

■ Provide supportive care (airway support so the patient can breathe).

■ Cool them down: cooling bed, antipyretics, cooled IV fluids.

■ Dantrolene (a muscle relaxant) is sometimes used but has been studied in recent years and not shown to be beneficial.

First Generation Antipsychotics (FGA)

DRUG	DOSING	SIDE EFFECTS/MONITORING/ CONTRAINDICATIONS
Chlorpromazine	300-1,000 mg/d	**SIDE EFFECTS** All are sedating and all cause EPS, however the lower-potency agents have ↑ sedation and ↓ incidence EPS (e.g. chlorpromazine), and the higher-potency agents have ↓ sedation (but still sedating!) with ↑ EPS (e.g. haloperidol).
Thioridazine BLACK BOX: QT prolongation	300-800 mg/d	
Loxapine	30-100 mg/d	Movement disorders include: Tardive dyskinesias (TD), which are facial movements. The risk is higher in elderly females. If TD occurs the drug should be stopped as soon as possible; TD can be irreversible.
Perphenazine	16-64 mg/d	
Fluphenazine Available in 2-wk decanoate (*Prolixin*)	5-20 mg/d	Dystonias, which are prolonged contraction of muscles (including painful muscle spasms) can occur during initiation. There is higher risk with younger males. Can consider use of centrally-acting anticholinergic (diphenhydramine, benztropine) for prophylaxis during therapy initiation.
Haloperidol (*Haldol*), see formulations to right Class: butyrophenone (and DA-blocker) Haloperidol is also used for tics and vocal outbursts due to Tourette syndrome.	Oral (tablet, solution): start 0.5-2 mg BID-TID, up to 100 mg/d IV: usually 5-10 mg Decanoate (monthly): IM only, for conversion from PO, use 10-20x the oral dose	Akathisia, which is restlessness with anxiety and an inability to remain still. Dyskinesias, which are abnormal movements, are possible however this is more of an issue with the Parkinson's drugs. Sexual dysfunction Cardiovascular Effects Orthostasis, tachycardia, QT prolongation
Trifluoperazine	15-50 mg/d	
Thiothixene	15-50 mg/d	

Second Generation (SGA) Antipsychotics

DRUG	DOSING	SIDE EFFECTS/MONITORING/ CONTRAINDICATIONS
Clozapine *(Clozaril, FazaClo ODT)* Only if failed to respond to treatment with 2 standard AP treatments, or had significant ADRs	300-900 mg/d, divided (start at 25 mg and titrate, also titrate off since abrupt discontinuation can cause seizures) Clozapine has ↓ risk EPS/TD	**SIDE EFFECTS** Clozapine is thought to be the most effective atypical, but use is limited due to the risk of agranulocytosis and seizures Myocarditis Orthostasis, with or without syncope Weight gain, ↑ lipids, ↑ glucose **MONITORING** REMS: Patient must register with *Clozaril* Registry. Only pharmacies using Registry can fill this drug: To start: WBC must be ≥ 3,500/mm³ and ANC must be ≥ 2,000/mm³. WBC and ANC weekly x 6 months, then Q 2 weeks x 6 months, then monthly. Monitor for metabolic effects; see counseling section.
Olanzapine *(Zyprexa)* and *Zydis ODT*, see injection to right	10-20 mg QHS IM Injection (acute agitation) *Relprevv* inj suspension lasts 2-4 weeks, restricted use REMS drug – can cause sedation (including coma) and/or delirium after injection	**SIDE EFFECTS** Sedation Weight gain, ↑ lipids, ↑ glucose EPS **MONITORING** For metabolic effects; see counseling section
Risperidone *(Risperdal)* **and Risperdal M-Tabs ODT**, see injection to right Also approved for autism	4-16 mg/d, divided **Risperdal Consta**, 2 week injection, 25-50 mg	**SIDE EFFECTS** Sedation EPS, especially at higher doses ↑ Prolactin – sexual dysfunction, galactorrhea, irregular/ missed periods Orthostasis Weight gain, ↑ lipids, ↑ glucose QT prolongation **MONITORING** For metabolic effects; see counseling section
Quetiapine *(Seroquel, Seroquel XR)*	400-800 mg/d, divided BID or XR QHS XR is taken at night without food, or light meal (food ↑ absorption)	**SIDE EFFECTS** Sedation, orthostasis An eye exam for cataracts is recommended at beginning of therapy Weight gain, ↑ lipids, ↑ glucose Little risk EPS – often used for psychosis in Parkinson disease **MONITORING** For metabolic effects; see counseling section

Second Generation (SGA) Antipsychotics continued

DRUG	DOSING	SIDE EFFECTS/MONITORING/ CONTRAINDICATIONS
Ziprasidone *(Geodon)*, see injection to right	40-160 mg/d, divided BID Acute injection: ***Geodon IM***: 10-20 mg	**SIDE EFFECTS** Sedation, respiratory tract infection **CONTRAINDICATIONS** Prolongs QT interval, contraindicated with QT risk
Aripiprazole *(Abilify, Abilify Discmelt ODT)*, see injection info to right	10-15 mg Q AM IM Injection	**SIDE EFFECTS** Anxiety, Insomnia Constipation No/less weight gain
Paliperidone *(Invega*, *Invega Sustenna* is long-acting monthly inj suspension) Similar SEs to parent compound risperidone	3-12 mg/d (3 mg if CrCl < 50 mL/min) Active metabolite of risperidone; OROS delivery, so dosed once daily	**SIDE EFFECTS** ↑ Prolactin – sexual dysfunction, galactorrhea, irregular/ missed periods EPS, especially at higher doses Tachycardia, HA, sedation, anxiety Prolongs QT interval, avoid use with QT risk Weight gain, ↑ lipids, ↑ glucose **MONITORING** For metabolic effects; see counseling section
Iloperidone *(Fanapt)*	12-24 mg/d	**SIDE EFFECTS** Dizziness, somnolence, orthostasis Prolongs QT interval, avoid use with QT risk Titrate slowly due to orthostasis/dizziness
Asenapine *(Saphris)*	10-20 mg/d SL No food/drink for 10 min after dose	**SIDE EFFECTS** Somnolence, tongue/mouth numbness EPS (5% more than placebo), prolongs QT interval, avoid use with QT risk
Lurasidone *(Latuda)*	40-80 mg/d	**SIDE EFFECTS** Sedation, EPS, dystonias, nausea, agitation Weight gain, ↑ lipids, ↑ glucose Prolongs QT interval, avoid use with QT risk

Antipsychotic Drug Interactions

- All antipsychotics can prolong the QT interval – note that some are considered higher risk than others. The higher risk QT SGAs are noted. Thioridazine (*Mellaril*) is a high risk FGA QT drug.

All Antipsychotic Counseling

- Dispense Med Guide and instruct patient to read it.

- This medication can decrease hallucinations and improve your concentration. It helps you to think more clearly and feel positively about yourself, feel less nervous, and take a more active part in everyday life.

- There may be a slightly increased risk of serious, possibly fatal, side effects when this medication is used in older adults with dementia. This medication is not approved for the treatment of dementia-related behavior problems. Discuss the risks and benefits of this medication, as well as other effective and possibly safer treatments for dementia-related behavior problems, with the doctor.

- Contact your doctor right away if you experience uncontrollable movements of the mouth, tongue, cheeks, jaw, arms, or legs.

- Contact your doctor immediately and seek immediate medical attention if you experience fever, sweating, severe muscle stiffness (rigidity) and confusion.

- Use caution when driving, operating machinery, or performing other hazardous activities. This drug may cause dizziness or drowsiness.

- Dizziness may be more likely to occur when you rise from a sitting or lying position. Rise slowly to prevent dizziness and a possible fall.

- To reduce the dizziness and lightheadedness that may occur when you first start to take this drug, your doctor will direct you to start taking it at a low dose and gradually increase the dose. Your doctor may direct you to start by taking the immediate-release form of this drug, then switch you to the sustained-release form when you are regularly taking the same dose.

- Avoid consuming alcohol during treatment with this drug. Alcohol may increase drowsiness and dizziness.

- Tell your doctor if your condition persists or worsens.

CLOZAPINE

- This medication can cause a serious immune system problem called agranulocytosis (low white blood cells). To make sure you have enough white blood cells, you will need to have a blood test before you begin taking clozapine and then have your blood tested regularly during your treatment.

- Clozapine can also cause seizures, especially in higher doses. Let your doctor or pharmacist know if you have ever had seizures. While taking this medication, avoid driving or other activities during which a sudden loss of consciousness could be dangerous (e.g., operating heavy machinery, swimming).

- This medication may rarely cause an inflammation of the heart muscle (myocarditis). Seek immediate medical attention if you have weakness, difficult/rapid breathing, chest pain, or swelling of the ankles/legs. Your risk is highest during the first month of treatment.

OLANZAPINE, CLOZAPINE, RISPERIDONE, PALIPERIDONE AND QUETIAPINE

- This drug has a risk of weight gain, and elevated lipids, blood pressure and blood glucose (hyperglycemia). These must be monitored, and treated if they occur. Talk to your doctor if you experience any signs of hyperglycemia including excessive thirst, frequent urination, excessive hunger, or weakness.

- Your doctor will order blood tests during treatment to monitor progress and side effects.

DIFFERENT TYPES OF ORAL FORMULATIONS

- *Asenapine*: Place the sublingual tablet under the tongue and allow it to dissolve completely. The tablet will dissolve in saliva within seconds. Do not eat or drink for 10 minutes. The tongue will feel numb afterwards.

- *FazaClo, Abilify Discmelt, Risperdal M-Tab, Zyprexa Zydis*: Immediately upon opening the foil blister, using dry hands, remove tablet and place in mouth. Do not push the tablet through the foil because it may crumble. Tablet disintegration occurs rapidly so it can be easily swallowed with or without liquid. Use liquid only if you need it.

- Most ODTs contain phenylalanine. Do not dispense ODTs to patients with PKU.

- *Risperdal* oral solution can be administered directly from the calibrated pipette, or mixed with water, coffee, orange juice, and low-fat milk; it is not compatible with cola or tea.

- *Quetiapine XR* is taken at night without food, or light meal. Food decreases the absorption significantly.

- Olanzapine is usually taken once daily at night (QHS), since it is long-acting and sedating.

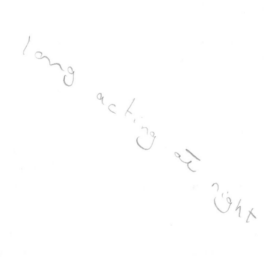

Practice Case

Ruby is a 24 year-old college student. Her parents have attempted to help Ruby over the past year. Her academic performance deteriorated and she began to look unkempt. About a month ago, her Mom was sure she saw Ruby mumbling to herself. Ruby began to call her mother "evil" and told her mother that she was destroying her life. Later, Ruby accused her mother of trying to feed her poisoned food. Ruby has dropped her old high-school friendships, except for one girl who her mother feels is more troubled than Ruby. When the mother went to talk to one of Ruby's instructors, they found out that Ruby had accused the teacher of changing what Ruby had written on an exam, and that the teacher had seen Ruby mumbling to herself in class. The teacher also complained that Ruby lacks attention in class, and reported that her work is sloppy and disorganized. The teacher had assumed there was difficulty at home, since Ruby told her that her mother is dying from cancer. This report from Ruby was not truthful.

The crisis in the family came to a head recently when Ruby stole a bottle of vodka from the local convenience store and was caught. Fortunately, the store manager knew the family and declined to press charges. However, later that night Ruby took some unknown medication and attempted to drown herself in the bathtub. She was taken by ambulance to the hospital.

The psychiatric team, after a brief visit with Ruby and a history taken from her family, gave Ruby a tentative diagnosis of schizophrenia. She received an injection of haloperidol and lorazepam, and is sleeping soundly. The psychiatric resident has come to the family to discuss treatment options.

No current medications; no known medical history. Height 5'5", weight 125 lbs.

QUESTIONS

1. The physician gave the patient an injection of haloperidol. This medication comes in the following formulations:

    a. Oral tablets

    b. IM injection

    c. Long-lasting (monthly) decanoate

    d. A and B

    e. All of the above

2. If Ruby is continued on haloperidol, she will be at risk for these side effects:

    a. Painful dystonic reactions (including painful neck and back muscle contractions)

    b. Tardive dyskinesias, or abnormal facial movements

    c. QT prolongation and possible arrhythmia risk

    d. A and B

    e. All of the above

3. If Ruby were to experience neuroleptic malignant syndrome while receiving haloperidol, what therapies would likely be administered in this emergency situation?

    a. Airway support

    b. Temperature cooling, such as ice beds

    c. Heating blankets

    d. A and B

    e. B and C

Questions 4-10 do not apply to the case.

4. Choose the potential adverse reaction/s from haloperidol which can be <u>irreversible</u> (and, if it occurs, the medicine should be stopped right away):

    a. Dystonic reaction

    b. Tardive dyskinesia

    c. Akathisia

    d. A and B

    e. B and C

5. A patient is started on olanzapine for psychotic symptoms. This agent puts the patient at high risk for the following side effects:

   a. Weight loss
   b. Elevated blood glucose
   c. Elevated blood lipids
   d. B and C only
   e. All of the above

6. A patient has been prescribed *Risperdal Consta*. Choose the correct statement:

   a. The medication lasts four weeks.
   b. The medication is given by slow IV infusion.
   c. *Risperdal Consta* is an orally-dissolving formulation for use with dysphagia.
   d. There remains a risk of EPS with this formulation.
   e. All of the above.

7. A patient has schizophrenia, with constant auditory hallucinations which have instructed the patient to harm himself and others. He has failed olanzapine and chlorpromazine. His other medications include sertraline for anxiety. His WBC ranges from 2.3-3.4 cells/mm³. He also has a low platelet count of 120. Which of the following statements is correct?

   a. He should begin clozapine therapy.
   b. Clozapine therapy is contraindicated due to his WBC count.
   c. Clozapine therapy is contraindicated due to his platelet count.
   d. Clozapine therapy is not indicated since he has not tried haloperidol.
   e. None of the above.

8. A patient with psychotic symptoms takes the following medications for chronic conditions: metoprolol, warfarin, amiodarone, lisinopril and insulin. His physician wishes to begin an antipsychotic. Which of the following agents represents the best option for this patient?

   a. Thioridazine
   b. Haloperidol
   c. Ziprasidone
   d. Risperidone
   e. Aripiprazole

9. A patient is using olanzapine in the morning. He takes 10 mg Q daily. He is tired all the time, but has trouble sleeping at night. Which option is best?

   a. Add temazepam at bedtime.
   b. Add zolpidem at bedtime.
   c. Move the olanzapine to bedtime.
   d. Add zaleplon at bedtime.
   e. Add mirtazapine at bedtime.

10. A physician wrote a prescription for *Abilify*. Which medication should be dispensed?

    a. Asenapine
    b. Olanzapine
    c. Aripiprazole
    d. Ziprasidone
    e. Thioridazine

ANSWERS

1-e, 2-e, 3-d, 4-b, 5-d, 6-d, 7-b, 8-e, 9-c, 10-c

BIPOLAR DISORDER

We gratefully acknowledge the assistance of Gollapudi Shankar, BPharm, MS, PharmD, CGP, BCPP, PhC, Western University College of Pharmacy, gshankar@westernu. edu, in reviewing this section.

Background

Bipolar Disorder (BD) used to be known as manic depressive disorder, but is now characterized primarily as bipolar I and bipolar II. There are two other minor types of bipolar in DSM IV – a milder form called cyclothymia and "bipolar disorder not otherwise specified."

Bipolar disease is a cyclical disorder, where the mood changes from one state to the other. Bipolar I is similar to what used to be the classic concept of manic-depressive disorder – manic or mixed episodes, alternating with major depression. The mania is severe and is the hallmark symptom of bipolar I. The person will act amazingly happy or high, irritable, restless, have grandiose behavior, and likely will have psychotic features such as hallucinations, delusions or paranoia. There is a decreased need for sleep and racing thoughts. At some point the mood darkens and depression occurs, which is severe and can last for weeks.

Bipolar II patients have "hypomania" and depression. Hypomania (or "euphoric mania") does not have psychotic symptoms and does not require hospitalization. It can be used to describe a "super happy" (or grouchy) person along with other symptoms such as talking fast, needing less sleep and engaging in risky behaviors. Both bipolar I and II have mania, but as a group the symptoms are less

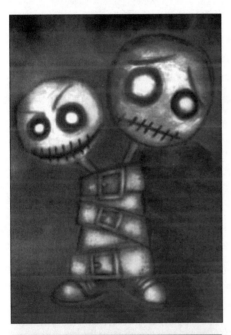

GUIDELINES

Diagnostic and Statistical Manual of Mental Disorders (DSM-IV-TR)

APA, Treatment of Patients with Bipolar Disorder, 2nd Ed., 2004. Available at: http://www.psychiatryonline.com/ pracGuide/pracGuideTopic_8.aspx.

VA/DOD, Management of Bipolar Disorder in Adults, 2010. Available at: http://www.healthquality.va.gov/bipolar/ bd_305_full.pdf

severe with bipolar II. However, although the symptoms are milder in bipolar II they are hard to treat. Bipolar II has about twice the incidence of bipolar I and is more common in women.

Bipolar disorder can be difficult to diagnosis since the high and low durations vary from weeks to months, and patients may come in for help only when in the depressed state. Medications can stabilize the mood swings and related symptoms, assuming the patient is using proper and continuous treatment. A challenge is that BD is often comorbid with a range of other mental disorders, such as ADHD, substance abuse and anxiety disorders.

Bipolar disorder (BD) is a severe mental disease that can lead to dangerous behaviors and ruined lives. It has a high rate of suicide.

DIAGNOSTIC CRITERIA

The criteria for a depressive disorder are listed in the depression section. The criteria for a manic episode include a distinct period of abnormally and persistently elevated, expansive, or irritable mood, lasting at least 1 week (or of any duration if hospitalization is necessary) and 3 or more of the following symptoms:

- Inflated self-esteem or grandiosity
- Decreased need for sleep
- More talkative than usual or pressure to keep talking
- Flight of ideas or subjective experience that thoughts are racing
- Distractibility
- Increase in goal-directed activity (either social, at work, at school, or sexually) or psycho-motor agitation
- Excessive involvement in pleasurable activities that have a high potential for painful consequences (e.g., buying sprees, sexual indiscretions, gambling)

PHARMACOTHERAPY

Historically, mood stabilizers (MS) and the first-generation antipsychotics were the mainstay of treating acute mania with psychotic symptoms. It is difficult to use the first-generation agents because bipolar patients are more susceptible to extrapyramidal symptoms (EPS) than those with schizophrenia.

In recent years, "atypical" or second-generation antipsychotic (SGA) agents have proved to be effective in the treatment of bipolar mania. The SGAs do not seem to induce depressive episodes, and some of them have antidepressant effects. The bipolar guidelines issued by the American Psychiatric Association are not current and have been in a (long) process of being updated. There are other guidelines and these vary in recommending either a MS first-line or SGA, or a combination of a MS and SGA. The benefit in using one agent first is that this enables the clinician to weigh the individual benefit and presentation and to identify the cause of adverse reactions. However, severe cases may warrant initiation with combination therapy.

If a MS is started first a SGA can be added. Or, if a SGA is started first a MS can be used, as needed. If psychotic features are present it makes sense to begin with a SGA. In deciding which SGA to use the clinician should consider if the primary treatment goal is control of acute mania or depression treatment. All the SGAs now have approvals for mania. Two of them have indications for mania <u>and</u> depression and thus can be useful to treat both stages of bipolar disorder: aripiprazole (*Abilify*) and quetiapine ext-rel (*Seroquel XR*) – this double-approval has led to a significant increase in the use of these agents to treat both phases of bipolar disorder. The side effects of the SGAs vary and are an important consideration in choosing an agent.

Lamotrigine can be useful for the treatment of the depressive stage but does not have benefit in mania. Lithium is also beneficial for depression – and for mania. This dual benefit makes lithium (an old, inexpensive drug) a treatment choice for many clinicians. Some patients on lithium will require augmentation with a second agent.

If an antidepressant is used there is risk of cycling. They may be used as adjunctive treatment in patients with refractory depression but the clinician will need to monitor for mania.

All antidepressants, anticonvulsants and antipsychotics require MedGuides.

Bipolar Medications and Pregnancy

Valproate, carbamazepine and lithium are pregnancy category D and have known fetal risk. The benefit must outweigh the risk. Lamotrigine (pregnancy category C) is often considered the safer option, relative to the other agents. During pregnancy if the risk is not well quantified an attempt should be made to avoid unnecessary drugs during the first trimester when organogenesis takes place.

- Lithium exposure in pregnancy is associated with an increase in congenital cardiac malformations.

- Valproate exposure in pregnancy is associated with increased risk of fetal anomalies, including neural tube defects, fetal valproate syndrome, and long term adverse cognitive effects. It should be avoided in pregnancy, if possible, especially during the first trimester.

- Carbamazepine exposure in pregnancy is associated with fetal carbamazepine syndrome. It should be avoided in pregnancy, if possible, especially during the first trimester. Carbamazepine has limited efficacy in treating bipolar but is occasionally used; see epilepsy section for a review of this agent.

- In addition, benzodiazepine use shortly before delivery is associated with floppy infant syndrome.

- If an antidepressant is used, paroxetine should be avoided. It is rated as pregnancy category D due to the risk of cardiac defects, particularly in the 1st trimester. Other SSRIs and SNRIs should be considered to have some degree of risk as well.

BIPOLAR MANIA OR ILLICIT DRUG USE?

A toxicology screen should be taken first (prior to start of treatment, and as-needed) to rule-out mania due to illicit drug use.

PRIMARY BIPOLAR MANIA AGENTS

DRUG	DOSING	SIDE EFFECTS/MONITORING/CONTRAINDICATIONS
Valproate or valproic acid (Depakene, Stavzor) solutions or liquid-filled capsules **Divalproex (Depakote)** Preg Categ D	**Initial** 125-250 mg BID **Maintenance** 15–45 mg/kg/day Serum levels: keep between 50-125 mcg/mL	**BLACK BOX WARNINGS (3)** Hepatic Failure; LFTs must be checked prior to start, frequently during the 1st 6 months, and periodically thereafter Teratogenicity, including neural tube defects (such as spina bifida) Pancreatitis, which has been fatal in children and adults **SIDE EFFECTS** GI upset, alopecia (treat with selenium and zinc), sedation, tremor, weight gain, thrombocytopenia [Cannot substitute *Depakote ER* for the delayed release tabs (*Depakote*); need to ↑ *Depakote ER* by 8-20%] **MONITORING** LFTs, CBC, platelets
Lamotrigine (Lamictal, Lamictal ODT [orally dispersable], Lamictal CD [chewable], Lamictal XR) Preg Categ C	Wk 1 and 2: 50 mg/day Wk 3 and 4: 100 mg/day Wk 5: 200 mg/day Wk 6: can ↑ by 100 mg every 1-2 wks, max 400 mg/d Divide BID, unless using XR	**BLACK BOX WARNINGS** Serious Skin Reactions, including SJS and TEN; ↑ risk with high starting doses, rapid increases, or co-administration of valproic acid, which ↑ lamotrigine levels > 2-fold. To ↓ risk of rash follow titration schedule – *Lamictal Starter Kit* and *Lamictal ODT Patient Titration Kits* provide the recommended titration schedule for the 1st 5 weeks. **SIDE EFFECTS** Diplopia, sedation, ataxia, headache (further review in seizure chapter)
Lithium (Eskalith, Lithobid) Preg Categ D Titrate slowly to help patient tolerate SEs Take with food (post-meal) to ↓ nausea, or split dosing If tremor/thirst/confusion may try QHS dosing	Start at 900 mg/d, divided Then 900-1,200 mg/d, divided **Therapeutic Range** 0.8-1.2 mEq/L (trough level) Acute mania may need up to 1.5 mEq initially	Cannot use with renal impairment: lithium is 100% renally cleared – and if not eliminated, toxicity will result **SIDE EFFECTS** GI upset (take with food in the stomach, can change to ER forms) Cognitive effects, cogwheel rigidity, fine hand tremor, weight gain Polyuria/polydipsia, hypothyroidism – must monitor, avoid co-admin with other serotonergic agents **TOXICITY** > 1.5 mEq/L (coarse hand tremor, vomiting, persistent diarrhea, confusion, ataxia) > 3 mEq/L (CNS depression, arrhythmia, seizures, irreversible brain damage, coma) **MONITORING** BMP, renal function, thyroid function (TSH, FT4)

VALPROIC ACID/DIVALPROEX DRUG INTERACTIONS

- VA can ↑ levels of amitriptyline, carbamazepine, lamotrigine, lorazepam, nortriptyline, paroxetine, phenobarbital, warfarin and zidovudine.

- Use special caution with combination of valproate and lamotrigine, due to risk of serious rash (combo is used in children, requires lower doses with slow titration and parent counseling).

- Salicylates may displace valproic acid from protein-binding site, leading to toxicity and valproate can displace phenytoin from albumin, resulting in phenytoin toxicity.

- Carbapenems can ↓ VA levels leading to seizures.

VALPROIC ACID COUNSELING

- Do not use if you have liver disease. In rare cases, this drug has caused liver failure. Notify your doctor if you develop severe fatigue, vomiting or loss of appetite. These could be early symptoms of liver damage.

- In rare cases, valproic acid has also caused severe, even fatal, cases of pancreatitis (inflammation of the pancreas). Some of the cases have progressed rapidly from initial symptoms to death. Cases have been reported soon after starting treatment with valproic acid, as well as after several years of use. Notify your doctor immediately if you develop nausea, vomiting, abdominal pain, or loss of appetite. These symptoms may be early signs of pancreatitis.

- Do not stop taking the medication even if you feel better.

- Do not crush, chew, or break the capsules because they may hurt the mouth or throat. Swallow them whole. *Depakene* capsules contain liquid which will cause irritation to the mouth and throat.

- Measure the liquid form of valproic acid with a special dose-measuring spoon or cup, not a regular eating spoon. If you do not have a dose-measuring device, ask your pharmacist for one.

- Valproic acid is FDA pregnancy category D. This means that it is known to be harmful to an unborn baby. Malformations of the face and head, heart, and nervous system have been reported. Do not take valproic acid without first talking to your doctor if you are pregnant or could become pregnant. This drug passes into breast milk. Tell your doctor if you are planning to breastfeed.

- Take each dose with a full glass of water. Take with food to help avoid stomach upset.

- Your doctor may want you to have blood tests during treatment. It is important for your doctor to know how much medication is in the blood and how well your liver is working.

LITHIUM DRUG INTERACTIONS

- These will ↑ lithium: ↓ salt intake, NSAIDs, ACE Is, ARBs, dehydration (and caution with diuretics), metronidazole.

- These will ↓ lithium: ↑ salt intake, caffeine, and theophylline.

- These will ↑ risk 5HT-syndrome if given with lithium: SSRIs, SNRIs, triptans, linezolid and other serotonergic drugs.

- ↑ neurotoxicity risk (ataxia, tremors, nausea) with lithium in combination with these drugs: verapamil, diltiazem, phenytoin and carbamazepine.

LITHIUM COUNSELING

- Call your doctor if you experience nausea, vomiting, diarrhea, slurred speech, extreme drowsiness, or weakness. These symptoms may indicate lithium toxicity.

- Do not crush, chew, or break any extended-release forms of lithium (e.g., *Lithobid, Eskalith CR*). They are specially formulated to release slowly in the body.

- Lithium may cause dizziness or drowsiness. Use caution when driving or performing other hazardous activities until you know how this medication affects you. If you experience dizziness or drowsiness, avoid these activities.

- Lithium is FDA pregnancy category D. This means that lithium is known to be harmful to an unborn baby. Do not take lithium without first talking to your doctor if you are pregnant or are planning a pregnancy. Lithium can pass into breast milk. Discuss with your doctor if you are breastfeeding.

- Maintain adequate fluid intake by drinking 8 to 12 glasses of water or other fluid every day while taking lithium. Vigorous exercise, prolonged exposure to heat or sun, excessive sweating, diarrhea, or vomiting may cause dehydration and side effects from lithium. Call your doctor if you lose a significant amount of body fluid as a result of sweating, diarrhea, or vomiting.

- Do not change the amount of salt you consume.

- Your doctor may order tests to monitor your lithium therapy.

- Do not stop taking this medication, even if you are feeling better.

LAMOTRIGINE DRUG INTERACTIONS

- Valproate, divalproex and strong inducers (including carbamazepine and others) increase lamotrigine levels significantly and increase rash risk. There are different (lower) titration schedules when using these drugs concurrently.

LAMOTRIGINE COUNSELING

- This medication may cause a mild or severe (and potentially life-threatening) rash. There is no way to tell if a mild rash will develop into a more serious reaction. A serious rash is more likely to happen when you start this medicine or within the first 2 to 8 weeks of treatment. But, it can happen in people who have taken this for any period of time. Children 2-16 years old have a higher chance of getting this serious skin reaction. The risk of getting a rash is higher if you:

  - Use this medicine with valproate (valproic acid, or *Depakene*) or divalproex (*Depakote*).

  - Use a higher starting dose than prescribed.

  - Increase your dose faster than prescribed.

- The dose must be increased slowly. It may take several weeks or months to reach the best dose for you and to get the full benefit from this medication.

- Take this medication regularly in order to get the most benefit from it. To help you remember, take it at the same time/s each day.

- A very small number of people may have worsened mental thoughts when using this medicine. Contact your doctor right away if you have recurrent thoughts of killing yourself or worsened depression or anxiety.

- Do not stop this medicine suddenly; if it is stopped it will need to be slowly decreased by your doctor.

- This medicine (very rarely) can cause aseptic meningitis, which is a serious inflammation of the protective membrane that covers the brain and spinal cord. You should get medical treatment immediately if you develop a severe headache, with fever, nausea and a stiff neck.

- Less serious side effects can include dizziness, sleepiness, blurred vision, nausea, upset stomach or diarrhea, headache, feeling uncoordinated and weight loss.

- If you have difficulty sleeping (insomnia) or get unusual dreams, please let your doctor know.

SECOND-GENERATION ANTIPSYCHOTICS USED IN BIPOLAR DISORDER

The 2010 VA guidelines list other second generation antipsychotics as treatment options. These are the agents with FDA approval.

DRUG	DOSING	SIDE EFFECTS/MONITORING/ CONTRAINDICATIONS
Aripiprazole (Abilify) Approved for manic & mixed symptoms, maintenance, +/- lamotrigine or valproate	15-30 mg QAM	These drugs can cause metabolic issues, including dyslipidemia, weight gain, diabetes Risk of Neuroleptic Malignant Syndrome Risk of Tardive Dyskinesia (TD) Risk of leukopenia, neutropenia, agranulocytosis All can cause orthostasis/dizziness
Olanzapine/fluoxetine (Symbyax) Approved for bipolar depression, 2nd line option due to metabolic effects from olanzapine	Usually started at 6 mg/25 mg capsule QHS (fluoxetine is activating, but olanzapine is more sedating), can ↑ cautiously. CI with pimozide, thioridazine, & caution with other QT prolonging drugs/conditions	**COMMON SIDE EFFECTS** **Abilify** Akathisia (esp in younger patients), restlessness, insomnia, constipation, fatigue, blurred vision **Olanzapine** Cognitive dysfunction, dry mouth, fatigue, sedation, ↑ appetite/weight, peripheral edema, tremor, blurred vision. ↓ CVD risk than other listed APs
Quetiapine extended-release (Seroquel XR) Approved for mania/maintenance with lithium or divalproex, and for bipolar depression	Bipolar mania/maintenance: 400-800 mg QHS Bipolar depression: 300 mg QHS	**Quetiapine** Sedation, dry mouth, constipation, dizziness, ↑ appetite/weight, nausea **Risperidone** Sedation, ↑ appetite, fatigue, insomnia, parkinsonism, akathisia, nausea, some QT risk
Risperidone (Risperdal) – has generic Approved alone or with lithium or valproate for acute mania or mixed episodes	Start at 2-3 mg/d, can ↑ to 6 mg In children start 0.5 mg/d Tablets, oral solution, M-tabs (ODT)	**Ziprasidone** QT risk, sedation, EPS, dizziness, akathisia, abnormal vision, asthenia, nausea **Asenapine** QT risk, numbs mouth, sedation, dizziness, weight gain (less than risperidone & olanzapine)
Ziprasidone (Geodon) Approved with lithium or valproate for maintenance, or alone for manic/mixed episodes	Start at 40 mg BID, can ↑ to 80 mg BID	ADA Screening/Monitoring Recommendations Patients being started on APs should first be screened for overweight and obesity, dyslipidemia and hyperglycemia, hypertension, and personal or family history of risk. While being treated, the patient should be monitored for treatment-emergent changes in weight, waist circumference, plasma lipid and glucose levels, and acute symptoms of diabetes (e.g., polyuria, polydipsia).
Asenapine (Saphris) Approved for acute manic or mixed episodes	5-20 mg Sublingual (SL) only: must dissolve under tongue, & no food/drink for 10 min after taking	

Note: Antipsychotic Drug Interactions & Counseling is in the Schizophrenia/Psychosis Section

Practice Case

Margie is a 65-year old female with a long history of bipolar I and hypertension. She has been reasonably controlled on lithium therapy for many years. Margie lives with her sister, who takes good care of her medical and social needs. Occasionally, her sister reports, Margie gets "back to her old thing" and becomes convinced that she is on a mission to "change the world." Margie is never quite sure what is involved with this mission.

Margie is brought to the clinic today by her sister. Her sister states that Margie has always had a fine hand tremor, but today her hand is visibly shaking. Margie is nauseous, and vomited the little she ate this morning. Her speech is slurred and confused. She appears to have difficulty walking into the examination room. She also appears to have a bad cold with nasal congestion.

Her medications include *Eskalith CR* 450 mg BID, metoprolol IR 50 mg BID, calcium carbonate 500 mg BID with meals and a B-complex tablet.

Previous labs, taken on 11/15/2007: BUN/SCr 14/0.7, lithium level 0.9 mEq/L

Labs taken (today), 10/1/2008: BUN/SCr 28/1.7, lithium level 1.8 mEq/L

QUESTIONS

1. The following factors are likely contributing to the current symptoms of GI distress, coarse hand tremor, ataxia and confusion:

   a. The use of a calcium supplement
   b. The patient's decline in renal function
   c. Lithium toxicity
   d. A and B
   e. B and C

2. Margie is using lithium. Describe lithium clearance:

   a. 100% renal clearance; no hepatic metabolism.
   b. 50% metabolized by 3A4, 50% excreted unchanged in the urine.
   c. 75% metabolized by 2D6, 25% excreted unchanged in the urine.
   d. 100% metabolized by 2C9, 100% metabolites cleared renally.
   e. Metabolized by 2C19, metabolites cleared renally.

3. Margie's sister helps with meal preparation. She is careful to keep this component of her diet constant, in order to keep the lithium level constant:

   a. Calcium
   b. Potassium
   c. Sodium
   d. Magnesium
   e. None of the above

Questions 4-10 do not apply to the case.

4. A patient has a history of two myocardial infarctions. He has bipolar II which is moderately controlled with the use of lithium monotherapy. He has been using lithium for many years. His physician wishes to use an antipsychotic as augmentation therapy. Considering ONLY cardiovascular risk, which of the following antipsychotics should be viewed as the safest option in this patient?

   a. Asenapine
   b. Risperidone
   c. Ziprasidone
   d. Thioridazine
   e. Olanzapine

5. Patient counseling for lithium should include the following points:

    a. You must keep the salt level in your diet around the same amount each day.

    b. You may notice that your hands develop a fine (light) tremor.

    c. If the tremor becomes worse, and you feel nauseated, contact the doctor at once.

    d. A and B

    e. All of the above

6. A patient is using valproate therapy. Black box warnings for this medication include:

    a. Hepatotoxicity

    b. Teratogenicity

    c. Pancreatitis

    d. A and B only

    e. All of the above

7. A patient has been diagnosed with bipolar II. Which of the following statement/s concerning bipolar II are correct?

    a. The mania symptoms are generally worse in bipolar II than in bipolar I.

    b. The depressive symptoms are generally worse in bipolar II than in bipolar I.

    c. Bipolar II is much less common than bipolar I.

    d. Bipolar II is much more common in men.

    e. None of the above.

8. A patient received a prescription for asenapine *(Saphris)*. Choose the correct statement concerning asenapine:

    a. Formulations of asenapine include an oral solution and tablets.

    b. Asenapine can make the mouth numb.

    c. Asenapine has little QT risk and can safely be used with cardiovascular conditions.

    d. A and B

    e. All of the above

9. In the past few years, drugs typically used for schizophrenia have been approved for bipolar disorder. Which of the following antipsychotics have indications for bipolar disorder, according to the FDA-indications?

    a. Aripiprazole and Tiagabine

    b. Thioridazine and Topiramate

    c. Risperidone and Quetiapine extended-release

    d. Lamotrigine and Levetiracetam

    e. All of the above

10. A physician wishes to use an atypical antipsychotic for a patient with early Parkinson Disease. Her medications include ropinirole, metformin, glipizide, and a daily aspirin. He chooses to use quetiapine extended-release. Which of the following benefits would likely be experienced with the use of this agent?

    a. Little risk of movement disorders

    b. Little risk of metabolic issues, such as elevated blood sugar and lipids

    c. Little risk of sedation, orthostasis or dizziness

    d. No risk of stroke or worsened mental state

    e. No risk of increased appetite or weight gain

ANSWERS

1-e, 2-a, 3-c, 4-e, 5-e, 6-e, 7-e, 8-b, 9-c, 10-a

PARKINSON DISEASE

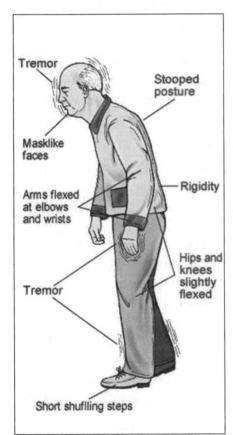

We gratefully acknowledge the assistance of Jack J. Chen, PharmD, FCCP, BCPS, CGP, Associate Professor of Neurology, Loma Linda University Schools of Medicine and Pharmacy in reviewing this section.

Background

Parkinson disease is a brain disorder. <u>It occurs when neurons in a part of the brain called the substantia nigra</u> die or become impaired. The cause of neuronal death is not well understood, but is multi-factorial. <u>Normally, these cells produce dopamine.</u> Dopamine allows smooth, coordinated function of the body's muscles and movement. When ~80% of the dopamine-producing cells are damaged, the symptoms of the disease appear. While this disease usually develops after the age of 65, 15% of those diagnosed are under 50. Initially (in what is called Stage I) the disease appears as tremor on one-side (unilateral) and eventually spreads bilaterally. Movement becomes more difficult. <u>Eventually, even with high doses of the two most effective classes of drugs (levodopa/carbidopa and the dopamine agonists), the "off" periods will increase</u> – this is among the most frustrating and challenging of the complications. An off episode is a period of time with muscle stiffness, slow movements, and difficulty starting movements. Eventually, the patient will be unable to walk and have difficulty feeding themselves and swallowing foods. There is a newer drug (apomorphine) that treats end-stage disease, but it is hard to take and provides increased movement for just about an hour.

GUIDELINES

Diagnosis and prognosis of new onset Parkinson disease (an evidence-based review): Report of the Quality Standards Subcommittee of the American Academy of Neurology. Neurology 2006 Apr 11;66(7):968-75.

PRIMARY SIGNS/SYMPTOMS

TRAP:

Tremor – seen during resting, usually worsened by anxiety

Rigidity – arms, legs, trunk and face (mask-like face)

Akinesia/bradykinesia – lack of movement or slow initiation of movement

Postural instability – poor balance, which may lead to frequent falls

Other Signs of Parkinson Disease
Small, cramped handwriting (micrographia)

Shuffling walk

Stiff facial expression, reduced eye blinking

Muffled speech, drooling, dysphagia

Depression, anxiety (psychosis in advanced dz)

Constipation, incontinence

DRUG-INDUCED PARKINSON DISEASE

Certain drugs can cause <u>Parkinsonism</u> due to their antagonism of dopamine receptors. These include <u>phenothiazines</u> (prochlorperazine, others), first generation antipsychotics (including <u>haloperidol</u>), second-generation antipsychotics [to a lesser degree- <u>risperidone *(Risperdal)*, at higher doses</u>, is considered high-risk for movement disorders], and the dopamine-blocking agent <u>metoclopramide</u> *(Reglan)*. Metoclopramide is most likely to produce Parkinsonism <u>when it is overdosed, which is not uncommon in the elderly since it must be reduced for renal dysfunction</u>. The cholinesterase inhibitors used for dementia such as donepezil *(Aricept)*, rivastigmine *(Exelon)*, and others can worsen Parkinson symptoms.

Therapy is directed at treating the symptoms. Medications can help improve movement, and may be used for related issues, such as psychosis and constipation.

Initial Therapy Selection

Levodopa, which is in the commonly used agent levodopa-carbidopa *(Sinemet)*, is the most effective agent and is sometimes better tolerated for initial treatment in the elderly than the dopamine agonists. Initial treatment of tremor in younger patients may be treated with an anticholinergic. The considerable side effects of the anticholinergics prohibit use in elderly patients. Amantadine is sometimes used for initial treatment of tremor, usually in younger patients. A monoamine oxidase inhibitor may also be used for a mild benefit as initial treatment.

As the disease progresses treatment will be directed at both reducing off periods and limiting dyskinesias.

DOPAMINE REPLACEMENT AGENTS & AGONISTS

DRUG	DOSING	SIDE EFFECTS/MONITORING/CONTRAINDICATIONS

Levodopa/Carbidopa MOA: Levodopa is a precursor of dopamine. Carbidopa inhibits dopa decarboxylase, preventing peripheral metabolism of levodopa

Carbidopa/Levodopa *(Sinemet, Sinemet CR)* Parcopa RapiTab rapidly dissolves on the tongue without water. Levodopa and carbidopa are available separately. If switching from levodopa to levodopa-carbidopa wait 12 hours and ↓ dose 25%.	Usual starting dose 25/100 TID IR: 10/100, 25/100, 25/250 mg tab SR: 25/100, 50/ 200 *Parcopa* comes in 10/100, 25/100 mg, 25/250 SR tab can be cut into half – do not crush or chew 70-100 mg of carbidopa is required to be effective and ↓ nausea	**SIDE EFFECTS** Nausea, vomiting, dry mouth, dizziness, orthostasis Dyskinesias (abnormal movements), dystonias (occasional, painful) ~1/3 of patients develop confusion, hallucinations, or psychosis Can cause brown, black or dark urine, saliva or sweat, and discolor clothing Possibility of unusual sexual urges, (rarely) priapism Response fluctuations after long-term use Separate from iron, possibly separate from protein (see counseling) May slightly increase uric acid

COMT-INHIBITOR: Used Only With levodopa to ↑ levodopa duration of action

Inhibits the enzyme COMT to prevent peripheral conversion of levodopa

Entacapone *(Comtan)* Levodopa/carbidopa + entacapone *(Stalevo)* Tolcapone *(Tasmar)* – not used much due to hepatotoxicity	200 mg with each dose of levodopa/carbidopa (max 1,600 mg/day)	**SIDE EFFECTS** Similar to levodopa: Nausea, dyskinesias Dizziness, orthostasis, hypotension Urine discoloration (brownish-orange), diarrhea

DA-AGONISTS – Act Similar to dopamine at the dopamine receptor

Pramipexole *(Mirapex, Mirapex ER)* Both dopamine agonists approved in IR formulations (not long-acting) for restless leg syndrome (dosed QHS)	Start 0.125 mg TID, titrate weekly to 0.5–1.5 mg TID ER: Start 0.375 mg daily, can ~5-7 d to max dose of 4.5 mg/d A slow dose titration (no more than weekly) is required due to orthostasis, dizziness, sleepiness	**SIDE EFFECTS** Drowsiness, including sudden daytime sleep attacks Nausea, vomiting, dry mouth, dizziness, orthostasis, peripheral edema Hallucinations, dyskinesias, impulse control disorders Renal ↓ pramipexole dose if CrCl < 60 mL/min
Ropinirole *(Requip, Requip XL)*	Start 0.25 mg TID, titrate weekly to 1–4 mg TID XL: Start 2 mg daily, can ~1-2 weeks to max dose of 24 mg/d	

Dopamine Replacement Agents & Agonists Continued

DRUG	DOSING	SIDE EFFECTS/MONITORING/CONTRAINDICATIONS

DA-agonist injection for advanced disease; a "rescue" movement agent

Apomorphine *(Apokyn)*	SC injection	**SIDE EFFECTS**
Lasts 45-90 minutes	Start 0.2 mL (this is 2 mg, but do not write in mg) and can increase to a maximum recommended dose of 0.6 mL (6 mg)	Severe NAUSEA and vomiting, hypotension; monitor BP
For hypomobility in advanced disease – SC injection restores temporary movement		Supine and standing blood pressure should be checked pre-dose and at 20, 40, and 60 minutes post dose
		Trimethobenzamide (*Tigan*) 300 mg PO TID or a similar antiemetic should be started 3 days prior to the initial dose of apomorphine and continued at least during the first two months of therapy
		Yawning, dyskinesias, somnolence, dizziness, QT-prolongation
		Contraindicated with 5HT-receptor antagonists, such as ondansetron, granisetron, dolasetron, palonosetron and alosetron, due to severe hypotension and loss of consciousness

LEVODOPA/CARBIDOPA *(SINEMET)* DRUG INTERACTIONS

- Contraindicated with non-selective MAO-Inhibitors (2 week separation).

- Do not use with dopamine blockers – which will worsen disease symptoms (see front section for complete list) – this includes phenothiazines, metoclopramide, etc.

- Iron can ↓ absorption.

- Protein-rich foods can ↓ absorption.

LEVODOPA/CARBIDOPA *(SINEMET)* COUNSELING   *Seprate From Fe/protein*

- Do not stop taking carbidopa and levodopa suddenly. It may take several weeks before you feel the full effects of this medicine. Stopping suddenly could make your condition much worse.

- Do not crush or chew any controlled-release forms of carbidopa and levodopa *(Sinemet CR)*. They are specially formulated to release slowly into your system. If necessary, the tablets can be split in half where they are scored, then swallowed without crushing or chewing.

- Use caution when driving, operating machinery, or performing other hazardous activities. Carbidopa and levodopa may cause dizziness or drowsiness. If you experience dizziness or drowsiness, avoid these activities.

- Call your doctor right away if you have uncontrollable movements of the mouth, tongue, cheeks, jaw, arms, or legs; fever; or increased body heat.

- Do not take carbidopa and levodopa if you are taking or have taken a monoamine oxidase inhibitor (MAOI) such as isocarboxazid *(Marplan)*, phenelzine *(Nardil)*, or tranylcypromine *(Parnate)* in the past 14 days.

- You may have unusual sexual urges – if this develops, discuss with your doctor.

- This drug may cause the urine to become darker, even dark brown, and can stain clothing.

- Iron can decrease absorption; separate doses.

- Foods high in protein may reduce absorption (however, protein intake is important and usually not reduced).

- For males, in the very unlikely event you have a painful or prolonged erection (lasting more than 4 hours), stop using this drug and seek immediate medical attention or permanent problems could result.

- The *Parcopa RapiTab* disintegrating tablet contains phenylalanine. If you have phenylketonuria, you should not use this medicine.

ROPINIROLE & PRAMIPEXOLE *(REQUIP & MIRAPEX)* COUNSELING

- This medicine can be taken with or without food. Taking it with food may lower your chances of getting nausea.

- Nausea and sleepiness are the most common side effects. If your ankles get swollen, let the doctor know.

- This medicine may cause you to fall asleep while you are doing daily activities such as driving, talking with other people, watching TV, or eating. If you experience increased drowsiness or dizziness, or episodes of falling asleep while performing daily activities, do not drive or participate in potentially dangerous activities and contact your doctor.

- This drug can cause dizziness, which may be more likely to occur when you rise from a sitting or lying position. Rise slowly and use caution to prevent a fall.

- Alcohol, sleep aids, antihistamines, antidepressants, antipsychotics, and other medicines that cause drowsiness may increase the drowsiness caused by this medicine, which could be dangerous. Do not use alcohol. Do not take other medicines without first talking to your doctor.

- Hallucinations may occur, and may be more common in elderly patients. Please tell your doctor if you experience hallucinations. There is medicine that may help, or the dose may need to be changed.

- It is likely that the doctor will increase the dose slowly, over time. This is normal, since the dose has to start low due to dizziness and sleepiness.

Apomorphine *(Apokyn)* Counseling

- Do not take with any of these drugs: ondansetron, dolasetron, granisetron, palonosetron, and alosetron or any drug of the $5HT_3$ antagonist class or group if using apomorphine.

- This drug causes severe nausea, and vomiting. A drug called trimethobenzamide *(Tigan)*, started before using this medicine and during treatment, will help reduce nausea.

- Other possible side effects include yawning, a runny nose, and swelling of your hands, arms, legs, and feet.

- Do not drink alcohol or any medicines that make you sleepy while you are using this medicine.

- Do not drive a car, operate machinery, or do anything that might put you or others at risk of getting hurt until you know how the medicine affects you.

- This medicine can cause dizziness or fainting. Do not change your body position too fast. Get up slowly from sitting or lying.

- Choose an injection site on your stomach area, upper arm, or upper leg. Change your injection site each time the medicine is used. This will lower your chances of having a skin reaction at the site where you inject.

- This medicine is given by subcutaneous (SC) injection. Never inject into a vein.

ADDITIONAL PARKINSON DISEASE MEDICATIONS

DRUG	DOSING	SIDE EFFECTS/MONITORING/ CONTRAINDICATIONS

Amantadine: dopamine reuptake inhibitor: Use for mild disease, or for dyskinesias in advanced disease

| Amantadine

(Symmetrel) | 100 mg BID-TID

↓ dose in renal impairment | **SIDE EFFECTS**
Most common are nausea, dizziness (lightheadedness) and insomnia

Toxic delirium (with renal impairment, ↓ dose)

Cutaneous reaction called *livedo reticularis* (reddish skin mottling – requires drug discontinuation) |

Selective MAO-B Inhibitors: used with levodopa or (Azilect) with levodopa or as initial therapy

| Selegiline

(Eldepryl)

Zelapar-ODT (rapidly dissolving oral formulation)

Rasagiline (Azilect)

Doses above max will become non-selective

Emsam (selegiline patch) is indicated for depression

May need to reduce levodopa dose when beginning therapy w/selective MAO-B Inhibitor--watch for side effects | Selegiline

5-10 mg daily

Zelapar

1.25-5 mg daily

Rasagiline

0.5-1 mg daily

Selegiline can be activating; do not dose at bedtime. If dosed twice, take 2nd dose at mid-day.

Selegiline only has benefit when used with levodopa

Rasagiline can be used as initial monotherapy or adjunctive with levodopa. | **SIDE EFFECTS**
Due to DA-excess, similar to levodopa

Rasagiline, when taken as monotherapy, can cause headache, joint pain and indigestion. If taken with levodopa, any of the side effects from dopamine excess are possible

Drug Interactions: meperidine (can be fatal), tramadol, methadone, propoxyphene, dextromethorphan, St. John's wort, mirtazapine, cyclobenzaprine

Tyramine interactions: Low risk, but possible, of hypertensive crisis if used with tyramine rich foods – see MAO Is in depression section

(Rasagiline is more risk with both drugs and tyramine-foods, selegiline has had interactions with mostly drugs--this is dose dependent, keep doses at SELECTIVE levels or drugs become non-selective.) |

Centrally-Acting Anticholinergics: used primarily for tremor in younger patients

| Benztropine

(Cogentin)

Trihexyphenidyl | 0.5-2 mg TID (start QHS)

1-2 mg TID (start QHS) | Used primarily for tremor; avoid use in elderly

SIDE EFFECTS
Dry mouth, constipation, urinary retention, blurred vision

Drowsiness, confusion, tachycardia, high incidence peripheral and central anticholinergic |

Practice Case

Benjamin, a 70 year-old male, has been using levodopa/carbidopa for 3 years. His current dose is 25/250 TID. For the past month, he reports he has had trouble eating his breakfast and has difficulty with "off" moments, mostly in the late afternoon before the evening dose. While Benjamin is talking, he is having difficulty keeping his arms still and occasionally rolls his head in a circular motion. He had started ropinirole after the last doctor's visit but found it made him so dizzy and sleepy that he couldn't drive safely. His wife does not drive, and the excessive sleepiness caused the couple much distress. He self-discontinued the ropinirole. The initial ropinirole prescription was written for 1 mg TID. He is asking for advice on the worsening disease.

CATEGORY	
Medications	Levodopa/carbidopa 25/250 mg TID
	Ropinirole 1 mg TID (not using, per patient)
	Ramipril 10 mg daily
	Amlodipine 10 mg daily
	Multivitamin daily

QUESTIONS

1. Choose the correct statement concerning the patient's levodopa/carbidopa therapy:

    a. The dose of carbidopa is too low.

    b. The dose of carbidopa is too high.

    c. The medication may make his urine turn brown.

    d. The medication will worsen his hypertension.

    e. The medication can cause severe rash.

2. When Benjamin started ropinirole, he found he could not tolerate the medicine due to excessive sleepiness. Choose the correct statement:

    a. The starting dose of ropinirole was too high.

    b. Pramipexole would be less sedating.

    c. The brand name of ropinirole is *Mirapex*.

    d. He should have been started on benztropine instead.

    e. He should have been counseled to increase his caffeine intake during therapy initiation.

3. Choose the correct titration schedule for ropinirole or pramipexole:

    a. Wait at least 2 days before increasing the dose.

    b. Wait about one week before increasing the dose.

    c. Wait at least two weeks before increasing the dose.

    d. Wait at least three weeks before increasing the dose.

    e. Wait at least four weeks before increasing the dose.

4. Benjamin is using levodopa therapy. He is taking carbidopa concurrently, in the combination medicine *Sinemet*. Choose the correct statement concerning carbidopa:

    a. Carbidopa inhibits decarboxylase and prevents the breakdown of levodopa outside the CNS.

    b. The dose of carbidopa should stay between 70-100 mg.

    c. Using carbidopa with levodopa will decrease nausea.

    d. A and B

    e. All of the above

5. Which of the following is a common side effect from ropinirole therapy?

   a. Brown urine
   b. Extreme hunger
   c. Somnolence
   d. Loss of consciousness
   e. Hyperglycemia

Questions 6-11 do not apply to the case.

6. A patient has been started on selegiline therapy. What is the mechanism of action of selegiline?

   a. Selective inhibitor of monoamine oxidase A
   b. Selective inhibitor of monoamine oxidase B
   c. Dopamine reuptake inhibitor
   d. Dopamine agonist
   e. Anticholinergic

7. Which of the following medications will require a dose reduction with renal disease?

   a. Rasagiline
   b. Pramipexole
   c. Benztropine
   d. Levodopa
   e. None of the above

8. Choose the drug which can be safely administered to a patient receiving *Azilect* therapy:

   a. Tramadol
   b. Meperidine
   c. Dextromethorphan
   d. Methadone
   e. None of the above

9. Which of the following side effects can occur with the use of benzotropine, a centrally-acting anticholinergic medication?

   a. Dry mouth
   b. Urinary retention
   c. Confusion, drowsiness
   d. A and B only
   e. All of the above

10. A patient is having a difficult time swallowing pills. Which of the following medications would be the best option for this type of patient?

    a. Comtan
    b. Cogentin
    c. Azilect
    d. Zelapar ODT
    e. Symmetrel

11. Which of the following medications can worsen or cause Parkinson-like symptoms?

    a. Metoclopramide, especially in a patient with renal insufficiency
    b. Risperdal, especially when dosed high (> 6 mg daily)
    c. Haloperidol
    d. A and B only
    e. All of the above

ANSWERS

1-c, 2-a, 3-b, 4-e, 5-c, 6-b, 7-b, 8-e, 9-e, 10-d, 11-e

ALZHEIMER'S DISEASE

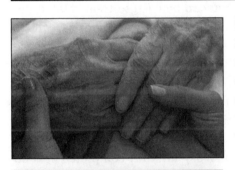

GUIDELINES

American Geriatrics Society. Guide to the management of psychotic disorders and neuropsychiatric symptoms of dementia in older adults. April 2011.

Qaseem A, Snow V, Cross T, et al. Current pharmacologic treatment of dementia: a clinical practice guideline from the American College of Physicians and the American Academy of Family Physicians. http://www.ncbi.nlm.nih.gov/entrez/query.fcgi?cmd=Retrieve&db=PubMed&list_uids=18316755&dopt=Abstract, Ann Intern Med 2008;148:370-8.

Background

Dementia is a group of symptoms affecting intellectual and social abilities severely enough to interfere with daily functioning. There are several types of dementia and Alzheimer's disease is the most common type and the type with well-defined treatment. Unfortunately, the treatments provide modest benefit.

DIAGNOSIS

Exams include the Folstein Mini-Mental State Exam (MMSE – a score < 24 indicates impairment), DSM IV criteria, National Institute of Neurological and Communicative Disorders and Stroke and the Alzheimer's Disease and Related Diseases Association (NINCDS-ARDA) criteria. If the diagnosis is a dementia that will progressively worsen over time, such as Alzheimer's disease, early diagnosis gives a person time to plan for the future while he or she can still participate in making decisions.

TREATMENT

Acetylcholinesterase inhibitors, such as donepezil, are the mainstay of therapy. These are used alone, or with memantine for more advanced disease. At best, one in twelve patients has improvement with these medications. However, for a family, this may mean that the patient who responds can feed themselves for a little while longer, or use the bathroom independently for several more months. Many others do not have noticeable improvement and likely experience side effects (nausea, diarrhea, dizziness).

A higher dose of donepezil *(Aricept)* was released in 2010 for advanced disease, however the benefit is very mild (2 point improvement on a 100-point cognition scale.) The motivation for

SYMPTOMS

Memory loss

Difficulty communicating

Inability to learn or remember new information

Difficulty with planning and organizing

Poor coordination & motor functions

Personality changes

Inappropriate behavior

Paranoia, agitation, hallucinations

Pathophysiology

Neuritic plaques & tangles in brain tissue; neuron signaling is interrupted

Alteration of neurotransmitters (e.g. decreased acetylcholine)

DRUGS THAT CAN WORSEN DEMENTIA

Peripheral anticholinergics (including incontinence & IBS drugs)

Central anticholinergics (benztropine, etc.)

Antihistamines & antiemetics

Antipsychotics

Barbiturates

Benzodiazepines

Skeletal muscle relaxants

Other CNS depressants

the release of this product was the availability of generic donepezil. If a prescriber writes for the higher dose the patient will need to purchase the brand medication. With acetylcholinesterase inhibitors the patient should be monitored for both improvement and side effects; if no improvement or intolerable side effects you can suggest stopping the drug – this may also be advisable if the dementia has advanced to the point where it is useless. However, it may not be acceptable to the family.

Antidepressants (e.g. sertraline, citalopram, escitalopram) can be used to treat related depression and anxiety. Antipsychotics can be used to treat delusion/anger, but they increase the risk of death in elderly patients (mostly due to an increased risk of stroke) and provide little benefit. Vitamin E is sometimes tried for dementia, but doses (> 150 IU) carry risk. *Ginkgo biloba* is commonly used for memory; a well-designed, 8-year study completed in 2008 did not find benefit for prevention of dementia with the use of ginkgo, but many patients still use it, and in some earlier studies the use of ginkgo provided modest benefit – for both dementia and in slowing age-related memory decline. At this point, the benefit is not well-defined. *Ginkgo* can increase bleeding risk. But remember, there is not much available to treat this disease and the patient and family want something to help.

Drugs to Treat Alzheimer's Disease

DRUG	DOSING	SIDE EFFECTS/MONITORING/ CONTRAINDICATIONS

Acetylcholinesterase Inhibitors (ACH Is) – Inhibits centrally-active acetylcholinesterase, the enzyme responsible for hydrolysis (breakdown) of acetylcholine, which results in ↑ ACh

DRUG	DOSING	SIDE EFFECTS/MONITORING/CONTRAINDICATIONS
Donepezil *(Aricept)* *Aricept ODT* 5 or 10 mg - disintegrating tablet Used alone or with memantine in more severe disease *Aricept 23 mg* used for advanced disease – minimal additional benefit	5-10 mg QHS for mild to moderate disease 23 mg QHS, for advanced disease Do not crush or chew	FOR MILD-MODERATE DISEASE (& IN COMBO FOR MODERATE-SEVERE AD) **SIDE EFFECTS** Bradycardia, fainting GI side effects (nausea, vomiting, loose stools) Donepezil given QHS to help with nausea
Rivastigmine *(Exelon, Exelon Patch)*	1.5-6 mg BID 4.6 & 9.5 mg/24 hr patch	Other oral formulations are BID or daily if long-acting Rivastigmine is with food – others without regards to meals
Galantamine ***(Razadyne, Razadyne ER)***	4-12 mg BID ER: start at 8 mg daily, then ↑ to 16-24 mg	Recommend *Exelon* patch or *Aricept* ODT to decrease GI side effects – if the cost difference is acceptable Hepatotoxicity *(Tacrine* only; contraindicated if history of tacrine-induced jaundice or bilirubin > 3 mg/dL)
Tacrine *(Cognex)* Not used much due to hepatotoxicity – if used, must monitor LFTs, clinical symptoms	10-20 mg BID	

Memantine – blocks NMDA (N-methyl-D-aspartate), which inhibits glutamate from binding to NMDA receptors & ↓ abnormal activation

DRUG	DOSING	SIDE EFFECTS/MONITORING/CONTRAINDICATIONS
Memantine *(Namenda, Namenda XR)* Approved for use alone or in combination with donepezil *(Aricept)* for moderate to severe AD Take XR with food or drink, IR with or without food	5-10 mg BID (titrate ~weekly) or 28 mg daily if XR (start at 7 mg daily and titrate not faster than weekly) XR caps can be opened & sprinkled in applesauce Oral Solution 2 mg/mL (10 mg = 5 mL)	FOR MODERATE-SEVERE DISEASE **SIDE EFFECTS** Dizziness, diarrhea, headache Rare SEs: flu-like symptoms, arthralgia, UTIs, urinary retention, small risk seizures Mostly excreted unchanged in urine; do not exceed 5 mg BID if CrCl < 30 mL/min

ACETYLCHOLINESTERASE DRUG INTERACTIONS

- Use caution with concurrent use of drugs that can lower heart rate (beta blockers, diltiazem, verapamil, digoxin, etc) and with drugs that cause dizziness (antipsychotics, antihypertensives, alpha blockers, skeletal muscle relaxants, hypnotics, opioids, etc.) due to the risk of dizziness and falls.

- Drugs that have anticholinergic effects can reduce the efficacy of this medicine (see previous table for drugs that can worsen symptoms).

ACETYLCHOLINESTERASE COUNSELING

- Tell patients that the drug dose may be increased, but is started low due to the risk of dizziness, falls, and nausea. Use caution when moving from a sitting to a standing position. Try not to use with other drugs that can lower your heart rate and make you feel dizzy. Try not to use alcohol when using this medicine.

- These medicines can cause nausea and stomach upset. If this remains a problem, talk to your doctor about changing to the longer-acting formulations, or the *Exelon* patch, which has the least nausea. Taking the medicine with food should help.

- Please tell the pharmacist about all medicine you purchase over-the-counter since some of these can worsen memory problems.

- Please make sure the pharmacist knows about all prescription drugs you are using. Some of them can worsen memory problems.

- Donepezil is started at 5 mg, at bedtime. It is taken at night to help with nausea. If you experience sleep problems (insomnia), you can take it in the morning. It may be increased to 10 mg. If you have trouble swallowing the medicine, there is a formulation that dissolves in your mouth that can be used instead. Your doctor may increase the dose after about 4 weeks.

- Rivastigmine is started at 1.5 mg twice daily, <u>with food</u>. Taking this medicine with food should help reduce nausea. Your doctor may increase the dose after about 4 weeks.

- Galantamine is started at 4 mg twice daily, with or without food. Your doctor may increase the dose after about 4 weeks.

Exelon patch application instructions

- Apply to the upper or lower back, upper arm, or chest; rotate applications site. Do not use the same site <u>within 14 days</u>. Do not apply to an area of the skin that is hairy, oily, irritated, broken, scarred, or calloused.

- Do not apply to an area where cream, lotion, or powder has recently been applied. Do not place the patch under tight clothing.

- Do not remove the patch from the sealed pouch until you are ready to apply it.

- Remove the protective liner from one side of the patch.

- Place the sticky side of the patch on the application site, then remove the second side of the protective liner.

- Press the patch down firmly until the edges stick well.

- After 24 hours, remove the used patch.

- Do not touch the sticky side. Fold the patch in half with the sticky sides together.

MEMANTINE COUNSELING (CAREGIVERS)

- Take this medication by mouth, with or without food. When you first start taking this medication, you will usually take it once daily. Your dose will be gradually increased to lower the risk of side effects. Once your dose increases to more than 5 milligrams per day, take this medication twice daily (5 mg twice daily, and then it usually increases to 10 mg twice daily).

- If you are taking memantine oral liquid, read the instruction sheet that comes with the bottle. Follow the directions exactly. Use the oral syringe that comes with the product to measure out your dose. Swallow the medication directly from the syringe. Do not mix it with water or other liquids. Rinse the syringe with water after each use.

- You may experience dizziness; use caution when moving from a sitting to a standing position. Try not to use with other drugs that can make you feel dizzy. Try not to use alcohol when using this medicine.

- If you become constipated from this medicine, please ask your pharmacist, who can recommend a stool softener (if the stool is hard) or a different type of laxative that is taken at bedtime. These are available over-the-counter. The laxatives come in chewable or liquid formulations.

MEMANTINE EXTENDED RELEASE *(NAMENDA XR)*

Same as above except:

- Take once daily with food or drink – if trouble swallowing can open capsule and sprinkle on applesauce (do not divide dose) but do not crush or chew the capsule.

- Start at 7 mg daily. Titrate weekly (as tolerated) to 28 mg daily.

50

ATTENTION DEFICIT HYPERACTIVITY DISORDER (ADHD) & STIMULANT AGENTS

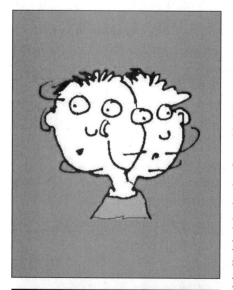

Criteria
Criteria set by DSM IV.

Treatment
Institute for Clinical Systems Improvement (ICSI) Health Care Guideline: Diagnosis and management of attention deficit hyperactivity disorder in primary care for school-age children and adolescents. April 2010.

American Academy of Child and Adolescent Psychiatry. Practice parameter for assessment and treatment of children and adolescents with attention-deficit/hyperactivity disorder. July 2007.

Background

The core symptoms of ADHD are inattention, hyperactivity, and impulsivity. People with ADHD often have difficulty focusing, are easily distracted, have trouble staying still, and frequently are unable to control impulsive behavior. Primary symptoms vary; some patients are more inattentive, and others are more impulsive.

The primary treatment for ADHD are stimulant medications, primarily methylphenidate formulations. The rationale behind using stimulants is to raise dopamine levels. In ADHD it is thought that there is a lack of dopamine, or a lack of functioning dopamine receptors or some defect in the dopamine pathway, in the brains of persons with ADHD. Providing medications is challenging because this condition, more than many others, is marked by a wide variation in treatment response and in optimal dosing range. The range in treatment response and dosing has led research into the hypothesis that genetic factors may underlie such differences. Due to the positive response from using methylphenidate, the primary focus of research is on the catecholamine system (dopamine is catalyzed to the two other primary catecholamines, epinephrine and norepinephrine.)

Keep in mind that a focus on genetics alone is a mechanistic view; it is possible that stressors alter the brains pattern of catecholamine use in some patients, which leads to ADHD symptoms. In the popular book *Scattered* (Gabor Maté, MD), the author focuses on altering the environment to help control symptoms. Environment, as well as genetics, is a determinant in brain chemistry and alterations in the environment can change the chemistry. However, some require medications even with strong social support.

ADHD causes a good deal of emotional response from those who feel stimulant drugs are over-used and, on the other side, from parents who rely on the drugs to help their children or from adults who use ADHD medications. As pharmacists, we should do our best to remain nonjudgmental and make sure that when medications are prescribed, they are used safely. Since the stimulants are C II, the prescriptions are for one month at a time, which makes it convenient to check blood pressure and heart rate (and weight and height, periodically.) We should offer empathy to the parents who have tried their best and have come to the use of medications as a last resort.

About 10% of school-aged children are using ADHD medications, with boys outnumbering girls. Many children do not outgrow ADHD; up to 80% of children continue to exhibit symptoms into adolescence and up to 65% of children will still exhibit symptoms into adulthood. Inattention and impulsivity often remain as the patient ages, and hyperactivity is decreased.

DSM-IV DIAGNOSTIC CRITERIA

At least 6 of 9 symptoms of inattention (trouble keeping attention, not listening, etc.) or at least 6 of 9 symptoms of hyperactivity/impulsivity (fidgeting, talking excessively, etc.):

- Symptoms must have been present for at least 6 months;

- Some symptoms were present before 7 years of age;

- Some impairment from the symptoms is present in 2 or more settings (e.g., at school or work and at home); and

- There is clinically significant impairment in social, academic or occupational functioning.

PHARMACOLOGICAL TREATMENT

First-line drug therapy for ADHD are stimulants. When stimulants do not work well enough (after trials of 2-3 agents), atomoxetine *(Strattera)*, a non-stimulant medication, can be tried next, or will be used first-line by prescribers who are concerned about the possibility of abuse by the patient or family.

The stimulant agent methylphenidate, which is available in various formulations, is tried first, or lisdexamfetamine *(Vyvanse)*, the pro-drug of dextroamphetamine. Longer-acting formulations are preferred for children who would otherwise need dosing at school (which would require a nurse's office visit) and to help maintain more steady symptom control. Other stimulant classes can be tried.

Guanfacine (approved in the ext-rel formulation *Intuniv*), clonidine (in the ext-rel formulation *Kapvay*) and antidepressants are sometimes used most often as adjunctive treatments. For example, it is common to see *Concerta* with *Intuniv*, or *Vyvanse* with *Kapvay*, or vice versa.

The guanfacine or clonidine formulation is being added-on to the stimulant after the stimulant was tried and provided some (but not enough) benefit. They are occasionally used alone.

Family therapy/psychotherapy may be required for an improved prognosis.

NATURAL PRODUCTS

Fish oils are a natural product increasingly used for a variety of psychiatric conditions, including ADHD. Fish oil supplements (which provide omega 3 fatty acids) with or without evening primrose oil (which provides omega-6 fatty acids) may be helpful in some patients. Fish oils are rated as "possibly effective" to improve cognitive function and behavior in children by the *Natural Medicines Database*. Check the dose prior to making a recommendation. The combo product used in the study that showed benefit used 6 capsules daily.

Stimulants for ADHD

Stimulants are C II; Instruct patients: DO NOT SHARE WITH OTHERS and store in safe place.

Stimulant Black Box Warning: The following have been reported with use of stimulant medicines:

Heart-related problems

- sudden death in patients who have heart problems or heart defects

- stroke and heart attack in adults

- increased blood pressure and heart rate

Instruct patients: Tell your doctor if you or your child have any heart problems, heart defects, high blood pressure, or a family history of these problems. Your doctor should check you or your child carefully for heart problems before starting this medicine. Your doctor should check you or your child's blood pressure and heart rate regularly during treatment.

Call your doctor right away if you or your child have signs of heart problems such as chest pain, shortness of breath, or fainting.

Mental (Psychiatric) problems

- All Patients: new or worse behavior and thought problems, new or worse bipolar illness, new or worse aggressive behavior or hostility.

Children and Teenagers

- New psychotic symptoms (such as hearing voices, believing things that are not true, are suspicious) or new manic symptoms. Instruct patients: Tell your doctor about any mental problems you or your child have, or about a family history of suicide, bipolar illness, or depression. Call your doctor right away if you or your child have any new or worsening mental symptoms or problems while taking this medicine, especially seeing, hearing things or believing things that are not real, or are suspicious.

DRUG	DOSING	SIDE EFFECTS/MONITORING/ CONTRAINDICATIONS

Methylphenidate

DRUG	DOSING	SIDE EFFECTS/MONITORING/ CONTRAINDICATIONS
Methylphenidate IR *(Ritalin, Methylin)*	2.5-20 mg tabs, and as oral solution and chewables BID-TID, 30 minutes before meals	**SIDE EFFECTS** Nausea, loss of appetite, insomnia, dizziness, headache, lightheadedness, irritability, blurry vision Stimulants ↑ BP ~2-4 mmHg, ↑ HR ~3-8 BPM, monitor), extreme caution with any CV disease
Methylphenidate long-acting *(Ritalin LA)* ½ IR, ½ SR in one capsule	10-40 mg LA caps	Exacerbation of mixed/mania episodes if bipolar disorder Withdrawal reactions (very hyper); do not stop suddenly; titrate both UP & DOWN Risk seizures (use caution with seizure history)
Methylphenidate sustained release *(Ritalin SR)*	20 mg SR tabs	**MONITORING** Blood pressure, heart rate (at least monthly), height and weight, symptom improvement, mood changes/worsening **CONTRAINDICATIONS** Glaucoma, history of tics, MAO-I use (current)
Methylphenidate ext-release *(Methylin ER, Metadate ER)*	10-20 mg ER tabs	*Focalin XR, Ritalin LA, Metadate CD* and *Adderal XR* can be taken whole or the capsules sprinkled on applesauce (if not warm and used right away, do not chew). *Concerta OROS* delivery
Methylphenidate IR – ext rel (Concerta) OROS system Somewhat harder to abuse (harder to crush)	18, 27, 36, 54 mg ER tabs	The capsule's outer coat dissolves fast to give immediate action, and the rest is released slowly. *Concerta, Metadate CD* and *Ritalin LA* are all QAM (IRs and some others are divided), and *Daytrana* patch is QAM, applied to alternate hip 2 hours before desired effect (or as soon as the child awakens so it starts to deliver prior to school).
Methylphenidate IR – ext rel *(Metadate CD)* Beads that dissolve at different rates	10- 60 mg ER caps	
Methylphenidate transdermal patch *(Daytrana)*	1.1 mg/hr (10 mg/9 hr)-3.3 mg/hr (30 mg/9 hr)	

Stimulants for ADHD Continued

DRUG	DOSING	SIDE EFFECTS/MONITORING/ CONTRAINDICATIONS
Dexmethylphenidate		
Dexmethylphenidate IR *(Focalin)*	2.5-10 mg tabs BID, 4+ hrs apart, with or without food	see Methylphenidate
Dexmethylphenidate ER *(Focalin XR)*	5-20 mg caps QAM	

DRUG	DOSING	SIDE EFFECTS/MONITORING/ CONTRAINDICATIONS
Dextroamphetamine and amphetamine		
Dextroamphetamine and amphetamine IR *(Adderall)*	5-30 mg scored tabs Given Q AM or BID without regard to meals. First dose on awakening, additional dose 4- 6 h later.	see Methylphenidate
Dextroamphetamine and amphetamine ER *(Adderall XR)*	5- 30 mg ER caps Q AM, with or without food	
Dextroamphetamine IR *(Dexedrine, Dextrostat)*	5-10 mg tabs QAM or BID, with or without food.	
SR and IR Dextroamphetamine *(Dexedrine Spansules)*	5, 10, 15 mg SR caps QAM, with or without food.	

DRUG	DOSING	SIDE EFFECTS/MONITORING/ CONTRAINDICATIONS
Lisdexamfetamine (prodrug of dextroamphetamine)		
Lisdexamfetamine *(Vyvanse)* Prodrug; may have ↓ risk abuse – cannot be injected or snorted	30, 50, 70 mg caps Can mix capsule contents with water, drink stat. QAM, with or without food	see Methylphenidate

PATIENT COUNSELING FOR STIMULANTS

- Dispense MedGuide and instruct parents/patient to read it. Stimulants should not be used in patients with heart problems or serious psychiatric conditions. Report at once if the child has chest pain, shortness of breath, or fainting. Report at once if the child is seeing or hearing things that are not real, believing things that are not real, or are suspicious.

- This is a controlled medication (C II). It has a potential to be abused. Do not share this medicine with anyone else. Store the medicine where it cannot be taken by the wrong person or stolen.

- Most side effects are minor and disappear when dosage levels are lowered. Discuss with your doctor if the side effects remain bothersome. Your child may experience decreased appetite. Children seem to be less hungry during the middle of the day, but they are often hungry by dinnertime as the medication wears off.

- Your child may have sleep problems. If a child cannot fall asleep, the doctor may prescribe a lower dose, or may move the dosing to earlier in the day, stop the evening dose or use a longer-acting formulation that can be dosed once-daily in the morning. Some children use the medication diphenhydramine, or a sedating antidepressant or the medicine clonidine to help them sleep if needed for sleep.

- Some children will complain of stomach upset and headaches. Nausea most commonly occurs when the medication is started or is being increased.

- The doctor will need to monitor the child's height, weight, blood pressure and heart rate.

- Less commonly, a few children develop sudden, repetitive movements or sounds called tics. These tics may or may not be noticeable. Changing the medication dosage may make tics go away. Some children also may appear to have a personality change, such as appearing "flat" or without emotion. Talk with your child's doctor if you see any of these side effects.

- If you are using a capsule formulation that can be mixed with applesauce *(Focalin XR, Ritalin LA, Metadate CD* and *Adderal XR)* and your child has difficulty swallowing the capsules, they can be sprinkled on applesauce (if not warm and used right away). The medicine, once mixed in applesauce, cannot be stored. Do not chew the applesauce. Use a small amount and swallow.

- If the child is using the medicine *Vyvanse*, the capsule contents can be mixed in water. It must be taken right away (you cannot store the water, or the medicine will dissolve and not work correctly).

DAYTRANA PATCH INSTRUCTIONS

- The patch is applied to the hip area in the morning (avoid waistline on pants may cause it to rub off) and apply 2 hours before the desired effect.

- Replace each morning.

- Alternate application site daily (left hip odd days, right hip even days).

- Hold patch on skin for 30 seconds and smooth down edges.

- When peeling off to discard, fold in half, put down the toilet or lidded trash can.

- The patch should stay on during bathing and swimming.

NON-STIMULANTS FOR ADHD – 2ND LINE AGENTS – NOT CONTROLLED

DRUG	DOSING	SIDE EFFECTS/MONITORING/ CONTRAINDICATIONS
Atomoxetine *(Strattera)*	40-80 mg caps Take daily, or can divide BID	**SIDE EFFECTS** Stomach upset, nausea, constipation, fatigue, loss of appetite, dry mouth, dizziness, trouble sleeping, menstrual cycle changes, mood changes, ↓ libido Do not open capsule – it's an irritant **BLACK-BOX WARNING** For risk of suicidal ideation in children Possibility liver injury, cardiovascular problems – monitor **CONTRAINDICATIONS** Glaucoma, pheochromocytoma, MAO-I use within past 14 days
Guanfacine ext-rel *(Intuniv)* Do not crush For patients using stimulants for additional benefit, or alone	1-4 mg tabs Daily, start at 1 mg Do not take with high-fat meal (↑ absorption)	**SIDE EFFECTS** Somnolence (high incidence), hypotension, bradycardia, headaches, fatigue, upper GI pain, nausea, ↑ lethargy, ↓ fainting 3A4 substrate; avoid use with 3A4 inducers/inhibitors Cannot interchange with other guanfacine formulations
Clonidine ext-rel *(Kapvay)* Do not crush For patients using stimulants for additional benefit, or alone	0.1-0.2 mg tabs Start 0.1 mg QHS, titrate weekly, using BID dosing	**SIDE EFFECTS** Bradycardia, dry mouth, drowsiness: start QHS Fatigue, lethargy, depression, psychotic reactions, nasal stuffiness, impotence, and exacerbation of Parkinson's Rebound hypertension (with sweating/anxiety/tremors), if stopped abruptly – do not become dehydrated Ext-rel formulation is supposed to have ↓ SEs

PATIENT COUNSELING FOR ATOMOXETINE

- Dispense MedGuide and instruct parents/patient to read it. Black-Box warning for risk of suicidal ideation in children.

- Less serious side effects may include stomach upset, nausea, constipation, fatigue, loss of appetite, dry mouth, dizziness, trouble sleeping, menstrual cycle changes, mood changes, ↓ libido.

- You may have suicidal thoughts or behavior while taking atomoxetine. Watch for symptoms of depression, unusual behavior, or thoughts of hurting yourself. Your doctor may need to check you at regular visits while you are taking this medication.

- The capsule cannot be opened. Do not use an open or broken capsule. If the medicine from inside the capsule gets into your eyes, rinse thoroughly with water and call the doctor.

- Atomoxetine can cause side effects that may impair your thinking or reactions. Be careful if you drive or do anything that requires you to be awake and alert.

■ Monitor for symptoms of liver damage, such as weakness, abdominal pain, yellowed skin, light colored stool or darkened urine.

STIMULANTS USED TO IMPROVE WAKEFULNESS IN ADULT PATIENTS WITH EXCESSIVE SLEEPINESS ASSOCIATED WITH NARCOLEPSY, OBSTRUCTIVE SLEEP APNEA/ HYPOPNEA SYNDROME, AND SHIFT WORK SLEEP DISORDER.

DRUG	DOSING	SIDE EFFECTS/MONITORING/CONTRAINDICATIONS
Modafinil *(Provigil)* C IV	200 mg daily	**SIDE EFFECTS** Common side effects include headache, dizziness, anxiety, agitation, nausea, diarrhea, insomnia, dry mouth, risk of severe rash. Both of these agents require a MedGuide due to risk of rash.
Armodafanil *(Nuvigil)* R-isomer of modafinil; similar drug C IV	150-250 mg daily	Similar side effects, similar drug to modafinil, including risk severe rash – give MedGuide

Note: Additional stimulants indicated for weight loss in weight loss/gain section.

51

ANXIETY

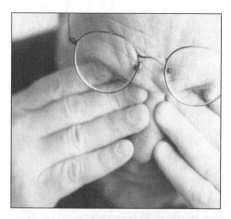

GUIDELINES

Diagnostic and Statistical Manual of Mental Disorders

Baldwin DS, Waldman S, Allgulander C. "Evidence-based pharmacological treatment of generalized anxiety disorder." *Int J Neuropsychopharmacol.* 2011 Jun;14(5):697-710.

(DSM-IV-TR)

Background

Anxiety occurs for everyone occasionally, when faced with problems or challenges at work, home or school. This is normal anxiety that dissipates when the problem is resolved. Fear and worry are the primary symptoms. Other symptoms include tachycardia, palpitations, shortness of breath, GI upset, pain (localized or generalized), chest pain, insomnia and fatigue.

Anxiety disorders are more serious than occasional anxiety and cause significant distress. Anxiety disorders interfere with the ability to lead a normal life. Common types of anxiety disorders include generalized anxiety disorder (GAD), panic disorder (PD), social anxiety disorder (SAD), obsessive compulsive disorder (OCD), post-traumatic stress disorder (PTSD) and specific phobias.

In all cases, lifestyle changes can improve symptoms [increasing physical activity, talk therapy (with friends or a trained therapist), helping others, community involvement, and other methods] to broaden the patient's outlook and reduce stress. Currently, financial stress and uncertainty about the future is causing considerable stress and anxiety in many people.

The anxiety disorders are primarily treated with SSRIs, SNRIs or tricyclic antidepressants. Although only some of the antidepressants carry specific indications (see chart), it is often the case that the agents are chosen based on the doctor's familiarity and/or the side effect profile. For example, although fluvoxamine was the first SSRI indicated for OCD, it is rarely used due to its drug interaction potential. Other SSRIs (prescribers tend to use the newer agents that have less drug interactions and smaller dosing ranges) are used instead. Specifics on the antidepressant drugs are located in the depression section.

ANTIDEPRESSANTS WITH ANXIETY INDICATION

Bupropion- SAD

Citalopram- OCD, PD

Escitalopram- GAD

Fluoxetine- OCD, PD

Fluvoxamine- OCD, SAD

Paroxetine- GAD, OCD, SAD, PD, PTSD

Sertraline- OCD (pedes and adults), PD, SAD

Duloxetine- GAD

Venlafaxine- GAD, PD, SAD

Doxepin- Anxiety

Imipramine- PD

COMMON MEDICATIONS THAT CAN WORSEN ANXIETY

Albuterol (if used incorrectly-swallowed)

Caffeine, in high doses

Stimulants

Decongestants (pseudoephed- rine and nasally inhaled agents)

Steroids

Bupropion

Fluoxetine

Illicit drugs, including cocaine, LSD, methamphetamine, others

Hydroxyzine *(Vistaril)* is occasionally used for short-term anxiety. This is a sedating antihistamine, and works by sedating the patient, rather than treating any underlying cause. It should not be used long-term.

Pregabalin *(Lyrica)* is sometimes used for anxiety, and can be especially useful if a patient has neuropathic pain. It is scheduled C-V since it is slightly euphoric – which can have a calming effect.

Quetiapine *(Seroquel)* is sometimes used for anxiety.

Propranolol *(Inderal,* others) is used to reduce symptoms of stage fright, or performance anxiety (tremor, tachycardia). It is dosed at 10-40 mg 1 hour prior to an event such as a public speech. Use caution with this approach since CNS effects (confusion, dizziness) may be present.

Buspirone *(Buspar)* is an option for anxiety for patients who do not respond to antidepressants or in a patient at risk of abuse with benzodiazepines, or in addition to other therapy. It is a commonly used agent.

Natural Products used for Anxiety

Natural products used for anxiety include valerian, lemon balm, glutamine, passion flower and hops (both as teas), chamomile tea, theanine and skullcap. Kava is used as a relaxant but can damage the liver and should not be recommended. Valerian may rarely be hepatotoxic (or some valerian products may have been contaminated with liver toxins); this is unclear at present. Passionflower is rated as "possibly effective" by the Natural Medicines Database. For most of the other agents evidence of efficacy is scant or poor but individual patients may get benefit from the various agents.

Benzodiazepine (BZD) Treatment for Anxiety

BZDs are often used for anxiety symptoms. They provide fast relief for acute symptoms. Situations in which BZDs are appropriate include short-term situations in which anxiety is acute and can cause extreme stress, prevent proper sleep, and disrupt life. This could be the recent death of a loved one, an earthquake, a motor vehicle accident, or other stressful situations. In such cases, they are used less than 1-2 weeks and can be discontinued. BZDs cover up, but do not treat, the causes of anxiety, and, in most cases, should not be used long-term.

However, benzodiazepines are often used chronically, including in the elderly, where they pose significant risk for confusion, dizziness and falls – the risk increases with concurrent use of other CNS depressants.

BENZODIAZEPINES

 Potentiate GABA, an inhibitory neurotransmitter, causing CNS depression.

DRUG	DOSING	SIDE EFFECTS/MONITORING/CONTRAINDICATIONS
Lorazepam (*Ativan*)	0.5-2 mg prn	C IV
		Potential for abuse
		Physiological dependence and tolerance develop with chronic use
		Drowsiness, dizziness, ataxia, lightheadedness
		Anterograde amnesia (some of the events that occur after taking the BZD cannot be stored as memories – forgetting what happens)
Alprazolam (*Xanax*)	0.25-2 mg prn	Withdrawal symptoms when discontinued: can include seizures, insomnia, mental/mood changes, increased reactions to noise/touch/light, N/V/diarrhea, loss of appetite, stomach pain, hallucinations, numbness/tingling of arms and legs, muscle pain, tachycardia, short-term memory loss, and very high fever
		L-O-T (lorazepam, oxazepam, and temazepam): these are considered less potentially harmful for elderly or with liver impairment since they are metabolized to inactive compounds (glucuronides)
Chlordiazepoxide (*Librium*)	5-25 mg prn	*Librium* and *Valium* also used for alcohol withdrawal and *Serax* has this indication. *Valium* is also used for muscle spasticity.
		Klonopin also used for seizures and *Tranzene* has this indication
Clonazepam (*Klonopin*)	0.125-2 mg prn	
Clorazepate (*Tranxene*)	3.75-15 mg prn	
Diazepam (*Valium*)	2-10 mg prn	
Oxazepam (*Serax*)	10-30 mg prn	

BENZODIAZEPINE DRUG INTERACTIONS

- Additive effects with sedating drugs, including most pain medicines, muscle relaxants, antihistamines, the antidepressant mirtazapine *(Remeron)*, trazodone, alcohol, among others.

BENZODIAZEPINE COUNSELING

- Only if used for insomnia: This medication should be taken before bedtime (for anxiety is taken prn).

- Common side effects include drowsiness, dizziness, unsteadiness on your feet, slow reactions, lightheadedness and difficulty remembering what happened after you had taken the medicine.

- This medication may cause dependence, especially if it has been used regularly for an extended time (more than 1-4 weeks), if it has been used in high doses, or if you have a history of alcoholism, drug abuse, or personality disorder. In such cases, if you suddenly stop this drug, withdrawal reactions may occur. Such reactions can include seizures, trouble sleeping, mental/mood changes, increased reactions to noise/touch/light, nausea, vomiting, diarrhea, loss of appetite, stomach pain, hallucinations, numbness/tingling of arms and legs, muscle pain, fast heartbeat, short-term memory loss, and very high fever. Report any such reactions to your doctor immediately.

- When stopping extended, regular treatment with this drug, gradually reducing the dosage as directed will help prevent withdrawal reactions. Consult your doctor or pharmacist for more details.

- Though it is unlikely to occur, this medication can also result in abnormal drug-seeking behavior (addiction/habit forming). Do not increase your dose, take it more frequently, or use it for a longer time than prescribed. Properly stop the medication when so directed. This will lessen the chances of becoming addicted.

- When used for an extended time, this medication may not work as well and may require different dosing. This is called "tolerance." Talk with your doctor if this medication stops working well. Do not increase your dose without first talking to your doctor.

- Do not take with other medicines that can make you sleepy, unless directed by your doctor. Do not use alcohol with this medicine.

- After taking this medicine, you should not be driving a car or using any dangerous machinery.

- This medicine is a federally controlled substance (C-IV) because it can be abused or lead to dependence. Keep the bottle in a safe place to prevent misuse and abuse.

Buspirone

5-HT$_1$ partial agonist: NOT CONTROLLED, NO ABUSE OR PHYSIOLOGICAL POTENTIAL – this, rather than a higher efficacy over BZDs, makes buspirone a widely used agent.

DRUG	DOSING	SIDE EFFECTS/MONITORING/CONTRAINDICATIONS
Buspirone *(Buspar)* Usually 20-30 mg/d (max 60 mg/d)	Start 7.5 mg BID Can increase by 5 mg/day Q 2-3 days until 30 mg/day, if needed	2-4 weeks for optimal effect No potential for abuse, tolerance or physiological dependence Nausea, dizziness, headache, lightheadedness, excitement Avoid use if severe kidney or liver dysfunction When switching from a BZD to buspirone, the BZD should be tapered slowly

BUSPIRONE DRUG INTERACTIONS

- Do not use with MAO Inhibitors.

- ↓ dose with erythromycin, diltiazem, verapamil; consider dose reduction with any 3A4 inhibitor.

- 3A4 inducers, including rifampin, may require an increase in the buspirone dose.

- Avoid consuming large amounts of grapefruit juice.

BUSPIRONE COUNSELING

- Buspirone comes in a *Dividose* tablet designed to make dose adjustments easy. Each tablet is scored and can be broken accurately on the score lines into thirds. It snaps into pieces with finger pressure.

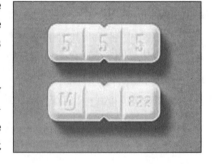

- Take this medication by mouth, usually 2 or 3 times a day or as directed by your doctor. You may take this medication with or without food, but it is important to choose one way and always take it the same way so that the amount of drug absorbed will always be the same.

- Grapefruit may increase the amount of buspirone in your bloodstream.

- Dosage is based on your medical condition and response to therapy. Use this medication regularly in order to get the most benefit from it. To help you remember, use it at the same times each day. When this medication is started, symptoms of anxiety (e.g., restlessness) may sometimes get worse before they improve. It may take up to a month or more to get the full effect of this medication.

INSOMNIA

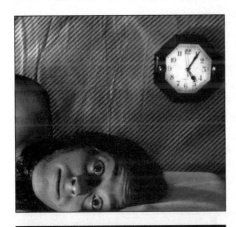

DRUGS LIKELY TO CONTRIBUTE TO INSOMNIA

Bupropion

Stimulants (methylphenidate, etc.)

OTC appetite suppressants

Decongestants (pseudoephedrine, etc.)

MAO-B Inhibitors, if taken late in the day

Fluoxetine, if taken late in the day

Caffeine

Steroids

Alcohol (initially induces sleep, but prevents deeper stages of sleep and causes nocturia)

Any drug that causes urinary retention or nocturia, including antihistamines and diuretics taken later in the day.

Background

Insomnia is having trouble falling or staying asleep. This is one of the most common medical complaints. A poor night's sleep reduces a person's ability to function well the following day, and can lead to depression and reduced quality of life. Most adults require seven to eight hours of sleep.

Poor "sleep hygiene" includes habits that contribute to insomnia and may be possible to reduce or stop, eliminating the need for drug therapy. For example, a retired, elderly person may have a daily routine that includes watching television and napping for much of the day. If the person can engage in a regular routine that reduces or eliminates daytime napping, they may not require a sleeping pill (a hypnotic).

Heart failure or any condition that causes shortness of breath can worsen sleep. Anxiety and depression cause insomnia; if the condition can be corrected by therapy, a prescription agent, or both, a hypnotic may not be required. When sleep hygiene issues or medical conditions cannot be corrected, or when a problem causing the insomnia has not been identified, hypnotics may be used to help provide a good night's rest.

NATURAL PRODUCTS USED FOR INSOMNIA

If insomnia is due to depression, taking St. John's wort may be helpful but this will interact with many prescription drugs. St. John's wort induces CYP 450 enzymes and lowers the concentration of many other agents. Chamomile tea taken in the evening helps many people feel calmer. Melatonin is useful for some patients. Valerian can be useful. There have been isolated reports of valerian causing liver toxicity; this risk is unclear at present. Check the Natural Medicines Database for doses and the current safety profile.

DRUG	DOSING	SIDE EFFECTS/CONTRAINDICATIONS/MONITORING
Non-benzodiazepines: Acts selectively at the benzodiazepine receptors to increase GABA		
Zolpidem *(Ambien, Ambien CR,* generic) C IV *Zolpimist-spray* C IV *Edluar SL tabs* C IV *Intermezzo SL* – for night-time awakening	5-10 mg QHS *Ambien CR*: 6.25-12.5 mg QHS *Zolpimist* 5 mg/spray QHS *Edluar* 5-10 mg QHS *Intermezzo SL* 3.5 mg males, 1.75 mg females	**SIDE EFFECTS** Potential for abuse and dependence Preferred over benzodiazepines for 1st line treatment of insomnia due to ↓ abuse, dependence and tolerance Do not take with fatty food, a heavy meal or alcohol Somnolence Dizziness, ataxia Lightheadedness "pins and needles" feeling on skin
Zaleplon *(Sonata,* generic) C IV	5-10 mg QHS	May cause parasomnias (unusual actions while sleeping – of which the patient may not be aware) Withdrawal symptoms if used longer than 2 weeks
Eszopiclone *(Lunesta)* C IV Not limited to short-term use (officially, although all 3 used long-term commonly) C IV	1-3 mg QHS 1 mg if difficulty falling asleep, 2 mg if difficulty staying asleep, 3 mg if helpful for longer duration	***Intermezzo SL*** Do not take unless planning to sleep 4+ more hours

Melatonin Receptor Agonist

Ramelteon *(Rozerem)* Not controlled	8 mg QHS	Melatonin receptor agonist Do not take with fatty food Somnolence, dizziness

Tricyclic Antidepressant

Doxepin extended-release *(Silenor)* Not controlled	6 mg QHS 3 mg if ≥ 65 years	This is an antidepressant and requires MedGuide for unusual thoughts/suicide risk Used for difficulty staying asleep (sleep maintenance) Somnolence, low incidence nausea and upper respiratory infections, possibility of anticholinergic SEs Requires 2 week washout for MAO Is

AMBIEN, SONATA AND *LUNESTA* DRUG INTERACTIONS

- Caution with the use of non-benzodiazepines with potent 3A4 inhibitors (e.g., ritonavir, indinavir, saquinavir, atazanavir, ketoconazole, itraconazole, erythromycin and clarithromycin).

- Additive effects with sedating drugs, including most pain medicines, muscle relaxants, antihistamines, the antidepressant mirtazapine *(Remeron)*, trazodone, alcohol and others.

AMBIEN, SONATA AND *LUNESTA* COUNSELING

- If using *Zolpimist*, spray directly into your mouth over your tongue (once for a 5 mg dose, twice for a 10 mg dose). Prime the bottle if 1st-time use. If using *Edluar* SL tablets, allow tablet to dissolve under tongue; do not swallow. For *Intermezzo*: this drug is not swallowed, it dissolves under the tongue. Do not take unless you are planning to sleep 4 or more hours.

- You should not eat a heavy/high-fat meal within 2 hours before taking this medication; this may prevent the medicine from working properly.

- Call your doctor if your insomnia worsens or is not better within 7 to 10 days. This may mean that there is another condition causing your sleep problem.

- Common side effects include sleepiness, lightheadedness, dizziness, "pins and needles" feeling on your skin and difficulty with coordination.

- You may still feel drowsy the next day after taking this medicine.

- This drug may (rarely) cause abnormal thoughts and behavior. Symptoms include more outgoing or aggressive behavior than normal, confusion, agitation, hallucinations, worsening of depression, and suicidal thoughts or actions. Some people have found that they get out of bed while not being fully awake and do an activity that they do not know they are doing.

- You may have withdrawal symptoms when you stop taking this medicine, if you have been taking it for more than a couple of weeks. Withdrawal symptoms include unpleasant feelings, stomach and muscle cramps, vomiting, sweating and shakiness. You may also have more trouble sleeping the first few nights after the medicine is stopped. The problem usually goes away on its own after 1 or 2 nights.

- Do not take with other medicines that can make you sleepy, unless directed by your doctor. Do not use alcohol with any sleep medicine.

- After taking this medicine, you should not be driving a car or using any dangerous machinery.

- This medicine is a federally controlled substance (C-IV) because it can be abused or lead to dependence. Keep the bottle in a safe place to prevent misuse and abuse.

SLEEP HYGIENE METHODS TO IMPROVE SLEEP

Keep the bedroom dark, comfortable, and quiet

Regular sleep schedule

Avoid daytime naps even after a poor night of sleep – or limit to 30 minutes

Reserve bedroom for only sleep and sex

Turn the face of clock aside to minimize anxiety about falling asleep

If unable to sleep, get up and do something to take your mind off sleeping

Establish a pre-bedtime ritual to condition your body for sleep

Relax before bedtime with soft music, mild stretching, yoga, or pleasurable reading

Avoid exercising right before bedtime

Do not eat heavy meals before bedtime

Do not take any caffeine in the afternoon

Benzodiazepines

Potentiate GABA, an inhibitory neurotransmitter, causing CNS depression.

DRUG	DOSING	SIDE EFFECTS/CONTRAINDICATIONS/MONITORING
Lorazepam (*Ativan*)	0.5-2 mg QHS	C IV Potential for abuse and dependence Drowsiness, dizziness, ataxia, lightheadedness Chronic use can lead to tolerance and dependence. Anterograde amnesia (some of the events that occur after taking the BZD cannot be stored as memories – forgetting what happens)
Temazepam (*Restoril*)	7.5-15 mg QHS	<u>Withdrawal symptoms when discontinued</u>: can include seizures, insomnia, mental/mood changes, increased reactions to noise/touch/light, N/V/diarrhea, loss of appetite, stomach pain, hallucinations, numbness/tingling of arms and legs, muscle pain, tachycardia, short-term memory loss, and very high fever <u>L-O-T</u> (lorazepam, oxazepam, and temazepam): these are considered less potentially harmful for elderly or those with liver impairment since they are metabolized to inactive compounds (glucuronides); <u>choose L-O-T if need BZD in elderly patient</u>
Estazolam (*Prosom*)		Cannot use with potent 3A4 inhibitors
Quazepam (*Doral*)		Caution when use in elderly due to its long half-life: risk of falls, fractures
Flurazepam (*Dalmane*)		Caution when use in elderly due to its long half-life: risk of falls, fractures
Triazolam (*Halcion*)		Associated with higher rebound insomnia and daytime anxiety; Tapering upon discontinuation. Contraindicated with efavirenz (*Sustiva*), delavirdine (*Rescriptor*), azole antifungals, and protease inhibitors

BENZODIAZEPINE DRUG INTERACTIONS

- Additive effects with sedating drugs, including most pain medicines, muscle relaxants, antihistamines, the antidepressant mirtazapine (*Remeron*), trazodone, alcohol and others.

BENZODIAZEPINE COUNSELING

- This medication should be taken before bedtime.

- Common side effects include drowsiness, dizziness, unsteadiness on your feet, slow reactions, lightheadedness and difficulty remembering what happened after you had taken the medicine.

- This medication may cause dependence, especially if it has been used regularly for an extended time (more than 1-4 weeks), if it has been used in high doses, or if you have a history of alcoholism, drug abuse, or personality disorder. In such cases, if you suddenly stop this drug, withdrawal reactions may occur. Such reactions can include seizures, trouble sleeping, mental/mood changes, increased reactions to noise/touch/light, nausea, vomiting, diarrhea, loss of appetite, stomach pain, hallucinations, numbness/tingling of arms and legs, muscle pain, fast heartbeat, short-term memory loss, and very high fever. Report any such reactions to your doctor immediately.

- When stopping extended, regular treatment with this drug, gradually reducing the dosage as directed will help prevent withdrawal reactions. Consult your doctor or pharmacist for more details.

- Though it is unlikely to occur, this medication can also result in abnormal drug-seeking behavior (addiction/habit forming). Do not increase your dose, take it more frequently, or use it for a longer time than prescribed. Properly stop the medication when so directed. This will lessen the chances of becoming addicted.

- When used for an extended time, this medication may not work as well and may require different dosing. This is called "tolerance." Talk with your doctor if this medication stops working well. Do not increase your dose without first talking to your doctor.

- Do not take with other medicines that can make you sleepy, unless directed by your doctor. Do not use alcohol with any sleep medicine.

- After taking this medicine, you should not be driving a car or using any dangerous machinery.

- This medicine is a federally controlled substance (C-IV) because it can be abused or lead to dependence. Keep the bottle in a safe place to prevent misuse and abuse.

Antihistamines

Compete with (block) histamine H1 receptors.

DRUG	DOSING	SIDE EFFECTS/CONTRAINDICATIONS/MONITORING
Diphenhydramine **(Benadryl,** Sominex, store brands)	25-50 mg QHS	**SIDE EFFECTS** Due to the side-effect profile, considered "DO NOT USE DRUGS IN ELDERLY" Significant anticholinergic side effects: Sedation Confusion (can exaccerbate memory/cognition difficulty) Peripheral anticholinergic side effects:
Doxylamine (Unisom)	25 mg QHS	Dry mouth Urinary retention (will make it very difficult for males with BPH to urinate, can slow down/delay urination in females) Dry/blurry vision, risk increased IOP Constipation Best to avoid use in BPH (will worsen symptoms) and glaucoma (can elevate IOP)

DIPHENHYDRAMINE *(BENADRYL)* COUNSELING (FOR ALL INDICATIONS – APPLIES TO OTHER SEDATING ANTIHISTAMINES)

- Diphenhydramine is an antihistamine used to relieve symptoms of allergy, hay fever and the common cold. These symptoms include rash, itching, watery eyes, itchy eyes/nose/throat, cough, runny nose and sneezing. It is also used to prevent and treat nausea, vomiting and dizziness caused by motion sickness. Diphenhydramine can also be used to help you relax and fall asleep. It is occasionally used for involuntary movements and muscle stiffness from Parkinson's disease.

- When using this medicine, you will become sleepy. It can also make you feel confused and make it difficult to concentrate.

- Do not take with other medicines that can make you sleepy, unless directed by your doctor. Do not use alcohol with any sleep medicine.

- This medicine should not be used by patients with an enlarged prostate, or BPH, without getting their doctor's approval. It will temporarily make urination more difficult.

- Do not use this medicine if you have glaucoma.

- If you have problems with constipation, this medicine will worsen the constipation.

- This medicine can cause your eyes to become dry and your vision to become blurry. It can also cause dry mouth.

- This medicine can make it difficult to urinate (it will take longer for the urine to come out).

- Although this drug is meant to be sedating, some children will experience excitability instead.

- After taking this medicine, you should not be driving a car or using any dangerous machinery.

- Take the tablet, capsule, or liquid form by mouth, with or without food. Diphenhydramine may be taken with food or milk if stomach upset occurs. If you are taking the suspension, shake the bottle well before each dose. Measure liquid forms of this medication with a dose-measuring spoon or device, not a regular teaspoon, to make sure you have the correct dose.

- The rapidly-dissolving tablet or strip should be allowed to dissolve on the tongue and then swallowed, with or without water. A second strip may be taken after the first strip has dissolved. The chewable tablets should be chewed thoroughly before being swallowed.

- To prevent motion sickness, take your dose 30 minutes before starting activity such as travel. To help you sleep, take your dose about 30 minutes before bedtime. If you continue to have difficulty sleeping for longer than 2 weeks, contact your doctor.

EPILEPSY/SEIZURES

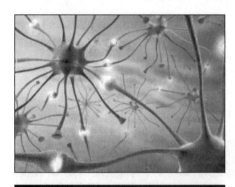

We gratefully acknowledge the assistance of Jack J. Chen, PharmD, FCCP, BCPS, CGP, Associate Professor of Neurology, Loma Linda University Schools of Medicine and Pharmacy.

GUIDELINES

Drugs for Epilepsy Treatment Guidelines, Medical Letter 2008 6(70):37-46

American Epilepsy Society (AES) and the American Academy of Neurology (AAN) Epilepsy Treatment Guidelines, 2004.

Practice Parameter Update: Management Issues for Women with Epilepsy – Focus on Pregnancy (an Evidence-Based Review): Obstetrical Complications and Change in Seizure Frequency.

Report of the Quality Standards Subcommittee and Therapeutics and Technology Assessment Subcommittee of the American Academy of Neurology and American Epilepsy Society, 2009.

Background

Epilepsy is a common neurological disorder, affecting up to 1% of the U.S. population. It is defined by unprovoked seizures, or abnormal "electrical storms" in the brain. Epilepsy more commonly occurs in children. Many patients do not have complete seizure control, even with current medications. This is unfortunate, since seizures damage and destroy neurons and can be life-threatening.

When anticonvulsants (or anticonvulsant epilepsy drugs, or AEDs) are used in women of reproductive age, it is important to consider teratogenicity and provide proper counseling. Carbamazepine, clonazepam, phenobarbital, phenytoin, topiramate and valproate are pregnancy category D – this means that there is known fetal risk, and the benefit must outweigh the risk. Health care providers should always consider that untreated or inadequately treated epilepsy or bipolar disorder during pregnancy increases the risk of complications in both the pregnant mother and her developing baby. Lamotrigine is pregnancy category C and may be safer than some of the others. Valproate and phenobarbital may have the highest risk of fetal harm. Weight gain is a primary reason why patients may be non-adherent; three of the seizure drugs can produce modest weight loss, which may be useful (topiramate, levetiracetam and zonisamide).

"CNS" side effects such as dizziness and cognitive dysfunction are common since these drugs have to penetrate the CNS to work. Many cause ataxia ("drunk-like", uncoordinated movement) and somnolence and some cause blurry vision (and diplopia if the drug is toxic). Side effects such as mental confusion and sedation can make it difficult for children to do well in school and will be an important consideration in drug selection.

Drug selection depends on the seizure type. A generalized seizure involves the entire brain and loss of consciousness. Types of generalized seizures include absence, clonic, myoclonic, atonic, tonic and tonic-clonic (grand-mal). Focal or partial seizures begin in one part of the brain and may or may not spread. If a partial seizure spreads, it is characterized as secondary-generalized. Never discontinue seizure medications abruptly due to seizure risk.

MedGuides

Most AEDs require MedGuides with a suicidality warning. Here is an example from the lamotrigine MedGuide: Like other antiepileptic drugs, LAMICTAL may cause suicidal thoughts or actions in a very small number of people, about 1 in 500.

TREATMENT OF CHOICE (VARIABLE, DEPENDING ON LITERATURE & CLINICIAN PREFERENCE)

SEIZURE TYPE	1ST LINE TREATMENT	ALTERNATIVES	PREG CATEGORY
Partial seizures	Carbamazepine Lamotrigine Levetiracetam Oxcarbazepine	Ezogabine Gabapentin Phenytoin Pregabalin Topiramate Valproate Zonisamide	**D – known fetal risk, benefit must outweigh risk** Carbamazepine Clonazepam Phenytoin Topiramate Valproate
Absence (petit-mal)	Ethosuximide Valproate	Clonazepam Levetiracetam Zonisamide	**C-possible fetal risk** Other AEDs
Atypical Absence, Myoclonic, Atonic	Lamotrigine Levetiracetam Valproate	Clonazepam Felbamate Topiramate Zonisamide	
Generalized Tonic-clonic	Lamotrigine Valproate Levetiracetam	Carbamazepine Oxcarbazepine Phenytoin Topiramate Zonisamide	

FIRST-LINE AND ALTERNATIVE AGENTS

DRUG	DOSING	SIDE EFFECTS/MONITORING/ CONTRAINDICATIONS
Phenytoin (PHT) *(Dilantin, generics)* **Mix injection in NS only;** max infusion rate 50 mg/min *– if faster, can cause severe bradycardia, hypotension* **Fosphenytoin** *(Cerebyx, generics)* **Pro-Drug of PHT (IV/IM)** Max 150 mg PE/min Fosphenytoin is dosed in phenytoin equivalents **(PE)** **1 mg PE = 1 mg PHT** Used to push drug faster, in acute cases. Benefit unclear, since conversion to active drug takes time. **Can mix FosPHT in NS or D5W** **Potent CYP 450 inducer**	**Usually dosed 100 mg TID, up to 600 mg/d** Saturable, or Michaelis-Menten kinetics; a small ↑ in dose can cause a big ↑ in serum level If the albumin is low (< 3.5 g/dL), the true phenytoin level will be higher than it appears **– adjust with this formula:** PHT correction = PHT measured/[(0.2 x alb) + 0.1] or can measure a free PHT level Therapeutic range **10-20 mcg/mL** Enteral feedings (tube feeds) may ↓ phenytoin absorption; must separate IV to oral ratio: 1:1 Phenytoin ER caps contain 8% less drug than chewable & suspension (dose adjust if changing formulations)	**SIDE EFFECTS** (note all significant) Sedation, cognitive impairment Toxicity symptoms (the drug level may be elevated) Ataxia/slurred speech Nystagmus (wobbly eye balls) Blurred vision, diplopia Lethargy, drowsiness, headache With chronic therapy: Skin thickening of facial features Lupus-like syndrome Connective tissue disorders, gingival hyperplasia Hirsutism Peripheral neuropathies Osteomalacia, osteoporosis Vitamin D, calcium deficiency – causes bone loss, folate deficiency – can cause anemia: consider supplementation of each **SERIOUS ADVERSE EFFECTS** Serious Skin Reactions, including SJS and TEN Behavior changes, blood dyscrasias, hepatotoxicity, "purple glove" syndrome if IV extravasates P: potent inducer, purple glove H: hirsutism (hair growth) E: enlarged gums (gingival hyperplasia), SLE N: nystagmus (wobbly eye balls if toxic) Y: yukky blood dyscrasias, yukky purple skin color/damage if drug extravasates T: teratogenicity, as with other AEDs O: osteomalacia, osteoporosis I: interference with folic acid absorption (anemia) N: neuropathies

First-Line and Alternative Agents Continued

DRUG	DOSING	SIDE EFFECTS/MONITORING/ CONTRAINDICATIONS
Carbamazepine *(Tegretol, Tegretol XR, Carbatrol, Epitol)* Indicated for many seizure types and trigeminal neuralgia Potent CYP 450 inducer and autoinducer – ↓ level of many other drugs, and ↓ CBZ level (itself)	Initial: 100–200 mg BID, or daily if XR Maintenance: 400-1,600 mg/day Therapeutic range **4-12 mcg/mL**	**SIDE EFFECTS** Nausea, dizziness, drowsiness, headache, fatigue, blurred vision, diplopia Occasional/Rare Hepatotoxicity; check LFTs Lupus-like syndrome SIADH/Low Na⁺ level **BLACK BOX WARNINGS** Serious Skin Reactions, including SJS and TEN: If of Asian ancestry MUST be tested for HLA-B 1502 allele prior to therapy; if positive, cannot be used (unless benefit clearly outweighs the risk). Aplastic Anemia and Agranulocytosis **MONITOR** LFTs, CBC, platelets
Oxcarbazepine *(Trileptal)* Partial seizures Potent 3A4 inducer	**300-600 mg BID** Reduce dose in renal impairment (CrCl < 30 mL/min); start 300 mg daily	**SIDE EFFECTS** Sedation, GI effects, diplopia, ataxia Serious Skin Reactions, including SJS and TEN (if rash with carbamazepine, 20-30% cross-sens with oxcarbazepine) Hyponatremia: Monitor serum Na⁺ levels esp during first 3 months, signs of CNS depression and seizure frequency
Valproate or valproic acid *(Depakene, Stavzor)* solutions or liquid-filled capsules **Divalproex** delayed release *(Depakote), extended release (Depakote ER)*, or sprinkle-filled capsules *(Depakote)* (125 mg) Indicated for many seizure types CYP 450 inhibitor with certain drugs, including lamotrigine	Initial: 125-250 mg BID Maintenance: 15-45 mg/kg/day Therapeutic range **50-100 mcg/mL** Cannot substitute *Depakote ER* for the delayed release tabs *(Depakote)*; need to ↑ *Depakote ER* by 8-20%	**SIDE EFFECTS** GI upset, alopecia (treat with selenium and zinc), sedation, tremor, weight gain Adverse reaction: thrombocytopenia **BLACK BOX WARNINGS (3)** **Hepatic Failure** LFTs must be checked prior to start, frequently during the 1ˢᵗ 6 months, and periodically thereafter **Teratogenicity** Including neural tube defects (such as spina bifida). **Pancreatitis** Which has been fatal in children and adults **MONITOR** LFTs, CBC, platelets

First-Line and Alternative Agents Continued

DRUG	DOSING	SIDE EFFECTS/MONITORING/ CONTRAINDICATIONS
Lamotrigine **(Lamictal, Lamictal ODT [orally dispersable], Lamictal CD [chewable], Lamictal XR)** Adjunct therapy for partial seizures, or conversion to primary therapy from older drugs Lamotrigine levels affected by both inducers and inhibitors. Preg Categ C; may be safer than some of the other anticonvulsants.	Wk 1 and 2: 50 mg/day Wk 3 and 4: 100 mg/day Wk 5: 200 mg/day Wk 6: can ↑ by 100 mg every 1-2 wks, max 400 mg/d Divide BID, unless using XR	**SIDE EFFECTS** Nausea, diplopia, sedation, ataxia, headache **BLACK BOX WARNING** Serious Skin Reactions, including SJS and TEN, ↑ risk with high starting doses, rapid increases, or co-administration of valproic acid, which ↑ lamotrigine levels > 2-fold. To ↓ risk of rash follow titration schedule! – *Lamictal Starter Kit* and *Lamictal ODT Patient Titration Kits* provide the recommended titration schedule for the 1st 5 weeks. 2010 FDA warning: ↑ risk aseptic meningitis
Ethosuximide *(Zarontin)* One of the DOCs for absence	Start 250-500 mg/d	**SIDE EFFECTS** Blood dyscrasias, SLE, effects on renal and hepatic function
Topiramate *(Topamax)* Adjunct therapy for partial seizures, or conversion to primary therapy from older drugs	Wk 1: 25 mg BID Wk 2: 50 mg BID Wk 3: 75 mg BID Wk 4: 100 mg BID Wk 5: 150 mg BID Wk 6: 200 mg BID Sprinkle capsules 15 and 25 mg	**SIDE EFFECTS** Oligohydrosis/hyperthemia (mostly in children) – try to limit sun, hydrate Nephrolithiasis (kidney stones) – keep hydrated Paresthesias, difficulty with memory, difficulty with concentration/attention, fatigue, dizziness, somnolence, nervousness, psychomotor slowing, and confusion FDA Safety Announcement 3/4/2011 Infants born with oral clefts to mothers taking topiramate during pregnancy Changed to Pregnancy Category D Weight loss – may be benefit for many patients Acute myopia and secondary narrow-angle glaucoma ↓ sodium bicarb concentrations – co-administration with valproate increases risk of hyperammonemia
Clonazepam *(Klonopin)* C IV Benzodiazepine	0.5 mg BID-TID, max dose 20 mg/d	**SIDE EFFECTS** Somnolence, dizziness/ataxia Cognitive impairment (try to limit other CNS depressants) Depression, mood changes, physiological dependence, tolerance Do not discontinue abruptly – seizures can result (applies to all anticonvulsants) – and with BZDs, panic attacks can occur if dosing interval missed

First-Line and Alternative Agents Continued

DRUG	DOSING	SIDE EFFECTS/MONITORING/ CONTRAINDICATIONS
Levetiracetam **(Keppra, Keppra XR)** Adjunct therapy for several seizure types	500-1,500 mg BID	**SIDE EFFECTS** Somnolence, dizziness, behavior changes, vomiting, anorexia Weight loss Hematologic abnormalities, hepatotoxicity (both rare) No significant drug interactions
Zonisamide *(Zonegran)*	Adjunct therapy for partial seizures 100-600 mg/d	**SIDE EFFECTS** Headache, confusion, somnolence Anorexia, weight loss Not to be used in patients with a sulfa allergy Serious Skin Reactions including SJS and TEN Oligohydrosis/hyperthemia (in children) – try to limit sun, hydrate Nephrolithiasis (kidney stones) – keep hydrated Metabolic acidosis Agranulocytosis, aplastic anemia

ANTICONVULSANTS NOT IN MEDICAL LETTER RECOMMENDATIONS

DRUG	DOSING	SIDE EFFECTS/MONITORING/CONTRAINDICATIONS
Phenobarbital *(Luminal, Barbital)* C IV Barbiturate MOA: Enhances GABA and ↑ seizure threshold PRIMIDONE *(Mysoline)* is pro-drug of phenobarbital Phenobarbital is a hepatic CYP 450 inducer	60-200 mg daily, or BID t½:~100 hrs Therapeutic range 20-40 mcg/mL in adults 15-30 mcg/mL in children	**SIDE EFFECTS** Somnolence (MAJOR sedation), cognitive impairment (try to limit other CNS depressants), dizziness/ataxia Depression, mood changes Osteoporosis Dependence, tolerance, hang-over effect Anemia Serious Skin Reactions, including SJS and TEN Do not discontinue abruptly – seizures can result (applies to all anticonvulsants) Pregnancy Category D
Tiagabine *(Gabitril)* Adjunct therapy for partial seizures	Start 4 mg daily Can ↑ to 32 mg BID	**SIDE EFFECTS** Worsening of seizures, and new-onset of seizures when used off-label for other indications. Somnolence, nausea, depression, dizziness

Anticonvulsants not in Medical Letter Recommendations Continued

DRUG	DOSING	SIDE EFFECTS/MONITORING/CONTRAINDICATIONS
Lacosamide *(Vimpat)* C-V	50 mg BID, max 400 mg/d Tablets and injection	**SIDE EFFECTS** Dizziness, somnolence, ataxia/shakiness, blurred vision, etc Scheduled C-V category – produces slight euphoria in a small number of patients Use cautiously in patients with cardiac conduction problems – Prolongs P-R interval; risk of arrhythmias; patients should get ECG prior to use
Pregabalin *(Lyrica)* Partial seizure, neuropathic pain C-V	Start 75 mg BID, up to 300 mg/d ↓ dose if CrCl < 60 mL/min	**SIDE EFFECTS** Slight euphoria, peripheral edema/weight gain, dizziness, somnolence, blurred vision Often used for neuropathic pain treatment
Vigabatrin *(Sabril)* Complex partial seizures and infantile spasms	Only available through SHARE distribution program (Support, Help and Resourses for Epilepsy) program	**BLACK BOX WARNING** Risk of permanent vision loss (25% in children, > 30% of adults). Vision testing at baseline and every 3 months
Ezogabine (*Potiga*) Partial onset seizures	Start at 100 mg TID, titrate weekly to 600-1200 mg/d	**SIDE EFFECTS** Urinary retention, confusion, dizziness, somnolence Psychotic symptoms, hallucinations QT prolongation
Rufinamide *(Banzel)* Indicated for Lennox-Gastaut seizures only (rare type of complex, childhood seizure)	Dosed by body weight in children: must dispense oral suspension with provided adapter and dosing syringe. Tablets for older patients	**SIDE EFFECTS** Headache, dizziness, fatigue, somnolence, nausea Shortens QT interval Drug Interactions – check prior to dispensing, including with valproate

STATUS EPILEPTICUS

Status epilepticus is generally defined as a continuous seizure lasting more than 5 minutes or 2 or more discrete seizures between which there is incomplete recovery of consciousness.

- It is a medical emergency

- 1st line agents used to treat are diazepam *(Valium)* or lorazepam *(Ativan)*. Chlordiazepoxide *(Librium)* is also used occasionally.

FAVORABLE FACTORS FOR WITHDRAWAL OF TREATMENTS

- Seizure-free for 2-4 yrs

- Complete seizure control within 1 yr of onset

- An onset of seizures after age 2 and before age 35

- Normal EEG

DRUG INTERACTIONS

Most drug interactions with clinically relevant anticonvulsants are due to 2 reasons:

- An anticonvulsant is increasing or decreasing the level of another anticonvulsant – often, patients with epilepsy need additional drugs for seizure control.

- Several of the anticonvulsants are strong inducers – and lower the concentration of many other drugs.

Phenytoin

- Phenytoin is a strong inducer of several CYP enzymes, including 3A4 and 2C9. It lowers the concentration of many drugs, including other anticonvulsants (carbamazepine, valproate, lamotrigine, as well as birth control pills, warfarin, etc).

- Caution for additive CNS depression with drugs with similar side effects.

- Phenytoin has high protein-binding (90-95%); it can displace other highly-protein bound drugs, and others can displace phenytoin, causing an increase in drug levels and potential toxicity.

- IV phenytoin can only be mixed with NS (fosphenytoin can use NS or D5W).

- Do not give with tube feeds. Hold tube feeds 2 hrs prior and 2 hrs after dosing. Calcium supplements should also be given at separate times.

Valproic Acid/Divalproex

- VA can ↑ levels of amitriptyline, carbamazepine, lamotrigine, lorazepam, nortriptyline, paroxetine, phenobarbital, warfarin and zidovudine.

- Use special caution with combination of valproate and lamotrigine due to risk of serious rash (combo is used in children, requires slow titration and parent counseling).

- Salicylates may displace valproic acid from protein-binding site, leading to toxicity and valproate can displace phenytoin from albumin, resulting in phenytoin toxicity.

- Carbapenems (imipenem, etc.) can ↓ the levels of valproic acid leading to seizures.

Carbamazepine

- Carbamazepine is a strong 3A4 inducer and auto inducer. It will ↓ the levels of many drugs, including oral contraceptives, other seizure medications which are 3A4 substrates (such as valproic acid), levothyroxine, warfarin and others.

- Carbamazepine is a 3A4 substrate. CYP 3A4 inhibitors will ↑ carbamazepine levels, and 3A4 inducers will ↓ carbamazepine levels.

- Avoid use of grapefruit products.

Oxcarbazepine

- Less drug interactions than carbamazepine.

- Weak inhibitor of 2C19 and weak inducer of 3A4/5. ↑ phenytoin levels at oxcarbazepine doses of ≥ 1,200 mg and ↓ levels of oral contraceptives (significant – do not use oral contraceptives with either carbamazepine or carbamazepine (will decrease lamotrigine concentration significantly.)

Lamotrigine

- ↑ lamotrigine levels when combined with valproic acid (hepatic metabolism inhibited).

- ↓ lamotrigine levels when combined with strong inducers, including phenytoin, phenobarbital, primidone, carbamazepine.

- Lamotrigine may induce own metabolism when used as monotherapy.

Ethosuximide

- Valproic acid can ↑ or ↓ ethosuximide.

- ↓ ethosuximide: strong inducers, including phenytoin, phenobarbital, primidone, carbamazepine.

Phenobarbital/Primidone

- Phenobarbital (primidone is the pro-drug) is a strong inducer of most CYP enzymes, including 3A4 – look for substrates. These two drugs will lower the levels of many drugs that are hepatically metabolized.

Levetiracetam

- No significant drug interactions.

Tiagabine, Zonisamide

- 3A4 substrate; look for 3A4 inducers and inhibitors.

Felbamate Drug Interactions

- Look at LFTs, or other hepatotoxic drugs and CBC – if it is being used in a case, there is likely a reason why it should not be used, this is a drug used by neurologists only for refractive cases.

Vigabatrin Drug Interactions

- Can ↓ phenytoin levels.

SIGNIFICANT TOXICITIES BY TYPE/AGENT

ADVERSE EFFECT	ASSOCIATED DRUGS
Teratogenicity Patients should be encouraged to enroll in the North American Antiepileptic Drug (NAAED) Pregnancy Registry if they become pregnant. This registry is collecting information about the safety of antiepileptic drugs during pregnancy. (aedpregnancyregistry.org)	Phenytoin Valproic acid (FDA black box warning) Carbamazepine Topiramate
Hepatotoxicity (FDA black box warning)	Valproic acid Felbamate
Caution in patients with hepatic dysfunction	Phenobarbital Phenytoin Carbamazepine Valproic acid Tiagabine
Caution in patients with renal failure	Gabapentin Topiramate Pregabalin
Significant cognitive impairment	Phenytoin Phenobarbital (and primidone) Clonazepam
Decrease effects of oral contraceptives	Felbamate Phenobarbital Phenytoin Carbamazepine Oxcarbazepine
Fatal pancreatitis (FDA black box warning)	Valproic acid
Aplastic anemia (FDA black box warning)	Carbamazepine Felbamate

Significant Toxicities by Type/Agent Continued

ADVERSE EFFECT	ASSOCIATED DRUGS
Skin rash (Stevens-Johnson Syndrome)	Phenobarbital
	Phenytoin
	Carbamazepine
	Oxcarbazepine
	Lamotrigine
	Valproic Acid
	Zonisamide
Oligohydrosis - inability to sweat, risk of heat stroke – highest risk in children	Topiramate
	Zonisamide
Nephrolithiasis (kidney stones)	Topiramate
	Zonisamide
Weight gain	Valproic acid
Weight loss	Levetiracetam
	Topiramate
	Zonisamide
Aseptic Meningitis	Lamotrigine

PATIENT COUNSELING

All Anticonvulsants

- <u>All require counseling regarding the risk of suicidal behavior/ideation.</u> Instruct patients/ family to report any changes in psychological behavior. Dispense MedGuide and instruct patient/family to read it.

- Seizure medications are not to be stopped suddenly; they require a taper or seizures can result.

- All have additive sedative/dizziness/confusion side effects with CNS depressants, including alcohol, hypnotics, benzodiazepines, skeletal muscle relaxants, etc. Avoid use of other CNS depressants drugs, if possible.

- Avoid St. John's Wort with all anticonvulsants. Evening primrose oil can ↓ seizure threshold. Avoid.

- Avoid use of drugs that can lower the seizure threshold or put patients at risk for seizures [e.g., bupropion, tramadol, meperidine (with poor renal function), PCNs, cephalosporins, carbapenems (in poor renal function), etc.]

- Use caution with different generic substitutions; try to stick to the same manufacturer. Small dosage variations can result in loss of seizure control.

Counseling for a Few of the Main Drugs

Carbamazepine

- You may experience dizziness and drowsiness, especially when starting therapy. Do not drive a car or operate any dangerous machinery until you feel safe.

- If you have nausea, take with food or ask your doctor to change to a long-acting formulation.

- Carbamazepine can rarely cause very serious (possibly fatal) skin reactions. If you are of Asian descent, you must have a blood test prior to using this medicine to determine if you are at greater risk. The serious skin reactions usually develop within the first few months of treatment. Seek immediate medical attention if you develop a serious skin rash or have blisters, peeling, itching or swelling.

- Carbamazepine has (rarely) caused a severe decline in bone marrow function, and has caused the conditions aplastic anemia or agranulocytosis. You will need to have your blood checked to make sure this is not occurring. Contact your doctor immediately if any of these rare but very serious side effects occur: signs of infection (e.g., fever, persistent sore throat), unusual weakness or fatigue, or easy bleeding or bruising.

- Carbamazepine is FDA pregnancy category D. This means that it is known to be harmful to an unborn baby. Do not take this drug without first talking to your doctor if you are pregnant or are planning a pregnancy.

- Avoid eating grapefruit or drinking grapefruit juice while being treated with carbamazepine.

- Some conditions (e.g., seizures) may become worse when the drug is suddenly stopped. If you plan to stop therapy, the dose should be gradually decreased.

Phenytoin Counseling

- This medicine can make you feel tired and confused, especially when you are starting therapy. Do not drive a car or operate any dangerous machinery until you feel safe.

- Patients should supplement with folic acid (particular women of childbearing age), calcium and vitamin D.

- Contact your physician immediately if a skin rash develops. If it looks serious, you should be seen right away.

- This medicine can damage the gums in your mouth. Brush and floss regularly; do not miss dental cleanings or appointments.

- Phenytoin is FDA pregnancy category D. This means that phenytoin is known to be harmful to an unborn baby. Do not take phenytoin without first talking to your doctor if you are pregnant or are planning a pregnancy. Phenytoin can pass into breast milk. Discuss with your doctor if you are breastfeeding.

- If using the suspension, shake the bottle well before each dose.

- Use this medication regularly in order to get the most benefit from it. It is important to take all doses on time to keep the amount of medicine in your body at a constant level.

- Do not stop taking this medication without consulting your doctor. Seizures may become worse when the drug is suddenly stopped. Your dose may need to be gradually decreased.

Lamotrigine Counseling

- Patients who experience headache, fever, chills, nausea, vomiting, stiff neck, rash, abnormal sensitivity to light, drowsiness, or confusion should contact their health care professional right away.

Valproic Acid Counseling

- Do not use if you have liver disease. In rare cases, this drug has caused liver failure. Notify your doctor if you develop severe fatigue, vomiting or loss of appetite. These could be early symptoms of liver damage.

- In rare cases, valproic acid has also caused severe, even fatal, cases of pancreatitis (inflammation of the pancreas). Some of the cases have progressed rapidly from initial symptoms to death. Cases have been reported soon after starting treatment with valproic acid, as well as after several years of use. Notify your doctor immediately if you develop nausea, vomiting, abdominal pain, or loss of appetite. These symptoms may be early signs of pancreatitis.

- Do not stop taking the medication even if you feel better.

- Do not crush, chew, or break the capsules because they may hurt the mouth or throat. Swallow them whole. *Depakene* capsules contain liquid which will cause irritation to the mouth and throat.

- Measure the liquid form of valproic acid with a special dose-measuring spoon or cup, not a regular table spoon. If you do not have a dose-measuring device, ask your pharmacist for one.

- Valproic acid is FDA pregnancy category D. This means that it is known to be harmful to an unborn baby. Malformations of the face and head, heart, and nervous system have been reported. In addition, children born to mothers taking valproate products while pregnant may have impaired cognitive development. Do not take valproic acid without first talking to your doctor if you are pregnant or could become pregnant. This drug passes into breast milk. Tell your doctor if you are planning to breastfeed.

- Take each dose with a full glass of water and take with food to help avoid stomach upset.

- Your doctor may want you to have blood tests during treatment. It is important for your doctor to know how much medication is in the blood and how well your liver is working.

Practice Case

Lucinda is a 35 year-old female who was in a motor vehicle accident and suffered a head injury. She suffered one seizure in the emergency room. She had two broken ribs and has a concussion. During her hospital stay, she was treated with fosphenytoin initially, and continued on phenytoin. Her only medications include *Loestrin*, for contraception. She does not smoke or drink.

Lucinda spent 2 weeks in the hospital recovering from the accident. She is being discharged on phenytoin 100 mg TID.

CATEGORY	
Laboratory Values	Phenytoin level at discharge 11.7 mcg/mL
	Albumin level 4.2 g/dL (normal albumin 3.5 - 5 g/dL)

QUESTIONS

1. Lucinda received fosphenytoin in the emergency room. What is the brand name for fosphenytoin?

   a. Celexa
   b. Celebrex
   c. Cerebyx
   d. Cefizox
   e. Suprax

2. The medical resident asks the pharmacist to explain when a phenytoin level needs to be adjusted for the albumin level. The pharmacist should give this response:

   a. The phenytoin level will appear artificially low if the albumin is low – and should be adjusted.
   b. The phenytoin level will appear artificially high if the albumin is low – and should be adjusted.
   c. The phenytoin level will appear artificially low if the albumin is high – and should be adjusted.
   d. The phenytoin level will appear artificially high if the albumin is high – and should be adjusted.
   e. Albumin levels have no effect on phenytoin levels.

3. Lucinda will be counseled to recognize symptoms of phenytoin toxicity. Which of the following should be included?

   a. Shakiness/walking unsteady
   b. Confusion
   c. Double vision
   d. Nystagmus
   e. All of the above

4. There is a serious drug interaction between Lucinda's birth control pills and phenytoin. Choose the correct counseling statement:

   a. Phenytoin will lower the amount of contraceptive medicine in her body.
   b. She will need to use a different type of contraceptive method.
   c. Phenytoin will increase the amount of contraceptive medicine in her body.
   d. A and B
   e. B and C

5. Patients using phenytoin are at risk for low bone density and folate deficiency. If Lucinda continues phenytoin long-term, which of the following medical conditions could result if she does not use proper supplementation?

   a. Osteoporosis
   b. Fetal damage, if she were to become pregnant
   c. Alopecia
   d. A and B
   e. All of the above

Questions 6-10 do not apply to the case.

6. A patient is going to receive a phenytoin injection. Choose the correct statement:

   a. Phenytoin has saturable kinetics.
   b. The maximum infusion rate is 100 mg/minute.
   c. The correct serum level is 3.5-5 mcg/ml
   d. Phenytoin should be mixed in dextrose only.
   e. The brand name of phenytoin is *Felbatol*.

7. A child has been receiving divalproex for seizure control. Unfortunately, the seizures are not well-controlled. The physician has ordered lamotrigine as adjunctive therapy, with a careful dose-titration. What is the reason that a slow titration is required when initiating lamotrigine?

   a. Risk of multi-organ hypersensitivity reaction
   b. Risk of cardiac myopathy
   c. Risk of fluid retention and heart failure
   d. Risk of severe, and potentially fatal, rash
   e. Risk of fulminant hepatic failure

8. What is the mechanism of action of phenobarbital?

   a. Enhances dopamine
   b. Enhances GABA
   c. Suppresses dopamine
   d. Suppresses GABA
   e. None of the above

9. Which of the following drugs decrease sweating and can cause heat stroke in children, and requires counseling to parents to help children avoid the sun and keep hydrated?

   a. Topiramate
   b. Zonisamide
   c. Felbamate
   d. A and B
   e. All of the above

10. Which of the following drugs can cause kidney stones and require counseling for adequate fluid intake?

   a. Topiramate
   b. Zonisamide
   c. Felbamate
   d. A and B
   e. All of the above

ANSWERS

1-c, 2-a, 3-e, 4-d, 5-d, 6-a, 7-d, 8-b, 9-d, 10-d

54

MULTIPLE SCLEROSIS

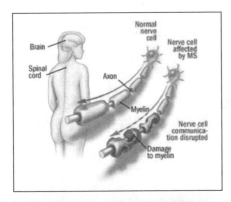

GUIDELINE

Disease Modifying Therapies in Multiple Sclerosis, TTA/AAN/MS Council, available at: http://advocacyforpatients.org/pdf/ms/ms_aan.pdf

Background

Multiple sclerosis (MS) is a chronic, progressive auto-immune disease in which the patient's immune system attacks the myelin peptide antigens, destroying the fatty myelin sheaths that surround the axons in the brain and spinal cord (CNS). As demyelination progresses, the symptoms worsen because the nerves can no longer properly conduct electrical transmission. Most patients experience periods of disease activity followed by intervals of remission. The presentation is highly variable with some patients having a much more aggressive course while others have occasional discrete attacks.

Early symptoms include weakness, tingling, numbness and blurred vision. As the condition worsens a variety of physical and psychological issues can make life very challenging, including deterioration of cognitive function, depression, fatigue, muscle spasms, pain, incontinence, depression, heat sensitivity, sexual dysfunction, difficulty walking and gait instability, weakness and visual disturbances. If left untreated about 30% of patients will develop significant physical disability. Up to 10% of patients have a milder phenotype in which no significant physical disability develops, although these patients may develop mild cognitive dysfunction. Male patients with primary progressive MS generally have the worst prognosis. Symptoms for MS are characterized as primary (due to demyelination, such as muscle weakness), secondary (which result from primary symptoms, such as incontinence due to muscle impairment) and tertiary, which involve psychological and social concerns, such as depression.

MS occurs in both sexes but is more common in women. The typical age of onset is between 20 to 40 years old. Regretfully this is not an uncommon condition; MS is one of the most frequent neurologic disorders in young adults. Over two million people suffer with MS around the world, with ~500,000 cases in the U.S.

The cause of MS is unknown. Current research is investigating whether certain viruses can be causative, or whether viruses were more likely to have occurred in patients who develop MS due to an immune system that was not functioning properly.

In addition to the personal suffering caused by this condition, MS inflicts a heavy financial burden on individuals and society. A primary goal of therapy must be prevention of disease progression; what is lost in neuronal function cannot be regained. The newer agents that can modify disease progression are costly. The beta interferons cost about $40,000/year. The newer oral immune modulator fingolimod costs about $48,000/year.

Pharmacological Treatment

In addition to using disease modifying drugs to prevent disease progression, the clinician must be focused on symptom control. The drugs used for various related symptoms are summarized at the end of this chapter, and detailed information on these agents can be found in other chapters of this text. Many chemotherapeutics are used in MS treatment off-label for anti-inflammatory properties, including cyclophosphamide, methotrexate, cladribine, alemtuzumab and rituximab (used for both cancer and RA).

Mitoxantrone is a chemotherapeutic agent that is sometimes used for MS and is approved for this condition; a review of mitoxantrone can be found in the oncology chapter. Steroids are used to help with exacerbations.

DISEASE MODIFYING DRUGS

Interferon beta formulations (*Betaseron, Avonex, Rebif, Extavia*) and glatiramer acetate (*Copaxone*) have been the mainstay of treatment for patients with relapsing forms of MS. Fingolimod (*Gilenya*) is the first oral disease-modifying agent and a second oral agent (*cladribine*) is expected to be approved in 2012.

Natalizumab (*Tysabri*) is a humanized monoclonal antibody that targets the α4-integrin, which interferes with the infiltration of activated T cells across the blood-brain barrier into the CNS. Results from clinical trials with natalizumab show a larger reduction in relapse rates, however it is used only in patients who could not tolerate or had poor response to other agents because it is associated with an increased risk of progressive multifocal leukoencephalopathy (PML), a rare, opportunistic, viral brain infection that can cause death or severe disability.

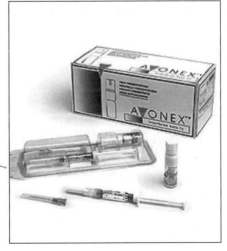
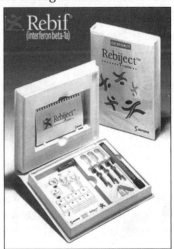

POINTERS FOR THE INJECTABLE IMMUNE MODULATORS

If hypersensitivity to a drug develops, further use is contraindicated (this is true for other drugs as well but these drugs cause more hypersensitivity). Consider varicella vaccination prior to the start of treatment. The patients should monitor for infections and for liver damage (see the counseling section). Note the injection information at the top of the dosing column. If you dispense a self-injectable counseling must instruct the patient how to store the medication, reconstitute it (if a powder) and where to inject (the SCs are the same sites for all; one of the MS injectables (*Avonex*) is IM and may be given by the patient or in a medical office). If the vial or syringe is kept refrigerated the patient should wait until the drug is at room temperature (cold injections are painful) but should not use external heat sources; holding the medication or slowly rolling it in the hand is acceptable.

If the drug is a powder that is reconstituted the drug powder may be required to be refrigerated or be kept at room temperature (they vary). If a drug is reconstituted it has to be used right away (at most within a few hours, a few reconstituted injections permit short storage in the refrigerator; others do not). Some of the powders that are reconstituted contain albumin and some patients will not wish to or cannot use albumin-containing products. Dispense MedGuides and instruct patients to read them. If pregnancy occurs during treatment the patient should be referred to the drug's pregnancy registry as the fetal effects of these newer drugs is not well known. Most are pregnancy category C and one (*Betaseron*) is pregnancy category X.

DRUG	DOSING	SIDE EFFECTS/ CONTRAINDICATIONS/MONITORING

Interferons: Have antiviral and antiproliferative effects. Reduces antigen presentation and T-cell proliferation, alters cytokine and matrix metalloproteinase (MMP) expression, and restores suppressor function.

DRUG	DOSING	SIDE EFFECTS/CONTRAINDICATIONS/MONITORING
Interferon beta-1a (Avonex), IM- glycosylated, more stable (weekly) Preg Categ C **Interferon beta-1a (Rebif)**-glycosylated, TIW Preg Categ C Interferon beta-1b (*Betaseron*) – more antibody development to drug (unclear if relevant) Preg Categ X Interferon beta-1b (*Extavia*) Preg Categ C	All: Do Not Shake All CI if hypersensitivity reaction has occurred to drug previously. For the SC injections Pinch skin, inject into SC tissue in abdomen, left arm, right arm, thighs, buttocks, rotate sites, see counseling. If refrigerated let stand to room temp prior to injection. Do not expel small air bubbles in pre-filled syringes because dose may be reduced. **Rebif** SC, TIW, refrigerate ready-to-use single-use syringe **Extavia** SC, every other day, keep at room temp, powder for reconstitution, contains albumin-some patients can't use. **Avonex** IM. 30 mcg in thigh or upper arm weekly with 1-1 ¼ syringe. Injection by medical staff or patient. Powder (for reconstitution, contains albumin – some patients cannot use) & pre-filled syringes require refrigeration.	**SIDE EFFECTS** Flu-like reaction following administration, usually lasting minutes or hours, usually dissipates with continued treatment. Some patients will take APAP or NSAIDs prior to injection. Injection site reactions: range from mild erythema to severe skin necrosis. Liver enzyme elevations, seizures, thyroid dysfunction, depression, suicidal ideation (monitor). **CONTRAINDICATIONS** Documented hypersensitivity, liver dysfunction, severe leukopenia, thrombocytopenia, lactation, *Betaseron* is pregnancy category X.

Pointers for the Injectable Immune Modulators Continued

DRUG	DOSING	SIDE EFFECTS/ CONTRAINDICATIONS/MONITORING

***Copaxone*: Immune modulator, mechanism not well-defined.**

Glatiramer acetate (*Copaxone*) Preg Categ B	20 mg SC daily, single use syringe, refrigerate.	**SIDE EFFECTS** Some get chest tightness, chest pain, palpitations, anxiety, and flushing following administration. Mild injection site reactions.

***Tsybari*: Recombinant humanized monoclonal antibody.**

Natalizumab *(Tsyabri)*	IV	**REMS DRUG** Due to possibility of progressive multifocal leukoencephalopathy – PML, an opportunistic brain viral infection, has TOUCH prescribing program, requires patient, physician and pharmacist registration. **CONTRAINDICATIONS** Hypersensitivity, history of PML

***Gilenya*: Oral Immune Modulators**

Fingolimod (*Gilenya*) Preg Categ C 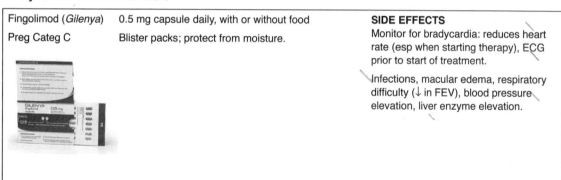	0.5 mg capsule daily, with or without food Blister packs; protect from moisture.	**SIDE EFFECTS** Monitor for bradycardia: reduces heart rate (esp when starting therapy), ECG prior to start of treatment. Infections, macular edema, respiratory difficulty (↓ in FEV), blood pressure elevation, liver enzyme elevation.

***Ampyra*: Potassium channel blocker, may increase nerve signal conduction.**

Dalfampridine (*Ampyra*) Preg Categ C Most do not respond; monitor for improvement, takes up to 6 weeks, if works primarily improves walking.	10 mg BID, extended-release tablets, if miss dose do not double-dose.	**SIDE EFFECTS** Urinary tract infections, insomnia, dizziness, headache, nausea, weakness, back pain Possibility of seizures **CONTRAINDICATIONS** History of Seizures, CrCl < 50 mL/min (renally cleared as unchanged drug)

INTERFERON COUNSELING

- Read the medication guide that comes with this medicine. You will be given a medication guide the first time you get the medicine, and with each refill.

- This medication may lower your ability to fight infections. This may make you more likely to get a serious (rarely fatal) infection or can make any infection you have worse. Tell your doctor immediately if you have any signs of infection such as a cough, night sweats or fever.

- This medicine has a possibility of causing liver damage. Call your doctor right away if you have any of these symptoms: feel very tired, skin or eyes look yellow, poor appetite or vomiting, pain on the right side of your stomach (abdomen).

- For injections: common side effects include injection site reactions such as redness, swelling, itching, or pain. If you have pain, redness or swelling around the injection site that doesn't go away or gets worse, call your doctor.

- (Refer to drug-specific administration/reconstitution instructions in the table. Do not shake the medicine.)

- Before using, check for particles or discoloration. If either is present, do not use the medicine.

- Before injecting each dose, clean the injection site with rubbing alcohol. It is important to change the location of the injection site each time you use this drug to prevent problems under the skin. New injections should be given at least 1 inch (2.5 centimeters) from the last injection site. Do not inject into areas of the skin that are sore, bruised, red, or hard.

- Some people have severe allergic reactions which can lead to trouble breathing and swallowing. Significant swelling of the mouth and tongue may occur with these severe allergic reactions. These reactions can happen quickly. Less severe allergic reactions such as rash, itching, skin bumps or minor swelling of the mouth and tongue can also happen. If you think you are having an allergic reaction, stop taking the drug and contact the doctor immediately.

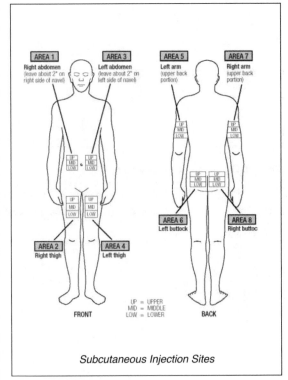

Subcutaneous Injection Sites

- If you become pregnant while taking this drug contact your doctor. (see specific agent risk above). If the drug has a pregnancy registry, please register. This is important for the public health.

DRUGS USED FOR SYMPTOM CONTROL

Patients with MS may be using a variety of medications for symptom control. The individual agents used can be found in the different chapters in this book. Commonly used symptom-control agents for MS include anticholinergics for incontinence, laxatives for constipation (or loperamide if diarrhea), skeletal muscle relaxants for muscle spasms/spasticity, or various pain agents for muscle spasms and pain. For localized pain and spasms botulinum toxin (*Botox*) injections can provide relief for up to three months. Propranolol can help with tremor. For depression many antidepressants are used; if an SNRI is chosen these may help both neuropathic pain and depression. Fatigue is often treated with modafinil or similar agents, or stimulants used for ADHD, such as methylphenidate. Meclizine and scopolamine are used for dizziness and vertigo. Acetylcholinesterase inhibitors, including donepezil, are used to help cognitive function. Erectile dysfunction can be treated with the phosphodiesterase inhibitors.

Notice that the drugs used for symptom control can worsen other symptoms. For example, anticholinergics can mildly worsen cognitive function (not all of them do, and this is patient-specific), but it happens. The vertigo agents can worsen cognitive function. Propranolol can worsen cognitive function, depression and cause problems with sexual performance. The SSRI and SNRI antidepressants will worsen sexual concerns, particularly by reducing libido or affecting the ability to sustain an erection or complete orgasm. Opioids, if used for pain, will worsen constipation, can decrease cognition and have dependence concerns. Managing the various medications used for MS requires competent pharmacists.

55

STROKE

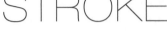
Hemorrhagic Stroke   Ischemic Stroke

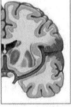

Hemorrhage/blood leaks into brain tissue   Clot stops blood supply to an area of the brain

GUIDELINES

Guidelines for the Early Management of Adults with Ischemic Stroke. AHA/ASA. Stroke 2007;38:1655-1711.

Guidelines for the Management of Spontaneous Intracerebral Hemorrhage. AHA/ASA. Stroke 1999;30:905-915.

Guidelines for the Management of Aneurysmal Subarachnoid Hemorrhage. AHA/ASA. Stroke 2009;40:994-1025.

Guidelines for Prevention of Stroke in Patients with Ischemic Stroke or Transient Ischemic Attack. AHA/ASA. Stroke 2006;37:577-617.

Background

A stroke or cerebrovascular accident (CVA) occurs when blood flow to an area of the brain is interrupted, by ischemia due to a clot (thrombus or emboli) or a ruptured blood vessel (hemorrhage). When a stroke occurs, it kills brain cells in the immediate area. When brain cells die, they release chemicals that set off a chain reaction that endangers brain cells in a larger, surrounding area of brain tissue (the penumbra). Without prompt medical treatment, this larger area of brain cells can also die. Acute ischemic stroke refers to stroke caused by thrombosis or embolism and is more common than hemorrhagic stroke. Intracerebral hemorrhage (ICH), subarachnoid hemorrhage (SAH) and subdural hematoma are all hemorrhagic strokes which indicate bleeding in the brain. Using agents that worsen bleeding can be harmful (and fatal) in these cases.

When brain cells die, the abilities controlled by that area of the brain can be lost or impaired. Some people recover completely from less serious strokes, while others lose their lives to severe ones. Stroke is the leading cause of disability and the 3rd leading cause of death in the U.S.

CLINICAL PRESENTATION & DIAGNOSIS

Signs and symptoms of a stroke can include:

- Sudden numbness or weakness of the face, arm or leg, especially on one side of the body (hemiplegia, hemiparesis)

- Sudden confusion, trouble speaking or understanding

- Sudden trouble seeing in one or both eyes

- Sudden trouble walking, dizziness, loss of balance or coordination

- Sudden, severe headache with no known cause

Diagnosis is based on the clinical presentation and computed tomography (CT) of the head. Sometimes, magnetic resonance imaging (MRI) may be used.

PHARMACOLOGICAL MANAGEMENT OF ACUTE ISCHEMIC STROKE

The goal of therapy is to maintain cerebral perfusion pressure (CPP) to the ischemic area, maintain normal intracranial pressure (ICP), control blood pressure and possibly remove the clot (MERCI device) or dissolve the clot with t-PA [alteplase *(Activase)*].

CAUSES OF STROKE
Hypertension is the most common cause of stroke and is thought to be the primary factor in up to 60% of cases.
Other risk factors include:
Gender
Ethnicity
Age
Cardiac Disease
Diabetes
Transient Ischemia Attack (TIA)
Prior history of stroke
Smoking
Hypercholesterolemia/Hyperlipidemia
Elevated Hematocrit

DRUG	DOSING	SIDE EFFECTS/CONTRAINDICATIONS/MONITORING

Thrombolytic therapy - recombinant tissue plasminogen activator (rt-PA) causes fibrinolysis by binding to fibrin in a thrombus (clot) and converts entrapped plasminogen to plasmin

Alteplase *(Activase, rt-PA)* Must confirm clot on head CT	Infuse 0.9 mg/kg (maximum dose 90 mg) IV over 60 minutes with 10% of the dose given as a bolus over 1 minute	**SIDE EFFECTS** Major bleeding (e.g. ICH), angioedema **CONTRAINDICATIONS** Active bleed, recent surgery, PLT count < 100,000/mm³, ↑ INR (> 1.7), ↑ aPTT, previous ICH, severe hypertension (> 185/110 mmHg), MI within the previous 3 months and many others. **MONITORING** Neurological assessments every 15 minutes during infusion, BP every 15 minutes for the first 2 hours, follow-up head CT at 24 hrs Treatment must be initiated within 3 hours of symptom onset (new data shows benefit up to 4.5 hrs but this is not FDA approved yet)

Pharmacological Management of Acute Ischemic Stroke Continued

DRUG	DOSING	SIDE EFFECTS/CONTRAINDICATIONS/MONITORING
Antiplatelet therapy - benefit appears to be reduction of early recurrent stroke		
Aspirin	325 mg PO daily	Oral administration within 24-48 hours after stroke onset is recommended in most patients Not recommended within 24 hours of thrombolytic therapy

DRUG	DOSING	SIDE EFFECTS/CONTRAINDICATIONS/MONITORING
Antihypertensive therapy – used to ↓ BP and possibly qualify patients for rt-PA; ↓ BP gradually		
Labetalol	10-20 mg IV over 1-2 min, titrate to effect	May repeat or double dose up to 300 mg (max dose)
Nicardipine *(Cardene)*	5 mg/hr IV infusion, titrate to effect	

PHARMACOLOGICAL MANAGEMENT OF INTRACEREBRAL HEMORRHAGE

Intracerebral hemorrhage (ICH) is more than twice as common as subarachnoid hemorrhage (SAH) and is much more likely to result in death or major disability than cerebral infarction or SAH. Vomiting is an important diagnostic sign.

DRUG	DOSING	SIDE EFFECTS/CONTRAINDICATIONS/MONITORING
Osmotic Diuretic - increases the osmotic pressure to reduce intracranial pressure (ICP) associated with cerebral edema		
Mannitol *(Osmitrol)*	Comes as 5%, 10%, 15%, 20%, 25% Mannitol 20% - 0.25-0.5 g/kg/dose IV; may repeat every 4 hrs PRN	**SIDE EFFECTS** Fluid and electrolyte loss, dehydration, hyperosmolar-induced hyperkalemia, hypernatremia, ↑ osmolar gap **CONTRAINDICATIONS** Severe renal disease and severe dehydration **MONITORING** Renal function, in's and out's, serum electrolytes, serum osmolality, CPP, ICP, and BP Maintain serum osmolality < 310 mOsm/L. Due to rebound phenomenon, use is recommended for ≤ 5 days

PHARMACOLOGICAL MANAGEMENT OF ACUTE SUBARACHNOID HEMORRHAGE

SAH is associated with a high incidence of delayed cerebral ischemia 2 weeks following the stroke. Vasospasm is thought to be the cause of the delayed ischemia and occurs 4-21 days after the bleed.

DRUG	DOSING	SIDE EFFECTS/CONTRAINDICATIONS/MONITORING
Dihydropyridine CCB		
Nimodipine *(Nimotop)*	60 mg PO Q4H for 21 days	**BLACK BOX WARNING** Nimodipine has been inadvertently administered IV when withdrawn from capsule into a syringe for subsequent nasogastric administration. Severe adverse events including death have occurred. **SIDE EFFECTS** Hypotension, headache, diarrhea **MONITORING** CPP, ICP, BP, HR, neurological checks Label syringes "For oral use only". Have pharmacy draw up to reduce medication errors.

Ischemic Stroke Prevention

Modifiable risk factors should be corrected.

- Hypertension - the use of ACE-Is, ARBs and diuretics have shown a reduction in the risk of stroke

- Hypercholesterolemia treated per the NCEP ATP III guidelines

- Tight glucose control in patients with diabetes to reduce risk of microvascular disease

- Lifestyle changes including smoking cessation, increased physical exercise (at least 30 minutes most days of the week), weight reduction if necessary (maintain BMI 18.5 - 24.9 kg/m² and a waist circumference < 35 inches for women and < 40 inches for men) and limit alcohol intake (≤ 2 drinks/day for males, ≤ 1 drink/day for females).

PRIMARY PREVENTION

Primary prevention is recommended for patients with atrial fibrillation only. See anticoagulation lecture for more detail.

SECONDARY PREVENTION

Patients with previous cardioembolic stroke should be placed on anticoagulant therapy for secondary stroke prevention. In patients with a previous non-cardioembolic stroke, the use of antiplatelet agents for secondary stroke prevention is recommended. Any of the 3 anti-platelet agents listed below are acceptable options for initial therapy.

ANTIPLATELET THERAPY

DRUG	DOSING	SIDE EFFECTS/CONTRAINDICATIONS/MONITORING
Aspirin	50 -325 mg daily	**SIDE EFFECTS** Dyspepsia, heartburn, GI upset, GI bleed/ ulceration, bleeding, renal impairment, hypersensitivity
Clopidogrel *(Plavix)*	75 mg daily	**BLACK BOX WARNING** Diminished Effectiveness in poor metabolizers Effectiveness depends on the activation to an active metabolite mainly by 2C19. Poor metabolizers exhibit higher cardiovascular events than patients with normal 2C19 function. Tests to check CYP 2C19 genotype can be used as an aid in determining a therapeutic strategy. Consider alternative treatment strategies in patients identified as 2C19 poor metabolizers. The CYP2C19*1 allele corresponds to fully functional metabolism while the CYP2C19*2 and *3 alleles are nonfunctional. **CONTRAINDICATIONS** Active pathological bleed (e.g. PUD, ICH) **SIDE EFFECTS** Bleeding, bruising, rash, TTP (rare) Rare, but serious – Thrombotic thrombocytopenic purpura (TTP): have patients report fever, weakness, extreme skin paleness, purple skin patches, yellowing of the skin or eyes, or neurological changes.
Dipyridamole ER/Aspirin *(Aggrenox)*	200 mg/25 mg BID	**SIDE EFFECTS** Headache (> 10%), dyspepsia, abdominal pain, nausea, diarrhea, and bleeding

DRUG INTERACTIONS

- Avoid use, if possible, with other agents that ↑ bleeding risk, including other antiplatelets (although clopidogrel is used with low-dose aspirin), NSAIDs, anticoagulants, ginkgo and others.

- Clopidogrel is a prodrug metabolized mainly by CYP2C19. Avoid concomitant use with strong or moderate 2C19 inhibitors (cimetidine, fluconazole, ketoconazole, voriconazole, fluoxetine, fluvoxamine and others). Omeprazole, a moderate 2C19 Inhibitor, has been shown to reduce the pharmacological activity of clopidogrel if given concomitantly or if given 12 hours apart. Consider using another PPI with less 2C19 inhibitory activity.

PATIENT EDUCATION

Identify and educate about modifiable risk factors. Call 911 immediately if you have any symptoms below:

- Sudden numbness or weakness of face, arm, or leg, especially on one side of the body

- Sudden confusion or trouble speaking or understanding speech

- Sudden trouble seeing in one or both eyes

- Sudden trouble walking, dizziness, or loss of balance or coordination

- Sudden severe headache with no known cause

ACT F.A.S.T (TEST TO LOOK FOR SIGNS/SYMPTOMS OF STROKE)	
Face	Ask the person to smile. Does one side of the face droop?
Arms	Ask the person to raise both arms. Does one arm drift downward?
Speech	Ask the person to repeat a simple sentence. Are the words slurred? Can he/she repeat the sentence correctly?
Time	If the person shows any of these symptoms, time is important. Call 911 or get to the hospital fast. Brain cells are dying.

56

GASTROESOPHAGEAL REFLUX DISEASE (GERD)

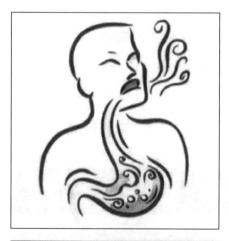

GUIDELINES

American Gastroenterological Association (AGA) Medical Position Statement on the Management of Gastroesophageal Reflux Disease. Gastroenterology 2008;135:1383-1391.

Updated Guidelines for the Diagnosis and Treatment of Gastroesophageal Reflux Disease. Am J Gastroenterology 2005;100:190-200.

Background

Gastroesophageal reflux disease (GERD) is a condition in which the stomach contents leak backward into the esophagus. Normally, gastric contents are prevented from backflow into the esophagus by a ring of muscle fibers called the lower esophageal sphincter (LES). In GERD, the LES pressure or muscle tone is reduced (or transiently relaxes) and allows for backflow of the stomach contents. Typical symptoms of GERD include heartburn, hypersalivation, regurgitation, and/or an acid taste in the mouth. Less commonly, symptoms can include recurrent cough, sore throat, hoarseness, and chest pain, which may be difficult to distinguish from cardiac pain. GERD can lead to esophageal erosion, strictures, bleeding, Barrett's esophagus, and esophageal cancer.

The stomach epithelial lining contains parietal cells which secrete hydrochloric acid and intrinsic factor, G cells that secrete gastrin, mucus-secreting cells, and chief cells that secrete pepsinogen. The parietal cells have receptors for histamine, acetylcholine, and gastrin, all of which stimulate HCl acid secretion. These substances activate the H^+/K^+ ATPase pump located in the parietal cell and represents the final common pathway for gastric acid secretion.

Treatment Principles

Patient-reported symptoms are used as initial diagnosis; invasive testing is not required in most cases. If there is a response to acid-suppressive therapy (generally PPIs), a diagnosis can be assumed. Patients with serious symptoms should be sent for further evaluation. Occasional and less bothersome symptoms may respond to antacids or H_2RAs. Caution should be used with chronic acid suppression from H$_2$RAs and PPIs due to recent concerns of increased fracture risk, increased risk of GI infections, increased risk of nosocomial pneumonia in hospitalized patients and increased risk of osteoporosis with long-term use.

Clinicians may follow "step-up" therapy – where they use OTC products 1st, and use Rx products only as necessary. Another approach is "step-down" therapy which starts with more intensive therapy (PPIs) and then therapy is tailored off as the symptoms decrease. In more serious conditions (where esophageal erosion is present), PPIs should be used first-line because they are the most effective agents at acid-suppression.

Misoprostol and sucralfate are difficult to use and seen infrequently. With these agents, there are a few important safety considerations to review. The American College of Gastroenterology (ACG) recommends against the use of metoclopramide as therapy for esophageal symptoms (risk outweighs benefit); however, it is still used commonly in the elderly, where it can pose significant risk of adverse events.

RECOMMENDED NON-PHARMACOLOGIC (LIFESTYLE) TREATMENT

- Avoid foods and substances that may reduce lower esophageal sphincter (LES) pressure or aggravate the condition including spicy foods, nicotine, coffee/caffeine/tea, alcohol, fatty foods, citrus, chocolate, and peppermint/spearmint.

- Decrease portion size (eat smaller and more frequent meals).

- Weight loss – best evidence in improvement, per AGA guidelines.

- Avoid or discontinue drugs, if possible, that can decrease LES pressure: anticholinergics, barbiturates, dihydropyridine calcium channel blockers, estrogen, nitrates, NSAIDs, theophylline and others.

- Do not eat before sleeping (last meal should be 2-3 hours before bedtime).

- Elevate the head of the bed 6-8″ (not with pillows, but with a wedge, or by elevating the head-side of the bed under the mattress).

- Avoid tight-fitting clothing.

Pharmacologic Therapy

ANTACIDS

Antacids work by neutralizing the gastric acid in a buffering reaction (producing salt and water), which raises pH. These agents are good for mild or infrequent symptoms or if the patient is in need of fast relief.

DRUG	DOSING	SIDE EFFECTS/CONTRAINDICATIONS/ MONITORING
Calcium *(Tums, others)* Aluminum *(AlternaGel)* **Magnesium [Phillips Milk of Magnesia (MOM)**, *others]* **Magnesium + (Aluminum or Calcium) combo *(Maalox, Mylanta, *Rolaids*, others)* **Mag-Al-Simethicone (anti-gas)** ***(Maalox Max, Mylanta Max* Strength**, others) Sodium bicarbonate *(Alka-Seltzer* Heartburn relief) *Gaviscon* contains antacids in combination with alginic acid which theoretically forms a barrier to combat reflux (efficacy?) Calcium carbonate, magnesium hydroxide, famotidine *(Pepcid Complete)*	Many formulations including suspensions, chewable tablets, capsules 10-30 mL or 2-4 tablets 4-6x/day	Onset of relief: < 5 minutes and lasts 1-2 hours. **SIDE EFFECTS** Aluminum causes constipation Magnesium causes diarrhea (Used together to counter-balance but still get loose stool) **RENAL** Aluminum and magnesium can accumulate with severe renal dysfunction. Use is not recommended in patients with a CrCl < 30 mL/min. Caution: *Maalox Total Relief* contains bismuth subsalicylate (for upset stomach and diarrhea – will darken stool, avoid in salicylate allergy – FDA expects name to be changed). *Pepcid Complete* provides immediate relief (antacid) and longer relief (H$_2$-RA) *Alka Seltzer* contains > 1 g Na$^+$ per serving; not generally used as an antacid any longer

ANTACID DRUG INTERACTIONS

- Separate 2 hours before or 4 hours after from quinolone and tetracycline antibiotics (reduced drug absorption due to chelation).

- Separate 2 hours before or 4 hours after from itraconazole, ketoconazole, calcium carbonate and iron, due to reduced absorption from increased pH.

ANTACID COUNSELING

- Use all lifestyle counseling points (from above).

- This medicine provides immediate relief, but lasts ~1-2 hours. If you need longer relief, a medicine such as famotidine will last longer (or PPI, but not used prn). If the symptoms remain bothersome, discuss with your doctor.

- If you are using this product more than 2 times per week, you may have a condition that requires stronger therapy. Discuss the symptoms with your doctor.

- Do not use aluminum or magnesium products if you have advanced kidney disease.

- If you experience constipation, discontinue use of aluminum-containing products.

- If you experience diarrhea, you may wish to discontinue use of magnesium-containing products.

- Do not use antacids that contain sodium if you are on a sodium restricted diet, have heart disease, high blood pressure, heart failure or kidney disease.

- Do not use sugar-containing antacids if you have diabetes.

- See a doctor immediately if you have bloody stools or "coffee-ground" like vomiting.

HISTAMINE$_2$-RECEPTOR ANTAGONISTS (H$_2$RAs)

H$_2$RAs reversibly inhibit the histamine-2 receptors on the gastric parietal cells inhibiting gastric acid secretion.

DRUG	DOSING	SIDE EFFECTS/ CONTRAINDICATIONS/MONITORING
	Given once or twice daily (or prn) depending on symptom severity	Onset of relief: 30-45 minutes and lasts 4-10 hours. Longer duration of action than antacids, but shorter than PPIs.
Famotidine **(Pepcid AC, Pepcid AC Max Strength)** **Pepcid Complete** - calcium carbonate, magnesium hydroxide, famotidine **Famotidine 26.6 mg + ibuprofen 800 mg (Duexis)**	Famotidine OTC *Pepcid AC* 10, 20 mg - Max Strength Famotidine Rx 20, 40 mg Powder for oral susp 40 mg/5 mL Injection 10 mg/mL	Occasionally may be appropriate with PPI if H$_2$RA is used at bedtime for nighttime reflux symptoms; otherwise, do not use H$_2$RAs with PPIs. **SIDE EFFECTS** Agitation/vomiting in children < 1 year Headache, dizziness, diarrhea, constipation
Ranitidine (Zantac)	Ranitidine OTC 75, 150 mg Ranitidine Rx 300 mg tablet 150 mg EFFERdose tablets (contains Na$^+$ and phenylalanine) Syrup 15 mg/mL Injection 25 mg/mL	May ↑ risk of GI infections and may ↑ risk pneumonia in hospitalized patients Cimetidine: CNS effects, gynecomastia (< 1-4%), impotence, uncommon: blood dyscrasias, ↑ LFTs, arthralgia, others. **Renal** Use lower doses in elderly and patients with ↓ renal function
Nizatidine (Axid)	Nizatidine OTC 75 mg Nizatidine Rx 150, 300 mg Susp 15 mg/mL	
Cimetidine *(Tagamet, Tagamet HB 200)*	Cimetidine OTC 200 mg Cimetidine Rx 300, 400, 800 mg Susp 300 mg/5 mL Injection 150 mg/mL	

H$_2$-RECEPTOR ANTAGONIST DRUG INTERACTIONS (ALL)

- CNS: Additive side effects, if elderly or reduced renal function; use lower doses.

- Avoid use with delavirdine and erlotinib. Caution with concurrent use of itraconazole, ketoconazole, calcium carbonate and iron due to reduced absorption from increased pH.

H$_2$RA-Blocker Drug Interactions (Cimetidine)

Cimetidine is a 3A4 inhibitor and weak-moderate inhibitor of other isoenzymes. Avoid use with clopidogrel, dofetilide, and thioridazine. Use caution with many other drugs including amiodarone, phenytoin, carbamazepine, quinidine, theophylline, citalopram, and others.

H₂-RECEPTOR ANTAGONIST COUNSELING (ALL)

- Use all lifestyle counseling points.

- This medicine provides fast onset (onset ~1 hour, lasts 4-10 hours). If you need longer relief, a medicine taken daily (such as omeprazole) may be more helpful. If the symptoms remain bothersome, discuss with your doctor.

- If you are using this product more than 2 times per week, you may have a condition that requires stronger therapy. Discuss the symptoms with your doctor.

PROTON PUMP INHIBITORS (PPIs)

PPIs block gastric acid secretion by irreversibly binding to the gastric H^+/K^+-adenosine triphosphatase (ATPase) pump in parietal cells. They block the final step in acid production. Since PPIs inhibit only proton pumps that are actively secreting acid, they are more effective when taken 30 minutes before a meal.

DRUG	DOSING	SIDE EFFECTS/CONTRAINDICATIONS/ MONITORING
	PPIs are taken daily, 30 minutes before breakfast. If this fails, BID (2nd dose before dinner) can be tried. For treating duodenal or gastric ulcers caused by *H. pylori*, dosing is usually BID.	Onset of relief: 2-3 hours and lasts 12-24 hours. PPIs are the most effective agents for severe disease/symptoms
Omeprazole *(Prilosec OTC, Prilosec, generic)*	20 mg (OTC), 10, 20, 40 mg (Rx) 2.5, 10 mg susp	**SIDE EFFECTS** Headache, dizziness (1-4%), diarrhea, constipation, vitamin B12 deficiency, hypomagnesemia (when duration of PPI use > 1 year), acid rebound
Omeprazole-Na⁺ Bicarb *(Zegerid, Zegerid OTC)*	20, 40 mg cap with 1.1 gram of Na⁺ bicarb 20, 40 mg powder for susp: both 1,680 mg Na⁺ bicarb (460 mg Na⁺) Omeprazole-Na⁺ Bicarb-Magnesium hydroxide 20, 40 mg tabs with 750 mg Na⁺ bicarb and 343 mg of Mag hydroxide	Can ↑ risk *C. diff* infections ↑ risk osteoporosis/fracture with long-term use – good reason to limit use! Can ↑ INR if using warfarin (monitor) Can ↑ risk pneumonia in hospitalized patients
Pantoprazole *(Protonix, generic)*	20, 40 mg tabs Granules for susp 40 mg/pk Injection *(Protonix* IV*)*, 40 mg	**MONITORING** Signs and symptoms of GERD
Lansoprazole *(Prevacid, Prevacid SoluTab. Prevacid 24H-OTC, generic)*	15 mg (OTC), 15, 30 mg (Rx) 15, 30 mg SoluTab (contains phenylalanine) Injection - discontinued	Dexlansoprazole, lansoprazole, esomeprazole and omeprazole capsules can be opened (not crushed) and mixed in apple sauce or acidic juice if patient cannot swallow pill or for NG tube delivery.
Dexlansoprazole *(Dexilant)* Lansoprazole-Naproxen *(Prevacid NapraPAC)*	30, 60 mg	Do not crush, cut, or chew tablets (pantoprazole and rabeprazole) or capsules
Esomeprazole *(Nexium)*	20, 40 mg caps Granules for susp 10, 20, 40 mg/pk Injection 20, 40 mg/mL	
Esomeprazole + naproxen *(Vimovo)*	20 mg + 375 or 500 mg naproxen	
Rabeprazole *(Aciphex)*	20 mg	

PPI DRUG INTERACTIONS

- Caution with concurrent use of drugs that require an acidic pH for absorption including itraconazole, ketoconazole, calcium carbonate, iron, and others.

- PPIs inhibit 2C19: Do not use with delavirdine, erlotinib, nelfinavir, and posaconazole. Do not use omeprazole (and possibly others) and clopidogrel concurrently. PPIs may ↑ levels of methotrexate, phenytoin, raltegravir, saquinavir, tacrolimus, voriconazole and warfarin.

PPI COUNSELING

- Use all lifestyle counseling points.

- Take 30 minutes before breakfast. If twice daily, take before breakfast and dinner.

- If taking long-term, ensure that calcium and vitamin D intake is optimal. Recommend calcium citrate formulations (improved absorption in basic pH).

- If you are planning to stop this medicine, you should "taper" the dose to avoid "acid rebound." Please discuss with your pharmacist (we should recommend decreased dose, then every other day, over at least a couple of weeks.)

- Do not use for occasional mild stomach upset. This can be effectively treated with an antacid (such as calcium carbonate) or a stronger medication such as famotidine (the generic for *Pepcid*).

- Effervescent and orally dissolving formulations contain phenylalanine. Do not use in patients with phenylketonuria (PKU).

- If you are using for more than 14 days and heartburn persists, consult your doctor.

- Do not crush or chew any capsules.

- *Prevacid SoluTab*: Do not swallow whole. Place on tongue and allow to dissolve (with or without water), then swallow.

CYTOPROTECTIVE AGENTS

Misoprostol is a prostaglandin E_1 analog that replaces the gut-protective prostaglandins removed by NSAIDs.

Sucralfate forms a complex by binding with positively charged proteins that protect the stomach lining against pepsin and HCl acid.

CYTOPROTECTIVE AGENTS

DRUG	DOSING	SIDE EFFECTS/CONTRAINDICATIONS/MONITORING
Misoprostol *(Cytotec)*	Start at 100 mcg right after dinner, increase (if tolerated) to 100 mcg QID or 200 mcg QID. Take right after meals and at bedtime.	**Black Box Warnings (2)** Not to be used to reduce NSAID-induced ulcers in women of childbearing potential unless she is capable of complying with effective contraceptive measures. Patients must be warned not to give this drug to others **Pregnancy Category X** Also used for medical termination of pregnancy with mifepristone (RU-486) **SIDE EFFECTS** Diarrhea, abdominal pain (both significant)
Sucralfate *(Carafate)*	1 g tablets QID <u>before</u> meals and at bedtime (usual), may be given 1 g Q4H (for treatment of active ulcer) Suspension 1 g/10 mL	**SIDE EFFECTS** Constipation Drug is in aluminum complex; can accumulate in severe renal disease (avoid)

MISOPROSTOL COUNSELING

- Do not use in women of childbearing age unless strict compliance with contraceptive measures.

- Can start with 100 mcg right after dinner (with food in stomach), attempt to increase as-directed. Use of psyllium *(Metamucil)* may help decrease diarrhea.

SUCRALFATE DRUG INTERACTIONS

- Avoid taking antacids within 30 minutes before or after taking sucralfate.

- Separate from many other drugs 2 hours before or 4 hours after (difficult to use).

SUCRALFATE COUNSELING

- Major side effect is constipation; drink adequate fluids and use laxatives if directed.

- Discuss other drugs, including OTC products you are using, with the pharmacist. This drug can decrease the absorption of other medicines.

Metoclopramide

<u>Metoclopramide is a dopamine antagonist</u>. At higher doses, it blocks serotonin-receptors in chemoreceptor zone of the CNS. It also enhances the response to acetylcholine in the upper GI tract causing enhanced motility and accelerated gastric emptying (peristaltic speed) and increases LES tone.

DRUG	DOSING	SIDE EFFECTS/CONTRAINDICATIONS/MONITORING
Metoclopramide *(Reglan)*	5 mg, 10 mg tabs, ODT 5 mg/mL injection, 5 mg/5 mL solution 10 mg QID 30 min <u>before meals</u> and at bedtime. – short duration of action (must be present in gut when food is present), and given at bedtime to control evening reflux symptoms – CrCl < 40 mL/min, ↓ dose 50%	**CONTRAINDICATIONS** GI obstruction/perforation, history of seizures **SIDE EFFECTS** CNS: Dizziness [somnolence and fatigue (up to 70%)], restlessness, akathisia, confusion, depression. CV – more common with IV dosing: AV block, bradycardia, fluid retention, CHF. Serious ADRs due to dopamine blockade: Extrapyramidal symptoms (EPS), including Parkinsonism (Parkinson disease-like symptoms), acute dystonic reactions, tardive dyskinesia (abnormal muscle moving, including facial twitches, tongue thrusting), and rarely, neuroleptic malignant syndrome. These symptoms are more common if the drug is not dose-adjusted with poor renal clearance (elderly) <u>and</u> in pediatrics. Wrong choice of drug in a patient with Parkinson disease.

METOCLOPRAMIDE DRUG INTERACTIONS

- Do not use in patients receiving medications for Parkinson disease (counter-effect).
- Caution for additive CNS effects, including dizziness, sleepiness, fatigue.

METOCLOPRAMIDE COUNSELING

- Use caution when driving, operating machinery, or performing other hazardous activities. This drug may cause dizziness or drowsiness.
- Dizziness may be more likely to occur when you rise from a sitting or lying position. Rise slowly to prevent dizziness and a possible fall.
- Avoid consuming alcohol during treatment with this drug. Alcohol may increase drowsiness and dizziness.
- Contact your doctor right away if you experience any unusual body movements, such as shakiness, stiffness, or uncontrollable movements of the mouth, tongue, cheeks, jaw, arms, or legs.
- Seek medical attention if you experience fever, sweating, severe muscle stiffness (rigidity) and confusion.

PRACTICE CASE

PATIENT PROFILE

Patient Name	Benjamin Specter								
Address	10 Pine Place								
Age	72	**Sex**	Male	**Race**	White	**Height**	5'6"	**Weight**	160lbs
Allergies	Aspirin (hives)								

DIAGNOSES

GERD	Seasonal allergies, occasional bronchodilator use
Prostate enlargement	Dyslipidemia, CHD, MI x 2 (last ~8 years ago)
Parkinson's disease	

MEDICATIONS

Date	No.	Prescriber	Drug & Strength	Quantity	Sig	Refills
6/23/09	35421	Cooper	Clopidogrel 75 mg	#30	1 PO daily	6
6/23/09	35422	Cooper	Protonix 40 mg	#30	1 PO daily	6
6/23/09	35423	Cooper	Pravastatin 20 mg	#30	1 PO BID	6
6/23/09	35424	Cooper	Sinemet 25/250	#120	1 PO daily	6
			Albuterol inhaler	#1	Occasional use	4
			Loratadine 10 mg		1 tablet, as needed	
11/1/09	42877	Kreinfeldt	Metoclopramide 10 mg	#120	1 PO QID	

LAB/DIAGNOSTIC TESTS

Test	Normal Value	Results		
		Date 5/12/09	Date	Date
Protein, T	6.2-8.3 g/dL			
Albumin	3.6-5.1 g/dL			
Alk Phos	33-115 units/L			
AST	10-35 units/L			
ALT	6-40 units/L			
CH, T	125-200 g/dL			
TG	<150 g/dL			
HDL	g/dL			
LDL	g/dL			
GLU	65-99 mg/dL			
Na	135-146 mEq/L			
K	3.5-5.3 mEq/L			
Cl	98-110 mEq/L			
C02	21-33 mmHg			
BUN	7-25 mg/dL	28		
Creatinine	0.6-1.2 mg/dL	1.9		
Calcium	8.6-10.2 mg/dL			
WBC	4-11 cells/mm^3			
RBC	3.8-5.1 mL/mm^3			
Hemoglobin	Male: 13.8- 17.2 g/dL Female: 12.1-15.1 g/dL			
Hematocrit	Male: 40.7-50.3% Female: 36.1- 44.3%			
MCHC	32-36 g/dL			
MCV	80-100 μm			
Platelet count	140-400 x 10^3/mm^3			
TSH	0.4-4.0 mIU/L			
FT4	4.5- 11.2 mcg/dL			
Hgb A1c	4-6%			

ADDITIONAL INFORMATION

Date	Notes
11/11/09	PCP (Cooper) on vacation. Reports bothersome heartburn. Reflux after eating dinner and during sleep. Eats dinner 8:30 pm, falls asleep 9:30-10 pm. Enjoys after dinner black tea with honey & pipe. Per discussion, symtpoms appear controlled.

QUESTIONS

1. The patient is using *Protonix* once daily. Which of the following is an appropriate substitution?

    a. Omeprazole
    b. Esomeprazole
    c. Pantoprazole
    d. Rabeprazole
    e. Lansoprazole

2. The patient is still experiencing symptoms despite his current therapy. The physician decided to add-on metoclopramide to control the reflux symptoms. Choose the correct statement:

    a. Inappropriate therapy; the physician should increase *Protonix* to 60 mg daily.
    b. Inappropriate therapy; the physician should either increase *Protonix* to BID dosing, or add ranitidine 75 mg at bedtime.
    c. Inappropriate therapy; the physician should add on magnesium citrate prn.
    d. Inappropriate therapy; the physician should start misoprostol 200 mcg QID.
    e. Metoclopramide is appropriate therapy; no change is required.

3. Benjamin can make several lifestyle changes that may help with his evening symptoms. Which of the following are correct counseling points the pharmacist can provide to the patient?

    a. Consider cessation of evening smoke
    b. Eat dinner at an earlier time
    c. Change his evening drink to a non-caffeinated, non-alcoholic option
    d. Elevate the head of his bead 6-8 inches
    e. All of the above

4. The substituting physician prescribed metoclopramide. Which of the following side effects may be present?

    a. Worsening of his Parkinson's disease symptoms
    b. Worsening of his prostate disease symptoms
    c. Dizziness, sleepiness
    d. A and B only
    e. A and C only

5. If the metoclopramide was to be used in a different patient with this degree of renal function, what would be the correct dose?

    a. 10 mg four times daily
    b. 10 mg twice daily
    c. 10 mg daily
    d. 5 mg four times daily
    e. 5 mg once daily

Questions 6-11 are NOT based on the above case.

6. An elderly female presents at the pharmacy. She does not have health insurance coverage. Which of the following PPIs is available over-the-counter?

    a. *Zegerid*
    b. *Prevacid*
    c. *Prilosec*
    d. A and C
    e. All of the above

7. A patient has entered the pharmacy and asked the pharmacy technician to help her locate the store-brand version of *Pepcid*. Which of the following medications should the technician select?

    a. Famotidine
    b. Cimetidine
    c. Ranitidine
    d. Omeprazole
    e. Lansoprazole

8. A physician has written a prescription for *Prevacid*. Which of the following represents an acceptable therapeutic substitution?

    a. Omeprazole
    b. Esomeprazole
    c. Rabeprazole
    d. Pantoprazole
    e. Lansoprazole

9. Which of the following proton pump inhibitors is available in an IV formulation?

    a. *Dexilant*
    b. *Nexium*
    c. *Protonix*
    d. *AciPhex*
    e. B and C

10. An elderly female patient has hypertension and heartburn. Her family states she has trouble swallowing large pills. She failed H$_2$-blocker therapy and has been well-controlled on a PPI. She is currently using *Nexium* 40 mg daily. Which of the following would be a better option?

    a. *Zantac EFFERdose*
    b. *NapraPAC*
    c. *Zegerid*
    d. *Prevacid SoluTab*
    e. *Maalox*

11. Proton pump inhibitors can increase the risk of:

    a. Bone fracture
    b. Heart attacks
    c. Stroke
    d. A and B
    e. All of the above

ANSWERS

1-c, 2-b, 3-e, 4-e, 5-d, 6-e, 7-a, 8-e, 9-e, 10-d, 11-a

PEPTIC ULCER DISEASE (PUD)

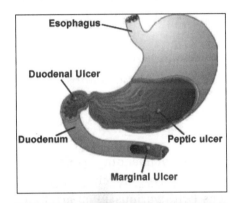

Background

Peptic ulcer disease (PUD) occurs from mucosal erosion within the gastrointestinal tract. Unlike gastritis and erosions, the ulcers in PUD extend deeper into the mucosa. Most ulcers occur in the duodenum but a small percent do occur in the stomach. The three most common types of PUD are *Helicobacter pylori (H. pylori)*-positive ulcers, nonsteroidal anti-inflammatory drug (NSAIDs)-induced ulcers and stress ulcers (from critical illness). *Helicobacter pylori (H. pylori)*, a spiral-shaped, pH sensitive, gram-negative bacterium that lives in the acidic environment of the stomach, is responsible for the majority of the peptic ulcers (~70-80%). Other, less common causes of PUD are hypersecretory states, such as Zollinger-Ellison syndrome (causes ↑ gastric acid), G-cell hyperplasia, mastocytosis, and basophilic leukemias.

Under normal conditions, a physiologic balance exists between gastric acid secretion and gastroduodenal mucosal defense. Mucosal defense and repair mechanisms include mucus and bicarbonate secretion, mucosal blood flow, prostaglandin synthesis, cellular restitution and regeneration, and epithelial cell renewal. These mechanisms protect the gastroduodenal mucosa from damage and irritation by noxious substances, such as NSAIDs (including ASA), *H. pylori*, acid, pepsin, and other factors. Mucosal injury and, thus, peptic ulcer disease occurs when the balance between the noxious mucosal irritants and the defensive mechanisms is disrupted.

Symptoms

The primary symptom of PUD is epigastric pain. Epigastric refers to the upper region of the abdomen. This pain can be associated with a burning or gnawing sensation and may awaken a patient if it occurs at night. If the ulcer is duodenal (usually caused by *H. pylori*), eating generally <u>lessens</u> the pain. With gastric ulcers (primarily from NSAIDs), eating generally <u>worsens</u> the pain. Other symptoms common to both types of ulcers include heartburn, belching, bloating, nausea and anorexia.

H. Pylori

H. pylori infection, if left untreated, can lead to cancer. If testing is positive for *H. pylori*, the infection should be treated. Common diagnostic tests include:

- Urea breath test (UBT): Breath test that identifies gas (CO_2) produced by the bacteria. False negatives can be due to the recent use of H_2RAs, PPIs, bismuth or antibiotics; discontinue H_2RAs and PPIs (1-2 weeks) and bismuth and antibiotics (4 weeks) prior to the test.

- Fecal antigen test: Detects *H. pylori* in the in stool. False negatives can be due to the recent use of H_2RAs, PPIs, bismuth, or antibiotics (to a lesser extent than the UBT); discontinue these drugs at least 2-4 weeks prior to test.

- Blood (serologic) test: Detects antibodies to the bacteria; cannot distinguish between a current or previous infection since patients can remain seropositive for 6 months - 1 year after *H. pylori* eradication.

TREATMENT

The American College of Gastroenterology guidelines have been recommending <u>triple therapy with an anti-secretory agent (preferably a PPI) + 2 antibiotics (clarithromycin and amoxicillin or metronidazole) for 14 days.</u> Several of the regimens (with various PPIs) are FDA-approved for a 10 day regimen. <u>Due to recent failures with triple therapy, many patients are currently receiving quadruple therapy.</u> This should be chosen if a patient has used a macrolide or metronidazole in the past, or if the local failure rates are known to be high. <u>Quadruple therapy consists of a PPI, bismuth, metronidazole, and tetracycline for 10-14 days</u> (can use *Helidac* or *Pylera*). Another option for resistant cases is "sequential therapy": a PPI and amoxicillin for 5 days, followed by a PPI, clarithromycin and tinidazole for 5 days.

Do not make drug substitutions in *H. pylori* eradication regimens. H_2RAs should not be substituted for a PPI, unless the patient cannot tolerate a PPI. Likewise, other antibiotics in the same class should not be substituted in *H. pylori* eradication regimens (for example, do not use ampicillin instead of amoxicillin).

FIRST-LINE *H. PYLORI* TREATMENT REGIMENS

DRUG	NOTES

Triple Drug Therapy – Take for 14 days

| PPI BID (esomeprazole is 40 mg daily) +

 Amoxicillin 1,000 mg BID +

 Clarithromycin 500 mg BID | <u>PCN or macrolide allergy</u>: replace amoxicillin or clarithromycin with metronidazole 500 mg BID in this regimen

 – or –

 can use alternative therapy below.

 See GERD chapter for PPI side effects and Infectious Disease section for more on the antibiotics |

Quadruple Therapy - Take for 10-14 days

(Use if failed above therapy, cannot tolerate above agents, have taken a macrolide or metronidazole in the past, or if high local resistance rates to clarithomycin)

| PPI BID +

 Bismuth subsalicylate 525 mg QID +

 Metronidazole 250 mg QID +

 Tetracycline 500 mg QID | **Alcohol use**
 Do not use metronidazole

 Pregnancy
 Do not use tetracycline

 Salicylate allergy/children
 Do not use bismuth subsalicylate (or tetracycline in children 8 years or less)

 If cannot tolerate a PPI, can substitute with H_2RA (e.g. ranitidine 150 mg BID, famotidine 40 mg daily, nizatidine 300 mg/d) |

Prevpac – BID x 14 days

Prevpac contains lansoprazole/amoxicillin/clarithromycin all on one blister card. One blister card is taken per day.

Pylera –QID x 10 days

Pylera contains bismuth subcitrate potassium/metronidazole/tetracycline in one capsule. Take 3 capsules QID. A PPI is obtained separately and given BID for 10 days.

Helidac – QID x 14 days

Helidac contains bismuth subsalicylate/metronidazole/tetracycline all on one blister card. One blister card is taken per day. A PPI is obtained separately. H_2RA is obtained separately and should be taken for a total of 28 days.

DRUG INTERACTIONS

- PPIs: Caution with concurrent use of drugs that require an acidic pH for absorption including itraconazole, ketoconazole, calcium carbonate, iron, and others. PPIs inhibit 2C19: Do not use with delavirdine, erlotinib, nelfinavir, and posaconazole. Do not use omeprazole (and possibly others) and clopidogrel concurrently. PPIs may ↑ levels of methotrexate, phenytoin, raltegravir, saquinavir, tacrolimus, voriconazole and warfarin.

- Clarithromycin is a 3A4 major inhibitor. See drug interactions chapter for more information.

- Tetracycline can chelate with aluminum, magnesium, calcium, iron and zinc leading to ↓ drug absorption. The administration time must be separated (2 hours before and 4 hours after). Monitor warfarin (may ↑ INR).

- Metronidazole: Avoid use of alcohol. Monitor warfarin (may ↑ INR).

■ Bismuth subsalicylate can ↑ risk of salicylate toxicity with other salicylates, including aspirin.

H. PYLORI COUNSELING

■ It is important to take all medication as directed and finish the complete course of therapy. Drink a full glass of water with each dose. These medications may upset your stomach and should be taken with meals.

■ Bismuth subsalicylate: The pink tablets are chewed while the other medications are swallowed. If taken with aspirin and ringing in the ears occurs, contact your doctor. Counsel on symptoms of bleeding. Bismuth subsalicylate may cause temporary and harmless darkening of the tongue and/or black stool.

■ Tetracycline: Do not use if pregnant or in children ≤ 8 years old. Oral contraceptives may be less effective. Use a back-up form of contraception, such as condoms, during antibiotic therapy. This medicine may make your skin more sensitive to the sun and you may burn more easily. Use sun protection such as light weight clothing and UVA and UVB sunscreen (SPF 30 or higher).

■ Metronidazole: Alcoholic beverages should be avoided during therapy with metronidazole and for at least one day afterward.

■ Clarithromycin may cause diarrhea, nausea and abnormal taste (each ~3%).

■ If *Helidac* or *Pylera*, take additional PPI *(Pylera)* or H$_2$RA *(Helidac)* for entire course of therapy, as directed. The H$_2$RA is recommended for an additional 14 days after the end of *Helidac* therapy.

■ If diarrhea or loose stools develop during use, contact your doctor immediately.

NSAID-Induced Ulcers (Primarily Gastric)

BACKGROUND

The use of high dose NSAIDs or chronic NSAID use greatly increases the risk for gastrointestinal (GI) ulcers. NSAIDs (including ASA) can cause gastric mucosal damage by 2 mechanisms; direct irritation of the gastric epithelium and systemic inhibition of prostaglandin synthesis (by inhibiting COX-1).

RISK FACTORS FOR NSAID-INDUCED ULCERS:

■ Age (> 65 years)

■ Previous ulcer

■ High dose NSAIDs

■ Concomitant use of steroids, anticoagulants, antiplatelets (aspirin, clopidogrel, prasugrel, ticagrelor), oral bisphosphonates and SSRIs

TREATMENT

Use of concomitant PPI therapy decreases ulcer risk. High risk patients should receive a PPI with chronic use of non-selective NSAIDs <u>regardless</u> of their previous history of GI ulcers. Alternatively, a COX-2 selective agent (e.g. celecoxib) can be used in high risk patients if they do NOT have cardiovascular risk factors. Generic NSAID agents that approach the selectivity of celecoxib are: meloxicam, nabumetone and etodolac.

If an ulcer develops, it would be best to discontinue the NSAID, if possible, and treat the ulcer with a PPI for ~ 8 weeks. If the NSAID therapy cannot be stopped, then reducing the NSAID dose, switching to acetaminophen or a nonacetylated salicylate or using a more selective COX-2 inhibitor should be considered. <u>In patients with cardiovascular risk, naproxen plus a PPI is recommended.</u> Misoprostol is also an option, but diarrhea and cramping along with its four times per day dosing regimen contribute to poor patient compliance.

Use caution with NSAIDs in any person with cardiovascular or renal disease for other reasons as well, including blood pressure elevation and decreased renal blood flow. If possible, avoid NSAIDs and celecoxib in patients with both <u>high GI and CV risk</u> and those at high risk of chronic kidney disease.

Patients who require antiplatelet therapy with a previous history of ulcers should be tested for *H. pylori* and treated, if positive.

PRACTICE CASE

PATIENT PROFILE

Patient Name	Edward Gilbert
Address	560 Milton Drive

Age	75	**Sex**	Male	**Race**	White	**Height**	5'10"	**Weight**	155 lbs

Allergies	Penicillin (severe rash)

DIAGNOSES

Shoulder/back pain, secondary to clavicle Fx 1/09	"Silent" MI, found on echo, no current Tx
Prostate CA	
Memory impairment	
Tremor	

MEDICATIONS

Date	No.	Prescriber	Drug & Strength	Quantity	Sig	Refills
8/11/09	77729	Sybell	Lupron 2 week-kit	#2	1 mg SC daily	
5/15/09	44825	Polonsky	Propranolol 20 mg	#90	1 TID	4
2/28/09	32187	Polonsky	Doxazosin	4 mg	1 PO QHS	7
5/15/09			Calcium carb+D 500-400	#120	1 PO BID	

LAB/DIAGNOSTIC TESTS

Test	Normal Value	Results		
		Date 5/12/09	Date	Date
Protein, T	6.2-8.3 g/dL			
Albumin	3.6-5.1 g/dL			
Alk Phos	33-115 units/L			
AST	10-35 units/L			
ALT	6-40 units/L			
CH, T	125-200 g/dL			
TG	<150 g/dL			
HDL	g/dL			
LDL	g/dL			
GLU	65-99 mg/dL			
Na	135-146 mEq/L			
K	3.5-5.3 mEq/L			
Cl	98-110 mEq/L			
C02	21-33 mmHg			
BUN	7-25 mg/dL			
Creatinine	0.6-1.2 mg/dL			
Calcium	8.6-10.2 mg/dL			
WBC	4-11 cells/mm³			
RBC	3.8-5.1 mL/mm³			
Hemoglobin	Male: 13.8- 17.2 g/dL Female: 12.1-15.1 g/dL			
Hematocrit	Male: 40.7-50.3% Female: 36.1- 44.3%			
MCHC	32-36 g/dL			
MCV	80-100 µm			
Platelet count	140-400 x 10³/mm³			

ADDITIONAL INFORMATION

Date	Notes
12/10/09	Patient's wife reports he is c/o severe epigastric pain for 2 weeks. Little relief with OTC antacids. Wife states she is giving spouse naproxen 250 mg #2 several times daily x 2-3 months for shoulder/back pain from his fall. Endoscopy report shows 1-cm gastric ulcer. A rapid urease test is negative. Evidence of anterior infarct reported during earlier hospital stay for cancer treatment. Family denies additional Rx or OTC medications.

QUESTIONS

1. Edward's wife is quite concerned about his severe gastric pain. Which change/s should be initiated?

    a. Discontinue naproxen
    b. Start PPI therapy
    c. Start antacid therapy
    d. Start *H. pylori* treatment
    e. A and B

2. Which of the following agents cause dizziness, syncope or fatigue and may have contributed to the fall that caused Edward to sustain a fracture?

    a. *Lupron*
    b. Propranolol
    c. Doxazosin
    d. Calcium+D
    e. A, B and C

3. Which of the following are risk factors present in Edward's case for the development of a gastric ulcer?

    a. Age
    b. High-dose, chronic use of non-selective NSAID
    c. Prostate cancer history
    d. A and B
    e. A, B and C

4. Eight weeks later, Edward has a follow-up endoscopy. The report states the ulcer has healed and the mucosa appears normal. PPI therapy is stopped. However, Edward is in pain, which he rates as a 4-5 on a pain scale. He states his back throbs when he sits or lies down. During this time, the oncologist has tried *Norco* and *Ultracet*, both of which did not offer much relief. Edward's wife asks if he can return to using naproxen, which was very helpful. Which is the most appropriate therapy at this time?

    a. Naproxen plus PPI therapy
    b. Celecoxib 400 mg once daily
    c. Piroxicam 20 mg twice daily
    d. Acetaminophen 325 mg, 1-2 as needed
    e. Fentanyl patch

Questions 5-8 are NOT based on the above case.

5. A female patient presents to the pharmacy with a prescription for lansoprazole 30 mg BID, bismuth subsalicylate 525 mg QID, metronidazole 250 mg QID and tetracycline 500 mg QID for 14 days. The patient's other prescriptions include hydrochlorothiazide and the combination oral contraceptive product *Lybrel*. Choose the correct counseling statement:

    a. You will need to use back-up contraception, such as condoms and foam, for the 14 days you are using this antibiotic therapy.
    b. You will need to use back-up contraception, such as condoms and foam, for the 14 days you are using this antibiotic therapy and for 1 week afterwards.
    c. You will need to use back-up contraception, such as condoms and foam, for the 14 days you are using this antibiotic therapy and for 2 weeks afterwards.
    d. You will need to stop the *Lybrel* and use an alternative form of contraception for the 14 days you are using this antibiotic therapy.
    e. It is acceptable to use alcohol in moderation during use of this regimen, as long as you do not exceed safe amounts.

6. A 16 year-old patient has the following allergies noted on her patient profile: ciprofloxacin, aspirin and erythromycin. The allergic reaction is not listed, and the patient is not available by phone. You wish to fill the prescription for *H. pylori* therapy, which includes rabeprazole, amoxicillin and clarithromycin. Choose the correct statement:

    a. It is safe to fill; most allergies to erythromycin are gastrointestinal.
    b. It is safe to fill; there is no cross-reaction with these agents.
    c. It is not safe to fill due to the use of amoxicillin in a patient with ciprofloxacin allergy.
    d. It is not safe to fill due to the patient's age.
    e. It is not safe to fill until the erythromycin "allergy" is clarified. It could be significant, or may be GI upset and not a true allergy to macrolide therapy. The physician should be notified of the discussion and his approval (if appropriate) of the use of clarithromycin noted on the prescription.

7. A 46 year-old man has received a prescription for lansoprazole 15 mg daily, amoxicillin 500 mg BID and clarithromycin 500 mg BID for *H. pylori* treatment. Choose the correct statement:

    a. Contact prescriber to correct dosages of lansoprazole.
    b. Contact prescriber to correct dosages of lansoprazole and amoxicillin.
    c. Contact prescriber to correct dosages of clarithromycin and amoxicillin.
    d. Contact prescriber to correct dosages of lansoprazole and clarithromycin.
    e. Fill as written.

8. A pharmacist is dispensing tetracycline. Which of the following are correct counseling points?

    a. Take this medication 2-4 hours before or after taking any products containing magnesium, aluminum, or calcium, including vitamins, supplements and dairy products.
    b. Do not use sunlamps while using this therapy.
    c. You should avoid getting pregnant while using this medicine.
    d. You may experience stomach upset, including loose stools and nausea.
    e. All of the above.

ANSWERS

1-e, 2-e, 3-d, 4-a, 5-a, 6-e, 7-b, 8-e

CONSTIPATION & DIARRHEA

BACKGROUND

Constipation is defined as infrequent or hard stools, or difficulty passing stools. More specifically, constipation may involve pain during the passage of a bowel movement, the inability to pass a bowel movement after straining or pushing for more than 10 minutes, requiring digital evacuation, or no bowel movements after more than 3 days.

- Look for offending drugs (see chart)

- Correct fluid intake (64 oz – caution with CVD)

- Limit caffeine & alcohol

- Replace refined foods with whole grain products, fruits and vegetables, beans

- Increase physical activity

- Don't delay going to the bathroom when the urge to defecate is present; may need to schedule time

Opioids and Constipation

Prevention: from <u>chronic opioids</u> – regular use of senna (<u>stimulant</u>) plus a stool softener (docusate), alone or in combo products is usually needed and a laxative should be recommended when a scheduled opioid is prescribed. What is needed depends on the patient and the drug (e.g., fentanyl is less constipating than morphine). The higher dose used, the more constipation will be

CONSTIPATION NOTES

Medical conditions where constipation is common

Cerebrovascular events	Irritable Bowel Syndrome (constipation-predominant)
Parkinson disease	
Spinal cord tumors	Anal disorders (anal fissures, fistulae, rectal prolapse)
Diabetes	
Hypothyroidism	
Multiple sclerosis	

Medications that are constipating

OPIOIDS	Iron (use docusate to avoid hard, compact stools)
Anticholinergic drugs	
Antihistamines, phenothiazines, tricyclic antidepressants, antispasmodics, urge incontinence drugs, especially darifenacin (*Enablex*)	Aluminum antacids (Mg often in combination with Al to counteract effect)
	Aluminum complex in other drugs (sucralfate [*Carafate*])
Non-DHP Calcium channel blockers, especially verapamil	Antineoplastics
Clonidine	Alkaloids, oxaliplatins, taxanes
Metals	
Bismuth	

present. Ask the patient how the bowel movements usually are, and you may be able to try docusate alone. If they are taking prn (e.g., *Vicodin*), they may need one or both as well, depending on how easily than can defacate.

Treatment: lactulose, sorbitol, MOM, mag citrate or *MiraLax*.

Fecal Impaction: Enema, may require digital evacuation.

LAXATIVES

CATEGORY	MECHANISM OF ACTION	ONSET OF ACTION / DOSE	POTENTIAL ADVERSE EFFECTS/ COUNSELING
Bulk laxative – *Usual First-Line Tx* Wheat bran **calcium polycarbophil (FiberCon)** **psyllium (Metamucil)** **methylcellulose (Citrucel)**	Creates gel-like matrix in stool – soaks up fluid in loose stool, adds bulk to hard stool	12 to 24 hours or more	Increased gas; bloating; bowel obstruction if strictures present; choking if powder forms are not taken with enough liquid Increase bulk in diet slowly Adequate fluid intake Take 2 hours before/after drugs (caution with other drugs that stick to fiber) Tart-like flavor; sugar-free forms avail
Emollients, lubricants (stool softeners) **Docusate Sodium (Colace)** Docusate Calcium, Mineral Oil	Lubricates and softens fecal mass	24 to 48 hours Typical dose: DSS 50-100 mg daily, or divided BID (up to 300 mg/daily)	Bitter taste with liquid only Do not use docusate with mineral oil Advise not to use more than 2 weeks without consulting physician (not that it's harmful, just to rule out more serious problem) Mineral oil – take a multivitamin at a different time
Stimulants and irritants **Bisacodyl** **(Dulcolax** – caution, this name can refer to doscusate, or bisacodyl tabs or supp) **Senna (Ex-Lax)** Cascara	Reduce water and electrolyte absorption by stimulating colonic neurons and irritating the colon mucosal lining	Rectals: 10 minutes Orals take 8-12 hours (generally used overnight so the bowel movement occurs the next morning, but can be BID) Bisacodyl OTC 5 mg	Stomach upset, cramping, electrolyte imbalance with overdose (e.g. eating disorders) Do not crush or chew bisacodyl tablets (are EC), do not take within 1 hr of milk or antacids – may require dose reduction with H_2RAs or PPIs.
Gut-Opioid-R Blocker **Methylnaltrexone (Relistor)**	Blocks opioid receptors in the gut – ONLY FOR USE WITH OPIOIDS	8 mcg if weight 38-61 kg, or 12 mcg if 62 kg+ Reduce dose 50% if CrCl < 30 mL/min Given SC every other day	Only for patients on opioids who have failed DSS + laxative (senna, bisacodyl). It is given SC every other day. Do not use routinely; can often ↑ laxative until the patient can excavate SE: abdominal pain, nausea, diarrhea Contraindicated if any GI blockage

Laxatives Continued

CATEGORY	MECHANISM OF ACTION	ONSET OF ACTION / DOSE	POTENTIAL ADVERSE EFFECTS/ COUNSELING
Osmotics Lactulose, **Magnesium salts (MOM)**, Sorbitol	Salts lead to retained fluid in the bowel lumen, with a net increase of fluid secretions in the small intestines	2 to 48 hours	Electrolyte imbalance; excessive gas; hypermagnesemia, hypocalcemia and hyperphosphatemia in patients with renal dysfxn; dehydration
Fleets Phospho-Soda	Causes reflex evacuation	Within 30 minutes These are OTC but the physician recommends use.	Dehydration DO NOT USE Phospho-soda in CHF, renal disease, ↓ Ca²⁺ or ↑ PO4
Nonabsorbable solutions **Polyethylene glycol (Golytely, MiraLax, Carbowax)** *NuLytely, Trilyte* are sulfate free *HalfLytely, MoviPrep* are less volume (2L)	Hyperosmotic *MiraLax* is OTC: Fill capful with powder, mix into a glass of water, drink. Add a little water to get the granules stuck to the side of the glass Almost tasteless	*Golytely*: Within 4 hours, directions: fill with water to line, shake well, refrigerate to improve taste, consume specified amount every 10 minutes until stool is watery & clear. Usually, no solid food should be eaten for at least 2 hours, and preferably 3-4 hours, before taking the solution and until procedure is complete.	Nausea, abdominal fullness, bloating
Glycerin supp *Babylax* is liquid in in rectal applicator (squeeze out liquid around stuck stool into rectum)	Suppositories come in pediatric and adult size Super, or highly osmotic, agent	Two sizes – pediatric and adult Insert rectally towards side of rectal wall (at side of stool), bowel movement within 20 minutes. (Usually in a minute or two). Can repeat x 1, if need > 1 week see physician.	Anal irritation, stomach cramping
Lubiprostone (Amitiza)	Activates chloride channels in the gut, leading to increased fluid in gut and movement	24 mcg capsule twice daily with food Can cut dose to once daily if nausea significant	Nausea, 30% Abdominal pain & distention Take with food

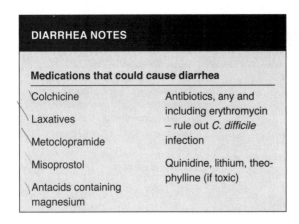

DIARRHEA NOTES

Medications that could cause diarrhea

Colchicine	Antibiotics, any and including erythromycin – rule out *C. difficile* infection
Laxatives	
Metoclopramide	
Misoprostol	Quinidine, lithium, theophylline (if toxic)
Antacids containing magnesium	

Diarrhea

BACKGROUND

Diarrhea occurs when there is an increase in the number of bowel movements or bowel movements are more watery and loose than normal. When the intestines push stools through the bowel before the water in the stool can be reabsorbed, diarrhea occurs. Abdominal cramps, nausea, vomiting, or a fever may occur along with the diarrhea.

TREATMENT

- Most cases are viral. Diarrhea can be idiopathic, caused by diseases, and is often caused by stomach flu or food poisoning. Drinking untreated water, not washing fruits/vegetables properly, using untreated ice for drinks, or unpasteurized dairy products can cause viral, bacterial, or parasitic infections. *E. coli* is the most common bacterial cause. The treatment of diarrhea caused by a bacterial infection is discussed in the ID chapter.

- If the infection is parasitical, most are caused by *Giardia lamblia* – if this is the cause, the diarrhea can develop 1 to 4 weeks after exposure. Giardia infections are a major diarrhea disease throughout the world, especially in places with poor sanitation. Lactose intolerance should be ruled out. Fluid and electrolyte replacement is essential. Besides *Giardia*, other parasites can include *Cryptosporidium parvum, Cyclospora cayetanensis, Entamoeba histolytica*, and *Dientamoeba fragilis*. Drugs used to treat giardia infections include metronidazole *(Flagyl)*, tinidazole *(Tindamax)* and nitazoxanide *(Alinia)*. Common treatment regimens are metronidazole 250-500 mg TID x 5-7 days (no alcohol, metallic taste, darkened urine) or tinidazole 2 g x 1 dose (same side effects). These drugs are taken with food to reduce stomach upset. (Technically, metronidazole is with or without food but is usually with food.)

TRAVELLER'S DIARRHEA PROPHYLAXIS/AVOIDANCE

- Prophylaxis with antibiotics for traveler's diarrhea (TD) is not recommended, except perhaps for short-term travelers who are high-risk (such as those who are immune-compromised) or who are taking critical trips during which even a short bout of diarrhea could impact the purpose of the trip. (If treatment is used for active infection, common agents currently are quinolones, azithromycin or rifaximin. Refer to the ID chapter.)

- Patients may choose to use prophylaxis with bismuth subsalicylate (BSS, *Pepto-Bismol)*. If an infection is present, treatment options are discussed above. BSS commonly causes blackening of the tongue and stool and may cause nausea, constipation, and rarely tinnitus. BSS should be avoided by travelers with aspirin allergy, renal insufficiency, and gout and by those taking anticoagulants, probenecid, or methotrexate. In travelers taking aspirin or salicylates for other reasons, the use of BSS may result in salicylate toxicity. Caution should be used in administering BSS to children with viral infections, such as varicella or influenza, because of the risk for Reye's syndrome.

- Care in selecting food and beverages for consumption will minimize the risk for acquiring TD. Travelers should be advised that foods that are freshly cooked and served piping hot are safer than foods that may have been sitting for some time in the kitchen or in a buffet. Care should be taken to avoid beverages diluted with nonpotable water (reconstituted fruit juices, ice, and milk) and foods washed in nonpotable water, such as salads. Other risky foods include raw or undercooked meat and seafood, and unpeeled raw fruits and vegetables. Safe beverages include those that are bottled and sealed or carbonated.

COUNSELING FOR ALL DIARRHEA CASES

- Do not self-treat if high fever or blood in stool; see physician if no improvement in 2 days (sooner for young children/infants)

- Diarrhea treatment should include fluid and electrolytes – this is important for all but especially so in young children or adults with chronic medical illness.

- For moderate-severe fluid loss, replacement is best accomplished with oral rehydration solutions (ORS), which are available at stores and pharmacies *(Pedialyte, Infalyte,* etc) in developed countries. Gatorade or similar products are used as alternatives.

- Caution with *Imodium* and *Lomitil* if a decrease in intestinal motility may be due to infection from *Shigella, Salmonella,* and toxigenic strains of *E. coli* – toxic megacolon (usually due to *E. coli* or severe IBS) may occur. These products are also NOT recommended in *C. difficile* infections – the patient's body must be able to rid itself of the toxin.

- If fever/cold symptoms are present, aspirin can rarely cause Reye's Syndrome in children and is avoided except under a doctor's care (it may rarely be used in a child with a heart condition, where benefit may outweigh risk). For fever or mild pain, the parent can treat the child with acetaminophen or ibuprofen but should not exceed recommended daily amounts of acetaminophen (10-15 mg/kg Q 4-6 hrs, maximum of 5 doses/24 hrs), or ibuprofen (10 mg/kg Q 6-8 hrs).

- Combination cough and cold products should not be used in children. Any combination product may contain additional amounts of acetaminophen or ibuprofen – the patient must be counseled to count all sources.

- RULE OUT lactose intolerance as a cause of the diarrhea by stopping use of dairy products. Physicians can confirm lactose intolerance by tests.

ANTIDIARRHEALS

CATEGORY	MECHANISM OF ACTION	DOSE	SIDE EFFECTS/COUNSELING
Psyllium	To soak up liquid. See constipation section.		
Bismuth subsalicylate (BSS or *Pepto-Bismol*)	Antisecretory and antimicrobial properties	1 oz of liquid or two chewable tablets every 30 minutes up to 8 doses	Black tongue/stool BSS should be used with caution in travelers on aspirin therapy or anticoagulants or those who have renal insufficiency Avoid in children with viral infections, such as varicella or influenza, because of the risk of Reye's syndrome Salicylate toxicity can present as tinnitus
Loperamide (Imodium)	Acts on intestinal muscles to inhibit peristalsis and to slow intestinal motility	4 mg PO after first loose stool initially; then 2 mg after each subsequent stool; not to exceed 16 mg/d	Don't self-treat for > 2 days Not for use in children < 2 ys old Avoid use if infection due to *C. difficile*, *Shigella*, *Salmonella*, and toxigenic strains of *E. coli* – otherwise, the toxins will stay in the gut as these agents considerably slow down gut motility. Same caution applies to diphenoxylate agents.
Diphenoxylate 2.5 mg with atropine 0.025 mg (*Lomotil*)	Drug combination that consists of diphenoxylate, which is a constipating meperidine congener, and atropine to discourage abuse	1 – 2 tab QID AC	May cause sedation, constipation, urinary retention, tachycardia, blurred vision, xerostomia, dizziness, or respiratory depression

INFLAMMATORY BOWEL DISEASE (IBD)

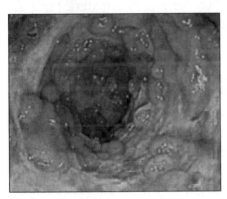

Background

Inflammatory Bowel Disease (IBD) is a group of inflammatory conditions of the colon and small intestine. The major types of IBD are <u>ulcerative colitis (UC)</u> and <u>Crohn's disease.</u> Symptoms include cramping, bloody diarrhea, fever and possible weight loss. Crohn's can cause malabsorption (vitamin deficiencies) and anal fissures. The treatment goal is to suppress inflammation to reduce symptoms. Acute symptom control (such as the use of antidiarrheals or antispasmodics), may be necessary. Symptoms increase when the patient is under stress or eats foods that may be disease triggers. Food triggers, in some patients, include beans, alcohol, lactose-containing dairy products, cabbage and broccoli.

ULCERATIVE COLITIS

UC affects only the rectum and colon with superficial ulcerations (in contrast to Crohn's, where the ulcers can be deep). The larger the affected area, the worse the symptoms. When the disease flares, patients are usually running to the bathroom often, with pain, which can significantly decrease quality of life. UC is characterized by abdominal pain, bloody diarrhea, weight loss and fever.

CROHN'S

Any part of the GI tract can be affected, although 2/3 of cases are in the ileum – the last part of the small intestine. The GI tract can get swollen and ulcerated. Crohn's is characterized by abdominal pain, diarrhea and weight loss. (Notice no fever and diarrhea is generally not bloody – which are present in UC).

TREATMENT

Both UC and Crohn's, in simpler cases, may only need antidiarrheal medicines, primarily loperamide (*Imodium*) 2 mg after each loose stool, up to 8 doses/day. Antispasmodics for UC may be useful. The most common antispasmodic is dicyclomine (*Bentyl*) given 10 mg AC and QHS. This is an anticholinergic with typical side effects (dry mouth, urinary retention, tachycardia, etc.)

With acute flare-ups of either condition, short courses of oral steroids (and occasionally, IV) are used. With more moderate symptoms, aminosalicylates (sulfasalazine or mesalamine) are used to control inflammation.

Crohn's, in moderate-severe cases, may require a stronger immunosuppressive agent (azathioprine [AZA], 6-mercaptopurine [6-MP], or methotrexate). In severe UC or Crohn's cases (fistula development or other severe symptoms), TNF-blockers (primarily infliximab) may be needed. Occasionally, IV steroids or cyclosporine are used.

Some patients find benefit with the use of rifaximin *(Xifaxan)*, an agent indicated for GI infections. There is no current FDA-indication for this purpose.

NATURAL PRODUCTS

Cascara and senna are "natural" stimulant laxatives since they are plant products and can be useful for patients with constipation. For diarrhea, psyllium (in *Metamucil* and many other formulations) or other "bulk-forming" fiber products can be useful. These agents are relatively well-tolerated but the patient should consider the standard safety considerations (see constipation/diarrhea section).

Peppermint (oil, sometimes teas) can be useful as an antispasmodic. Some use chamomile tea. The probiotic *Lactobacillus* or *bifidobacterium infantis* may help reduce abdominal pain, bloating, urgency, constipation or diarrhea in some patients. Antibiotics and probiotics are not taken together; separate the dosing by at least two hours. Fish oils (for the EPA and DHA, omega fatty acid components) are being used, although the evidence for benefit is contradictory. Indian frankincense gum resin taken TID may be beneficial for UC, based on preliminary studies.

Watch for avoidable problems: Sorbitol is used as a sweetener in some diet foods and is present in various drugs. It can cause considerable GI distress in some patients with IBS. Sorbitol has laxative properties.

And: Check if the IBS patient is lactose-intolerant. Lactose is not only in dairy products; it is also used in some oral drugs as an excipient.

Both sorbitol and lactose are classified as excipients (or binders); they help hold tablets together.

COMMON AGENTS USED FOR ACUTE SYMPTOM CONTROL: DIARRHEA, CRAMPING/GI SPASMS

DRUG	DOSING	SIDE EFFECTS/MONITORING/CONTRAINDICATIONS

Antidiarrheals

DRUG	DOSING	SIDE EFFECTS/MONITORING/CONTRAINDICATIONS
Loperamide (*Imodium*)	2 mg tab, cap, liquid	Don't self-treat for > 2 days
	4 mg PO after first loose stool initially; then 2 mg after each subsequent stool; not to exceed 16 mg/d	Not for use in children < 2 yrs old
Bismuth subsalicylate (*Pepto-Bismol, BSS*)	2 tbsp or 2 tablets Q hr, up to 8 doses/day, max 2 days	Black tongue/stool BSS should be used with caution in travelers on aspirin therapy or anticoagulants or those who have renal insufficiency Avoid in children with viral infections, such as varicella or influenza, because of the risk of Reye's syndrome Salicylate toxicity can occur if used excessively.
Diphenoxylate **2.5 mg with atropine** **0.025 mg** (*Lomotil*)	1 – 2 tabs QID AC	Sedation, constipation, urinary retention, tachycardia, blurred vision, xerostomia, dizziness, or respiratory depression

Antispasmodic

DRUG	DOSING	SIDE EFFECTS/MONITORING/CONTRAINDICATIONS
Dicyclomine (*Bentyl*)	10 mg AC and QHS	Anticholinergic Dry mouth, urinary retention, dry/blurry vision, constipation Confusion, tachycardia

STEROIDS TO DECREASE SEVERITY OF ACUTE ATTACKS

DRUG	NOTES	SIDE EFFECTS/MONITORING/ CONTRAINDICATIONS
Prednisone 5-60 mg/d **Budesonide** (*Entocort EC*-do not crush) 9 mg/d (~15x more potent – if changing from prednisone, allow a 2-week overlap) Budesonide preferred if disease is in ileum or ascending colon May be using ADT (Alternate Day Therapy or QOD) to ↓ adrenal suppression	Acute flares – steroids are not supposed to be used long-term – however, some patients use chronically due to severe condition. If used long-term assess bone density, consider use of bisphosphonates, optimize calcium and vitamin D intake. If used longer than 2 weeks, taper dose off to avoid withdrawal symptoms.	Use until acute flares resolve or weight is regained. Side effects (systemic steroid treatment) Short-term: Fluid retention, emotional instability (euphoria, mood swings depression, insomnia), if high dose acute rise in blood glucose, possible rise in blood pressure. Long-term: Adrenal suppression/ Cushing's syndrome, impaired wound healing, hypertension, hyperglycemia, cataracts, osteoporosis, etc.

BUDESONIDE DRUG INTERACTIONS

- Budesonide is a 3A4 substrate; potent inhibitors (ketoconazole, itraconazole, ritonavir, etc.) will require a budesonide dose reduction.

- Avoid the use of grapefruit products when using this medication.

Maintenance Therapy

DRUG	NOTES	SIDE EFFECTS/MONITORING/ CONTRAINDICATIONS
Mesalamine *(Apriso, **Asacol, Asacol HD, Pentasa** and **Lialda** are all long-acting orals, **Canasa** – supp, **Rowasa** – enema)* 1 g rectally QD or 1 g 3 x/ week Enema 2-4 g/d 1.5-4.8 g/d orally Sulfasalazine *(Azulfidine, Sulfazine, Azulfidine EN-tabs, Sulfazine EC)* 4-6 g/d Can cause <u>yellow-orange</u> coloration of skin/urine <u>Impairs folate absorption</u>, may give 1 mg/d folate supplement Take with food and 8 oz of water to prevent cystalluria *Asacol* 400 mg x 2 is not interchangeable with *Asacol HD* 800 mg	<u>Enema or rectal mesalamine suppositories are 1st line for UC mild-mod distal disease</u> (over oral agents – these may be used in some patients, alone or with topical) <u>Crohn's requires oral therapy w/mesalamine or sulfasalazine for mild-mod cases.</u> Oral sulfasalazine is 1st line in UC mild-mod <u>extensive disease</u> Mesalamine or sulfasalazine can be used for Crohn's.	**SIDE EFFECTS** **Mesalamine** <u>If oral formulation</u>: headache, nausea, abdominal pain, flatulence. Pancreatitis CI: Hypersensitivity to salicylates or any component of the formulation; avoid concomitant use with antacids, H2-RAs, or PPIs **Sulfasalazine** CI in patients with sulfa or salicylate allergy, GI or GU obstruction <u>HA, GI upset, loss of appetite, N/V/D, photosensitivity</u> (> 10%), rash 5-aminosalicylic acid derivative

If Failed Above Therapy Or In Combo With Above

Azathioprine (AZA or *Imuran*) 50 mg tablet or 100 mg IV Purine antimetabolite Protect tablets from light	"Steroid-sparing"	Black Box Warnings (2) Chronic immunosuppression, ↑ risk of neoplasia Hematologic toxicities (leukopenia, thrombocytopenia) and mutagenic potential
6-Mercaptopurine (6-MP)		Bone marrow toxicity: anemia, leukopenia, thrombocytopenia
Methotrexate (*Rheumatrex*) Dose is 7.5 – 20 mg/week Preg. Category X Antidote: leucovorin or levoleucovorin – for chemo doses or in overdose Monitor CBC, LFT's		<u>MANY Black Box Warnings</u> – liver, renal, pneumonitis, BMS, mucositis/stomatitis, dermatologic reactions, etc. – most pertain if using higher doses as in cancer CI in patients with active infectious disease or pneumonitis, myelodysplasia, WBC < 3,000/mm³, PLT < 50,000/mm³, elevated LFTs, CrCl < 30mL/min, pregnancy and breastfeeding Side effects: nausea, diarrhea, mucositis/stomatitis, skin reactions, etc.

If Failed Above Therapy: Monoclonal antibodies to TNF

Remicade: Chimeric monoclonal antibody *Humira*: Humanized monoclonal antibody (may have ↓ antibody development and ↓ resistance) *Cimzia*: PEG-linked humanized monoclonal antibody *Tsyabri*: Humanized monoclonal antibody that inhibits α4-integrin

Maintenance Therapy Continued

DRUG	NOTES	SIDE EFFECTS/MONITORING/ CONTRAINDICATIONS
Infliximab *(Remicade)* IV only Acute: 5 mg/kg x 1, then same at weeks 2 and 6 Q 8 weeks for maintenance – some patients will eventually need 10 mg/kg dose (due to tolerance)	Alternative 1st line in mod-severe Crohn's or UC Alone, or with AZA Drug should be used within 3 hrs of reconstitution and dilution Infusion requires a filter	All TNF inhibitors carry a black box warning for risk of serious infections, including tuberculosis, and invasive fungal and other opportunistic infections. All patients should be evaluated for TB before starting these drugs. Patients with latent TB should start prophylactic treatment. Monitor for infectious diseases throughout the course of therapy and possibly longer. Precautions: TNF inhibitors can cause neurological reactions, demyelinating disease, malignancies, hepatitis B reactivation, HF, auto-immunity (lupus), and immunosuppression. They should not be used with *Anakinra*, other TNF inhibitors, or live vaccines. Infusion rxns: hypotension, fever, chills, pruritis, (may benefit w/pre-treatment w/APAP, antihistamine, steroids) Delayed HSN 3-10 days after admin (fever, rash, myalgia, HA, sore throat) INFECTION: All TNF-blockers get CBC (for WBC), TB test prior to admin (and annually), monitor S/Sx infection, WBC HF exacerbation: CI in NYHA III/IV and max 5 mg/kg dose in milder HF. Bone marrow suppression Hepatitis, monitor LFTs, reactivation of Hep B Antibody induction: ↓ usefulness of drug

If failed above therapy these are next line options

DRUG	NOTES	SIDE EFFECTS/MONITORING/ CONTRAINDICATIONS
Certolizumab *(Cimzia)* 400 mg SC, then 400 mg weeks 2 and 4, then 400 mg Q 4 weeks	Crohn's Good response if CRP > 10 mg/L Pegylated formulation Vials refrigerated, reconstituted vials are good for 24 hrs if in refrigerator or 2 hrs at room temp.	Similar side effects to infliximab
Adalimumab *(Humira)* 40 mg pre-filled syringe, SC admin (higher doses for acute attack)		Similar to infliximab, however humanized so may have ↓ antibody development
Natalizumab *(Tysabri)* Discontinue if no response by week 12.	Must be enrolled in manufacturer TOUCH prescribing program. Cannot be used with other immunosuppressants	Black Box Warning Risk for progressive multifocal leukoencephalopathy (PML) – monitor mental status changes Hepatotoxicity, infection, infusion-related reactions (observe for 1° after infusion)

MESALAMINE COUNSELING

■ Do not crush or chew long-acting formulations. You may see a ghost tablet in the feces *(Asacol HD)*.

- *Rowasa* enema: Remove bottle from pouch and shake well. Remove the protective sheath from the applicator tip. Hold the bottle at the neck so as not to cause any of the medicine to be discharged. Best results are obtained by lying on the left side with the left leg extended and the right leg flexed forward for balance. Gently insert the lubricated applicator tip into the rectum to prevent damage to the rectal wall, pointed slightly toward the navel. Grasp the bottle firmly, and then tilt slightly so that the nozzle is aimed toward the back, and squeeze slowly to instill the medication. Steady hand pressure will discharge most of the medicine. After administering, withdraw and discard the bottle. Remain in position for at least 30 minutes, or preferably, all night.

- *Canasa* suppository: For best results, empty your rectum (have a bowel movement) just before using. Detach one suppository from the strip. Carefully peel opens the plastic at the pre-cut line to take out the suppository, trying to touch as little as possible since your hands will melt the medicine. Insert the suppository with the pointed end first completely into your rectum, using gentle pressure. For best results, keep the suppository in your rectum for 3 hours or all night, if possible. You may put a little bit of lubricating gel on the suppository.

BUDESONIDE *(ENTOCORT EC)* COUNSELING

- Take this medication with a full glass of water before a meal. Do not crush, chew or break open the capsule.

- Tell your doctor if you have changes in the shape or location of body fat (especially in your arms, legs, face, neck, breasts, and waist), high blood pressure, severe headache, fast or uneven heart rate, blurred vision), or a general ill feeling with headache, tiredness, nausea, and vomiting.

- If using this medication long-term, you should have your blood pressure monitored on a regular basis. The blood pressure should remain in a healthy range.

- If using this medication long-term, you should have your blood glucose ("blood sugar") monitored on a regular basis. The blood glucose should remain in a healthy range.

- Do not use grapefruit products with this medication. If you have been using grapefruit juice or fruit do not change the amount without discussing this with your doctor or pharmacist.

- Avoid being near people who are sick or have infections.

SULFASALAZINE COUNSELING

- Do not use if you have an allergy to sulfa or salicylates.

- You may experience loss of appetite, headache, nausea, stomach pain or upset or a rash.

- Patients with any of these symptoms should see their physician immediately: sore throat, pale or yellowed skin or fatigue.

- Use protection if you are out in the sun (clothing, sunscreen) as you will burn more easily.

- This medicine may make the urine or skin turn an orange-yellowish color.

PRACTICE CASE

PATIENT PROFILE

Patient Name	Frank Clough
Address	1020 Darby

Age	Sex	Race	Height	Weight
75	Male	White	5'5"	148lbs

Allergies Penicillin (severe rash)

DIAGNOSES

Ulcerative Colitis

MEDICATIONS

Date	No.	Prescriber	Drug & Strength	Quantity	Sig	Refills
5/15/09	76740	Greer	Atenolol 100 mg	30	1 PO daily	3
5/15/09	76743	Greer	Mesalamine 1 g supp	30	1 pr QHS	3

LAB/DIAGNOSTIC TESTS

Test	Normal Value	Results
Protein, T	6.2-8.3 g/dL	
Albumin	3.6-5.1 g/dL	
Alk Phos	33-115 units/L	
AST	10-35 units/L	
ALT	6-40 units/L	
CH, T	125-200 g/dL	
TG	<150 g/dL	
HDL	>50 g/dL	
LDL	g/dL	
GLU	65-99 mg/dL	
Na	135-146 mEq/L	
K	3.5-5.3 mEq/L	
Cl	98-110 mEq/L	
C02	21-33 mmHg	
BUN	7-25 mg/dL	
Creatinine	0.6-1.2 mg/dL	
Calcium	8.6-10.2 mg/dL	
WBC	4-11 cells/mm³	
RBC	3.8-5.1 mL/mm³	
Hemoglobin	Male: 13.8- 17.2 g/dL Female: 12.1-15.1 g/dL	
Hematocrit	Male: 40.7-50.3% Female: 36.1- 44.3%	
MCHC	32-36 g/dL	
MCV	80-100 μm	
Platelet count	140-400 x 10³/mm³	

ADDITIONAL INFORMATION

Date	Notes
12/10/09	Well-controlled on mesalamine supp x 5 months. Comes in today for acute flare; reporting 5-6 diarrhea episodes/day x 3d. Bloody today only. Rx prednisone 10 mg #28, 1 QID x 7 days, return to clinic in 1 week.

QUESTIONS

1. The patient was originally prescribed mesalamine suppositories for distal disease classified as mild-moderate. Which of the following statements is correct?

    a. Oral therapy is preferred for initial treatment.

    b. Mesalamine is available in oral and rectal (suppositories, enema) formulations.

    c. Sulfasalazine is preferred over mesalamine for distal disease.

    d. Mesalamine cannot be used in a sulfa allergy.

    e. Mesalamine is not 1st-line therapy for distal disease.

2. Mesalamine rectal suppository counseling should include the following points:

    a. Peel open the plastic and remove suppository prior to use.

    b. Handle unwrapped suppository as little as possible.

    c. Should be kept in the rectum for 3 hours, or longer.

    d. Lubricating gel may be used to ease application.

    e. All of the above

3. The physician prescribed prednisone therapy for the acute flare-up. Which of the following are <u>short-term</u> side effects that may occur and should be conveyed to the patient?

    a. Elevated blood glucose

    b. Elevated blood pressure

    c. Changes in mood

    d. A and B

    e. A, B and C

4. ACG guidelines recommend against steroid treatment for long-term control of IBD symptoms; however, many patients use budesonide (or prednisone) daily. Which of the following are LONG-TERM side effects that may occur and should be conveyed to the patient?

    a. Decreased bone density

    b. Poor wound healing

    c. Fat redistribution

    d. Adrenal suppression

    e. All of the above

Questions 5-12 are NOT based on the above case.

5. A female patient has failed her initial therapy for Crohn's disease, which included etanercept and methotrexate. Her symptoms are described as severe. She is prescribed infliximab. Which of the following statements is CORRECT?

    a. She can use *Enbrel* instead.

    b. She should have been prescribed *Tysabri* prior to use of infliximab.

    c. Infliximab should be used 1st in suppository formulation.

    d. This medication comes in an IV formulation only and cannot be self-administered.

    e. This medication can suppress TB activation.

6. A patient has heart failure NYHA stage III. She is taking the following medications: lisinopril, carvedilol, amlodipine, atorvastatin and aspirin. She has failed mesalamine and azathioprine therapy. The doctor wishes to start infliximab. Which of the following statements is CORRECT?

    a. Infliximab is contraindicated in this patient.

    b. Infliximab can be used if the atorvastatin is stopped.

    c. Infliximab can be used if the carvedilol is stopped.

    d. A and C.

    e. None of the above.

7. A patient has been prescribed infliximab. Which of the following tests should be ordered prior to the start of therapy?

    a. WBC

    b. TB

    c. TSH and FT4

    d. A and B

    e. None of the above

8. Which of the following describes the mechanism of action of infliximab?

    a. Chimeric monoclonal antibody against integrin
    b. Chimeric monoclonal antibody against interleukin-1
    c. Chimeric monoclonal antibody against TNF
    d. Fully humanized monoclonal antibody against integrin
    e. Fully humanized monoclonal antibody against TNF

9. Which of the following can occur with the use of infliximab?

    a. Infusion related reactions (hypotension, fever, pruritis, chills)
    b. Reactivation of latent TB infection and/or severe systemic infections
    c. Antibody induction
    d. Liver inflammation
    e. All of the above

10. A physician has ordered infliximab. The pharmacist calls the prescriber to ask if she wished to pre-medicate with acetaminophen, antihistamine and steroids. Which of the following statements is CORRECT?

    a. This may be used for infusion-related reactions from infliximab therapy.
    b. This may be used for infusion-related reactions from amphotericin therapy.
    c. This may be used for infusion-related reactions from fluconazole therapy.
    d. A and B
    e. All of the above

11. A physician has written a prescription for *Entocort EC*. Choose the appropriate therapeutic interchange:

    a. Prednisone EC
    b. Budesonide EC
    c. Azathioprine EC
    d. Mesalamine suppository
    e. Sulfasalazine EC

12. A physician has written a prescription for *Asacol*. Choose the appropriate therapeutic interchange:

    a. Prednisone
    b. Budesonide
    c. Azathioprine
    d. Mesalamine
    e. Sulfasalazine

ANSWERS

1-b, 2-e, 3-e, 4-e, 5-d, 6-a, 7-d, 8-c, 9-e, 10-d, 11-b, 12-d

ERECTILE DYSFUNCTION

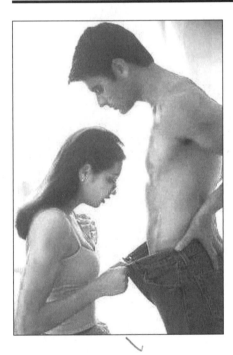

Background

The most common direct cause of erectile dysfunction (ED) is reduced blood flow to the penis, which is commonly caused by diseases, including diabetes, hypertension, heart disease, and nerve damage (most commonly due to diabetes). Hormone imbalances (such as low testosterone), psychological issues (including stress) and neurological illness can also cause ED. Some men will need testosterone replacement therapy in order to sustain an erection. In these cases, they are likely to have other signs of low testosterone. See the hormone therapy chapter for more information on testosterone.. Some men have more than one contributing factor contributing to ED. Also, select drugs can cause ED.

More common drugs that can cause sexual dysfunction include:

- Blood pressure medications – especially beta blockers, clonidine, methyldopa

- Antipsychotics – including haloperidol, chlorpromazine, fluphenazine and thioridazine

- Antidepressants – particularly SSRIs and SNRIs

- The BPH drugs finasteride, dutasteride and silodosin

- Chemotherapeutic agents that ↓ sex hormone levels, leuprolide *(Lupron)*, etc.

- Cimetidine – which blocks androgenic hormones

- Opioids, especially methadone

- Nicotine (smoking – the guy in the picture is a smoker)

Drug Therapy

The phosphodiesterase Type 5 (PDE5) Inhibitors are the primary drugs used for ED in males. We are not discussing female ED since there is not, at present, drugs with an indication for this condition. If a patient cannot tolerate PDE5 I's (or has a contraindication) there are a few other less effective options discussed at the end of this section.

Note that the PDE5-Is are used under different names for pulmonary arterial hypertension (PAH) – do not use same drugs under different names concurrently (duplicate therapy). For PAH:

Viagra

- Sildenafil *(Revatio)* is dosed at 20 mg three times a day (TID), taken approximately 4-6 hours apart, with or without food.

- Tadalafil *(Adcirca)* is dosed at 40 mg (two 20 mg tablets) taken once daily with or without food. *Cialis*

PHOSPHODIESTERASE TYPE 5 (PDE5) INHIBITORS

Following sexual stimulation (which is required), PDE5 inhibitors increase blood flow to the penis, causing an erection.

DRUG	DOSING	SIDE EFFECTS/MONITORING/ CONTRAINDICATIONS
Sildenafil (*Viagra*)	25, 50, 100 mg Start at 50 mg, taken ~1 hour before intercourse In elderly patients (age > 65) start with 25 mg	Sildenafil and Vardenafil: Best when taken on an empty stomach, avoid with fatty food (tadalafil is with or without food). For All: May cause dizziness or a sudden drop in blood pressure. Common adverse effects include headache, dyspepsia, flushing, runny nose, stomach pain, back pain *(Cialis).* Priapism (< 2%) – if erection lasts for > 4 hours (and is painful), get medical help right away.
Vardenafil (*Levitra*, *Staxyn ODT*)	5, 10, 20 mg Start at 10 mg, taken ~1 hour before intercourse In elderly patients (age > 65) start with 5 mg. Use this lower starting dose for patients with moderate hepatic impairment.	Sudden vision loss in one or both eyes – seek medical help right away. May cause permanent vision loss. Other visual problems (blurred vision, increased sensitivity to light, bluish haze, or temporary difficulty distinguishing between blue and green) may occur. Sudden decrease or loss of hearing have been reported, usually in one ear. Tinnitus is another rare, but possible, side effect.
Tadalafil (*Cialis*)	2.5, 5, 10, 20 mg Start at 10 mg, with or without food, taken ~ 1 hour before intercourse or 2.5-5 mg daily (for men who use Cialis > 2 times per week). ↓ dose to 5-10 mg with renal impairment. Do not exceed 10 mg with hepatic impairment. ALL 3 DRUGS: use lower doses if concurrent 3A4 Inhibitor; these drugs are 3A4 substrates.	

Drug Interactions

PDE5-Is Are Contraindicated With Nitrates!

- Concurrent use of nitrate medications (for example, nitroglycerin *[NitroQuick, Nitro-Bid, Nitro-DUR, Nitroderm, Nitrogard, Nitrolingual, Nitrostat]*, isosorbide mononitrate [ISMO], or isosorbide dinitrate *[Isordil, ISDN, Sorbitrate])* increases the potential for excessively low blood pressure. Taking nitrates is an <u>absolute contraindication</u> to the use of these medicines. These include the illicit drugs such as amyl nitrate and butyl nitrate ("poppers").

- If a patient with ED has taken a PDE5 inhibitor and then develops angina, nitroglycerin should not be used until after 24 h for sildenafil or vardenafil and after 48 h for tadalafil. Other anti-anginal and anti-ischemic therapies may be used - such as beta blockers, calcium channel blockers, aspirin, morphine, statins and percutaneous coronary intervention. (Sometimes nitrates are used in an acute emergency, despite this warning, with careful monitoring.)

Caution with PDE5-I and Concurrent Alpha Blocker Therapy
(tamsulosin – *Flomax*, doxazosin – *Cardura*, etc)

- Wording from the PI, which is the same for all 3:

- Caution is advised when PDE5 inhibitors are co-administered with alpha blockers. PDE5 inhibitors and alpha-adrenergic blocking agents are both vasodilators with BP lowering effects. When vasodilators are used in combination, an additive effect on BP may be anticipated. In some patients, concomitant use of these two drug classes can lower BP significantly leading to symptomatic hypotension (e.g. dizziness, light headedness, fainting).

- The precaution goes on to suggest that patients should be on stable alpha-blocker therapy before PDE5 inhibition and that lowest doses of the PDE5 inhibitors be used to initiate therapy. Conversely, if a patient is already taking an optimal dose of PDE5 inhibitor and an alpha blocker needs to be started, the alpha blocker should be started at the lowest dose, and preferably the alpha-1a selective agents are chosen (tamsulosin, silodosin).

If a person cannot or will not use PDE 5 Is, there are several alternatives, however they have methods of delivery that limit the acceptance of these options.

ALTERNATIVE AGENTS

DRUG	ROUTE	SIDE EFFECTS
Intracavernosal alprostadil *(Caverject)* Refrigerate vials, reconstitute prior to use	Injected via syringe into penis	Penile pain; hematoma; priapism Causes erection 5-10' after injection, lasts ~1 hr, max 3x/week and 1x/day
Transurethral alprostadil *(MUSE)* Refrigerate	Inserted into urethra	Penile pain
Tri-Mix gel (papaverine, phentolamine, and alprostadil) – compounded – not FDA approved	Inserted into urethra doses of 500 mcg	Penile pain

Practice Case

Jim is a 60 year-old male patient who has presented to his physician with complaints of impotence. He cannot sustain an erection. This has caused performance anxiety, which has worsened the situation. The patient's medical conditions include hypertension, anxiety/low mood, obesity and prostate enlargement. The physician has written him a prescription for sildenafil 50 mg to be taken 1 hour prior to sexual activity.

viagra

CATEGORY	
Medications	⍺ Tamsulosin 0.4 mg daily
	βᵦ *Inderal LA* 160 mg daily
	ᴬᶜᴱ Fosinopril 10 mg BID
	ˢˢᴿᴵ Sertraline 100 mg daily
	Vitamin D 200 IU daily
	Aspirin 325 mg daily
Vitals	Height 5'9", weight 210 lbs.

QUESTIONS

1. Is sildenafil contraindicated in this patient?

   a. Yes, the combination of tamsulosin and sildenafil is contraindicated.

   b. No, but he must be cautioned about dizziness, light headedness and fainting.

   c. No, but he has to begin sildenafil at 12.5 mg once daily.

   d. The tamsulosin should be changed to doxazosin; this is a safer combination.

   e. None of the above.

2. Which of the following medications could be contributing to Jim's problem with erectile dysfunction?

   a. *Inderal LA*

   b. Sertraline

   c. Vitamin D

   d. A and B only

   e. All of the above

3. The pharmacist should call the physician and recommend possible medication changes that could reduce or eliminate the ED problem. These suggestions should include:

   a. Change the sertraline to a medication that is not in the SSRI or SNRI class.

   b. Change propranolol to a different class of medication, or try a trial with metoprolol.

   c. Change the fosinopril to losartan.

   d. A and B only.

   e. None of the above.

4. If Jim begins sildenafil therapy, he should be counseled concerning the risk of priapism. Choose the correct counseling statement:

    a. If you sustain an erection that lasts more than 4 hours, you should stop using the medicine. The erection will go away in about 24 hours.

    b. If you sustain an erection that lasts more than 4 hours, you should stop using the medicine and take 25 mg of over-the-counter diphenhydramine. The erection will go away in about 24 hours.

    c. If you sustain an erection that lasts more than 4 hours, you should stop using the medicine and rest in bed until the erection goes away, which takes about 4-6 hours.

    d. If you sustain an erection that lasts more than 4 hours, you will need to get medical help right away. Priapism must be treated as soon as possible or it can cause lasting damage to the penis.

    e. None of the above.

Questions 5-10 do not apply to the above case.

5. A patient is using tadalafil three times weekly. He uses 10 mg, taken 1 hour before sexual intercourse. He has asked the physician to change him to the daily form of the medicine, since he uses it more than twice weekly. Choose the correct dosing range for daily tadalafil:

    a. 0.125-2.5 mg daily
    b. 2.5-5 mg daily
    c. 5-10 mg daily
    d. This medicine cannot be used daily
    e. None of the above

6. The PDE5 Is require lower doses, and in some cases avoidance, when a patient is using any of these drugs: ritonavir, indinavir, saquinavir, atazanavir, ketoconazole, itraconazole, erythromycin and clarithromycin. This is due to the following reason:

    a. These are potent CYP 3A4 inducers; they could cause the PDE5 I level to decrease to a dangerous level.

    b. These are potent CYP 3A4 inhibitors; they could cause the PDE5 I level to increase to a dangerous level.

    c. These are potent CYP 3A4 inducers; they could cause the PDE5 I level to increase to a dangerous level.

    d. These are potent CYP 3A4 inhibitors; they could cause the PDE5 I level to decrease to a dangerous level.

    e. There is no interaction between PDE5 Is and these medications.

7. Jon is a 58 year-old male with dyslipidemia, type 2 diabetes, hypertension and coronary heart disease. His medications include insulin glargine 40 U QHS, metformin 1 g BID, lisinopril-HCT 20-12.5 mg Q daily, vardenafil 10 mg as-needed, clopidogrel 75 mg Q daily and aspirin 81 mg EC Q daily. He went to his doctor with several medical complaints, including a dry, intermittent cough. The physician discontinued the lisinopril-HCT and gave him prescriptions for valsartan-HCT, *Restasis* and nitroglycerin SL 0.4 mg, as instructed. Which of the following action should the pharmacist take?

    a. Do not fill nitroglycerin SL
    b. Do not fill *Restasis*
    c. Do not fill valsartan-HCT
    d. A and B only
    e. A and C only

8. A young man is having difficulty sustaining an erection because he does not find his girlfriend to be sexually arousing but he does not wish to leave her because she has a lot of money. He has not had a problem with sexual dysfunction previously. Is sildenafil indicated in this case?

   a. Sildenafil is not indicated; the most likely problem is a lack of sexual desire.
   b. Yes, the drug will work, but he should break up with this woman.
   c. Yes, the drug will work but at a higher dose.
   d. He would be better off using tadalafil, since it is a more effective agent.
   e. None of the above.

9. A physician has written a prescription for *Levitra*. Which of the following represents an acceptable therapeutic substitution?

   a. Sildenafil
   b. Vardenafil
   c. Tadalafil
   d. Alprostadil
   e. Lansoprazole

10. A physician has written a prescription for *Cialis*. Which of the following represents an acceptable therapeutic substitution?

    a. Sildenafil
    b. Vardenafil
    c. Tadalafil
    d. Alprostadil
    e. Lansoprazole

ANSWERS

1-b, 2-d, 3-d, 4-d, 5-b, 6-b, 7-a, 8-a, 9-b, 10-c

61

BENIGN PROSTATIC HYPERPLASIA (BPH)

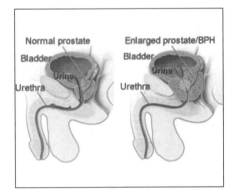

Background

The prostate is a walnut-sized gland that forms part of the male reproductive system. The prostate surrounds the urethra and squeezes fluid into the urethra as sperm moves through during sexual climax, energizing sperm and forming semen.

Both testosterone and estrogen contribute to prostate growth. The prostate has two main periods of growth. The first occurs early in puberty, when the prostate doubles in size. At around age 25, the gland begins to grow again. As the prostate enlarges, the layer of tissue surrounding it stops it from expanding, causing the gland to press against the urethra like a clamp on a garden hose. The bladder wall becomes thicker and irritated. The bladder begins to contract even when it contains small amounts of urine, causing more frequent urination. Eventually, the bladder weakens and loses the ability to empty itself, and some urine remains in the bladder. Interestingly, there is not a direct linear correlation between prostate size and symptoms; some men are more bothered even with a smaller prostate size, while others with a larger prostate are not as symptomatic. The enlargement does not usually cause problems until later in life. Over half of men in their 60's and as many as 90% in their 70's and 80's have symptoms of BPH.

SYMPTOMS/COMPLICATIONS

- Hesitant, interrupted, weak stream of urine

- Urgency and leaking or dribbling

- More frequent urination, especially nocturia (urination at night)

BPH rarely causes more severe symptoms – but if the blockage is severe, the urine could back up into the kidneys and result in acute renal failure. Urinary tract infection can also present, but is uncommon.

DIAGNOSIS

Prostate cancer symptoms may be similar to BPH and the Digital Rectal Examination (DRE) and Prostate Specific Antigen (PSA) can be used to rule out cancer as a cause of the symptoms. PSA, a protein produced by prostate cells, is frequently ↑ in prostate cancer – however, it can also increase from other conditions, including BPH. Note that the recommendations for routine prostate cancer screening have changed (they will be done less frequently than in the past); see oncology chapter.

DRUGS THAT WORSEN BPH SYMPTOMS

Combination cold medicines, decongestants, antihistamines and medications with anticholinergic side effects will worsen symptoms. Diuretics, if they must be used, should be dosed early in the day. Caffeine, if used (and it is a diuretic) should not be taken later in the day as it will worsen nocturia (night-time urination).

Treatment

Treatment for BPH depends primarily on the patient's perception of how bothered they are by the symptoms. A scoring system called the International Prostate Symptom Score (IPSS) is used, which is determined by the man's answers to questions on a scoring sheet. This is used to determine how bothersome the symptoms are to the patient. The mass of the prostate, as estimated by the physician, will also be used in therapy considerations. Initially, alpha blockers are used, alone or in combination with the 5-alpha-reductase inhibitors. In 2011 tadalafil *(Cialis)* was approved for mild symptom improvement in BPH (it primarily decreases urinary frequency). Concurrent use with alpha blockers will require careful dosing/caution for additive hypotension. The benefit from tadalafil is mild, but the use might also help men with concurrent erectile dysfunction and might provide a way to obtain insurance coverage for the ED drug. Some men will require non-pharmacological options, such as surgery.

NATURAL PRODUCTS

Saw palmetto is used for BPH, but it is rated as "possibly ineffective" by The Natural Medicines Database. If men wish to try saw palmetto, they should be counseled to be seen first to rule out the possibility of prostate cancer and to receive treatment, if needed. Pygeum is another natural product, and may be useful. Do not recommend a pygeum product unless it has been harvested ethically; ripping the bark off the trees to extract pygeum is not sustainable. Another natural product that may be useful is beta-sitosterol, which comes as supplements, in margarine substitutes, in African wild potato extract products, in pumpkin seed and in soy and red clover. Rye grass pollen is also used, including in Europe. (Lycopene is used for prostate cancer prevention, however there is not good evidence for taking supplements for this purpose.)

ALPHA BLOCKERS RELAX THE SMOOTH MUSCLE OF THE PROSTATE AND BLADDER NECK TO IMPROVE URINE FLOW.

DRUG	DOSING	SIDE EFFECTS/MONITORING/ CONTRAINDICATIONS

Non-Selective Alpha Blockers

DRUG	DOSING	SIDE EFFECTS/MONITORING/ CONTRAINDICATIONS
Terazosin (Hytrin)	Start at 1 mg, up to 2-10 mg daily (titrate slow), usually at bedtime	There are 3 types of alpha receptors: 1A (prostate primarily has these receptors), 1B, and 1D; terazosin and doxazosin are non-selective and this results in more orthostasis/dizziness/fatigue/HA than the selective agents Both classes of agents start to work right away, but efficacy may take weeks to months, they do not shrink the prostate and do not change PSA levels. **SIDE EFFECTS** Orthostatic hypotension, dizziness, fatigue (much less with selective agents) – can titrate Q 3-4 weeks, as-needed (to reduce dizziness/hypotension)
Doxazosin (Cardura)	Start 1-2 mg, up to 4-8 mg daily (titrate slow), usually at bedtime	The non-selective agents are often given QHS to help with the initial "first dose" effect of orthostasis/dizziness. This requires careful counseling (see below) as the man likely has nocturia, and getting up at night to use the bathroom with dizziness and orthostasis can be dangerous.

Selective Alpha Blockers

DRUG	DOSING	SIDE EFFECTS/MONITORING/ CONTRAINDICATIONS
Tamsulosin (Flomax, generic) + dutasteride (Jalyn)	0.4 mg (usually), can ↑ 0.8 mg	**SIDE EFFECTS** Tamsulosin, alfuzosin and silodosin are selective for 1A, with significantly ↓ incidence and severity of OH, dizziness, however they can still cause dizziness/fatigue/hypotension/HA – must include in counseling Do not use alfuzosin in patients at risk for QT prolongation – extends QT-interval Silodosin can cause retrograde ejaculation (stops with drug discontinuation) (28%)
Alfuzosin (Uroxatral)	10 mg ER, after same meal daily	Renal Caution with alfuzosin in CrCl < 30 mL/min Silodosin dosed at 4 mg if CrCl 30-50 mL/min, and CI if CrCl < 30 mL/min, or in severe liver disease Note that you may see alpha blockers in women – used for bladder outlet obstruction.
Silodosin (Rapaflo)	8 mg	Some men may also be using 5-a-reductase inhibitors to prevent prostate cancer (controversial at present)

ALPHA BLOCKER DRUG INTERACTIONS

- Caution is advised when PDE5 inhibitors *(Viagra/Revatio, Cialis/Adcirca, Levitra)* are co-administered with alpha blockers. PDE5 inhibitors and alpha blockers are both vaso-dilators with BP lowering effects. When they are used in combination, there will be an additive effect on BP. In some patients, concomitant use of these two drug classes can lower BP significantly leading to symptomatic hypotension (e.g., dizziness, light headedness, fainting). Patients should be stable on alpha-blocker therapy before PDE5 inhibition and the lowest doses of the PDE5 inhibitors should be used to initiate therapy. Conversely, if a patient is already taking an optimal dose of a PDE5 inhibitor and an alpha blocker needs to be started, the alpha blocker should be started at the lowest dose, and the selective agents will be preferred (over non-selective).

- Use caution with any low BP condition or with other drugs that lower BP.

- Alfuzosin and silodosin are hepatic substrates-can increase with potent 3A4 inhibitors (ritonavir, itraconazole, ketoconazole, clarithromycin, others) – use with potent 3A4 inhibitors is contraindicated.

- Silodosin cannot be used with strong P-gp inhibitors, such as cyclosporine.

- Alfuzosin: can cause QT-prolongation; do not use with other QT-prolongating agents.

ALPHA BLOCKER COUNSELING

- You should see an improvement of your symptoms within 1 to 2 weeks. In addition to your other regular checkups you will need to continue seeing your doctor regularly to check your progress regarding your BPH and to monitor your blood pressure.

- Especially for NON-selective agents, such as doxazosin: This medicine can cause a sudden drop in blood pressure. You may feel dizzy, faint or "light-headed," especially after you stand up from a lying or sitting position. This is more likely to occur after you have taken the first few doses or if you increase your dose, but can occur at any time while you are taking the drug. It can also occur if you stop taking the drug and then restart treatment. When you get up from a sitting or lying position, go slowly and hold onto the bed rail or chair until you are steady on your feet.

- Your blood pressure should be checked when you are sitting or lying down and standing.

- If you take the medicine at bedtime, but need to get up from bed to go to the bathroom, get up slowly and cautiously.

- You should not drive or do any hazardous tasks until you are used to the effects of the medicine. If you begin to feel dizzy, sit or lie down until you feel better.

- This medicine can cause side effects that may impair your thinking or reactions. Be careful if you drive or do anything that requires you to be awake and alert.

- Drinking alcohol can make the dizziness worse, and increase night-time urination if taken close to bedtime.

- Taking cold medicine such as decongestants and antihistamines can make your symptoms worsen. Discuss what to use with your pharmacist if you need assistance.

ALFUZOSIN

- Do not crush, chew, or break the alfuzosin tablets. Swallow them whole.

- Take immediately after the same meal each day (food increases absorption)

SILODOSIN

- Possibility of retrograde ejaculation (stops with drug discontinuation).

- Take with food.

5-α REDUCTASE INHIBITORS INHIBIT THE 5-α REDUCTASE ENZYME, WHICH BLOCKS THE CONVERSION OF TESTOSTERONE TO DHT

DRUG	DOSING	SIDE EFFECTS/MONITORING/CONTRAINDICATIONS
Finasteride (Proscar) Used for hair loss (*Propecia* 1 mg daily)	5 mg daily	Pregnancy Category X Pregnant women should not handle nor take these meds: can be absorbed through skin, can be detrimental to fetus, semen of male taking this drug may present a danger **SIDE EFFECTS** ↓ libido (0-3%), ↓ ejaculation (0.1-2.9%), impotence (0-4.4%) – sexual SEs ↓ with time; and approach placebo levels at one year of use
Dutasteride (Avodart) + tamsulosin (*Jalyn*) Affects both types of 5-α-receptors (types 1 and 2), may have better efficacy; not proven.	0.5 mg soft gel daily	6 months of treatment may be required for maximal efficacy Usually used in men with larger prostate size (40+ grams) or more severe symptoms; due to the slow-onset, often given with α-blocker 5-α reductase inhibitors SHRINK the prostate and ↓ PSA levels

PDE5 INHIBITORS: MILD EFFECTIVENESS FOR BPH SYMPTOM IMPROVEMENT IS THOUGHT TO BE DUE TO EFFECT ON CGMP, BUT IS NOT WELL ESTABLISHED

DRUG	DOSING	SIDE EFFECTS/MONITORING/CONTRAINDICATIONS
Tadalafil (Cialis)	5 mg daily, same time each day CrCl 30-50 mL/min 2.5 mg, if CrCl < 30 mL/min, do not use. Use 2.5 mg at start if using 3A4 inhibitor, or alpha blocker concurrently (due to additive hypotension)	**SIDE EFFECTS** Dizziness, drop in blood pressure, headache, flushing, runny nose, stomach pain, back pain, indigestion Priapism (< 2%) – if erection lasts for > 4 hours, get medical help right away Sudden vision loss in one or both eyes – seek medical help right away. May cause permanent vision loss Other visual problems (blurred vision, increased sensitivity to light, bluish haze, or temporary difficulty distinguishing between blue and green) may occur Sudden decrease or loss of hearing have been reported, usually in one ear. Tinnitus is another rare, but possible, side effect

5-α REDUCTASE INHIBITOR DRUG INTERACTIONS

- Dutasteride is a CYP 3A4 and 3A5 substrate; potential for interactions; not studied.

- Do not use finasteride in a patient using *Propecia* for hair loss; refer to prescriber.

5-α REDUCTASE INHIBITOR COUNSELING

- Women who are or may become pregnant should not handle the tablets. (These drugs can cause birth defects to a developing male fetus – Preg. Categ. X). The semen of males using the medicine may also be harmful.

- Your doctor may perform blood tests or other forms of monitoring during treatment with finasteride. One of the tests that may be performed is called PSA (prostate-specific antigen). This drug can reduce the amount of PSA in the blood.

- Tell your doctor if you experience any of these side effects: decreased sex drive, decreased volume of ejaculate, impotence, breast tenderness or enlargement.

- Taking cold medicine such as decongestants and antihistamines can make your symptoms worsen. Discuss what to use with your pharmacist if you need assistance.

For drug interactions/counseling for tadalafil, please refer to Erectile Dysfunction chapter.

OVERACTIVE BLADDER

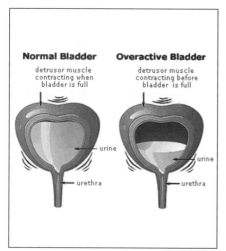

Normal Bladder
detrusor muscle
contracting when
bladder is full
urine
urethra

Overactive Bladder
detrusor muscle
contracting before
bladder is full
urine
urethra

Background

Overactive bladder (OAB) is a common, disabling urinary disorder that affects many people (1 in 6 people or over 33 million Americans). It is not a normal sign of aging. In overactive bladder, the detrusor muscle contracts frequently and before the bladder is full, leading to the classic symptoms of:

- urinary urgency with or without urge incontinence

- urinary frequency (voiding ≥ 8 times in a 24 hour period), and

- nocturia (≥ 2 awakenings to void per night)

Overactive bladder can lead to urinary incontinence. About 1/3 of patients have incontinent episodes (OAB wet) and the other 2/3 of patients do not have incontinence (OAB dry).

Implications of Overactive Bladder

Many co-morbidities exist in patients with OAB including falls and fractures, skin infections, UTIs, depression, and sexual dysfunction. Due to embarrassment of their condition, there are many social implications that go along with OAB including low self-esteem, lack of sexual intimacy, social and physical isolation, sleep disturbances, limits on travel, and dependence on caregivers (e.g. nursing home). Many patients become dehydrated because they limit their fluid intake. The cost of pads and adult diapers can be a huge financial burden.

FORMS OF URINARY INCONTINENCE

Functional incontinence

- There is no abnormality in the bladder, but the patient may be cognitively, socially, or physically impaired thus hindering him or her from access to a toilet (e.g. patients in wheelchairs)

Overflow incontinence

- Leakage that occurs when the quantity of urine stored in the bladder exceeds its capacity

- Benign Prostatic Hyperplasia (BPH) is the most common cause

Stress incontinence

- Urine leaks out during any form of exertion (e.g. exercise, coughing, sneezing, laughing, etc.) as a result of pressure on the bladder

Urge incontinence

- Patient cannot hold in urine long enough to reach the toilet

- Associated with neuropathy: often found in those who have diabetes, strokes, dementia, Parkinson's disease, or multiple sclerosis (although people without co-morbidities are affected also)

- Can be warning sign of bladder cancer

Mixed incontinence

- Combination of urge and stress incontinence

Approximately 1/3 of incontinence is stress, 1/3 is urge and 1/3 is mixed.

RISK FACTORS FOR OVERACTIVE BLADDER

- Age > 40 years

- Diabetes

- Restricted mobility

- Obesity

- Prior vaginal delivery

- Neurologic conditions (e.g. stroke, Parkinson's disease, dementia)

- Hysterectomy

- Concurrent use of certain medications (e.g. diuretics, bethanechol, cholinesterase inhibitors, alpha antagonists)

- Pelvic injury

NON-PHARMACOLOGICAL THERAPY

Behavioral Therapy: Kegel exercises

- These are exercises done to strengthen the pelvic floor muscles; can improve or diminish signs and symptoms of urinary incontinence

- Proper technique is key and this means finding the correct muscles. Imagine that you are trying to stop yourself from passing gas. Squeeze the muscles you would use. If you sense a "pulling" feeling, those are the right muscles for pelvic exercise.

- Pull in the pelvic muscles and hold for a count of 3. Then relax for a count of 3. Work up to 3 sets of 10 repeats. Be patient. Do not give up. It takes just 5 minutes, three times a day to strengthen the muscles and reduce wetting incidents.

Additional therapies

- Bladder diary, bladder training, education about lifestyle interventions, regulate fluid intake, eliminate bladder irritants, and maintain bowel regularity.

PHARMACOLOGICAL THERAPY

Anticholinergic drugs are muscarinic receptor antagonists that compete with acetylcholine, thus blocking contractions of the detrusor muscle.

DRUG	DOSING	SIDE EFFECTS/CONTRAINDICATIONS/MONITORING
Oxybutynin *(Ditropan)* **Oxybutynin XL *(Ditropan XL)*** Oxybutynin patch *(Oxytrol)* Oxybutynin 10% topical *(Gelnique)*	5 mg PO BID-TID 5-30 mg PO daily 3.9 mg daily (patch is dosed 2x/week) Apply contents of 1 sachet to intact, dry skin (gel)	**SIDE EFFECTS** Dry mouth, constipation, dry eyes/blurred vision, urinary retention, somnolence, dizziness, cognitive impairment (especially with oxybutynin and tolterodine)
Tolterodine *(Detrol)* **Tolterodine ER *(Detrol LA)***	1-2 mg PO BID 2-4 mg PO daily	**CONTRAINDICATIONS** Urinary retention, bladder outlet obstruction, gastric retention, decreased gastric motility and uncontrolled narrow angle glaucoma
Trospium *(Sanctura, Sanctura XR)*	20 mg BID or 60mg XR daily and take on empty stomach	↓ dose in renal impairment (CrCl < 30 mL/min) with fesoterodine, solifenacin, tolterodine, and trospium (do not use Trospium XR formulation in these patients) Extended-release formulations have less incidence of dry mouth than their IR counterparts
Solifenacin *(Vesicare)*	5-10 mg PO daily	Oxybutynin patch and gel causes less dry mouth and constipation than oral forms. Darifenacin may cause more constipation
Darifenacin *(Enablex)*	7.5-15 mg PO daily	
Fesoterodine *(Toviaz)*	4-8 mg PO daily	

DRUG INTERACTIONS

- All of the anticholinergics may have additive effects with other medications that have anticholinergic side effects.

- Tolterodine – do not exceed 2 mg/day when administered with potent 3A4 inhibitors.

- Solifenacin – do not exceed 5 mg/day when administered with potent 3A4 inhibitors.

- Darifenacin – do not exceed 7.5 mg/day when administered with potent 3A4 inhibitors.

- Fesoterodine – do not exceed 4 mg/day when administered with potent 3A4 inhibitors.

PATIENT COUNSELING

Overactive Bladder Drugs (e.g. *Detrol LA*)

- This medication is used to treat symptoms of an over-functioning bladder

- Certain medications can interact with this medication. Tell your doctor or pharmacist of the medications you are currently taking including any over the counter products, vitamins and herbal supplements.

- Take directly as prescribed by your doctor.

- Swallow the capsules whole.

- Can be taken without regards to meals (except trospium which needs to be taken on an empty stomach).

- If you miss a dose, forget it. Just take your next scheduled dose. Do not take 2 doses within the same day.

- This medicine can cause dry mouth. Some formulations of incontinence medicines cause more dry mouth than others (the longer-lasting forms tend to cause less dry mouth). If dry mouth is bothersome, please discuss with your doctor. Using sugar-free lozenges and sucking on ice chips may be helpful. And, remember to take good care of your teeth since dry mouth contributes to tooth decay.

- Another possible side effect of this medicine is constipation. Some formulations of the incontinence medicines cause more constipation than others [darifenacin *(Enablex)* may cause the most]. Your diet should be rich in fibers, including vegetables and whole-grains. Make sure to consume adequate fluids. A stool softener, such as docusate, may be helpful. If not, a laxative such as senna may be helpful. You may need to discuss this with your doctor. If you have any type of serious constipation or "GI" problems currently, you should let your doctor know.

- Other side effects can include dizziness or drowsiness. Do not operate any dangerous machinery (or cars) until you know how this medicine affects your concentration and coordination.

- Doing pelvic floor muscle (Kegel) exercises in combination with this medicine will work better than taking the medicine alone. You should get instructions on how to do this correctly, and do them for a few minutes three times daily, so you can slowly build up these muscles.

Oxytrol **Patch**

- The patch has fewer anticholinergic side effects such as less dry mouth.

- Apply one patch to dry, intact skin on the abdomen, hip, or buttock.

- The patch is changed every 3 to 4 days (2 times weekly).

- Try to always change the patch on the same 2 days of the week to help you remember.

- Open the pouch and remove the protective liner from the patch to expose the adhesive.

- Press firmly to be sure the patch stays on.

- Apply to an area of skin that is under clothing and protected from sunlight. Avoid applying the patch on your waistline, since tight clothing may rub the patch off, or on areas where sitting may loosen it.

- Do not apply the patch to areas of skin that are irritated, oily, or to where lotions or powders have been applied.

- The patch must be removed prior to having a MRI procedure.

- Contact with water (e.g., swimming, bathing) will not change the way the drug works. Avoid rubbing the patch area during these activities.

- If the area around the patch becomes red, itchy, or irritated, try a new site. If irritation continues or becomes worse, notify your doctor promptly.

Oxybutynin topical *(Gelnique)*

- This formulation causes less anticholinergic side effects (e.g., less dry mouth).

- Each packet of oxybutynin gel is for one use only.

- Apply to abdomen, upper arm/shoulders, or thighs. Rub into skin until dry. Use a different site each day (cannot use the same site two days in a row.)

- Do not shower for 1 hour after application.

- Cover treated area with clothing.

- Oxybutynin gel is flammable. Avoid using near open flame, and do not smoke until the gel has completely dried on your skin.

GLAUCOMA, ALLERGIC CONJUNCTIVITIS, OTHER OPTHALMICS & OTICS

ABBREVIATION	MEANING	CAUTION
AD, AS, AU	Right Ear, Left Ear, Each Ear	These directions can be mistaken (interchanged) for each other & may mean other things: know how to interpret them but it is safer to write them out: use right eye, left eye, each eye, right ear, left ear, each ear.
OD, OS, OU	Right Eye, Left Eye, Each Eye	
Memory tip: <u>A</u> is from the Latin for ear (auris), <u>O</u> is from eye (oculus), <u>D</u> is from right (dextra) and <u>S</u> is from left (sinistra).		

- Eye drops and ear drops are either solutions or suspensions.

- <u>Suspensions</u> require <u>shaking</u> prior to use.

- Use Aux Labels: "For Use in the Eye" or "For Use in the Ear"

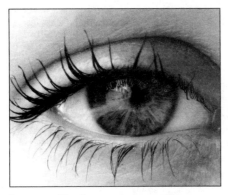

Background

Glaucoma is an eye disease caused by an increase in intraocular pressure (IOP). If left untreated, glaucoma can result in damage to the optic nerve and gradual loss of vision. There may be no symptoms felt by the patient, although some may experience eye pain, headache, or decreased vision.

There are two main forms of glaucoma. Angle-closure, or closed-angle glaucoma is treated in the hospital and is a medical emergency. The more common type, open-angle glaucoma, is most commonly treated with eye drops.

Risk Factors

Include family history, increased age, African Americans and nearsightedness (myopia). A history of eye surgeries and diabetes can be contributory.

DRUGS THAT MAY INCREASE IOP &/OR SHOULD BE AVOIDED IF POSSIBLE IN PATIENTS WITH GLAUCOMA

- Cough/cold/motion sickness medications (antihistamines)

- Anticholinergics (e.g., oxybutynin, tolterodine, benztropine, trihexyphenidyl, tricyclics)

- Chronic corticosteroids, especially eye drops such as prednisolone and others

- Beta-agonists (e.g. albuterol)

- Topiramate *(Topamax)*

PHARMACOLOGICAL TREATMENT

Before latanoprost *(Xalatan)*, the first prostaglandin analog (PA) to become available, beta blockers (most commonly timolol) were used as first-line agents to lower IOP. Now, PAs are often used 1st (they lower IOP more than beta blockers and are approved for initial use), and beta blockers are often used afterwards, if needed. Beta blockers are used initially most commonly when only one eye needs to be treated, as it would be distasteful to cause iris darkening in one eye only.

Be careful since the beta blockers used for glaucoma are non-selective agents and can be poorly tolerated in some patients. Often, a multiple drug regimen is necessary to adequately control glaucoma and many of the medications come in combination formulas. Pharmacists should make sure patients are inserting eye drops or gel appropriately in order to get the most benefit from the medication. If you ask, you will find that most patients do not hold the lacrimal duct down (closed) for an adequate time period (if at all) after inserting the medication.

GLAUCOMA MEDICATION THERAPY

DRUG	DOSING	SIDE EFFECTS/CLINICAL CONCERNS
Beta Blockers, Nonselective: reduce aqueous humor production		
Timolol 0.25% and 0.5% **(Timoptic, Timoptic-XE)** Levobunolol *(Betagan)* Carteolol *(Ocupress)* Metipranolol *(OptiPranolol)* Betaxolol *(Betoptic, Betoptic S)*	*Timoptic* is QD or BID *Timoptic-XE* is a gel taken QD	**SIDE EFFECTS** Can cause burning, stinging or itching of the eyes or eyelids, changes in vision, increased sensitivity of the eyes to light These are all non-selective beta blockers (except for betaxolol); although most medicine stays local, it is best to try and avoid in asthma, COPD, chronic bronchitis, emphysema, or advanced cardiac disease – some patients will have exacerbated symptoms – especially if used incorrectly Some contain sulfites, which can cause allergic reactions

Glaucoma Medication Therapy Continued

DRUG	DOSING	SIDE EFFECTS/CLINICAL CONCERNS

Prostaglandin Analogs: increase aqueous outflow

Travoprost *(Travatan Z)* **Bimatoprost** *(Lumigan)* **Latanoprost** *(Xalatan)* Unoprostone *(Rescula)* **Latanoprost**: store unopened bottles in refrigerator	All once daily at night, except *Rescula* is BID Cannot be administered with contact lenses – remove and wait 15 min prior to re-insertion (most given QHS so this is not an issue but tell patient)	**SIDE EFFECTS** An increase in brown pigment in the iris and gradual changes in eye color may occur; eyelash growth and pigmentation may increase; skin on the eyelids and around the eyes may darken Eyelash changes: ↑ length, thickness, number (goes away when drug discontinued) Eye redness (ocular hyperemia), tearing, eye pain, or lid crusting Bimatoprost *(Latisse)* is indicated for eyelash hypotrichosis (to↑ eyelash growth) – do not use concurrently with same class for glaucoma without MDs approval (using PAs more frequently ↓ effectiveness) *Travatan Z* does not contain benzalkonium chloride (BAK), instead has different preservative. This may be helpful to some with reaction to BAK or dry eye, but most people are fine with the much less expensive, generic latanoprost.

Miotics: increase aqueous outflow

Carbachol *(Carbastat, Isopto Carbachol, Miostat)* Pilocarpine *(Pilocar, Piloptic, Pilostat)*	*Isopto, Pilocar* are dosed 1-2 drops, up to 6 times daily	Use with caution if history of retinal detachment or corneal abrasion

Carbonic Anhydrase Inhibitors: reduce aqueous humor production

Acetazolamide *(Diamox)* Brinzolamide *(Azopt)* **Dorzolamide** *(Trusopt)* **Dorzolamide HCl/ timolol** *(Cosopt)*	*Azopt, Trusopt* are TID	Bitter or unusual taste 5-10%

Adrenergics: increase aqueous outflow, reduce production

Apraclonidine *(Iopidine)* **Brimonidine** *(Alphagan)* Dipivefrin *(Propine)*	*Iopidine, Alphagan* are dosed TID Brominidine+Timolol *(Combigan)*	Can cause macular edema (swelling of the macula, the center part of the retina) and eye irritation

Patient Counseling (eye drops)

- Wash your hands.

- Before you open the bottle, shake it a few times.

- Bend your neck back a little so that you're looking up. Use one finger to pull down your lower eyelid. It is helpful, at least initially, to use a mirror.

- Without letting the tip of the bottle touch your eye or eyelid, squeeze one drop of the medicine into the space between your eye and your lower eyelid. If you squeeze in more than one drop, you are wasting medicine.

- After you squeeze the drop of medicine into your eye, close your eye. Then press a finger between your eye and the top of your nose. Press for at least one full minute (or longer if instructed by your doctor). This way, more of the medicine stays in your eye. You will be less likely to have side effects.

If you need to take more than one glaucoma medicine:

- Put a drop of the first medicine in your eye. Wait at least 10 minutes to put the second medicine in your eye. If you're taking three medicines, wait 10 more minutes before putting the third medicine in your eye. If you don't wait 10 minutes between medicines, some of the medicine may run out of your eye. If the medicine runs out of your eye, it does not help.

- If someone else puts your medicines in your eye for you, remind that person to wait 10 minutes between each medicine.

Prostaglandin Analog Counseling Specifics

- Remove contact lenses before using this medication because it contains a preservative that can be absorbed by the lenses, and cause them to become discolored. Wait at least 15 minutes after using this medication before putting your lenses back in.

- You may experience an increase in brown pigment in the iris and gradual changes in eye color (for this reason, they are not usually administered to patients with light eyes who have glaucoma in one eye only). Eyelash growth and pigmentation may increase (which is often pleasing to the patient). The skin on the eyelids and around the eyes may darken.

- This medicine is well-tolerated, but occasionally a patient can experience excessive tearing, eye pain, or lid crusting. If this occurs, please discuss with your doctor.

- Latanoprost (Xalatan) unopened bottles should be stored in the refrigerator.

- Do not use this medicine if you are also using Bimatoprost (Latisse), to increase eyelash growth, without your doctor's approval. Latisse may reduce the effectiveness of the glaucoma medicine.

Timolol (Timoptic) Counseling Specifics

- Common side effects from beta blockers include burning/stinging or itching of the eyes, and possible light sensitivity

- Timolol is a non-selective beta blocker, and although proper application should keep most of the medicine local, it is <u>best to avoid in patients with asthma, COPD, chronic bronchitis, emphysema, or advanced cardiac disease</u>. The medicine might exacerbate the disease symptoms. If you have any of these conditions, please discuss if this medicine is safe to use.

- <u>If dispensing the drops in the *Ocudose* dispenser</u>: To open the bottle, unscrew the cap by turning as indicated by the arrows on the top of the cap. Do not pull the cap directly up and away from the bottle. Pulling the cap directly up will prevent your dispenser from operating properly.

- Invert the bottle, and press lightly with the thumb or index finger over the "Finger Push Area" until a single drop is dispensed into the eye.

- If dispensing the gel *(Timoptic XE)*: Turn the container upside down once and shake the contents prior to use (the gel is a suspension and needs to be mixed). The gel is used once daily.

Other Ocular Conditions

COMMON AGENTS KNOWN TO CAUSE VISION CHANGES/DAMAGE

- Amiodarone (corneal deposits, optic neuropathy)

- Digoxin (yellow/green vision, blurriness, halos)

- Ethambutol, linezolid *(Zyvox)* (optic neuropathy, especially with chronic use)

- Hydroxychloroquine *(Plaquenil)* (retinopathy)

- Isoniazid (optic neuritis)

- Isotretinoin (↓ night vision which may be permanent, dry eyes/irritation)

- Sildenafil *(Viagra)* and other PDE5-Inhibitors used for ED and PAH (greenish tinge around objects, possible permanent vision loss in one or both eyes)

- Tamoxifen *(Nolvadex)* (corneal changes, decreased color perception)

- Voriconazole *(Vfend)* (abnormal vision, color vision change, photophobia)

ALLERGIC CONJUNCTIVITIS TREATMENT

OVER THE COUNTER (OTC)

Antihistamine/Decongestant

Naphazoline/pheniramine *(Naphcon-A, Opcon-A, Visine-A)*

Antihistamine

Ketotifen *(Zaditor, Alaway)*

PRESCRIPTION

Antihistamine

Levocetirizine *(Xyzal)*

Emedastine *(Emadine)*

NSAID

Ketorolac *(Acular, Acular PF)*

Mast Cell Stabilizer

Cromolyn

Lodoxamine *(Alomide)*

Nedocromil *(Alocril)*

Pemirolast *(Alamast)*

Antihistamine/Mast Cell Stabilizer

Azelastine *(Optivar)*

Epinastine *(Elestat)*

Olopatadine *(Patanol)*

Steroids: Short term use, caution for ↑ IOP

Dexamethasone Na+

Loteprednol *(Alrex, Lotemax)*

Medrysone *(HMS Liquifilm)*

Prednisolone acetate 1%

ALLERGIC CONJUNCTIVITIS

Background

A clear, thin membrane called the conjunctiva covers the eyeball and inside of the eyelids. If something irritates this covering, the eyes can become red, swollen and may itch. This is called conjunctivitis, or sometimes "pink eye." Common irritants include bacteria, viruses or allergens (animal skin or secretions, pollen, perfumes, air pollution, smoke).

Pharmacological Treatment

Different classes of medicines are used. Two are OTC – naphazoline/pheniramine *(Visine* and others) and the antihistamine ketotifen *(Zaditor, Alaway)*, a beneficial more recent addition to the OTC arsenal.

Counsel patients to remove contact lenses prior to use (true for most eye drops) and wait 15 minutes afterwards before reinserting. Many eye drops cause a slight temporary burning or stinging when used.

If a corticosteroid is prescribed watch out for chronic use: these can cause glaucoma, or further raise intraocular pressure (IOP).

If any eye condition worsens after a few days or does not improve refer to the physician.

DRY EYES

Background

Dry eyes can be caused by medications (primarily anticholinergics/antihistamines), environmental triggers (such as pollution, smoke) and an imbalance in tear production.

Pharmacological Treatment

The use of artificial teardrops is the primary treatment for dry eye. Popular artificial teardrops available over the counter are *Systane, Refresh, Clear Eyes* and *Liquifilm*.

It may be necessary to try a couple of different OTC eye drops before finding one that provides the most comfort. If the preservative is irritating (likely benzoyl peroxide) most artificial tear drops come in individual use containers that are preservative-free. If the eyes dry out while sleeping an ointment may be preferable.

In 2002 the FDA approved cyclosporine eye drops *(Restasis)* for patients who did not get satisfactory relief from other measures, including ductal occlusion (lacrimal duct plugs). *Restasis* provides benefit for a small percentage of users and is expensive – patients should be instructed to monitor for benefit. This is by a reduction in symptoms AND a reduction in the use of OTC drops.

CYCLOSPORINE EMULSION EYE DROPS

DRUG	DOSING	SIDE EFFECTS/FORMULATIONS/CONTRAINDICATIONS
Cyclosporine Emulsion Eye Drops (Restasis)	1 drop to each eye twice daily (~12 hours apart)	REQUIRES MEDGUIDE WHICH STATES: The emulsion from one individual single-use vial is to be used immediately after opening for administration to one or both eyes, and the remaining contents should be discarded immediately after administration. Do not allow the tip of the vial to touch the eye or any surface, as this may contaminate the emulsion. Do not administer while wearing contact lenses. (may be reinserted 15 mins afterwards.) **SIDE EFFECTS** (unusual) Burning, stinging, redness, pain, or itching eye Blurred vision, feeling as if something is in the eye, or eye discharge may also occur

ANTIBIOTIC EYE DROPS FOR BACTERIAL CONJUNCTIVITIS (PINK EYE) & OTHER EYE INFECTIONS

Common eye drops: pharmacists should know what is in them and be able to counsel for temporary stinging and reporting if situation worsens – and to limit contact lens use during an infection. Since these are antibiotics the patient should complete the duration of therapy. Some patients will have an allergic reaction to the eye drop and will need to return to the doctor if the condition worsens.

- Azithromycin *(Azasite)* – stored in refrigerator, 14 days at room temp.
- Moxifloxacin *(Vigamox)*
- Besifloxacin *(Besivance)*
- Tobramycin/Dexamethasone (Antibiotic/Steroid)

Other common antibiotic eye drops

- Ciprofloxacin *(Ciloxan)*, ofloxacin *(Ocuflox)*, gentamicin *(Garamycin)*, tobramycin *(Tobrex)*, erythromycin, sulfacetamide *(Bleph-10, Sulamyd)*, trimethoprim/polymyxin *(Polytrim)*, neomycin/bacitracin/polymyxin *(Neosporin)*.

Common antibiotic ointments used for blepharitis (eyelid inflammation)

- Note that treatment does not always warrant medication use – warm compresses such as a washcloth to the outer eyelids, gentle cleansing and gentle massage may be all that is required and is considered first-line. Occasionally, medications are used and in some patients blepharitis can be chronic and cause considerable distress.
- Bacitracin or erythromycin ointment, applied BID to QID.

OTICS

Swimmer's ear, otitis media pain

- Antipyrine and benzocaine (*A/B Otic, Auralgan*)

- Benzocaine (*Americaine Otic*)

Ear drops with antibiotics may also be used for outer ear infections. A few common products:

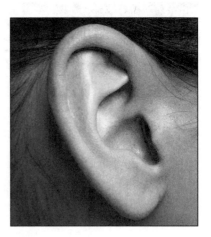

- Ciprofloxacin and hydrocortisone *(Cipro HC)*

- Ciprofloxacin and dexamethasone (*Ciprodex*)

- Ciprofloxacin (*Floxin Otic, Floxin Otic Singles*)

- Neomycin and hydrocortisone (*Cortisporin-TC*)

Ear wax (cerumen) removal

- Carbamide peroxide (*Debrox*)

- Triethanolamine (*Cerumenex*)

- A ntipyrine and benzocaine (*Auralgan*)

OTIC MEDICATION APPLICATION

- If cold hold the bottle for 1 or 2 minutes to warm the solution. Ear drops that are too cold will be uncomfortable and may cause dizziness.

- Lie down or tilt the head so that the affected ear faces up.

- Gently pull the earlobe up and back for adults (down and back for children) to straighten the ear canal.

- Administer the prescribed number of drops into the ear canal. Keep the ear facing up for about 5 minutes to allow the medicine to coat the ear canal.

- Do not touch the dropper tip to any surface. To clean wipe with a clean tissue.

Ear wax removal: flush ear with warm water after you have used the medicine for 2-3 days. (This may be done in doctor's office.)

MOTION SICKNESS

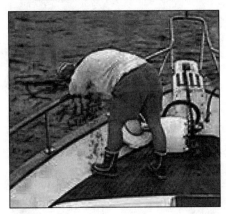

Background

Motion sickness (kinetosis) is also called seasickness or airsickness. Symptoms are nausea, dizziness and fatigue. People can get motion sickness on a moving boat, train, airplane, car, or amusement park rides. This is a common condition.

Nonpharmacological Treatment

Some patients find benefit with a wrist band that presses on an acupuncture point located on the inside of the wrist, about the length of 2 fingernails up the arm from the center of the wrist crease. One popular brand is *Sea-Band*.

NATURAL PRODUCTS

Ginger, in teas or supplements, is used most commonly. Peppermint may be helpful.

Pharmacological Treatment

Medications for motion sickness are anticholinergics and may cause drowsiness and may impair judgment. Pilots, ship crew members, or anyone operating heavy equipment or driving a car should not take them.

Scopolamine *(Transderm Scop)* is the most commonly prescribed medication for motion sickness. It is not more effective than generically-available OTC agents but is applied topically (behind the ear) and is taken less frequently (apply 4-6 hours prior to need, lasts three days, do not cut patch, alternate ears, wash hands afterwards).

Antihistamines used for motion sickness include cyclizine (*Marezine*), diphenhydramine *(Benadryl)*, dimenhydrinate *(Dramamine)* or Meclizine *(Bonine)*.

Promethazine is used and is prescription only. Do not use promethazine in children. All promethazine products carry a black box warning contraindicating use in children less than 2 years and strongly cautioning use in children age 2 and older. The FDA advises against the use of promethazine with codeine cough syrups in children less than 6 years of age, due to the risk of respiratory depression, cardiac arrest and neurological problems.

All of the antihistamines have anticholinergic effects similar to scopolamine. Make sure the oral agents are taken prior to travel (30-60 minutes prior) and ensure that the patient knows they will get tired. Instruct them not to consume alcohol or other CNS depressants.

DRUG	DOSING	SIDE EFFECTS/FORMULATIONS/CONTRAINDICATIONS
Scopolamine 3-day patch *(Transderm Scop)* Applied behind ear Q 72 hrs, rotate ears	1.5 mg, patch placed behind ear (hairless), 4-6 hours before needed (or evening before AM surgery – remove 24 hours after surgery) Primarily for motion sickness and occasionally used inpatient. Do not cut patch, wash hands after application.	**SIDE EFFECTS** Dry mouth, dizziness, stinging eyes (if touch eyes after handling patch), pupil dilation Confusion (can be significant in elderly, frail) **RARELY** Hallucinations, tachycardia Remove patch prior to MRI
Meclizine *(Antivert)*	12.5-25 mg 30-60 minutes before needed.	1st generation antihistamine: see diphenhydramine in allergies or insomnia chapters for complete discussion and counseling. Drug is highly sedating and causes anticholinergic side effects (dry mouth, urinary retention, constipation, dry/blurry vision, tachycardia) Will worsen BPH symptoms, can elevate IOP (glaucoma), and worsen cognition (elderly)
OTHER ANTIHISTAMINES USED Cyclizine Diphenhydramine Dimenhydrinate Promethazine [Rx-do not use in children due to (primarily) risk of respiratory depression.]		

TRANSDERM SCOP COUNSELING

- Wear only one patch at any time.

- No alcohol. Try to avoid other drugs that make you tired – this drug causes significant drowsiness. Do not use in children.

- The most common side effect is dryness of the mouth. Other common side effects are drowsiness, temporary blurring of vision and dilation (widening) of the pupils may occur, especially if the drug is on your hands and comes in contact with the eyes.

- Remover prior to an MRI procedure or the patch will burn your skin.

- Infrequently, some people get disoriented, and others can get confusion, hallucinations or heart palpitations. If any of these occur remove the patch and contact your doctor.

HOW TO USE

- Peel off the clear backing from the patch and apply <u>it to a clean, dry, hairless area of the skin behind the ear.</u> <u>Press firmly for at least 30 seconds</u> to make sure the patch sticks well, especially around the edges. The patch will slowly release the medication into your body over 3 days. Do not use the patch if it appears broken, cut, or damaged. <u>Apply at least 4 hours before activity that will cause motion sickness.</u>

- Be sure to <u>wash your hands thoroughly with soap and water immediately after handling the patch,</u> so that any drug that might get on your hands <u>will not come into contact with your eyes.</u>

- Also wash the area behind the ear where the patch was removed.

COMMON SKIN CONDITIONS

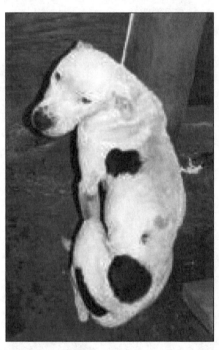

Guidelines

There are various conditions presented in this section and treatments for each are presented below. It can be difficult to determine the type of skin condition – which are often presented by the patient to the community pharmacist. *The Handbook of OTC Drugs* has pictures of common conditions, and many more are available at www.dermnet.com. If recommending OTC treatment it is important to tell the patient to be seen by a physician if the condition does not improve or worsens. You should be able to recognize a blemish that could be skin cancer; see the pictures and description in the oncology section.

Aloe is a natural product produced from the aloe vera plant that is used for many skin conditions, including sunburn and psoriasis. It has little proven efficacy but if used as a gel or lotion it may provide a soothing effect.
Tea tree oil is used for a variety of skin conditions. It can be useful for treating acne. It may be helpful for onychomycosis symptoms (depending on the dose and application schedule), but is not useful in eradicating the infection in most patients. Tea tree oil may also be useful for athlete's foot symptoms if the 10% oil is used (not tea tree cream). Higher concentrations (25 or 50%) can cure the infection in up to half of patients, but are not as effective as the recommended antifungal agents. This efficacy data is from the Natural Medicines Database. Help your patients choose a reputable product.

CONDITION	NOTES	SAFETY/COUNSELING

Acne: Recommend test dose of any product 1ˢᵗ to check for irritation. Continue treatment for full trial period (requires time to work).

Retinoids 1ˢᵗ line agents Tretinoin cream *(Retin-A)* Slower-release, less skin irritation with: ■ Microsphere gel *(Retin-A Micro)* ■ Polymerized cream or gel *(Avita)* -**Adapalene *(Differin)*** cream, solution well tolerated with little to no skin irritation. Combo drug: Adapalene+BPO *(Epiduo)* Tazarotene *(Tazorac)* Dapsone gel *(Aczone)* (new formulation, 2009, not in guidelines) Tretinoin *(Retin-A Micro)* is a gel, and comes pre-formulated in a tube or pump dispenser and does not require refrigeration. Retinoids are popular and there are many other products, such as clindamycin + tretinoin gel *(Ziana)* and others. **Birth control pills + antibiotics** When used, regular counseling applies.	Retinoids and Pregnancy There have been case reports of birth defects occurring in infants of mothers who used topical retinoids during pregnancy. For this reason, retinoids are not recommended for use during pregnancy or breastfeeding. Tretinoin and adapalene are pregnancy category C; tazarotene is pregnancy category X. Retinioids can cause some burning and irritation, especially in the early weeks of therapy. The formulations *Retin-A, Avita* and *Differin* ("retinoid-like") are less irritating (alcohol-based gels are generally more irritating than a cream-based product). There are other similar formulations.	Limit sun exposure; your skin will burn more easily. Begin with a reduced frequency of application (every second or third day) and shorter duration of contact (washing off the application after a period of time), to improve tolerance. A pea-sized amount is sufficient (for facial application); it should be divided into 4 equal parts and smoothed over the entire surface of the face. Should not be used as "spot" therapy. Use of salicylic acid scrubs or astringents while starting a retinoid will cause worse irritation. Wash only with mild soap twice daily. Takes 4-12 weeks to see response.
Benzoyl peroxide (most effective OTC agent), salicylic acid is alternative OTC (many products) including *Benoxyl, Benzac, Clearasil*, If needed with retinoid. *Benzamycin* (BPO + 3% erythromycin) ***BenzaClin*** (BPO + 1% clindamycin) (combo preferred) **Clindamycin+BPO topical gel *(Duac)***	Antibiotics should be used with a retinoid and discontinued when no longer needed (usually 6-8 weeks) ***Duac*** Dispense with 60 day expiration. Apply QHS to affected areas. Can store at room temp, do not freeze. Limit sun exposure!	BPO can bleach clothing, hair Limit sun exposure; skin will burn more easily. ***Benzamycin and BenzaClin:*** Add indicated amount of purified water to the vial (to the mark) and immediately shake to completely dissolve medication. If needed, add additional purified water to bring level up to the mark. Add the solution in the vial to the gel and stir until homogenous in appearance (1 to 1½ minutes). *Benzamycin* is kept refrigerated. *BenzaClin* is kept at room temp. Place a 3 month expiration date on the label following mixing.

Skin Condition Treatment Notes Continued

CONDITION	NOTES	SAFETY/COUNSELING
Oral Isotretinoin (*Amnesteem, Sotret, Claravis* is generic) Only for the treatment of severe recalcitrant nodular acne 0.5–1.0 mg/kg/day, divided BID with food (to ↑ absorption) for 15-20 weeks. Comes as 10, 20, and 40 mg capsules. Counseling about contraception and behaviors associated with ↑ risk of pregnancy must be repeated on a monthly basis. Two forms of birth control are required with taking this medication (not the mini-pill). DRYNESS! Carry bottled water, eye drops and lip balm.	Female patients must sign patient information/informed consent form about birth defects that contains warnings about the risk of potential birth defects if the fetus is exposed to isotretinoin. Must have had 2 negative pregnancy tests prior to starting treatment. Cannot get pregnant for one month before, while taking the drug, or for one month after the drug is stopped. Do not breast feed or donate blood until at least one month has passed after the drug is stopped. Do not use with vitamin A supplements, tetracyclines, steroids, progestin-only contraceptives, or St. John's wort.	Pregnancy Category X Can only be dispensed by a pharmacy registered and activated with the pregnancy risk management iPLEDGE program. **BLACK BOX WARNING** Women who are pregnant or trying to get pregnant should never take this drug due to severe birth defects or miscarriage. **SIDE EFFECTS** Arthralgias, skeletal hyperostosis, osteoporosis, psychiatric issues (such as depression, psychosis, and ↑ risk of suicide), ↓ night vision (may be permanent), difficulty wearing contact lens (dry eyes/irritation), dry skin, chapped lips, ↑ cholesterol and blood glucose, transient chest pain and hearing loss, and photosensitivity.

Commonly used Oral Antibiotics

Extended-release Minocycline (*Solodyn*) 12 years and older, dosed by weight	Like other tetracyclines can cause fetal harm if administered during pregnancy. May cause permanent discoloration in teeth.	See column to left. Photosensitivity, rash.

Dandruff

Dandruff, sometimes due to yeast overgrowth Treat with hypo-allergenic shampoo such as selenium sulfide (*Selsun Blue*), zinc pyrithone (*Head & Shoulders*), or coal tar shampoos.	Ketoconazole (*Nizoral*) is available as a non-prescription shampoo called *Nizoral A-D*. Previously, this shampoo required a prescription. *Nizoral A-D* is applied twice weekly, for up to 8 weeks. Not more effective than less-expensive options for most patients.	Rub shampoo in well and leave in for 5 minutes, then rinse out. Do not use if open sores on scalp. Can cause propecia (hair growth), skin irritation

Skin Condition Treatment Notes Continued

CONDITION	NOTES	SAFETY/COUNSELING

Fungal Infections

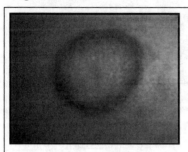

IF the infection looks like this recommend an antifungal, such as clotrimazole, etc.

Terbinafine (*Lamisil AT* cream and solution) – most effective OTC

Butenafine (*Lotrimin Ultra* cream)

Clotrimazole (*Lotrimin* cream, lotion, solution, *Desenex*)

Miconazole (*Monistat-Derm, Lotrimin* powder and spray)

Miconazole+petrolatum (for moisture barrier, used in geriatrics) *(Baza)*

Monistat Derm cream

Tolnaftate (*Tinactin* powder, cream, spray)

Undecylenic acid (*Cruex, Desenex*)

Rx

Ketoconazole (cream), ketoconazole foam *(Extina)*

Fungal infections are called tinea capitas (scalp), tinea cruris (jock itch, or groin), tinea corporis (body), tinea pedis (foot) and tinea unguium (fingernails or toenails).

Creams work best.

Solutions for hairy areas.

Powders do not work well for treatment but may be used for prevention.

If infection is large and looks severe, patient should not be self-treating – refer for systemic therapy – or in fingernails/toenails: griseofulvin, terbinafine, azole antifungals

Fingernails 6 WEEKS Tx

Toenails 12 WEEKS Tx

Topicals used to treat onychomycosis (terbenafine-*Lamisil*, and ciclopirox-*Penlac*) do not work as well as oral medicines. Not usually recommended, however they may be used in patients with liver disease. It takes a long time for the nail bed to look better – sometimes up to a year in toenails. Toenails take longer to treat than fingernails, and are more commonly infected. Recurrence is common. Keep the nails dry. Practice proper foot care. Keep blood glucose controlled. Don't smoke.

Apply medicine 1-2 inches beyond the rash.

Use for at least 2-4 weeks, even if it appears healed.

Reduce moisture to the infected area

If foot infection, do not walk barefoot (to avoid spreading it)

Wear sandals in public showers (to avoid catching it)

Nail infections (onychomycosis, *tinea unguium)* and scalp infections *(tinea capitas)* usually require systemic Tx: see duration (left column)

If using systemic therapy for nail infection, test with KOH smear 1st, monitor for hepatotoxicity, patient must complete long duration of Tx.

Oral therapy with azole antifungal (often ketoconazole) or terbinafine, sometimes griseofulvin

When used systemically, ketoconazole is a CYP 3A4 inhibitor. Use caution with other drugs given concurrently.

Instruct patients to report unusual fatigue, anorexia, nausea and/or vomiting, jaundice, dark urine or pale stools.

If ketoconazole oral stop acid suppressing agents

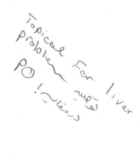

Skin Condition Treatment Notes Continued

CONDITION	NOTES	SAFETY/COUNSELING

Eczema (atopic dermatitis)

Tx: topical or oral steroids, antibiotics, antihistamines Treat first with topical steroids, only use these agents if failed steroids: **Tacrolimus (Protopic)** Pimecrolimus (Elidel) *Avoid use in children younger than 2 years of age Keep skin moisturized Eczema is a combination of dry skin and allergies. In addition to providing lubrication with a moisturizer such as Aquaphor, Eucerin, Keri or store brands (and maintaining humidity in the home) it may be possible to eliminate the allergan. Allergans are often detergents (including dish soap, clothes detergent – use mild, dye-free detergents, use liquid detergent, rinse twice, avoid bubble bath), and avoid scented lotions. Cotton clothing/sheets can help. Ask the patient to think about what may have irritated their skin.	1% of patients on CCBs may have eczema; see if problem stops if CCB is stopped For *Protopic* and *Elidel* Dispense MedGuide-calcineurin inhibitors carry cancer risk Apply a thin layer only to the affected skin areas, twice a day. Use the smallest amount needed to control symptoms Wash your hands after application.	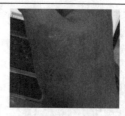 Warnings for *Elidel* and *Protopic*: Associated with cases of lymphoma and skin cancer; use only as second-line agents for short-term and intermittent treatment of atopic dermatitis (eczema) in patients unresponsive to, or intolerant of other treatments. Do not bathe, shower or swim right after applying cream. You can use moisturizers (petrolatum, lanolin, mineral oil-based) with the cream – dry skin worsens eczema. Limit sun exposure; your skin will burn more easily. Takes weeks to work; continue to apply.

Lice

Permethrin is OTC DOC for lice *(Nix, RID, Triple A,* etc)-treat as soon as possible after seeing lice, and follow-up with a 2nd treatment 7-10 days later. Spinosad *(Natroba)* – newer agent, works well, expensive. 4 yrs+ (use after agents above) If the 2nd Tx fails, refer for Rx therapy [malathion *(Ovide),* Benzyl Alcohol Lotion *(Ulesfia)* Lindane is no longer routinely recommended; high risk neurotoxicity/ seizures, requires MedGuide *Ovide* is flammable. The lotion and wet hair should not be exposed to open flames or electric heat sources, including hair dryers, electric curlers or other heat devices.	Occurs most commonly in elementary school age children. Wash clothes and bedding in hot water, followed by a hot dryer. If you can't wash something seal it in an air-proof bag for 2 weeks. Vacuum the carpet well. Soak combs and brushes in hot water for 10 minutes. Make sure to check other children in the household.	Check all family members. In addition to OTC treatment, remove the live lice and nits by inspecting the hair in 1-inch segments and using a lice comb. Without removing live lice and nits, the OTC product will not work. Nits are "cemented" to the hair shaft and do not fall off after treatment. Nit removal requires multiple efforts, which should be continued for two weeks after treatment.

Skin Condition Treatment Notes Continued

CONDITION	NOTES	SAFETY/COUNSELING

External genital warts

Imiquimod cream *(Aldara)* Apply 3 x per week to to external genital/perianal warts until there is total clearance or for the max time of 16 weeks. *Aldara* is also approved for superficial basal cell carcinoma and actinic keratosis. *See immunization section for use of HPV vaccine.*		Apply to entire treatment area before bedtime and rub in until the cream is no longer visible. Use only 1 packet per application. Wash off after 8 hours. Wash hands before and after application. Do not touch eyes, lips or nose. Local skin reactions are common. *LCO*

Topical Inflammation due to various conditions/rashes

Topical steroids (see full chart at end of section) OTC steroids are low potency: Hydrocortisone 0.5% (infants) and 1% for mild conditions, thin skin (groin area, elderly) and for children. *Aquanil* HC 1% lotion HC 2.5% is Rx only	Ointments often more potent than creams; use ointments for thick or dry skin. Use lotions, gels and foams for hairy skin. No evidence for use of topical diphenhydramine – can use systemic (25 mg) but caution due to anticholinergic effects, avoid in BPH, glaucoma, elderly. Skin should be lubricated (moisturizers). Camphor, menthol, local anesthetics (often in combo creams with HC) can help relieve itching.	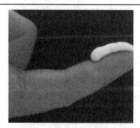 The "finger-tip" unit is used to estimate amount required: the amount that can be squeezed from the fingertip to the 1st joint covers one adult hand (about ½ g) Topical steroid over-use can cause thinning of skin, striae in skin folds and worsen acne. Do not apply to face for longer than 2 weeks. Encourage patient not to use more than directed. Apply high potency Rx steroids once daily – Apply OTC/lower potency 1-2x daily. Severe rash needs oral steroids for 1-2 wks.
antihistamine Hydroxyzine *(Atarax)* 25 mg TID-QID	Used for general urticaria (hives) which itch badly	Anticholinergic: primarily sedation and dry mouth

Skin Condition Treatment Notes Continued

CONDITION	NOTES	SAFETY/COUNSELING

Diaper Rash

Desitin (contains zinc oxide, a dessicant that can decrease moisture) and petrolatum *A&D Ointment*, or plain petrolatum, or store-brands.	If due to candida, can use topical (OTC) antifungals (physician will recommend) or miconazole+zinc oxide+petrolatum *(Vusion)*. May also be due to bacteria and require a topical antibiotic.	Recommend: frequent changes, clean well (do not rub hard), do NOT use baby wipes that contain alcohol or propylene glycol, AIR dry well, do not use plastic pants over cloth diapers. Provide physical barrier with product. If worsens, could be fungal or bacterial infection or combination – see doctor.

Minor cuts/abrasions

The triple antibiotic ointment **(*Neosporin*, generics) contains polymyxin, bacitracin and neomycin**. It is used to prevent infections from minor cuts, scrapes or burns. Some patients have an allergic reaction to the neomycin component. *Polysporin* contains bacitracin and polymixin, and *Bacitracin* contains just bacitracin. **Mupirocin *(Bactroban)* is an Rx antibiotic cream or ointment; very good staph and strep coverage.** Make sure tetanus vaccine is current (Q 10 years for adults). If large/dirty, infected cut, refer out. If wound looks like abuse, contact authorities if able.	To apply topical antibiotics: Clean the affected area and apply a small amount of medication (an amount equal to the surface area of the tip of a finger) to the affected area 1 to 3 times daily. The wound may be covered with a sterile bandage if it is in a place that could get dirty.	Leaving a wound uncovered helps it stay dry and helps it heal. If the wound isn't in an area that will get dirty or be rubbed by clothing, don't cover it. If area can get dirty (such as a hand) or be irritated by clothing, cover with an adhesive strip (e.g., *Band-Aid*) or with sterile gauze and adhesive tape +/- Abx ointment. Change daily. Certain wounds, like large scrapes, should be kept moist and clean to help reduce scarring and speed healing. Bandages used for this purpose are called occlusive or semi-occlusive bandages. They are available OTC.

Poison Ivy/Oak/Sumac

Ivy Block (bentoquatam) or other barrier blocks *Zanfel* is supposed to bind urushiol (this is the toxin) – low evidence for efficacy Aluminum acetate solution *(Burrow's)* Colloidal oatmeal *(Aveeno)* Calamine lotion - *Caladryl, IvaRest* are calamine + topical analgesics Topical or oral steroids will help (oral needed in severe rash) Cold compresses can help	Rash due to allergic reaction to uroshiol-wash off with soap and water ASAP Poison ivy/oak – eastern states Poison sumac – western states (note red stem)	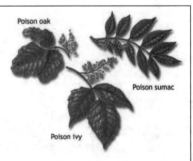

Skin Condition Treatment Notes Continued

CONDITION	NOTES	SAFETY/COUNSELING

Psoriasis

Coal tar, in many products, including *Neutrogena T, Denorex* Keratolytics (salicylic acid, sulfur), combo with cold tar *(Sebutone)* Retinioids (see acne above) Anthralin *(Anthranol*, others) Calcipotriene *(Dovonex*, a vit D analog) **Calcipotriene and betamethasone ointment (*Taclonex, Taclonex scalp suspension*)** If topicals are not effective, can use: Oral steroids Psoralens+UV therapy Acitretin *(Soriatane)* (severe cases only) – see biologic use next column.	Chronic, inflammatory condition with silvery scales (plaques) with clear edges. Lesions can cover large areas. If combined with arthritis (swollen, inflamed joints), called psoriatic arthritis – treat with RA drugs *Taclonex* If suspension shake well Do not use > 4 weeks Do not use > 100 g ointment weekly	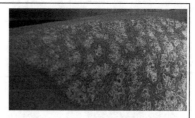 *DermaZinc* is a psoriasis product that contains zinc pyrithione (OTC), which can be compounded with a steroid (powder), usually betamethasone or clobetasol. It comes as a spray, cream and shampoo. Compounded products have 6 months stability. With spray and shampoo: shake well prior to use.

Alopecia (Hair Loss)

Finasteride *(Propecia)* 5-alpha reductase type 2 inhibitor 1 mg daily Check that drugs are not contributing to hair loss (valproate, warfarin, levonorgestrel) or zinc or vitamin D deficiency.	Do not dispense with someone on finasteride *(Proscar)* for BPH	Preg Categ X: females should not handle – can damage male fetus. Only for men Must be used indefinitely or condition reappears. **SIDE EFFECTS** Lower dose than *Proscar*, lower risk of sexual side effects
Minoxidil topical OTC 2% and 5% – 5% solution more effective, but more facial hair growth.	Rx tablets indicated for hypertension only (very rarely used)	For men and women Must be used indefinitely or condition reappears.
Bimatoprost solution *(Latisse)* For thinning eyelashes (hypotrichosis)	Apply nightly to the skin at the base of the upper eyelashes only (do not apply to the lower lid). Use the applicator brush. Blot any excess. Dispose of the applicator after one use. Repeat for other eye.	May cause itchy eyes and/or eye redness. If discontinued, lashes eventually return to previous appearance. Eyelid skin darkening may occur which may be reversible. Hair growth may occur in other skin areas that the solution frequently touches. Do not use concurrently with PG analogs used for glaucoma.

Skin Condition Treatment Notes Continued

CONDITION	NOTES	SAFETY/COUNSELING

Sunscreens

CONDITION	NOTES	SAFETY/COUNSELING
Many products, choose one with UVA and UVB coverage, SPF 15+. Two new interesting ones that have UVA coverage: *L'Oreal Anthelios SX* (contains ecamsule) *Neutrogena Helioplex* (contains avobenzone)	UVA: Blocks aging (A for aging – wrinkles). Ingredients that block UVA: ecamsule, avobenzone, oxybenzone, sulisobenzone, titanium dioxide, zinc oxide (zinc and titanium are common barrier agents). UVB: Blocks burning (B for burning). Broad spectrum – blocks both UVA and UVB. Water resistant – means resistant for 40-80 minutes. SPF (sun exposure factor) – measures how long it takes to burn versus not using sunscreen (measures UVB only). An SPF of 15 takes 15 times longer for skin to redden than without the sunscreen.	All sunscreens wash off; reapply after going in the water and at least every 2 hours. Avoid peak sun (10AM-4PM), even if overcast. Wear protective clothing. Consider vitamin D deficiency-if avoiding sun or little sun exposure may need supplementation. Avoid ingredients that are known allergans, particularly in children with sensitive skin: para-aminobenzoic acid (PABA) and benzephenones (dioxybenzone, oxybenzone, sulisobenzone). UVA and UVB exposure increases risk of skin cancer, including most common type (squamous cell) Some dermatologists recommend SPF 15 and others recommend SPF 30. The key is to apply liberally and at least every two hours. The American Academy of Pediatrics says to keep all babies less than 6 months old out of the sun.

Cold Sores (herpes simplex virus (HSV), usually type 1)

CONDITION	NOTES	SAFETY/COUNSELING
OTC Docosanol cream *(Abreva)* Rx Acyclovir /Hydrocortisone *(Xerese)* Acyclovir *(Zovirax)* cream, penciclovir *(Denavir)* cream, or oral antivirals	*Abreva*: apply 5 x/day until sore healed, max 10 days *Zovirax* cream, 5 x daily x 4 days *Denavir* cream, Q2H during day x 4 days	Cold sores are not canker scores (these are inside mouth). Cold sores are on the lips. Highly contagious (from kisses, toothbrushes, glasses), kids often contract, > 50% population infected. Sores brought on by triggers, primarily stress.

POTENCIES OF TOPICAL STEROID PRODUCTS

PRODUCT	ACTIVE NGREDIENT

Very High Potency

Clobex Lotion/Spray/Shampoo, 0.05%	**Clobetasol propionate**
Cormax Cream/Solution, 0.05%	**Clobetasol propionate**
Diprolene Ointment, 0.05%	Betamethasone dipropionate
Olux E Foam, 0.05%	**Clobetasol propionate**
Olux Foam, 0.05%	**Clobetasol propionate**
Temovate Cream/Ointment/Solution, 0.05%	**Clobetasol propionate**
Ultravate Cream/Ointment, 0.05%	Halobetasol propionate
Vanos Cream, 0.1%	Fluocinonide
Psorcon Ointment, 0.05%	Diflorasone diacetate
Psorcon E Ointment, 0.05%	Diflorasone diacetate

High Potency

Diprolene Cream AF, 0.05%	Betamethasone dipropionate
Elocon Ointment, 0.1%	**Mometasone furoate**
Florone Ointment, 0.05%	Diflorasone diacetate
Halog Ointment/Cream, 0.1%	Halcinonide
Lidex Cream/Gel/Ointment, 0.05%	**Fluocinonide**
Psorcon Cream, 0.05%	Diflorasone diacetate
Topicort Cream/Ointment, 0.25%	**Desoximetasone**
Topicort Gel, 0.05%	**Desoximetasone**

Medium Potency

Cutivate Ointment, 0.005%	Fluticasone propionate
Lidex-E Cream, 0.05%	Fluocinonide
Luxiq Foam, 0.12%	Betamethasone valerate
Topicort LP Cream, 0.05%	Desoximetasone

Medium-Low Potency

Cordran Ointment, 0.05%	Flurandrenolide
Elocon Cream, 0.1%	**Mometasone furoate**
Kenalog Cream/Spray, 0.1%	**Triamcinolone acetonide**
Synalar Ointment, 0.03%	Fluocinolone acetonide
Westcort Ointment, 0.2%	Hydrocortisone valerate

Potencies of Topical Steroid Products Continued

PRODUCT	ACTIVE NGREDIENT
Capex Shampoo, 0.01%	Fluocinolone acetonide
Cutivate Cream/Lotion, 0.05%	Fluticasone propionate
DermAtop Cream, 0.1%	Prednicarbate
DesOwen Lotion, 0.05%	**Desonide**
Locoid Cream/Lotion/Ointment/Solution, 0.1%	Hydrocortisone
Pandel Cream, 0.1%	Hydrocortisone
Synalar Cream, 0.03%/0.01%	Fluocinolone acetonide
Westcort Cream, 0.2%	Hydrocortisone valerate

Mild Potency

Aclovate Cream/Ointment, 0.05%	Alclometasone dipropionate
Derma-Smoothe/FS Oil, 0.01%	Fluocinolone acetonide
Desonate Gel, 0.05%	**Desonide**
Synalar Cream/Solution, 0.01%	Fluocinolone acetonide
Verdeso Foam, 0.05%	Desonide

Low Potency

Cetacort Lotion, 0.5%/1%	Hydrocortisone
Cortaid Cream/Spray/Ointment	Hydrocortisone
Hytone Cream/Lotion, 1%/2.5%	Hydrocortisone
Micort-HC Cream, 2%/2.5%	Hydrocortisone
Nutracort Lotion, 1%/2.5%	Hydrocortisone
Synacort Cream, 1%/2.5%	Hydrocortisone

WEIGHT LOSS

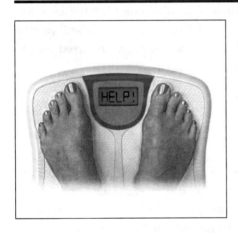

Background

Overweight and obesity is a national health threat and a major public health challenge. Data from the CDC (2008) estimates obesity at 72.5 million adults in the U.S., with many more falling into the overweight category. Overweight puts patients at increased risk for coronary heart disease, hypertension, stroke, type 2 diabetes, certain types of cancer, and premature death. In addition to health risks, overweight reduces quality of life and causes social stigmatization and discrimination. This is sadly true for adults, and for children.

Weight loss is successful only when the patient (and usually the family) is able to make permanent changes in diet and exercise habits. Fad diets may cause an acute weight drop but do not contribute to long-term weight loss and can have harmful health consequences. Calories count: many people think they are just "born fat" or have low metabolism. Children become overweight (and grow into overweight adults) due to poor eating habits in the family and community. If low metabolism is an issue it will show up on lab tests (as hypothyroidism) and will be treated.

A HEALTHY WEIGHT: VALUE AND ACHIEVEMENT

The Body Mass Index BMI is used to find the healthy weight range. The BMI calculation is in the calculations section. A healthy (normal) BMI is between 18.5 to 24.9. The bottom line is that calories have to be cut and the nutritional quality of the food will need to be increased.

Diet plans do not work long-term, but rather the patient will need education and to embrace healthy eating as a lifestyle. They will need to move gradually away from low-fiber (refined) foods towards nutrient-rich foods including fruits, vegetables and whole grains. In addition keep in mind that meat intake is high for many Americans and a move towards healthier protein sources should be encouraged.

A 500 kcal decrease per day equals 1 pound weight lost per week (3500 kcal/pound). By adding modest physical activity, this can be increased to 2 pounds weekly. A faster rate of weight loss typically reverses – usually with more weight than at the start. Exercise should be encouraged. If the patient is able, the recommendation is for 30- 60 minutes of moderately intense activity daily.

Please note: the "calorie in, calorie out" concept is the currently accepted method to lose weight and maintain weight loss. In this model, patients are instructed to expend more calories than consumed. However, cutting back food intake does not work for the majority of overweight patients. Current research is focusing on ideas that go beyond the "calorie-in, calorie-out" concept. It is possible that eating a carbohydrate-based diet may increase hunger more than a diet heavily weighted toward protein and fat. When health care providers began to encourage patients to eat according to the food pyramid (which is carbohydrate based, including the new "plate" design), obesity increased. It is also complicated by cost: carbohydrates are cheaper than protein-rich food sources. If the cheaper food makes one heavier, we need to find ways to subsidize healthier options. Keep your eye focused on research as weight loss recommendations may change.

WEIGHT LOSS DRUGS: OTC AND RX

OTC

OTC weight loss drugs commonly contain stimulants, such as the ephedra alkaloid bitter orange or related compounds, along with excessive amounts of caffeine. Caffeine is packaged under different names – including as yerba mate, guarana or concentrated green tea powder. Tolerance develops quickly with the use of these agents, requiring higher doses. In patients with cardiovascular risk – which is often present in overweight patients – they carry significant risk. A newer OTC product called *Fastin* (the name is taken from the previous Rx drug phentermine) is being marketed as a "thermogenic intensifier." It contains stimulants, including synephrine and caffeine. For CVD-risk patients it should be viewed as a potential heart-attack-in-a-bottle. OTC weight loss agents should not be recommended unless it is *Alli*, which contains a lower dose of the prescription agent orlistat (*Xenical*). This may be useful for patients who wish to provide a motivation to reduce fat intake, but use caution since *Alli* has tolerability problems, including flatulence, and is expensive. It would be better to help the patient just cut down on fat by replacing fatty foods with healthier options. This is required for long-term benefit.

RX

Prescription drugs should be used only in addition to changes in diet and increased physical activity and only for use in patients with higher BMIs – above 27 with health complications or above 30 without. Prescription agents are not appropriate for patients with small amounts of weight to lose. This chart does not contain sibutramine (*Meridia*) which was pulled from the US market in October, 2010.

DRUG	DOSING	SIDE EFFECTS/WARNINGS

Short term appetite suppressants – controlled, C III agents

| Phentermine *(Adipex-P)* | 15-37.5 mg, before or after breakfast, or in divided doses | Dizziness, tremor, agitation, tachycardia, blood pressure elevations, insomnia, cardiovascular complications, dependence, psychotic symptoms possible

Used for 3-4 weeks to "jump-start" a diet. |
| Diethylpropion *(Tenuate)* | 25 mg IR, TID 1 hour before meals and mid-evening

75 mg SR, once in midmorning | ↑BP
Tachy
dizzy |

Long-term lipase inhibitor

| Orlistat Rx *(Xenical)* | 120 mg w/each meal containing fat

Both orlistat formulations must be used with a low-fat diet plan. | GI (flatus with discharge, fecal urgency, fatty stool)

~13 lbs in 1 year

Reduces 1/3 dietary fat

Take multivitamin with A, D, E, K and beta carotene at bedtime or separated by 2+ hours from *Xenical*. Do not use with cyclosporine. Separate levothyroxine by 4 hours.

Must stick to dietary plan for both weight improvements and to help moderate side effects |

OTC

| Orlistat OTC *(Alli)* | 60 mg w/each meal containing fat | Same as *Xenical* (above) for counseling, vitamin and diet/fat intake, and drug interactions.

~5 pounds in 6 months

Reduces 1/4 dietary fat |

APPENDIX

Top Selling Drugs

This data is from 2010, the latest available.

BRAND TOP SELLERS	
RANK	DRUG
1	Lipitor
2	Nexium
3	Plavix
4	Singulair
5	Lexapro
6	Crestor
7	Synthroid
8	ProAir HFA
9	Advair Diskus
10	Cymbalta
11	Diovan
12	Ventolin HFA
13	Diovan HCT
14	Actos
15	Seroquel
16	Levaquin
17	Lantus
18	Nasonex
19	Viagra
20	Lyrica

BRAND TOP SELLERS	
RANK	DRUG
21	Celebrex
22	Concerta
23	Spiriva
24	Premarin Tabs
25	Effexor XR
26	Tricor
27	Zetia
28	Vytorin
29	OxyContin
30	Abilify
31	Tri-Sprintec
32	Loestrin 24 Fe
33	Vyvanse
34	Cialis
35	Suboxone
36	Aricept
37	Benicar
38	Januvia
39	Lunesta
40	Ambien CR

BRAND TOP SELLERS	
RANK	DRUG
41	Niaspan
42	Xalatan
43	Levoxyl
44	Benicar HCT
45	Flovent HFA
46	NuvaRing
47	Ocella
48	Lovaza
49	Yaz
50	NovoLog
51	Budeprion XL
52	Combivent
53	Namenda
54	Detrol LA
55	Ortho Tri-Cyclen Lo
56	Sprintec
57	Lantus SoloSTAR
58	Fluvirin
59	Proventil HFA
60	Aciphex

BRAND TOP SELLERS	
RANK	DRUG
61	Endocet
62	Avapro
63	Bystolic
64	Adderall XR
65	Symbicort
66	Zyprexa
67	Trilipix
68	Boniva
69	Avodart
70	Glipizide XL
71	Pristiq
72	Lidoderm
73	Humalog
74	Vigamox
75	Evista
76	Aviane
77	Flomax
78	Chantix
79	Avalide
80	Protonix

Top Selling Drugs Continued

RANK	DRUG
81	Cozaar
82	Vivelle-DOT
83	Vesicare
84	Prempro
85	Avelox
86	Focalin XR
87	Strattera
88	Xopenex HFA
89	Actonel
90	Travatan Z
91	Levemir
92	Lumigan
93	Apri
94	Levitra
95	Geodon Oral
96	Micardis
97	Exforge
98	Coumadin Tabs
99	Janumet
100	Ciprodex Otic
101	Valtrex
102	Restasis
103	Seroquel XR
104	Micardis HCT
105	Junel FE
106	Methylin
107	Actonel 150
108	Lotrel
109	Tussionex
110	Prometrium

RANK	DRUG
111	AndroGel Pump
112	Kariva
113	Patanol
114	Afluria PF 2010-2011
115	Voltaren Gel
116	Hyzaar
117	Thyroid, Armour
118	Dexilant
119	Nasacort AQ
120	Coreg CR
121	Qvar
122	Cryselle
123	Morphine Sulfate CR
124	Pataday
125	Xyzal
126	Humulin N
127	Vagifem
128	Toprol XL
129	Byetta
130	NovoLog Mix 70/30
131	Low-Ogestrel
132	Necon 1/35
133	Veramyst
134	Azor
135	Caduet
136	Welchol
137	Jantoven
138	Morphine Sul Non Inj
139	Actoplus Met
140	Provigil

RANK	DRUG
141	Epipen
142	Aggrenox
143	Dilantin
144	Enablex
145	Alphagan P
146	Premarin Vaginal
147	Xopenex
148	Uroxatral
149	Asmanex
150	Prevacid SoluTab
151	Moviprep
152	Avandia
153	Tekturna
154	Propecia
155	Hydromet
156	Ortho Evra
157	Solodyn
158	Fluzone PF 2010-2011
159	Humulin 70/30
160	Lanoxin
161	Asacol
162	Prevacid
163	Atacand
164	Nitrostat
165	Combigan
166	Halflytely Bowel Pre
167	Relpax
168	Novolin 70/30
169	Femara
170	Tamiflu

RANK	DRUG
171	Zovirax Topical
172	Camila
173	Trivora-28
174	Lovenox
175	Errin
176	Zymar
177	Maxalt
178	Estrace Vaginal
179	Fluzone Split
180	Exelon Patch
181	Intuniv
182	Allegra-D 24 Hour
183	Nortrel
184	Astepro 0.15%
185	Influenza A(H1N1)Mon
186	Maxalt MLT
187	Arimidex
188	Amitiza
189	Doryx
190	Levora
191	Differin
192	Clarinex
193	Lotemax
194	Astelin
195	Transderm-Scop
196	Humulin R
197	Levothroid
198	Advair HFA
199	Truvada
200	Nuvigil

Top Selling Drugs Continued

GENERIC TOP SELLERS			
RANK	DRUG	RANK	DRUG
1	Hydrocodone/APAP	31	Cephalexin
2	Lisinopril	32	Trimethoprim/Sulfa
3	Simvastatin	33	Fexofenadine
4	Levothyroxine	34	Amoxicillin/Pot Clav
5	Amoxicillin	35	Ciprofloxacin HCl
6	Amlodipine Besylate	36	Pravastatin
7	Azithromycin	37	Trazodone HCl
8	Alprazolam	38	Lovastatin
9	Hydrochlorothiazide	39	Triamterene w/HCTZ
10	Omeprazole	40	Carvedilol
11	Metformin	41	Alendronate
12	Furosemide Oral	42	Ranitidine HCl
13	Metoprolol Tartrate	43	Meloxicam
14	Atenolol	44	Diazepam
15	Sertraline	45	Naproxen
16	Metoprolol Succinate	46	Propoxyphene-N/APAP
17	Zolpidem Tartrate	47	Vitamin D
18	Oxycodone w/APAP	48	Fluconazole
19	Citalopram HBR	49	Methylprednis Tabs
20	Gabapentin	50	Doxycycline
21	Ibuprofen	51	Paroxetine
22	Prednisone Oral	52	Oxycodone
23	Tramadol	53	Clonidine
24	Lisinopril/HCTZ	54	Amitriptyline
25	Fluoxetine	55	Allopurinol
26	Lorazepam	56	Enalapril
27	Warfarin	57	Carisoprodol
28	Clonazepam	58	Acetaminophen w/Cod
29	Fluticasone Nasal	59	Klor-Con
30	Cyclobenzaprine	60	Pantoprazole

GENERIC TOP SELLERS			
RANK	DRUG	RANK	DRUG
61	Potassium Chloride	91	Potassium Chlorid ER
62	Temazepam	92	Phentermine
63	Promethazine Tabs	93	Mirtazapine
64	Glimepiride	94	Hydroxyzine
65	Albuterol Neb Soln	95	Estradiol Oral
66	Tamsulosin HCl	96	Valacyclovir HCl
67	Folic Acid	97	Diclofenac Sodium SR
68	Spironolactone	98	Ntrofrntin Mnohy Mcr
69	Amlodipine Besy/Benz	99	Verapamil SR
70	Amphetamine Salt Cmb	100	Venlafaxine ER
71	Metformin HCl ER	101	Mupirocin
72	Triamcinln Acet Top	102	Buspirone HCl
73	Digoxin	103	Gemfibrozil
74	Lamotrigine	104	Amphetmn Salt Cmb SR
75	Cefdinir	105	Ondansetron
76	Diltiazem CD	106	Famotidine
77	Benazepril	107	Sumatriptan Oral
78	Topiramate	108	Promethazine/Codeine
79	Isosorbide Mono ER	109	Propranolol HCl
80	Ramipril	110	Terazosin
81	Risperidone	111	Polyethylene Glycol
82	Glyburide	112	Meclizine HCl
83	Penicillin VK	113	Acyclovir
84	Lansoprazole	114	Fentanyl Transdermal
85	Clindamycin Systemic	115	Methotrexate
86	Bupropion XL	116	Finasteride
87	Metronidazole Tabs	117	Ferrous Sulfate
88	Glipizide	118	Benzonatate
89	Divalproex Sodium	119	Bupropion SR
90	Losartan Potassium	120	Methadone HCl Non-In

Top Selling Drugs Continued

GENERIC TOP SELLERS		GENERIC TOP SELLERS		GENERIC TOP SELLERS		GENERIC TOP SELLERS	
RANK	DRUG	RANK	DRUG	RANK	DRUG	RANK	DRUG
121	Cheratussin AC	141	Bisoprolol/HCTZ	161	Atenolol Chlorthal	181	Cyanocobalamin
122	Tizanidine HCl	142	Glybrid/Metfrmin HCl	162	Labetalol	182	Oxybutynin Chl ER
123	Quinapril	143	Nabumetone	163	Cefuroxime Axetil	183	Promethazine DM
124	Butalbital/APAP/Caf	144	Hydroxychloroquine	164	Hydrocortison Top Rx	184	Terbinafine HCl
125	Metoclopramide	145	Benztropine	165	Morphine Sulfate ER	185	Fexofenadine/Pseudo
126	Clotrimazl/Betamthsn	146	Ropinirole HCl	166	Fluocinonide	186	Ondansetron ODT
127	Doxazosin	147	Minocycline	167	Clindamycin Topical	187	Hydromorphone HCl
128	Methocarbamol	148	Trinessa	168	Nystatin Systemic	188	Diltiazem SR
129	Clobetasol	149	Phenazopyridine HCl	169	Prenatal 1+1	189	Ergocalciferol
130	Nifedipine ER	150	Phenytoin Sodium Ext	170	Tramadol HCl/APAP	190	Pramipexole Dihydroc
131	Aspirin,Enteric-Coat	151	Ketoconazole Topical	171	Etodolac	191	Medrxyprgsterone Tab
132	Fenofibrate	152	Hydroxyzine Pamoate	172	Indomethacin	192	Carbamazepine
133	Levetiracetam	153	Prednisln Sd Phs Orl	173	Diphenoxylate w/Atro	193	Benazepril/HCTZ
134	Nitroglycerin	154	Hydralazine	174	Phenobarbital	194	Prednisolne Acet Oph
135	Chlorhexidine Glucon	155	Colchicine	175	Oxcarbazepine	195	Lithium Carbonate
136	Baclofen	156	Nortriptyline	176	Diltiazem	196	Multivits w/Flur Chw
137	Glipizide ER	157	Nystatin Topical	177	Carbidopa/Levodopa	197	Hydrocodone/Ibprofen
138	Losartan Pot/HCTZ	158	Bupropion ER	178	Gianvi	198	Sodium Fluoride
139	Dicyclomine HCl	159	Venlafaxine	179	Amiodarone	199	Dexamethasone Oral
140	Clarithromycin	160	Oxybutynin Chloride	180	Felodipine ER	200	Prochlorperaz Mal

We gratefully acknowledge the assistance of SDI Health, Inc., in providing the top sellers list for inclusion in this text.

Common Laboratory Values

The range may change slightly depending on the laboratory that has issued the report.

ITEM	VALUE		
Albumin	3.5 - 5.0 g/dL		
Alkaline phosphatase	33 - 131 IU/L		
AST	8 - 48 IU/L		
ALT	7 - 55 IU/L		
Bilirubin, direct	0.1 - 0.3 mg/dL		
Bilirubin, total	0.1 - 1.2 mg/dL		
BUN	7 - 20 mg/dL		
Creatinine	0.5 - 1. 3 mg/dL		
	Male		Female
Hemoglobin (g/dL)	13.5 - 16.5		12.0 - 15.0
Hematocrit (%)	41 - 50		36 - 44
RBC's (x 106/mL)	4.5 - 5.5		4.0 - 4.9
MCV	80 - 100 micrometer^3		
MCH	26 - 34 pg/cell		
MCHC	31 - 37 g/dL		
Platelets	150,000 to 450,000/mm^3		
WBC	4,000 - 11,000/mm^3		

Electrolytes

Calcium	8.5 - 10.5 mg/dL
Calcium, ionized	4.5 - 5.6 mg/dL
Chloride	95 - 107 mEq/L
Magnesium	1.6 - 2.5 mEq/L
Phosphate	2.5 - 4.5 mg/dL
Potassium	3.5 - 5.0 mEq/L
Sodium	135 - 145 mEq/L

Diabetes

Estimated Average Glucose	< 154 mg/dL
Hemoglobin A1C	< 7%
Preprandial blood glucose	70-130 mg/dL
Postprandial blood glucose	< 180 mg/dL (ADA)

Common Laboratory Values Continued

ITEM	VALUE

Lipids

Cholesterol, total	< 200 mg/dL
HDL, low	< 40 mg/dL
HDL, optimal	≥ 60 mg/dL
LDL, optimal	< 100 mg/dL, or < 70 mg/dL
LDL, normal	100-129 mg/dL
Triglycerides	< 150 mg/dL

Thyroid Function

Free thyroxine (FT4)	0.8-1.7 mcg/dL
TSH	0.3 – 3.0μIU/mL

Iron

Iron	65 - 150 mcg/dL
Total iron binding capacity (TIBC)	250 - 420 mcg/dL
Transferrin	> 200 mg/dL

Uric Acid

Uric acid (male)	3.5 - 7.2 mg/dL
Uric acid (female)	2.0 - 6.5 mg/dL

Inflammation

C-Reactive Protein	Normal: < 0.8 mg/dL
	High risk: > 3.00 mg
Rheumatoid Factor, serum	< 40 IU/mL
Erythrocyte Sed Rate (ESR)	Male: ≤ 20 mm/hr
	Female: ≤ 30 mm/hr

Common Medical Abbreviations

Medical safety warning: Use only the approved list in your institution; the meaning of abbreviations varies.

ABBREVIATION	MEANING
AAA	abdominal aortic aneurysm
A&O	alert & oriented
ABG	arterial blood gas
ACTH	adrenocorticotropic hormone
ADH	anti-diuretic hormone
ADR	adverse drug reaction
AF	atrial fibrillation, or Afib
ANA	antinuclear antibody
ANS	autonomic nervous system
ARDS	acute respiratory distress syndrome
APTT	activated partial thromboplastin time
ARF	acute renal failure
BEE	basal energy expenditure
BMP	Basic Metabolic Panel
BP	blood pressure
BPH	benign prostatic hypertrophy
BUN	blood urea nitrogen
C&S	culture and sensitivity
CA	cancer
CABG	coronary artery bypass graft
CAD	coronary artery disease
CBC	complete blood count
CC	chief complaint
CF	cystic fibrosis
CH	cholesterol
CHF	congestive heart failure
CI	cardiac index
CMV	cytomegalovirus
CNS	central nervous system
CO	cardiac output
C/O	complaining of
COPD	chronic obstructive pulmonary disease
CP	chest pain or cerebral palsy
CPAP	continuous positive airway pressure

Common Medical Abbreviations Continued

ABBREVIATION	MEANING
CPK	creatine phosphokinase
CPR	cardiopulmonary resuscitation
CrCL	creatinine clearance
CRF	chronic renal failure
CRP	C-reactive protein
CSF	cerebrospinal fluid
CT	computerized tomography
CVA	cerebrovascular accident
CXR	chest X-ray
D/C	discontinue or discharge
D5W	5% dextrose in water
DJD	degenerative joint disease (osteoarthritis)
DKA	diabetic ketoacidosis
DM	diabetes mellitus
DOE	dyspnea on exertion
DVT	deep venous thrombosis
Dx	diagnosis
ECG	electrocardiogram
ETOH	ethanol
FBS	fasting blood sugar
FEV	forced expiratory volume
FT4	free thyroxine (T4) enzyme
fxn	function
F/U	follow-up
GFR	glomerular filtration rate
GI	gastrointestinal
GTT	glucose tolerance test
HA	headache
HBV	hepatitis B virus
HCG	human chorionic gonadotropin
HCT	hematocrit
HCV	hepatitis C virus
HDL	high density lipoprotein
Hgb	hemoglobin
HIV	human immunodeficiency virus
HJR	hepatojugular reflex
H/O	history of

Common Medical Abbreviations Continued

ABBREVIATION	MEANING
HPI	history of present illness
HR	heart rate
HSV	herpes simplex virus
HTN	hypertension
Hx	history
I&O	intake and output
ICU	intensive care unit
IM	intramuscular
INR	international normalised ratio
IV	intravenous
LDH	lactate dehydrogenase
LDL	Low-Density Lipoprotein
LFTs	Liver function tests
LVH	left ventricular hypertrophy
MAO	monoamine oxidase
MCH	mean cell hemoglobin
MCHC	mean cell hemoglobin concentration
MCV	mean corpuscular volume
MI	myocardial infarction
MRI	magnetic resonance imaging
MRSA	methicillin resistant staph aureus
MS	multiple sclerosis or morphine sulfate (don't use for morphine – dangerous)
MSSA	methicillin-sensitive staph aureus
MVA	motor vehicle accident
MVI	multivitamin injection
NG	nasogastric
NKA	no known allergies
NKDA	no known drug allergies
NPO	nothing by mouth
NSAID	nonsteroidal anti- inflammatory drugs
NSR	normal sinus rhythm
N/V	nausea and vomiting
PAP	pulmonary artery pressure
PCWP	pulmonary capillary wedge pressure
PE	pulmonary embolus, or physical exam
PKU	phenylketonuria
PMH	past medical history

Common Medical Abbreviations Continued

ABBREVIATION	MEANING
PPD	purified protein derivative
PRBC	packed red blood cells
PRN	as needed
PT	prothrombin time, or physical therapy
Pt	patient
PTCA	percutaneous transluminal coronary angioplasty
PTH	parathyroid hormone
PUD	peptic ulcer disease
RA	rheumatoid arthritis
RBC	red blood cell
R/O	rule out
ROS	review of systems
RSV	respiratory syncytial virus
Rx	treatment, prescription
rxn	reaction
SCr	serum creatinine
SIADH	syndrome of inappropriate antidiuretic hormone
sig	write on label
SLE	systemic lupus erythematous
SOAP	subjective, objective, assessment, plan
SOB	shortness of breath
SQ	subcutaneous
STAT	immediately
Sx	symptoms
TB	tuberculosis
TG	Triglycerides
TIA	transient ischemic attack
TIBC	total iron binding capacity
TPN	total parenteral nutrition
TSH	thyroid stimulating hormone
TTP	thrombotic thrombocytopenic purpura
Tx	treatment
UA	urinalysis
UFH	unfractionated heparin
URTI	upper respiratory tract infection
UTI	urinary tract infection
VRE	vancomycin-resistant enterococcus
VT	ventricular tachycardia
WBC	white blood cell or count
WNL	within normal limits
y/o	years old
yr	year